The
Treatment
of
Stuttering

THE
TREATMENT
OF
STUTTERING

CHARLES VAN RIPER
Western Michigan University

PRENTICE-HALL, INC., ENGLEWOOD CLIFFS, NEW JERSEY

Library of Congress Cataloging in Publication Data

VAN RIPER, CHARLES GAGE
　The treatment of stuttering.

　Includes bibliographies.
　1. Stammering.　2. Speech therapy.　I. Title.
[DNLM:　1. Stuttering—Therapy.　WM 475 V274t　1973]
RC424.V32　　　616.8′554′06　　　72-13087
ISBN 0-13-930594-7

© 1973 by **Prentice-Hall, Inc., Englewood Cliffs, New Jersey**

PRINTED IN THE UNITED STATES OF AMERICA

10　9　8　7　6　5　4

Prentice-Hall International, Inc., LONDON
Prentice-Hall of Australia, Pty. Ltd., SYDNEY
Prentice-Hall of Canada, Ltd., TORONTO
Prentice-Hall of India Private Limited, NEW DELHI
Prentice-Hall of Japan, Inc., TOKYO

To all who seek the untangling of tongues

Contents

OUR OWN THERAPY

Preface

In these pages will be found an account of the valiant efforts of many men and women to solve the age-old mystery of stuttering. Since, using a variety of methods, they both succeeded and failed, it is possible that somewhere in this book the key to the ancient puzzle may be found. The author hastens to add however that he has never been able to grasp that key with the fine assurance of his many predecessors (and some contemporaries) who, claiming to have found the cure, have so often yelped a loud Eureka. Nevertheless, since he has worked long and hard with many stutterers and with some success, he adds to his description of the other therapies his own approach. By doing so, he becomes equally vulnerable to the useful criticism that represents the stutterer's only hope that someday we will have a kind of treatment that will provide permanent relief for all who seek it. The mysterious forest of stuttering is full of old trails. Though we have tried to identify them and to blaze a better one, we are certain that easier, quicker routes will yet be discovered. They are there!

The Treatment of Stuttering

HISTORICAL
AND CURRENT APPROACHES
TO THERAPY

One of the sad things about stuttering, that sad disorder of the human race, is that its victims far too often find themselves in the hands of a *naive* rather than an incompetent therapist. It is truly unfortunate that stuttering can be temporarily ameliorated by so many different kinds of treatment, since the sporadic successes seem to generate a host of blind enthusiasts who make vast claims that eventually are disproved. Each new generation of therapists seems to have to rediscover the same old methods, alter them slightly, give them a new rationale, and then apply them to a new crop of stutterers. There are many vicious circles in stuttering but certainly this is one of the most tragic ones. If we are to interrupt this sad cycling, someone should bring together the pertinent information and subject it to critical scrutiny and this we have tried to do.

Nevertheless, we do not wish to imply that these therapeutic methods of the past and present are completely valueless. We are certain that each of them has freed some stutterers from their communicative disabilities and has produced improvement in others. Our task is to sift out the grains and nuggets of therapeutic gold from the large amount of gravel and sand, and be very wary of the iron pyrites—the fool's gold. At the present time, the treatment of stuttering is far from satisfactory. We have much to learn about the basic nature of the disorder as well as about its therapy.

Perhaps this quotation from Wendell Johnson (1939) will reinforce the point we are making:

> The longer I work with stutterers, the more tolerant I become of anyone who has any therapeutic ideas at all concerning it. . . . There is no such thing as *the* method for treating stuttering, and the fact that so many differing methods are more or less successful is of more than incidental interest. (p. 170)

Desiring to emphasize in this account what therapists actually do with stutterers, we find some strange fellows in the same bed. Our chapter on punishment and reinforcement therapies, for example, contains both a contemporary Dr. Goldiamond and that ancient Dr. Frank who advocated that stutterers be given a good flogging. The chapter on suggestion and persuasion runs the gamut from Mesmer to Wendell Johnson. All treatments could have been included in the chapter on suggestion. A chapter heading should therefore be viewed merely as a convenient indicator of a dominant clinical feature of a group of therapies that may differ markedly in other ways. For the most part we have emphasized what these clinicians have done with, or done to their stutterers rather than why they did what they did. It will become apparent that many clinicians do the same things for different reasons and different things for the same reason and that some clinicians seem to have no reasons at all to justify the odd things they ask the stutterer to do. We will try to find some order in this chaos.

Suggestion, Distraction,

and

Persuasion Therapies

We feel it appropriate to begin this exploration of the many kinds of treatment experienced by stutterers of the past and present by considering the role played by suggestion, distraction, and persuasion in the various therapies. Indeed, if there is any commonality in the stuttering therapies it resides in these. This of course is not surprising since we find suggestion and persuasion permeating all forms of therapy including those practiced in medicine. No patient will go to a physician unless he has some hope that his distress may be thereby alleviated. No stutterer will seek help from a clinician without similar expectations, nor will he continue in therapy unless those expectations are fostered. All physicians and all therapists know this well and so, directly or indirectly, deliberately or unconsciously, some kind of suggestion and persuasion seems to be inherent in any therapeutic relationship. Certainly it seems evident with regard to stuttering that in one way or another, all therapists seek to influence their clients to unlearn old maladaptive responses and to learn better ones, and much of that influence depends upon how well they stimulate the client's favorable expectations. The essential core of this suggestion and persuasion is that if the sufferer puts himself into the hands of the practitioner and does what the latter asks him to do, he will get better.

What is more significant, he may get better no matter what he is told to do or what the practitioner does to him. The days of faith healing are not dead. Indeed, as Frank (1961) and King (1962) have shown, they are very much alive and there is a bit

3

of shaman in every successful physician. While we shall deal extensively with the placebo effect in a later section of drug therapy, let us say here that at least with the psychosomatic disorders inactive placebos have often led to cure or marked improvement when they were accompanied by suggestion. Platonov (1959) in Russia reports a wide variety of disorders being treated successfully by direct or indirect suggestion and persuasion, and there are numerous reports in our own literature which offer other evidence that the outcome of treatment often depends upon the patient's belief in its efficacy. The role of suggestion is to enhance this belief.

In many respects, the disorder of stuttering, at least in its advanced forms as shown by adults, seems almost expressly designed for therapies stressing suggestion and persuasion. First of all, it is intermittent. It comes and goes; it appears and disappears. No one stutters on every word of every conversation. Secondly, when present it is highly variable in form. Rarely does it present a monosymptomatic picture. Thirdly, its severity in terms of frequency and duration is also highly variable being influenced by a host of conditions, some of which increase and others which decrease the severity. Fourthly, spontaneous recoveries, especially in childhood, have been commonly reported. Fifthly, temporary fluency can be easily established. Finally, in most adult stutterers we find evidence of morbid negative suggestion, the person constantly thinking about his speech difficulty, expecting to have it displayed, and planning strategies for coping with its appearance or threat. Any disorder with such characteristics should be highly amenable to suggestion and it is, as the following quotation from Blanton (1936) demonstrates:

I tried out one summer, with a group of intelligent young people, a method of curing stuttering by stroking the vagus nerve by running the hand back of the ear down to the neck and also of relaxing the tongue and the vocal cords by running the finger from the chin back to the larynx. I informed the young people that this method relaxed the vagus nerve which controls the vocal cords and also relaxed the glossopharyngeal muscles which became tense. These exercises, along with some mental hygiene talks, eliminated the symptom of stuttering in several of these young people, and yet there was no truth whatever in the theory that I presented to them about the vagus nerve and the glossopharyngeal muscles, but they believed me and were helped. I therefore should like to reemphasize the fact that the power of suggestion and the influence of the transfer of emotion from patient to teacher and teacher to patient must be considered in every type of treatment. (p. 29)

Suggestion comes in various forms. It may be direct or indirect. It may involve hypnosis or autosuggestion. The therapist may use it very deliberately or quite without awareness that he is doing so. The stutterer may be actively persuaded by the therapist that if he does certain specific things or follows certain specific procedures he will then become more fluent; or the same suggestion can be produced by subtle implication. No therapeutic procedure is free from the influence of suggestion. Our perceptions, our emotions, our belief systems can be altered by the self-statements we make and when these self-statements echo or are influenced by the therapist the impact of suggestion can be discerned.

Direct suggestion

As the advertising agencies know all too well, the efficacy of direct suggestion depends upon the frequency and intensity of its repetition, on its appeal to the person's desires, and in part on the prestige of the person making the suggestion. All of these approaches have been and are still being used in stuttering therapy. Many of the older books in the field were full of direct exhortations, the stutterers being told over and over again (often in capital letters) that *if* they followed THE METHOD (whatever it might happen to be) they could be and would be cured. The horrible fate lying in wait for them if they rejected the suggestion was also painted in vivid colors. Eloquent testimonials from preachers, bankers, officials, and from persons reputed to have undergone treatment with astonishing success are found throughout these old pages. Let us give just one illustration from a book by Beasley (1897):

> For instance, I had a pupil who visited me daily for about a week only; he could not possibly remain longer. A month after he returned home he wrote me as follows: "One month only has elapsed since I first commenced under your system, and in that short period I have acquired a freedom of speech beyond my most sanguine expectations. I can now speak with mental tranquillity and self control." . . . Another remarkable case was that of a boy of nearly eighteen, who was with me not quite a fortnight, but worked so well and got such a grasp of my system that he not only cured himself, but cured also a younger brother who was afflicted in the same manner. (p. 35)

Over and over again, we find these authors telling how they cured themselves by discovering some new technique—though they rarely reveal all their secrets. A bit of mystery often aids suggestion. This quotation from Yearsley (1909) is fairly typical in its assurance of successful outcome:

> After diligent study and research, my efforts were crowned with wonderful success. In the remarkably short period of two weeks, I had eradicated every trace of my impediment. The news of my cure quickly spread, and medical men of high standing who knew how severely I had been afflicted, showered upon me their congratulations. A well known specialist, who has practiced for twenty-five years in the treatment of speech defects, imediately acknowledged my abilities by offering me a partnership in his business. . . . (p. 20)

If this passage appears dated and quaint in its attempt to create the prestige which facilitates suggestion, we can refer the reader to the book by Reichel entitled *Stop Stammering and Stuttering* published in 1964 in our own country or to that by Mathur (1958) in India which carries on its frontispiece the following: "Congratulations, Mr. Mathur, on your logical and helpful advice on a particularly troublesome problem. You have proved from your own experience the value of your methods, which I am sure should be of equal value to others afflicted with this disorder."

At the present time, few therapists employ such blatant varieties of self-advertisement to establish their authority, preferring instead the indirect approach or perhaps autosuggestion. Nevertheless we still find direct suggestion being currently used in the form of hypnosis.

Hypnosis

Though hypnosis had been known and practiced for centuries, especially in India and China, it was Anton Mesmer in the eighteenth century who first demonstrated clearly that by putting persons into a trance he could cause some of their undesired symptoms to disappear dramatically. Though his theory of animal magnetism and his methods for inducing hypnotic states were soon challenged, Mesmer may certainly be said to have given some impetus to the whole field of modern psychotherapy. Braid, Liebault, Bernheim, Charcot, Breuer, and Freud all used hypnosis and the psychoanalytic movement grew out of their experiments. As might have been expected, stuttering soon came to the attention of the hypnotists.

Hypnotic phenomena are still not completely understood. For example, electroencephalographic studies have shown clearly that, under hypnosis, the hypnotized person is not truly asleep; his cortical brain waves are indistinguishable from those of his waking states. On a subcortical level however there seems to be some evidence that the filtering and buffering function of the ascending reticular system may be involved in hypnosis. The Russians tend to view hypnosis as resulting from partial cortical inhibition, a condition produced by the secondary signal system (language). It is partial because it is characterized by "sentinel points" which remain disinhibited and functional. They explain hypnotic phenomena as somewhat akin to the selective attention which enables a mother to jump up out of a deep sleep to attend to the faintest cry of her infant, yet to fail to respond to much louder noises.[1]

Other explanations view hypnosis as merely an extreme instance of the vulnerability to suggestion which all of us show (Hull, 1933). The psychoanalysts view the hypnotic state as one of identification and transference. By some authors hypnosis is considered a transitory psychosis.

Still others (Sarbin, 1950) see hypnosis as role-taking behavior akin to that shown by actors who momentarily but completely identify with the character they play. Finally, the hypnotic state has been considered similar to the kind of situation which occurs under extreme sensory deprivation. Chertok (1967) probably sums up what we know about hypnosis as well as anyone: "The interesting attempts at synthesis during the past few years have not yet provided an adequate explanation of the interplay of psychological and physical factors involved in hypnosis."

In the past, almost all hypnosis was accomplished by very authoritarian methods, but today, though these are not always inappropriate, most modern practitioners of hypnosis avoid them though they still use strong direct suggestion. Descriptions of the various techniques are available elsewhere.[2] Here we wish to say only that not all persons are equally vulnerable, that some are completely resistant, and that even with those stutterers who are easily hypnotized the results in terms of symptom remission have not been particularly impressive.

Review of the literature on hypnosis and stuttering. It is difficult to evaluate the literature concerning hypnosis and stuttering. Many of the references do not describe, for example, the type of stuttering exhibited, the techniques used, the depth of the trance, or provide any data concerning follow-up. Typical is the article by Donath (1932) who simply tells us that two sutterers were "completely cured" by hypnosis. Richter (1928) in the same year gives a more complete account of how he used hyp-

---

[1] For a less cursory statement of the Russian position, see Razran (1961), Winn (1957), and Platonov (1959).

[2] See Hilgard (1965), Gordon (1966), and, for some very practical information and cautions, the book by Meares (1957).

nosis. The stutterer was first placed in a hypnotic sleep, then told first to repeat simple words, then simple sentences, speaking slowly and carefully until no stuttering occurred. (Most stutterers of course would be able to repeat fluently after the therapist even if they were not hypnotized!) This practice of repetition in the trance had to be continued for some time to produce effective results. Richter stressed that the simple posthypnotic suggestion, "Now you do not have to stutter any more," is not sufficient in itself but must be prefaced by much training in fluent utterance. Negative posthypnotic suggestion that the person will *not* stutter seems to be not only unwise but dangerous. This author remembers very well the extreme anxiety attack he experienced when subjected to this sort of posthypnotic negative suggestion and then had to speak before a class of medical students.

Vogel (1934) reported the successful use of hypnotism with hospitalized marines but he used it mainly to explore the past history of the "psychic trauma" presumably underlying their stuttering. In the trance, these stutterers were told that they would recall the incidents which caused the onset of the disorder. Then the suggestion was made that upon awakening they would now know the cause and would be able to overcome the stuttering. Vogel cites the case of one individual who could not remember the causative incident before being hypnotized but readily related it under hypnosis and was able to recall it to mind after being awakened. (It was that he had been severely whipped at the age of seven years!) This patient was "cured in three sessions though he lost control and stuttered 'slightly' under excitement."

This account is fairly typical of many of those reported earlier in the literature and anyone who has any sophistication about hypnosis will recognize the possibility that the patient will often invent the kind of an incident which he surmises the hypnotist desires (a phenomenon which, by the way, is not confined to hypnosis). Freud found the same invention of imaginary traumatic incidents in his early explorations of psychoanalysis.

Scattered throughout the older literature are occasional reports of stutterers who did become fluent as the result of hypnotherapy. Bramwell (1930) reviews these cases as well as two of his own, one of whom (after two years of hypnotic treatment) was "practically well" and the other "improved." A few of the writers he reviews, Von Corm, Osgood, and Hamilton, had reported individual case successes but others like Forel were discouraged by the results. H. Gutzmann (1898) expressed himself rather eloquently on the subject:

The hypnotic treatment of stuttering has been an abject failure. Forel, the chief advocate of hypnotic therapy, has so attested. What success has been obtained has only been in conjunction with other training. No competent physician doubts that a stutterer could be calmed by hypnotic suggestion and to speak rather well when so relaxed, but he would doubt that this tranquil mood would last. (p. 394)

We also have some relatively recent reports of successful hypnotherapy. Levbarg (1941) describes his work with a rather paranoid accountant who began to stutter severely at the age of 50 when he was about to be called upon to testify before a grand jury. Within a week of daily sessions, the stuttering disappeared and at the end of a further five weeks it had not returned. Schneck (1959) used hypnotherapy with a 17-year-old boy stutterer, finding initial improvement and then relapse. Rehypnotized, he improved again but Schneck seems to be guarded in his statement of prognosis. Nao (1964), a Japanese, claimed that three out of five of his stutterers were completely cured by hypnosis. A study which describes the hypnotic treatment of stuttering in some detail is found in a reference by Watkins (1949) describing the hypnotic treatment of a soldier who, under 'battle stress, had experienced a recurrence of his childhood stuttering. Rosen (1953) also gives a play-by-play account of 37 hypnotic sessions with a 21-year-old woman, based primarily upon age regression and catharsis, in which she came to realize that her stuttering had sexual implications. Subsequent to this experience she became fluent and returned to college and for four months was free from stuttering. She then suffered a mild relapse, returned to Rosen for another hypnotic session, and remained fluent thereafter for at least six years.

Most of the material available in the literature consists of these individual case reports. In most of them we do not find anything about the severity of stuttering nor its symptomatology or history, nor how well the stutterers fared in other speaking situations. Careful follow-ups are lacking. Nor do we know how many other stutterers were hypnotized and showed no improvement. It is also interesting that many of these reported hypnotic successes were individuals who had begun to stutter relatively late in childhood or as adults, perhaps thereby indicating the kind of problem termed "hysterical stuttering" by Freund (1966). Luchsinger and Arnold (1965) state

that "hypnosis is of help only in acute traumatic cases of stuttering."

We have at least two studies which involved the hypnotizing of a substantial number of stutterers. The first by Wetterstrand, which we find reported in Bramwell (1930), was done long ago. Of the 45 stutterers he hypnotized, 15 were reported as having been cured (of these all but 2 were children between the ages of five and twelve). According to Bluemel (1931) who also cites the study, Wetterstrand "admits ignorance as to whether or not many of his cures were permanent." The other major study was performed by Moore (1946). Of 40 subjects, only 8 spoke fluently under hypnosis, carried out posthypnotic suggestions fluently, and reported easy and relaxed speech for two or three days. Eleven others spoke fluently to audiences while under hypnosis and were able intermittently to carry out posthypnotic suggestion to speak relaxedly. Twelve others did all right when hypnotized but were unable to carry out posthypnotic commands to speak fluently. Nine could not be hypnotized. No extensive follow-up was done. Despite his findings, Moore concluded that hypnosis should not be used alone but only in conjunction with other therapy.

In another review of hypnotherapy, McCord (1955) states that few modern practitioners of hypnosis now recommend the use of the simple posthypnotic suggestion that the individual will be able to talk without stuttering. His survey indicates that hypnosis should be used primarily as hypnoanalysis to produce age regression or to facilitate ventilation and catharsis. In a later review of the literature, Rousey (1961) concluded that when hypnotherapy is used, it should be employed as an adjunct to speech therapy, and that it is likely to be effective only when the patient can be deeply hypnotized.

Some renewed interest in hypnosis has resulted from the work of Wolpe (1958) who induces relaxation and then presents a hierarchy of imagined stress situations for desensitization. This use of hypnosis is described and recommended in the text by Brutten and Shoemaker (1967). We also have an interesting report from Japan: Takeyama (1963) put his stutterers into a trance, trained them to relax, and then gave them the post-hypnotic suggestion to stutter openly and easily in feared situations.[3] To conclude this survey of the literature, we should mention Falck (1964) who reviews some of the literature and makes a plea for better reporting of the type of stuttering demonstrated, the techniques used, and the effectiveness of improvement after a lapse of time—a plea that we would heartily echo.

Our own exploration of hypnosis has been partially reported elsewhere (Van Riper, 1958). Having been hypnotized himself several

times without obtaining successful relief from his stuttering, the author may have lacked the necessary faith in the process to be completely effective. Nevertheless, we found that though we could easily produce fluency when the stutterer was deeply hypnotized, the posthypnotic suggestion that the stutterer would be able to speak without any stuttering failed consistently to produce more than momentary fluency. We also used hypnotic training to induce relaxation while speaking (nothing was said about stuttering) and then used the posthypnotic suggestion that the stutterer would speak in the same relaxed way upon awakening. This produced a marked increase in fluency and a decrease in the severity of stuttering without accompanying anxiety. However, the effect soon wore off. We then rehypnotized the stutterers, finding again the same relief but it soon became apparent that more and more hypnotic booster sessions were being required to maintain the relaxed way of speaking and so this procedure too was discontinued.

Next we sought in the trance to train the stutterers to respond to their stuttering first by cancellation and then by "pull-outs." (See Van Riper, 1971, for a description of these procedures.) We were surprised to find how easily the stutterers learned to react more appropriately to fear or experience of their stuttering since normally such techniques are not mastered without some difficulty. Elated at this discovery we felt that at least we were close to a solution of the old problem. Unfortunately, very soon the amount of fluency the stutterers had previously possessed was fast disappearing. They were cancelling per-

---

[3] This approach is one which we also used for a short time and Gardner (1960) also provides an illuminating commentary:

I wish to relate to you an incident. I had a stutterer about 30 referred to me and a psychiatrist. Knowing how long and difficult it is to break down the many manifestations of stuttering and the related fears, I suggested that he aid the process by hypnosis. . . . The man went under and the doctor began to talk to him about his stuttering, that he said a lot of sounds that were not necessary and that perhaps he would be able to smooth out his speech when he woke up so that it would not appear so odd to other people. The stutterer spoke right out of his sleep and said, "But, Doctor, I don't want to stutter!"

fectly and pulling out of their blocks beautifully but their speech was becoming infested with more and more cancellations and pullouts. The severity had decreased but the frequency had ballooned. When one stutterer whose stuttering had previously been usually confined to the first words of phrases or sentences began to have to cancel or pull out of every single word he uttered, we rehypnotized him and suggested very strongly that he would never do either of them again.

Another of our attempts involved the suggestion that the stutterer would "try" to do some voluntary stuttering when entering a specified feared situation. This led to some very long combinations of both voluntary and involuntary stuttering behaviors and so this too was soon discarded.

The one truly successful result of our hypnotic experimentation concerned the facilitation we achieved in getting three stutterers to stop avoiding or postponing and to inhibit a particular instrumental behavior such as a head jerk. For example, one suggestion was that the stutterer would "try to hold his head steady while stuttering and to say any word he feared without pausing first." It seemed to us that these stutterers unlearned these instrumental behaviors much more swiftly than we would have expected. At any rate we finally concluded that we did not know enough about hypnosis to make it a regular part of our therapy with stutterers. There always were too many individuals whom we could not hypnotize and those that we could seemed to become too dependent upon us. Moreover, when our suggestions failed, we found it very difficult to regain any useful rapport again with those stutterers.

Anything we could do under hypnosis, we found we could do without it, though at times it seemed to take longer. We wanted to make our cases strong and free from us, not weak and dependent. So with some regret we discarded hypnotic therapy many years ago though we have since referred an occasional patient elsewhere for hypnoanalysis. Perhaps this quotation from Kline (1965) sums up the current view of hypnotherapy as well as any:

At the present time, little work is being done with hypnosis in its historical therapeutic role, namely suggestive therapy with the utilization of posthypnotic suggestion as the major source of behavioral change. Rather we see the emergence of hypnosis as a dynamic tool for gaining access to many facets of personality and behavioral reactions. (p. 1289)

Many of the adult stutterers who come to us ask if they should try to get cured by hypnosis. We tell them no!

Autosuggestion

We know of no other disorder for which self-suggestion has been so often recommended as for stuttering. We find it in the admonitions of parents and teachers: "Now just tell yourself to stop stuttering. Insist that you will speak smoothly. Tell yourself to relax. Make up your mind not to stutter. Use your will power." These naive self-commands constitute the bulk of the advice every stutterer receives from his associates—and most stutterers have tried in vain to follow them. A few former stutterers tell us that they overcame their disorder by such self-statements and, as we shall see, some current therapies are expressly designed to exploit autosuggestion.

Let us provide some examples. Wedberg (1937) tells us in his autobiography how often he consciously and unconsciously suggested to himself that he would stutter and how he had to learn to oppose them with positive self-suggestions.

The following suggestions are most effectively applied just before falling asleep at night and during a short period of relaxation after awakening in the morning. Think them first. Vary them to fit your individual case by attacking the attitudes which have disturbed you the most, and repeat them aloud: "I have never felt so calm and peaceful. When I am calm within, my speech pours out freely. All talking can be just lilke this, smooth and free . . ." (and so on!) (p. 16)

Something very similar is provided by Robbins (1926):

You can overcome this fear of stammering by autosuggestion provided you select the time when your brain is most suggestible, which has been found to be when you feel an inclination to sleep. Just before dropping off to sleep, breathe slowly and deeply through your nose, relax every muscle in your body, dismiss all worries from your mind and concentrate your thought upon the words: "I can speak fluently." It is not enough merely to think these words; you must believe them. (pp. 96–97)

When the writer was a young man, Coué, the famous French advocate of autosuggestion, was at the acme of his influence. He was reported to have dramatically cured a severe stutterer by suggestion before a large audience (Heltman, 1943).[4] Everyone had heard of Coué's famous formula: "Every day in every way I am getting better and better!" Even complete strangers offered it

gratis to us when they heard us stutter. We got rather tired of hearing the nonsense and so appreciated the following passage from Boome and Richardson's book, *The Nature and Treatment of Stammering* when it was published in 1932:

It should hardly be necessary to mention that negative suggestion does more harm than good; "I will not stammer," for instance, generally has the effect of enhancing the trouble. A child of nine informed us when he first came that he had already had "thought treatment," which consisted in the formula; "Every day and in every way my stammer gets better and better." If "better" stood for "bigger," the formula was having excellent results! We find that even Coué's well-known phrase, which we used for several years, may defeat its own ends—with stammerers at any rate—by being too positive. At times it is all too evident to a severe case that he is *not* "getting better and better" at the moment. (p. 100)

We find this sort of self-suggestion to be very widespread. In Japan, Mochizuki (1965) tells of stutterers having to repeat to themselves over and over, "My stuttering is cured. My stuttering is cured. I can read and speak smoothly," and he calls this common procedure unwise and unscientific. In India, the homeland of Yoga, such self-suggestion is a very prevalent practice. Mathur (1960) has his stutterer sit in a silent corner and then say to himself, "I do not stammer. I have cured it. I know where the mischief lay. I have cured it and will cure it completely." He should add to his will daily and whenever an (evil) autosuggestion comes he should then and there give a countersuggestion, "No I do not stammer," and say confidently "I will not stammer (p. 72)." In England we find Brook (1957) offering this formula: "A change is taking place

<hr />

[4] The stutterer relapsed within a week and was worse than before.

in my attitude toward speaking. I am calm and my speech is easy. The picture of ease and stillness often comes to me during the day so that my speech flows more easily. I look out for this feeling every time I talk. I feel calm and confident and I enjoy this effortless speech." But perhaps the pinnacle of this mountain of autosuggestive formulae is found in a book published in our own country by Wilton (1950). "There is a definite procedure by which you may strengthen your faith, and that is what I call the Priceless Affirmation." Chapter 10 of Wilton's book is devoted to this Priceless Affirmation and we hope we are not sullying it by quoting it here. Anything so precious should not be lost. This is Wilton's Priceless Affirmation:

I am calm. I have a feeling of calmness throughout my body. This calmness of my body calms my mind. I feel at peace. I possess peace. I am at peace with every thing around me. This peace is so deep that it makes everything that surrounds me peaceful too. In calmness is borne strength. In calmness is born freedom. In calmness is born free action. From my present state of calmness I can begin to function freely. And all of my actions shall be calmly done. (pp. 72–73)

Autogenic therapy. This type of therapy, very prevalent in Europe, is used in treating a wide range of psychosomatic illnesses, and stuttering is only one of the many disorders to which it has been applied. The basic concepts were devised by Dr. J. H. Schultz, an eminent psychiatrist and neurologist in Berlin, who in turn had been influenced by the writings of Oskar Vogt during the early years of this century. Schultz, dissatisfied with the usual methods of hypnosis since the hypnotized patient tended to become too passive and dependent, explored various autosuggestive methods including Yoga and finally developed a rather sophisticated system of exercises which would create a relaxed autogenic state (said to be similar but not identical to sleep or hypnosis). Under the direction of a physician, the patient, by passively concentrating his attention on certain self-statements, comes to achieve normalization of his body processes. The patient reclines or sits droopingly in a chair with eyes closed. There are six standard exercises, each with its key self-statement to be repeated over and over again to oneself. The series deals in turn with heaviness, warmth, cardiac regulation, breathing, abdominal warmth, and cooling of the forehead. We offer this brief quotation from Luthe and Schultz (1959) to illustrate one of the first exercises:

Trainee, lying down on a couch, relaxes in typical training posture and closes eyes. Doctor (in calm voice): "My right arm is heavy. (I am at peace) . . . My right arm is heavy. . . . My right arm is heavy. . . . My right arm is heavy. . . . " Trainee continues with passive concentration on "My right arm is heavy" for about 20 seconds.
Doctor: "Well, I think it's time to terminate."
Trainee: (a) flexes his arms vigorously, (b) breathes deeply, (c) open his eyes. (p. 25)

Since the same routine training must be done for the left arm, legs, and other parts of the body, numerous sessions are required even to master the first standard exercise of heaviness. Some of the self-suggestion formulae for the other standard exercises are: "My arms and legs are warm. . . ." "heartbeat calm and regular. . . ." "My solar plexus is warm. . . ." "My forehead is cool" and "It breathes me. . . ." This last phrase, so ungrammatical in English translation, refers to the passive awareness of the regularity and ease of respiration Luthe and Schultz (1968) give a daily play-by-play account of 112 sessions of this autogenic training during which time only the six standard exercises were mastered by the patient.

Only when the patient has become proficient in the standard exercises, may he be given the second series, the Meditative Exercises. These entail the imagining of various visual patterns, beginning with simple uniform colors, and progressing through a series of seven stages to the imagining of emotional scenes in which the patient participates. For some patients, these meditative exercises are omitted and they are given certain "intentional formulae" which pertain more directly to their problem. On these they must concentrate, as earlier they concentrated upon sensations of weight and temperature. One of those used for stuttering is called a neutralizing formula: "Talking does not matter." Another is: "My brain talks automatically." The training program ends with abreacting and ventilating methods for neutralizing emotional disturbances. This cursory account does not do justice to the elaborate and Germanic complexity of autogenic training or the dynamics involved, but it at least outlines the major features.[5] Autogenic training is not recommended for child stutterers younger than nine years and some of the more difficult older cases are said to need preliminary hypnosis before undergoing

the training. Brankel (1958) in his evaluation of autogenic training says, "Autogenic training is of value in that it induces a calm state of the respiratory and articulatory apparatus prior to phonation thus reducing the harsh impact of acoustic, visual, and emotional factors upon the onset of the speech (p. 118). Perhaps a sentence from Luthe and Schultz (1968) will summarize the purpose of autogenic therapy: "In cases of stuttering, autogenic therapy aims primarily at inducing a more passive and casual attitude toward the disturbed speech by emphasizing that the neuromuscular system functions at its best when left alone (p. 134)." To this author it seems that an awful lot of labor is needed to achieve such a goal.

The methods of Fernau-Horn. Among the European workers who use suggestion, we find Helene Fernau-Horn (1969). Her theory and methods have had considerable influence, especially in Germany. She adopts Schultz's view that stutterers have two kinds of neuroses. The first (Kern) is a "core" or primary neurosis in which the stuttering is symptomatic of some basic conflict. Stutterers with *Kern* neuroses require deep psychotherapy, since they do not really desire to talk fluently. The second type, the *Rand* neuroses, are what we might term secondary or expectancy neuroses, the stutterer having become convinced, through some traumatic speaking experiences, that he cannot speak without difficulty.[6]

Although either *Kern* or *Rand* neuroses or both may be present in a given stutterer, most of Fernau-Horn's therapy (1969) seems to be

---

[5] The best English source is the series of six volumes by Luthe and Schultz entitled *Autogenic Therapy*, New York: Grune and Stratton, 1968.

[6] Freund (1966, pp. 128–29) has clarified these concepts of the depth of neurosis according to Schultz and has also provided a useful critical reference by Jaspers.

devoted to helping those of the latter type, since according to Hanicke and Leben (1964) she feels that the *Rand* type is present in from 80 to 90 percent of all stutterers. Fernau-Horn views the basic difficulty as consisting of respiratory arrest due to the factors above mentioned. The neurotic blocking or freezing of breathing (and as a consequence, phonation) becomes part of a self-reinforcing chain of circles and spirals of inhibition which are almost as automatic as a Pavlovian conditioned reflex. These vicious circles and spirals must be interrupted and replaced by what she calls the *Aublaufzirkel*—a term which is hard to translate into English but which seems to refer to the normal timing and parallel flow of breath and sound in the synergies which underlie all normal speech.

Freund (1966) classifies Fernau-Horn's method as one of the auto-suggestive techniques and from her writing it is easy to see why. She begins by trying immediately to persuade the stutterer that his neurotic fears of speaking have no basis in reality, and to give him some fluent speech at the very first sitting. She wants him to think, "Ich habe keine Sprechsterung. Ich siehe nur die Sprech-bremset." (I have no disorder of speech. I am merely putting on my speech brakes.) The patient usually lies on a cot with the therapist hovering over him and he is put through a series of breathing exercises to lessen abdominal pressure and to produce relaxation by short inhalations and prolonged exhalations as he repeats after her such sentences as these: "My breath flows like the waves." "My tone flows like the waves." "My speech flows like the waves. I hear, feel, know that I can speak. I can say anything if I am calm. My confidence grows from day to day." Visual and auditory imagery are emphasized in these verbalizations (They are sometimes tape recorded.) and the procedure comes close to being hypnotic in its suggestiveness. The breathing exercises are primarily designed to promote relaxation and serenity since it is in these conditions that the *Ablaufzirkel* or normal synchronization of utterance can come to replace the evil circles and spirals of inhibition. Fernau-Horn, however, does not seek a complete relaxed state but rather a balanced tonicity of the respiratory musculatures sufficient to produce calm and rhythmic speech.

The training is controlled firmly by the therapist, the patient being placed in a rather passive role at least until he has mastered calm, relaxed, confident speech in the therapy room. He is given prescribed speaking tasks to effect a transition into everyday life where, whenever anxiety threatens, he must have recourse again to the relaxed calming procedures he has learned. The therapy seems to us to be highly stereotyped, a bit mystical, and rather rigidly based upon suggestion.

Schilling's signal training. Many European logopedists (speech therapists) have not been content to follow either Fernau-Horn or Schultz exactly. Many modifications are made; combinations of these procedures with others, such as Froeschels' breath chewing techniques, are common. One of the most successful of these modifications (according to his own report) was that devised by Anton Schilling (1965). In essence it consists of a preliminary period of standard autogenic training which is then followed by relaxed speech exercises a la Fernau-Horn. Then both are integrated by means of Schilling's signal training. In essence, some stimulus (a hand gesture, a sensation of warmth on the hand, a slight facial gesture, a tone or snatch of melody, etc.) is repeatedly paired with the formula-induced autogenic state and also with relaxed breathing and phonation (Fernau-Horn's therapy) until it comes to serve as the conditioned stimulus for the evocation of these states. Schilling writes, "This gesture, comparable to the gesture which one executes almost automatically in a joyous greeting, is combined with an almost-smiling inhaled flow of air through the slightly opened lips, and this leads automatically to deep abdominal breathing and the sensations of soft utterance." Schilling says that this signal can be conditioned to a visual image or to one of the autogenic intentional formulae and that when it is so conditioned it will enable the stutterer to become calm and integrated in a fraction of a second—even under stress. Schilling makes clear, however, that this signal training must be rigorous: "Only if this (conditioning) is adequately established will transfer occur to all speaking situations."

Indirect suggestion

Thus far most of the procedures we have been describing have involved fairly direct suggestion whether administered by the therapist or by the stutterer himself. We wish to make clear however that the use of indirect suggestion has always been more prevalent. We find it historically and we find it today. Essentially what happens is that the stutterer becomes convinced that he will stop stuttering and become fluent. The source of that conviction however is not necessarily the therapist, though he may manipulate the forces which underlie it. Instead, the suggestion may stem from the stutterer's desperate hope for relief, or the sheer amount of labor he invests in the therapeutic activities, or the magical properties of a distractor, a prosthesis or apparatus, or a novel way of speaking, or an identification with a charismatic therapist, or a hundred other such factors. Needing to believe, he comes to believe. He rejects his doubts. He tells himself privately and repeatedly that what he does in therapy will help him. He collects every scrap of confirmation that he can find. The author remembers vividly this process as it occurred during his own treatment at some of the stuttering institutes he attended as a young man. Some of the fool things he had to do were incredibly silly but because of his desperate need for hope, he brainwashed himself into a strong belief in their efficacy. Moreover, with that faith came some temporary though not complete relief. We are certain that some suggestion of this sort takes place in all stuttering therapy and that some of the milder stutterers have found freedom thereby, no matter what kind of treatment was being experienced.

Speech drills and logopedic exercises

It was apparent to the earliest observers that stutterers had breathing abnormalities, that they had difficulties at times in beginning to phonate, and that they often exhibited abnormal articulatory postures during the stuttering act. A natural inference was that stutterers had some basic weakness in the muscles that performed these acts and therefore needed exercises to strengthen these muscles. Thus Demosthenes practiced speaking while climbing mountains with lead plates upon his chest and shouted against the roar of the surf. Celsus, the famous Roman physician, prescribed various physical and breathing exercises for his stutterers. As we read these old writings, it is almost amusing to find the authorities of the past arguing about the location of the weakness—Itard (1817) insisting that it was in the laryngeal muscles, McCormac (1828) claiming that the respiratory muscles were those chiefly involved, and many others blaming the tongue. In addition, other old authors, recognizing that no real weakness was present in these musculatures but still impressed by their unruliness, attributed the disorder to neurologic spasms of the glottis, the breathing apparatus, or the articulators. One of them called stuttering the "St. Vitus Dance (chorea) of the tongue." Again, the chief method that they recommended for counteracting these spasms was highly conscious training in how to breathe, how to produce voice and how to articulate the various sounds. A third school viewed stuttering as a simple bad habit that could be broken by intensive practice of normal speech. Amman as early as 1700 writes:

Stammering is almost a perpetual blundering of utterance, which arises as much as anything from a bad habit. It consists, for the most part, in so labored an anxious repetition of the explosive letters that the face of the stammerer appears livid and suffused with blood from the constant struggle to speak, and the consequent diminution of inhaled air. I recommend to persons so affected to read much with a distinct and loud voice, to relate narratives lately read to a friend, to commit something to memory daily, and often to repeat it, and never to speak but with slowness and premeditation.

We find a clear illustration of this pedagogical training in the speech exercises of the Brosterian method in England (1827) and in the vocal gymnastics which accompanied the use of the mouth pad in the American Method so well promoted by Madame Leigh.[7] As an example of the sort of therapy based upon these beliefs, we might provide an outline of Schmalz's (1846) program. First of all Schmalz stressed that the stutterer should have a quiet mind, self-security and a belief in the method's infallibility and then should perform all these exercises daily for a long enough time:

1. Prolong the inhalation and exhalation before speech begins;
2. Relaxed breathing and articulation movements;
3. Use a low-pitched voice;
4. Speak softly, not loudly;
5. Begin speaking with air in lungs;
6. Concentrate on contracting the abdomen;
7. Shift the attention from the articulation to the voice and stress the tone;
8. Speak the sentences without interruption.

The stutterers were to practice reading and speaking until they could fulfill these requirements.

These speech drills became very popular in the 1800s. They kept the stutterers busy and involved. They could be practiced without triggering much stuttering, thus fostering the indirect suggestion that they were curative. They were easy for thera-

[7] A good description of Madame Leigh's method is given in the article by Schoolfield (1938).

pists to administer and they doubtless produced some temporary relief for many stutterers and cures for a few. The most influential advocate of pedagogical retraining through speech exercises was Gutzmann (1898) whose system dominated speech therapy for stutterers for many years. The set of exercises that he devised was usually carried out by the stutterer under rigid supervision in a home, hospital, or institution. The stutterer had to learn the correct way of coordinating his speech muscles and to speak highly consciously rather than automatically. Beginning with intensive breathing exercises and some training in vocalization, he then proceeded to practice first simple sounds, then syllables, then words and finally sentences. In the latter phase, all words had to be spoken on the voluntary exhalation of the breath and the vowels of those words had to be prolonged.[8]

Gutzmann's therapy was relatively easy to carry out even by untrained individuals. In the typical German fashion, it was systematic and thoroughly defined. The exercises were spelled out in complete detail. His writings were authoritative and had the heady smell of science. It was so easy to follow that some normal speakers or stutterers (who had gained some fluency by undergoing the treatment) set up institutes or stammering schools usually in private homes thereby controlling the stutterer's environment almost totally. In these homes, stuttering was of-

ten "verboten." You followed the method. You did the exercises. You obeyed the commands. Many stammering institutes flourished in this country during the first 30 years of the present century and in many other parts of the world. Even today we find places where such exercise treatments are still being employed and we find a vestige of them given in a recent book by Anderson (1970).

Usually, when a stutterer first entered one of these stammering schools or institutes he was placed "on silence" for a period which might last for as long as two weeks. He was impressively told that this was necessary to weaken his bad speaking habits before the new ones could be built through the proper exercises. As one who experienced these silence periods, the author can state they were extremely traumatic at first but also that as the days went by, the hope came up that when at last he could begin to speak again, he would be more fluent. The use of a silence period enforced a commitment; it provided an opportunity to sign the invisible contract which always exists between a therapist and his client. If you broke your silence, you had not signed. And what happened in this event is that more days of silence were added onto the quota as a penalty. In certain stammering centers, it was possible to speak during the silence period but only during the recitations and exercises in unison or while beating time or using other rhythmic aids. Since the stutterer was usually fluent in such activities, they became invested with almost magical potency. Yearsley (1909) wrote this:

Silence, so far as relating to the cure, means not to attempt conversation with

---

[8] According to Freund (personal communication), Gutzmann's method was originally developed by Emil Gutzmann, a teacher of deaf mutes, though it was given scientific respectability and promotion by his son Herman Gutzmann a physician and professor. It owed much to such earlier workers as Denhardt, Kussmaul, and Klencke.

anyone under any circumstance, and this must be observed!) for a period of at least ten days. A much longer period would in many cases be to the pupil's advantage. He should not, during this stage, converse even in the most limited degree. Even the usual "Good Morning" and "Good Evening" must be avoided. In the presence of others he must be dumb. . . . A week's silence would have the effect of restoring his mind to its normal condition. There would be no constant fear of approaching failure and disaster so far as conversation is concerned. He would simply resign himself to a week's peace and quietness, undisturbed by any thought of speech or criticism. . . . All that the pupil requires is to make a firm resolution that he will not be tempted into conversation. (p. 17)

More recently, we have this account by DeHirsch and Langford 1950):

Prolonged periods of silence have been used by therapists, chiefly, we believe, in speech institutes where patients can live in. Stutterers who have been through this procedure testify that it does aid relaxation, and tends to break the bad habit, for, whatever the origin of stuttering, there is no question that a stuttering habit is established. During the period of silence, rhythmic exercises, breathing exercises, and so on may be undertaken as additional aids to relaxation. When silence is finally broken, it is broken first in rather controlled simple speech situations. Many stutterers derive tremendous encouragement from finding that after a period of silence of two or three weeks, they are able to say words quite well, sometimes with no stuttering whatever. Such an experience gives the stutterer a feeling of making a new start which is very helpful in coping with his long-standing problem. (p. 938)

As we have said, and as these authors knew well, the effect of suggestion depends not only on the prestige of the suggester, or upon the massed repetition of the message, but it also depends upon the stimulus intensity. Weak suggestion has little effect. We provide an example of strong suggestion in a speech drill therapy session observed in France by Rigmor Knudsen (1946):

The stutterers start out the day at nine o'clock by getting electric massage in the face and throat presumably to loosen the tension of these muscles. Then the adults practiced breathing exercises in a respiratory apparatus under the supervision of the assistants. Then followed the "psycho-neuro-motor exercises" which were directed by Madame P. herself. They last from 9:30 to 11 A.M. and take place in a rather large room in which the stutterers of all ages sit on little chairs arranged in a row. Mme. P. who is no longer young but has white hair which stands out like foam on the head, confronts the class and yells with a forceful voice what the students must do. "It is energy that is necessary," she explained to me, "and I have it." They started with silent exercises. "Ouvrez la bouche!" Mme. P. yelled, and it was fantastic to watch forty people forcing their mouths open. "Try to create resistance in the jaw!" the commando shouted, and I have never dreamt of seeing tensions like these. But it was the exercises with voice that were most remarkable. They were all to be shouted as loudly as possible. "Without energy, no result!" Mme. P. stated triumphantly. There was for instance the exercise on "kra-rra-rra;" this was repeated an immense number of times with different vowels, without stopping, and with increasing speed. At the same time Mme. P., like a tamer of wild beasts, was exciting the students to use more and more force: "Give everything! Louder! Still more!" Finally, after a series of exercises which seemed interminable, and at the loudest intensity, sentences like "J'arriverai a l'amelioration avec de l'energie" were used and the class finished by answering questions in unison. (One course of this sort of therapy lasts at least fourteen months.) At the end of the class, Mme. P. turned triumphantly to me and said, "Every day the same energy! Don't say I haven't got energy!" And I could not help but answer, "Madame, only now I understand Napoleon!" She took it for a compliment and invited me to come again every day so that I could learn the method and import it into Denmark but I thanked her and escaped. (pp. 15–16)

On the assumption that some stutterers were helped by such a routine, the question arises again as to what might be the healing components in such practices. We might consider any of the following: the use of assertive behavior to reciprocally inhibit the stutterer's anxiety; the modeling effect through identification; the possible integration of the basic synergies of voice, articulation, and respiration; the presence of masking noise; the prosodic and timing effects of unison speaking. But, more potent than any of these presumed influences, is the very evident use of both direct and indirect suggestion in these exercises.

As one looks through many of the old books and manuals of stuttering therapy, one is struck by the number of them that contain not only phonetic drills and sentences but also long passages to be read orally or memorized and recited. Were the long hours spent by the large host of homeless, forgotten stutterers in such activities entirely in vain? Is suggestion the basic reason for any effectiveness which this labor had? Is it not possible that large doses of normal reading and speaking (however procured) might overcome the tendency to stutter? If the normal speech can be strongly reinforced by massed practice, will this not weaken its competing stuttering response to the same verbal cues? Many of our forerunners in the field of speech pathology certainly believed that it would.

Let us try to explain why these exercises were used so widely. Oral reading, at least in the clinical situation, is for many stutterers less stressful than speaking if only because they are not burdened by the need to formulate messages. The same can be said for memorization. Through the use of choral (unison) reading and speaking, or relaxation, or other methods, most stutterers can readily produce good fluency in these activities. In memorized material the adaptation effect soon reduced the stuttering. The prime concern of our predecessors was to get the stutterer to be fluent as soon as possible and here were activities which certainly helped them do so. Anything which worked so quickly and worked so well must be good! Perhaps it was because they believed so strongly in the efficacy of giving the stutterer repeated and prolonged experiences in normal speaking that they resorted to so many dubious practices to attain it.

Presumably there are always rewards and positive reinforcements which follow the normal speech thus produced. Some of them come from the therapist, some from the listener and many more from the stutterer himself. Unfortunately, this normal speaking does not occur in the contexts linked with the stuttering behavior since the communicative situation is usually different. In the therapy room the stress is lessened; fear and frustration are prevented. Though the words may appear to be the same as those on which the stutterer usually had trouble, they are perceived differently and so it is difficult to get much transfer into live communication. Stuttering is not a disorder of pronunciation. Much of the improvement shown as a result of long sessions in practicing normal speaking is probably due more to the increase in the stutterer's self-esteem due to his involvement. He is making a commitment. He is working on his speech by doing all this reading and speaking. Surely these long hours of labor must be helping him. So runs the indirect suggestion and so down goes the anxiety and stuttering for the time being. Besides, if the stutterer is spending his time practicing, he does not need to be out in the evil world of threat. Perhaps he would do as well by spending his time in singing or talking to himself or copying the reading passages in script. But one real advantage accrues; it sets the therapist free if not the stutterer as evidenced by this old cry from Appelt (1929):

> I slaved my life out over breathing, vocal, and articulatory exercises by the aid of books; but, however much I pondered over the cause of the suffering and watched its different symptoms, all my pains proved futile, nor was I spared the disheartening realization that those fetters did but strengthen the more I worked to rid myself of them. . . . I came to the conclusion that by far the largest percentage (at least 90 percent) of those who have been discharged as "cured" are, in reality, only seemingly cured, and, when my investigations led me to discover that dread of speaking and inner psychic resistances are the cause of the complaint, I knew that mechanical exercises would not remove such subtle difficulties, and that a real and lasting cure was yet to be found. (pp. v–vi)

There has been a tremendous amount of this busy work in the treatment of stuttering. Since we assume that some few stutterers have been cured and some improved by such practices even if all the rest were not benefited, we feel that most of the change can be attributed to sugges-

tion. Boome and Richardson (1932) say it clearly:

> The majority of exercises devised for group work have their greatest value as vehicles for suggestion. The younger the children the more necessary it is to give them definite occupation. But with older children it is possible to explain to a certain extent in simple language that the trouble is psychological, and that the alteration of their habits of thought is a more important part of the treatment than the actual exercises, which are only a means to that end. (p. 96)

Commercial stuttering schools

Perhaps a glimpse into the functioning of the old stuttering institutes might be of value in evaluating the treatment in terms of suggestion since in them stutterers could be found practicing their exercises night and day. As we have said earlier, treatment usually began with a period of complete silence for several weeks, during which time the stutterer was subjected to intense verbal suggestion. Methods were secretive. Often the stutterer was sworn never to reveal the method. Testimonials (often solicited and paid for from people who had never stuttered) covered the walls, and were read silently or aloud as part of the daily ritual. Once the silence period was over, the speech work was done in groups, the stutterers breathing, chanting, timing their syllables with their arms or fingers in unison with the instructor or marching about the room beating their chests to his baton.

In his younger days the author attended several of these commercial stammering institutes and, from what he has read, they were typical of most of the others that exploited stutterers in the early years of this century. Each institute had its own minor variations in the treatment but all of them employed direct and indirect suggestion constantly. One used arm swinging, another the swaying of eyes or hands or body, the third a lalling rhythmic form of continuous utterance in which all words were joined and all consonants were slurred. In each one of these insti-

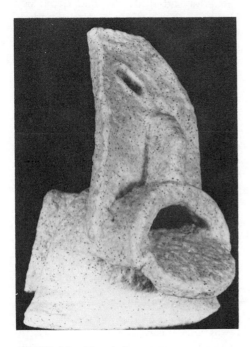

FIGURE 1.1 The author as a young man. (Courtesy Woodruff Starkweather.)

tutes we chanted slogans full of suggestion, such as the following: "I will; I will; I WILL!" "I shall be strong; I'll not be weak; I shall not stutter; Hear me speak!" or "I will be cured now that I have found the way." And at each one we had the same interminable breathing exercises: lying down, sitting, standing up; chest breathing rituals, "costal" breathing exercises, diaphragmatic

ones, abdominal ones. (Our chests were measured each week to see if they were benefitting from the practice!) We phonated single vowels in unison, then double vowels, then triplets and quadruplets. Then we ran them together always watching and controlling our breathing. Then we repeated words and sentences after the instructor timing this utterance with simultaneous swings of our arms or dumbells or Indian Clubs or the pinching of fingers. As we chanted the suggestive sentences after the instructor woe be unto any poor soul who stuttered then. He was banished from the group, fined, sentenced to spend hours in complete silence or assigned great numbers of pages of reading to oneself, or held up to shame before his peers.

These old quack practitioners knew all about contingencies and positive and negative reinforcement. They were controlling and shaping behavior in stutterers long before Skinner was born. Half starved in the boarding houses, we were given extra beans and hominy for faithful work and success—or privileges such as being allowed to leave the premises to go for a walk or to buy razor blades or peanuts, etc., but to gain these we had to earn them. Tokens in the form of stamped paper chits (tokens) served as the currency of that autocratic kingdom. We remember selling a sweater once for eight pieces of such paper, and using the privilege obtained thereby (seven chits worth, with one left for the supper's extra dish of beans) to get down to the corner store for the first ice cream in months. Any stutterer who so much as expressed any hint of doubt concerning the possibility that THE METHOD was not going to aid him was shamed or expelled. We held morning prayers as a group, chanting our faith and belief as we swung our arms.

At one of the institutes, kangaroo courts were held regularly each week on Friday. All of us dreaded that day for anyone of us might be summoned before the judge, accused of failing to do the necessary work or of not using the prescribed form of utterance or, what was worse, of stuttering. The prosecutor summoned witnesses who testified against the accused, who, poor devil, was his own lawyer and had to conduct his defense. Under that stress it was difficult to use the method or to keep from stuttering so the culprit was usually found guilty and sentenced to severe penalties. Often he was required to go back three grades and work up, with each grade necessitating at least a week of hard, boring speech labor. The system was ingeniously contrived to keep the stutterers there in the institute as long as possible since we not only had to pay board and room but also extra tuition by the week. But there was always hope held out to us—lovely, shining hope, based on faith, hard work and sacrifice. If the bedbugs bit too hard at night, we could always get up and do more exercises, and we did them.

In rereading this, 40 years later, the author finds it hard to believe that he could have endured the charlatanry, but when one stutters terribly and there is no other recourse in the world, one will put up with any folly and endure anything for the hint of hope. And indeed there was hope. It was brainwashed into us by probably fraudulent but highly fluent strangers who came each week and gave their testimonials of having been cured. (They often seemed memorized.) Hope was engendered

also by the suggestive phrases we chanted, by the material we read, yes, even by the air we breathed in and out during our respiratory exercises. And fear, the dragon, was also often invoked to spur us on. Each time a stutterer managed to escape or was expelled, the teacher or director called a meeting and painted in vivid hues the fate which lay before the poor sad soul who had departed. Under such a regime and confined to quarters, most of us improved. We saw each other getting fluent and this too was highly suggestive and impressive.

Elsewhere we have written (Van Riper, 1971):

The quacks of that day were excellent operant conditioners. We lived (almost imprisoned) in the institute and were manipulated like Skinnerian pigeons in a laboratory. Occasionally by immense effort and concentration I was able to get enough metrical fluency to smell the cheese of hope but too often even in my metronomic singsong I would block severely with my arm frozen in the air and my fingers glued together. Gluency not fluency was my lot when finally my funds ran out and I was unceremoniously booted out of that institute. There were 64 other stutterers there at the same time I was and I corresponded with each of them afterward. Only one of them said he had gained anything from the training; most were worse than when they entered. This surprised me because most of them had not had the difficulty in mastering metronomic speech that I had experienced. They had become fluent there at the institute and upon their departure they had signed testimonials to the fact that they were cured. I later met the one man who was the exception and found him speaking without stuttering but at the rate of about two measured monotonous syllables per second. He sounded like a zombie, the living dead.

Many of the stutterers with whom I worked in my early professional years

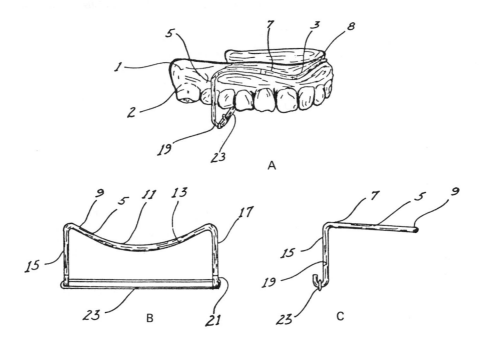

FIGURE 1.2 Freed Stammercheck to slow speech and require conscious articulation. (U.S. Patent 2, 818,065 [1955].)

had had similar experiences. Then for a couple of decades, with the advent of our new profession and the disappearance of the commercial stuttering schools, the use of time beating methods seemed to have died out but now here they are again all fancied up in behavior modification terminology. Doubtless another crop of disillusioned stutterers and herapists will need to be harvested before we can hope for further progress in devising a truly adequate therapy for stuttering. (pp. 12–13)

The use of prostheses and appliances

Often the speech training exercises were performed in conjunction with various prosthetic appliances. These provided some of the corroboration which suggestion always needs if it is to be effective. They also served as distractors. The alteration of stimulus configurations which is produced by having your mouth filled with strange objects or wearing

a laryngeal harness around your neck or having to operate a breathing belt in a certain way when you talk does reduce word fears and so, temporarily, the stuttering. Again in them we find the magic of suggestion at work. They have been used for centuries and we find them being sold today. Itard, a French physician (1765–1838), placed little gold or ıvory forks under the stutterer's tongue to overcome its presumed spasmodic weakness. Another early prosthesis is described by Schilling (1965):

Columbat's Muthonom was a small instrument of silver and ivory which, when slid under the tongue and attached to the lower incisors, had the task of elevating and retracting the tongue. Other devices sought to achieve just the opposite effect, to thrust the allegedly short tongue near the lower incisors. One of these was a thin silver plate duplicating the teeth designed by Hervez de Chegoin in 1830. (p. 368)

Other appliances impeded abdominal breathing and still others such as the Bates devices had springs which exerted pressure on the Adam's Apple, and there were also several weird assemblies of wire to be worn inside the mouth. Robinson (1964) describes one which was recently patented in this country:

As recently as 1957, for example, patent number 2,818,065 was issued for the FREED STAMMERCHECK, an oral apparatus to slow tongue movement and thus assist in the reduction of stammering (stuttering) symptoms. The patent account states, "When the device is properly fitted in the mouth of a stutterer an immediate improvement in his speech has been observed, and with only intermittent wearing, the reflex habit has been broken." (p. 14)

McCarthy (1970) says that there are over 50 such patents for curing stutterers currently registered in the United States Patent Office. They also exist in Japan. There Sato (1954) describes an apparatus consisting of a thin celluloid shield to be attached to the teeth of stutterers, reporting that the results in 18 of 69 cases were excellent, 32 very good, 17 good, 2 were fair, and none was bad. Clark (1959) tells of wire appliances called "Zonds" used in Russia to alter tongue positions of stutterers.

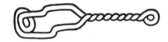

FIGURE 1.3   A Zond.

In his miserable youth, the author of this text did not have such devices

but found that he could speak more easily with pebbles (a la Demosthenes) or, preferably, hard candies, in his mouth—though not for long—and he wondered why they helped reduce his stuttering. Alexander Melville Bell (1853), the inventor of visible speech for the deaf, provided one answer. He wrote:

The Stammerer has undoubtedly high authority and ample precedent for trying the effect of pebbles in his mouth; but he may perhaps be satisfied to spare himself the chance of a fit of indigestion should he swallow one of them, when we tell him that he would find pebbles in his mouth useless.

Demosthenes did not cure himself by pebbles but by indomitable energy and perseverance. If the pebbles had at all assisted him, it would be by keeping his teeth open. Perhaps he had the Stammerer's snappish habit of jerking his jaws close at every articulation and a pebble between the teeth would be of service in correcting this. At all events, let the Stammerer not trust to anything out of himself—to any mechanical assistance or unusual expedient—for the working of his cure. (p. 49)

One of the more ingenious appliances comes from Japan in the form of Idehara's "Stuttering-curing apparatus" (1937) which consists of a little whistle located within the mouth cavity and fastened by bands to the upper teeth. The object of the device assures feedback from airflow, a most pertinent procedure in terms of modern servotherapy. Though others cannot hear the tiny whistle, the stutterer certainly can, and so he learns to whistle as he talks. At the base of the whistle, a sharp point projects sufficiently to punish the stutterer for excessive tongue pressure.

We also have contemporary col-

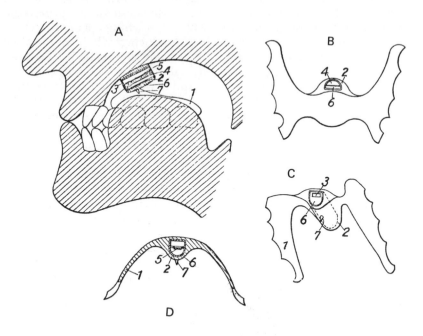

FIGURE 1.4   Idehara (Izuhara) stutter-cure device. (British Patent 501,779 [1939].)

leagues who strongly recommend the electric metronome worn behind or in the ear like a hearing aid, but more of that in a later section. We now may smile at Itard's forks or Columbat's Muthonome but modifications of these are being sold today. We might wonder why the Prussian government could ever pay so much money for Madame Leigh's secret cure [9] and make it the official treatment for stuttering. Yet we marvel less when we think of some of the modern methods and devices used in

retraining tongue thrust and reversed swallowing. Sometimes it seems that progress is always circular!

Distraction

If suggestion is to be truly effective, it needs some corroboration. We resist suggestions that are obviously implausible or invalid; we more readily accept those that seem appropriate or true. Since workers who use hypnosis know this well, they may ask a subject to fixate his eyes for some time upon a light or object held or waved above his head before they suggest that his eyelids are growing heavy and that he is about to go to sleep. Told that he will soon be falling backwards into

[9] The secret: Bring the tongue far forward in the mouth and talk while keeping its tip on the upper gum ridge in contact with the teeth. At night keep a small roll of linen under the tongue so the position will become habitual.

the safe arms of the hypnotist, the subject finds that he is indeed swaying when his hair is stroked and so he believes the suggestion, not realizing that there is always some body sway when one stands rigidly erect and that the hypnotist is timing his stroking with the rhythm of that sway. Told that he will be unable to open his tightly locked fingers, the subject finds that holding them in that position for several minutes does indeed make them difficult to unfold, and so the suggestion gets the corroboration it needs to be accepted.

We find the same process occurring in stuttering therapy. Indeed many common therapeutic techniques were found and used by stutterers themselves long before they were ever exploited systematically by therapists It has been fascinating to observe how many untreated stutterers discover the same identical ones: changing the tempo of their utterance, varying the way they articulate, adopting unusual inflection patterns, and so on. What is important is that we recognize that since these ways of coping with stuttering do offer some temporary but real relief from stuttering, this relief provides the partial corroboration which any effective suggestion requires.

Long ago, in a German article that impressed this author greatly when he first translated it and which still does today, Henry Freund (1932) classified these speech-modifying techniques and showed why they helped reduce or prevent stuttering. Prominent among them were the methods that distracted the stutterer from his pathological attention to verbal and situational cues signifying danger in speaking. Freund showed that many workers had sought to divert the attention of the stutterer from his articulation by

techniques which forced him instead to concentrate upon adopting a novel way of breathing, phonating, accenting, producing syllables, or altering the tempo and melodic features of his talking. In Freund's view, such methods were a far cry from the old suggestive speech gymnastics and strengthening exercises since they directly attacked the expectancy core of the expectancy neurosis involved in stuttering and so he still recommends their judicious use. If distraction techniques can break up the vicious self-reinforcing cycles of negative suggestion and abnormal perception, why not use them? Dr. Freund, a wise and kind man, feels that the stutterer's use of any of these methods or even an occasional avoidance such as the use of synonyms is "still preferable to the feelings of complete failure and frustration which accompany actual stuttering."

It is at least certain that stutterers have been using distracting devices and behaviors for years to ease their distress. And so have their therapists. Over a century ago, Schulthess (1830) insisted that it was very important that the stutterer be given ways of diverting his morbid attention from his speaking difficulties. Many modern workers, seduced by the temporary increments in fluency produced by some of these ancient methods, have rediscovered them and justify their use by impressive modern rationales while denying their utility as distractors. The old therapists were not so naive. Potter (1882) provided a long list of distractors ranging from drawling and sniffing to syllable-timed speech and rate control and he had some reservations about their use:

The whole subject of tricks and mechanical contrivances may be dismissed in a very few words. Any one of them will be found useful while the novelty to the patient, serving to concentrate his attention and to exercise his will, by constituting an additional obstacle to his speech, rouses the whole latent will power to overcome it. Thus, in conquering the new and greater obstacle, the older and for the time being lesser one is surmounted at the same time. But when by usage the organs become habituated to the trick, the will is freed from the necessity of exertion, the stammer returns with the same severity as before, the patient curses the quack who victimized him. and relapses into despair. (pp. 95–96)

About 50 years later Fletcher (1928) made a similar comment in a very long sentence:

Placing corks or wedges between the teeth, shrugging the shoulders, tapping with the feet, pinching with the fingers, whistling or counting before speaking, and numerous similar therapeutic expedients, all of which have been known to be effective in certain cases, seem to owe their efficacy to the fact that they distract the attention of the stutterer from his difficulty, and that, in consequence, they afford him a relief from the morbid inhibitions by which his speech is hindered. (p. 125)

Consider for a moment how distracting were the Bates appliances which we briefly mentioned in our section on prostheses. Potter (1882) tells of his own sad experiences with them:

The Bates appliances were extensively advertised for the cure of stuttering a few years ago and have made many victims. They cost $35, are patented, and consist of three articles, (1) a coin-silver instrument in the form of a small flattened bedpan, worn in the mouth with the handle projecting between the lips, for the purpose of giving access to air and egress to the breath in labial stuttering; (2) a small gold tube to be at-

tached by a rubber band to one of the teeth for the relief of the dental form of stuttering; (3) a larynx compressor, capable of increased pressure by tightening up a screw and a buckle, attached to a band for the neck, to be worn by those who have difficulty in enunciating the gutterals. As nearly every serious case presents all the forms mentioned, the simultaneous use of the three appliances would be necessary in order to be prepared for any emergency. The folly of expecting benefit from such contrivances for any length of time is known by experience to the writer, who gave the above mentioned sum for a set of these toys at a time when he had to deny himself the necessaries of life in order to pay for them. (pp. 93–94)

An old account by Gutzmann (1898) may demonstrate how a distraction can alter the speaking situation so that the usual stimuli controlling stuttering become ineffective. He applied a weak faradic electric current to the neck of some stutterers at the level of the larynx and found that some of them became remarkably fluent. However, he also found that some of them also became fluent when the electrodes were put on but no current was sent through the wires. They were simply thinking more about the shock than the possibility of stuttering. Some stutterers report that they can speak more easily when swimming or driving an automobile or performing other activities. While some of this effect, as in swimming or dancing, may be due to the facilitation of timing, some of it, as in driving the car, must be due to the need to scan the road more than their speech. One of the most vivid illustrations of this novelty effect is to be found in a little article by Geniesse (1935) in which it was found that stutterers at the University of Michigan were able to speak fluently when on hands and knees.

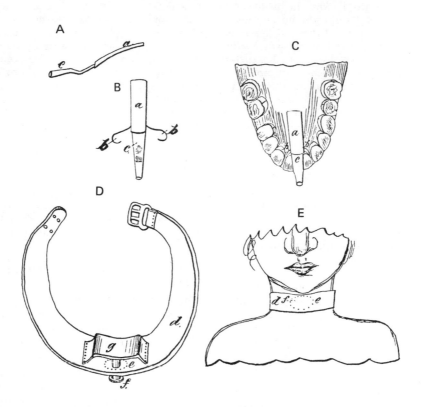

FIGURE 1.5   The Bates appliances. (U.S. Patent 8, 394 [1851].)

(This author developed a silly theory about temporary dilatation of the precentral cortical capillaries.) Fitz (1961) gives a modern illustration of another way in which suggestion and distraction are employed today:

> During the course of treatment 15 of the most severe stutterers were individually exhibited before speech therapists in a home for children who were unfit for school. Their initial speech breakdowns weakened immediately when they were subjected to *elastic vibration exercises.* In half an hour the demonstration was concluded because all of them spoke freely for an average of at least two minutes each. (p. 263)

In his youth, the author of the present text was once subjected to the visualization therapy advocated by Swift (1931), a very famous physician who specialized in speech disorders. Locating the cause of stuttering in the cuneus and attributing it to a failure in visual imagery, Swift trained his patients to improve this function. If we said "green chair" we had to see it in our mind's eye. If we had to say an abstract sentence, then we visualized it written in orange script on a "field of blue." Unfortunately for the theory and method (which did help us temporarily) Bluemel (1931) pointed out that congenitally blind people didn't stutter any more than those with normal sight. Some wild claims were made for the validity of the visualization method but its major claim to fame was that it was probably the purest form of distraction ever invented.

Novel ways of speaking

Mackay (1969) found that normal speakers experienced much less disruption and stuttering under delayed feedback when they spoke in a nasal voice. By attending to the tone, they could ignore the delay. We are not surprised. Stutterers discovered long ago that if they adopted an unfamiliar manner of speaking that they could become more fluent for a time though the effect usually did not last. Kingdon-Ward (1942) is only one of many authors who have made the observation, for example, that the severity and frequency of stuttering decreases suddenly and dramatically when they speak with a foreign or regional dialect. Bloodstein (1969) provides such an illustration:

Distractions rarely continue to be effective if they are used repeatedly. One stutterer, newly arrived in New York City from a small town in the Midwest and anticipating an exceptional amount of difficulty speaking, adopted the habit of talking in a Texas "drawl" and spoke quite fluently for about a month in this way. He began to stutter again, however, as soon as the drawl became an accustomed manner of speaking. (p. 198)

The old therapists also discovered this phenomenon and exploited it thoroughly. Some of them trained their stutterers to speak in a monotone, others stressed the use of abnormal inflections. One of the latter techniques was Scripture's "octave twist," the stutterer being taught to raise his pitch by an eye-popping octave the moment he found himself stuttering on a word. A sing-song type of speaking was also recommended by many other workers with every other word or syllable being uttered at a different pitch level. Arnott's method, first developed in 1864, was very popular for many years and we find some therapists using it still today. It consisted of requiring the stutterer to prefix the short vowel ɛ before the first word of every sentence or feared word. Many varieties of the Arnott technique have been employed with schwa vowels or nasals or the aspirate "h" being used alternatively as the prefixed starting sounds. Since for a short time this prefixing will undoubtedly distract the stutterer's attention away from his usually feared sounds (since the words no longer start with them), the technique can produce some temporary fluency. Eventually however the prefixed sound becomes a feared sound itself by contiguity of association, or else the distraction wears out as it becomes habituated and then the poor devil's problem is doubled. The former King of England, George VI, was taught by the therapist Leary of Australia to start all sentences, phrases and feared words with the schwa vowel and to speak very slowly. We have heard that monarch speaking via radio to an empire on which the sun then never set. He was gallant but there were times when his technique failed him.

Another very common technique required the stutterer to use a lalling way of speaking, the tongue being anchored either to the lower or upper teeth. All plosive consonants were to be "slighted," that is, to be produced with very low pressure or even to be almost omitted. Fluency was produced thereby but certainly at the expense of intelligibility. The same could be said about the demand that all speaking should be done very softly, almost in a breathy whisper. Therapists seem to have used every possible variation of the characteristics of speech in the treatment of stuttering, altering the pitch, intensity, and quality to produce novel forms of utterance. They have also altered the tempo but we shall consider syllable-timed speech, abnormally slow speech and rate control, in another chapter. What we must remember is that these unusual ways of talking to produce temporary fluency are not new. Thousands of stutterers now dead have spent hours, days, months, and years chasing the will o' the wisp of fluency by adopting a novel way of talking. Though for a time little stuttering occurred when they spoke in these strange ways, only rarely did any of them remain fluent when they once again tried to talk like a human being. It is very difficult to "shape" such an abnormal manner of talking into normal speech because the moment the stutterer speaks in his natural manner the distractive value is lost and the cues that precipitate stuttering once again raise their ugly heads.

There is doubtless some distraction inherent in all forms of stuttering therapy. Even in psychotherapy, the stutterer's attention is directed away from his speech difficulty and toward his other more basic problems of adjustment. We well remember L. E. Travis' off-hand remark when chivvied about simultaneous talking and writing owing its effectiveness merely to distraction: "If so, it's a very good one." Not even operant conditioning procedures are free from the suspicion of distraction. Indeed, Biggs and Sheehan (1969), in their replication of the operant study by Flanagan, Goldia-

mond, and Azrin (1958), insist that their data show clearly that the reduction in stuttering resulting from contingent application of an aversive tone of 108 decibels was probably due to the distraction effect. Any serious student of the disorder when contemplating any presentation of therapy must take this effect into account and so must researchers and clinicians.

Stutterers themselves have long used various kinds of distractive behaviors to free themselves from the tyranny of their fears and to gain some temporary fluency. Unfortuately, most of those which have been employed are neither "good" ones (in Travis' sense) nor are they able to yield any permanent relief. The following quotation from Greene (1931) makes the point very vividly:

At one period we took a group of 25 stutterers and purposely tried out every trick of distraction we ever heard of and besides improvised a few new ones for the occasion. The results were positively bad, for as soon as they discarded their temporary crutch they went back to their old style of stuttering speech. Two cases did show decided improvement and stayed so, but those were the ones which get better anyway with very little persuasion of any kind. They are the highly impressionistic cases that occasionally appear and immediately improve no matter what treatment they receive, as long as it is considered treatment by them. We found that tricks, distractions of any kind, interfere with the orderliness of the stutterer's thoughts causing him to talk mechanically and interfering with his ability to concentrate on what he is talking about. (p. 173)

That distraction can indeed ameliorate stuttering temporarily is indisputable, as Bloodstein's (1969) review has shown. But surely we should do more than give this factor a name. Why does a distractor distract? Why does the stutterer speak better when he chants in a sing-song fashion, or uses an odd form of breathing, or is bombarded with electric shocks or blasts of noise, or interjects "Hey" before a feared word (Dixon, 1957), or any number of similar conditions?

Newman (1968) attributes the distraction effect to the novelty of the stimulus events, a novelty which so alters the speaking situation that the old cues to which the stuttering behaviors were linked are either not present or occur in weaker strength or are not perceived as being linked to stuttering. He proposes two hypotheses: (1) By bringing novel stimuli into the speaking situation, the latter deviates so far from what is typical for the stutterer that stimulus generalization does not occur and so the cues which precipitate stuttering are no longer attended to, and (2) The unusual nature of the distraction situation so changes the perceptions of the stutterer that the conditioned stimuli which formerly elicited the stuttering are themselves significantly altered.

We should like to add two other explanations: first, under distraction the stutterer is less aware of the possible unpleasant consequences of his stuttering; and secondly, but more importantly, when attending to the distracting stimuli, he just does not assume his usual preparatory sets with their covert rehearsal of abnormality which so often lead to overt stuttering behaviors. He does not assume the abnormal postures which trigger tension and tremors. He is too busy coping with the pebbles in his mouth or performing the prescribed odd ways of talking or thinking about how to breathe or phonate or articulate, or getting set

for an expected electric shock or the blast of intense white noise. Perhaps, by his selective attention to these other things, he cannot visually scan his listeners for cues signifying impatience or other forms of possible rejection, or listen for the expected gaps and abnormalities in his speech. His usual perceptions are thereby altered. It is even possible that by concentrating on the slow pacing of his syllables or on the expectation of punishment, he will allow more proprioceptive information to be used in the automatic monitoring of his speech, thereby enabling him to bypass any dysfunction in his auditory processing system.

Persuasion

A common bit of lay advice that stutterers are often offered very freely may be expressed in any of the following ways: "There's nothing really wrong with you; why don't you stop that stuttering?" "See, you can talk all right if you really put your mind to it." "It's just a habit and you've got to break it." "It's all in your head!" These comments and exhortations reflect an ancient and widespread belief that the stutterer can stop stuttering if he really wants to do so. They also imply that the stutterer can be persuaded that he need not stutter. Over a hundred years ago, Wyneken (1868) expressed the sentiment very clearly: "We must deprive the stutterer of his doubt and replace it with conviction, that is to say by faith in his ability to speak. If once we succeed in convincing the stutterer of the certainty of a method of cure, he will speak well so long as he believes it."

Although persuasion is closely related to suggestion and probably represents one of its special cases, its major feature is the use of logic and reasoning to create belief. When used in therapy, the clinician usually first verbalizes the beliefs of his client and then presents his own contrasting beliefs. Next there follows an interchange in which the evidence in favor of the clinician's beliefs is strongly stated while that supporting the client's is minimized or shown to be faulty. In persuasion, there is always the appeal to reason, to logic, or perhaps to authority. The client's experiences are interpreted in such a way as to sway him to accept the therapist's assumptions and to act upon them. Most of the persuasion therapies used with the stutterer have tried to convince him that he could speak normally and had no real reason to continue to struggle or to avoid.

One of the well known therapies based upon persuasion is that described by Froeschels (1964) in a long series of publications. It has also been known as the breath chewing method. Stuttering, according to Froeschels, was a hyperfunctional disorder with its struggle and tension being due to misevaluation. Froeschels believed that the child, in responding to his normal disfluencies and speech hesitations, makes what he calls "a logical error." This error is the belief that speaking is difficult. To persuade the stutterer that he is wrong in this false conviction, Froeschels used breath-chewing or ventriloquism to convince him that his fears are groundless, that he can speak without struggling, and that therefore he has no need for avoidance or struggle. To quote Froeschels directly with respect to breath-chewing:

The method should be used in the following way. First, an explanation of the identity of chewing and speaking movements is given the patient. Then he should be asked to chew in his ordinary manner, with closed lips but with the mouth empty, and to observe his tongue moving constantly during the act of chewing. Immediately afterward he is asked to "chew like a savage," that is to say, by opening his mouth and using extensive movements of his lips and tongue. . . . Subsequently the patient must give voice during the act of chewing. If the chewing is performed correctly, a great variety of sounds will escape from his mouth. If uniform sounds like "ham-ham-ham" are heard, the lips and tongue do not move sufficiently. Correctly performed, chewing gives the impression of a foreign language. In this way the patient may learn how easy it is to speak. (1964, p. 67)

Froeschels felt that most of the logopedic training methods of drilling the stutterer in normal speech were wrong and that any success procured through their use was due to suggestion. "In addition," he writes, "it seems to me that these methods may confirm the opinion of the patient that speech is difficult." Froeschels admits that breath-chewing is a "surface method" but he feels that for most cases deep psychotherapy is entirely unnecessary. In turn, Kastein (1947), who in her advocacy of breath chewing states that "Half the battle is to convince the stutterer of the ease of speech" also feels constrained to say, "The well trained therapist will always consider the personality of the patient as a whole, and that, in addition to using the chewing method or any other method for that matter, the therapist will contribute constructively to rebuilding the patient's injured personality (p. 195)." Froeschels felt that breath chewing should, in any case, precede any psychotherapy. If the method seems far too simple, one might consider Rothe's position (1928). This writer praised the chewing method precisely because it was a pure form of treatment and avoided the therapy-salad approach. However, its simplicity may disguise its real sophistication. Hollingsworth (1939) showed that chewing had a tranquilizing effect; Despert (1942) viewed vocalized chewing as an abreactive activity, saying, "The chewing-speaking games reproduce the early eating-speaking situation and give an opportunity for the reliving (abreacting) of a traumatic psychomotor experience on better affective terms;" and Van Riper (1957) discusses its psychotherapeutic effectiveness as a form of reassurance: "Unlike some of the more bizarre suggestive techniques such as rate control, the octave twist, speaking in a monotone, syllable tapping, the activity of chewing is a familiar one to every patient. Used discreetly it has no more additional abnormality than chewing gum while speaking (p. 220)."

Froeschels noted however that some of his patients had difficulty accepting the persuasion that, by learning to chew their breath as they talked, they could always speak without stuttering. For these he recommended ventriloquism as an alternate procedure: "With patients who are not cooperative in using the practical application of the chewing idea, ventriloquism is offered as another way of demonstration (that they can indeed speak without stuttering) although it is more of an indirect approach than the chewing method."

In teaching ventriloquism the therapist authoritatively and impressively instructs the stutterer concerning the importance of articulatory movements as they modify phonation and then he manipulates the patient's lips to produce different vowels. The stutterer is told that voicing and sighing are identical and that if he has trouble phonating he should merely sigh. Next he is required to read aloud "with opened mouth but to move neither the lips or tongue," and then to speak as a ventriloquist would, using only minimal movements of articulation. Singing is sometimes used to effect a gradual transition into normal speech. Both the breath-chewing and ventriloquistic techniques are used basically to prove to the stutterer that he can speak fluently. Essentially they are methods of persuasion and suggestion. Though they have been used very little in the United States, they are still being used fairly widely in Europe.

Semantic therapy

It will seem strange to some readers to find the therapy advocated by Wendell Johnson, Dean Williams, and others of the so-called Iowa School included among the persuasion therapies. Nevertheless, if we ignore for a moment the theory, and focus instead upon the methodology, a good case can be made for this categorization. Like Froeschels, Johnson believed that stuttering originated in faulty perception, primarily that of the parents of a normally nonfluent child, parents who had mistakenly viewed and labeled the child's normal speech hesitations as stuttering. Johnson felt that when these parental misevaluations were accepted by the child he would tend to respond by anticipatory struggle and avoidance reactions. As these became learned and automatized, the stuttering would become worse and worse. But the core of the problem, according to Johnson, consisted of the stutterer's mislabeling of his normal disfluencies as "stuttering" and of himself as a "stutterer." The task of therapy accordingly was to change these wrong assumptions about the nature of his disorder.

Bloodstein (1969) provides this picture of Johnson's therapy:

His basic clinical procedure became one of training the stutterer to be conscious of the inappropriateness of the language he tended to use in talking about his problem. In group or individual discussions the person was taught to examine carefully what he meant when he referred to himself as a "stutterer," as though assuming that there was something about him which marked him as basically different from other people, or when he referred to what he did when he talked about as his "stuttering" or "it" as though his problem was not what he did when he talked but a thing inside of him which he needed to manage, or stop, or control in some way. (p. 249)

Wendell Johnson was one of the most charming and persuasive persons we have ever met and the many stutterers with whom he worked held the same opinion. His basic approach was the dialogue (often Socratic in nature). The stutterer was led by skillful questioning and challenges to believe that there was nothing essentially wrong with him except his assumptions and the language in which they were couched. General semantics theory as expounded by Korzybski (1941) provided the rationale for the verbal analysis of the stutterer's report of his feelings and speaking experiences. Stutterers were sent out to observe how often normal speakers could be disfluent without reacting by misevaluation or avoidance. They were urged to talk more and react less. They were persuaded to talk and think descriptively rather than evaluatively. This routine of constant questioning, observing, testing, analyzing, re-evaluating was designed to help the stutterer gain the

conviction that he was basically a normal speaker.

Williams (1957) has also insisted that the stutterer's assumption that he is in some way different from the normal speaker is entirely incorrect and is due to the kind of language he uses in referring to his difficulties.

There is the tendency, then, to talk as if (and to approach the problem as if) a "something" were there. In this sense, his stuttering is an entity, an animistic "thing" that lies inside him. This is fundamentally a belief in magic. He talks and acts as though he believes either that there exists a little man inside him eager to grab certain words, or that certain words are possessed of physical properties such that they get stuck in his throat. "When I talk, I try to hide it." "I feel like it is going to happen." " 'It' stops me from talking." . . . As long as one functions as though an "it" makes things happen, he is not motivated to observe cause and effect relationships in his behavior, for "it" is both cause and effect. (p. 391)

When the actual process of this therapy is scrutinized, we find the therapist challenging the stutterer's language and persuading him to change it to a more descriptive, analytical type. The stutterer, in this treatment, is reasoned with, is shown the folly of his "animistic thinking," and, it is hoped, becomes convinced that he is merely a normal speaker who has learned some erroneous ways of thinking about himself and has reacted to them improperly. Bloodstein (1958) boils it all down to one sentence: "Stuttering has one cause, the child's assumption that it is necessary for him to struggle to speak," a statement which Froeschels would certainly accept.

Sander (1970) shows that the actual process of therapy poses some problems:

What makes the principles of semantic reorientation so elusively difficult to apply is that one must first unlearn less appropriate ways of talking about the stuttering problem. For that reason, a descriptive-behavioral language as applied to stuttering therapy can probably best be taught by citing examples of unfortunate language usage and by learning to revise such statements according to broadly prescribed rules. (p. 252)

Sander states that the stutterer must use a descriptive language which will confront him with his actual behavior; it should be a verb language, not a noun language, a "do" language, not a "have" language; it should be positive, not negative. He stresses that the therapist must also use this way of talking about stuttering but he points out that it is not easy. "These are not overly-difficult skills; but six years of teaching has convinced me that they are more difficult to acquire than I had first thought." In our opinion, probably biased, they are even harder for the stutterer to acquire. When a whole culture insists that you stutter and that you have an impediment in your speech, and when you have felt the penalty and frustration of not being able to speak fluently, it is very hard to follow Johnson's (1961) suggestion that the stutterer should work to change his self-image as a deviant, and to act as though he were a normal speaker. Examining the actual practices dispassionately, we feel that semantic reeducation belongs, at least in part, in the category of persuasion and suggestion therapies.[10]

As we come to the end of this rather sad account of suggestion, distraction, and persuasion in stuttering therapy, the need for a different approach to the problem seems clear. It is discouraging to find many of the same old outworn techniques appearing again and again, often cloaked in new rationales but producing the same old outcomes. When will therapists learn that it is easy to get the stutterer to speak fluently? When will they really confront the fact that stutterers already know how to speak fluently? When will they understand that what the stutterer does not know is what to do when he does stutter or expects to?

[10] We shall consider semantic therapy again in other chapters.

Bibliography

AMBROSE, G., Technique and value of hypnosis in child psychotherapy, *British Journal of Medical Hypnotism*, 1 (1950), 7–10.

AMMAN, J. C., *A Dissertation on Speech.* London: Low, Marston and Searle, 1873. Originally printed in Latin by John Wolters, Amsterdam, 1700.

ANDERSON, E. G., *Therapy for Young Stutterers: The Kopp Method.* Detroit: Wayne State University Press, 1970.

APPELT, A., *Stammering and Its Permanent Cure.* London: Methuen, 1911.

BEASLEY, B., *Stammering: Its Treatment,* 17th ed. Birmingham: Hudson, 1897.

BELL, A. M., *Observations on Defects of Speech, The Cure of Stammering and Principles of Elocution.* London: Hamilton, Adams, 1853.

BIGGS, B. E. and J. G. SHEEHAN, Punishment or distraction? Operant conditioning revisited, *Journal of Abnormal Psychology*, 74 (1969), 254–57.

BLANTON, S., The treatment of stuttering, *Proceedings of the American Speech Correction Association,* 6 (1936), 23–31.

BLOODSTEIN, O., *A Handbook on Stuttering.* Chicago: National Easter Seal Society for Crippled Children and Adults, 1969.

————, Conditions under which stuttering is reduced or absent: A review of the literature, *Journal of Speech and Hearing Disorders,* 14 (1949), 295–. 301.

————, Stuttering as an anticipatory struggle reaction, in Jon Eisenson (ed.), *Stuttering: A Symposium.* New York: Harper & Row, 1958.

BLUEMEL, C. S., *Stammering and Cognate Defects of Speech.* New York: Stechert, 1913.

————, Stammering as an impediment of thought, *Proceedings of the American Speech Correction Association,* 1 (1931), 27–32.

BOOME, E. J. and M. RICHARDSON, *The Nature and Treatment of Stammering.* New York: Dutton, 1932.

BOSTOCK, J., A case of stammering successfully treated by the long continued use of cathartics, *Medical-Chirurgical Transactions,* (London), 16 (1830), 72–77.

BRADY, J. P., A behavioral approach to the treatment of stuttering, *American Journal of Psychiatry,* 25 (1968), 843–48.

BRAMWELL, J. M., *Hypnotism: Its History, Practice and Theory.* Philadelphia: Lippincott, 1930.

BRANKEL, O., Sinn and grenzen des autogenen trainings in rahman der stotter-behandling, *Folia Phoniatrica,* 10 (1958), 112–19.

BROOK, F., *Stammering and Its Treatment.* London: Pitman, 1957.

BROSTER, J., *Rise and Progress of the Brosterian System.* London: 1827.

BRUTTEN, E. J. and D. J. SHOEMAKER, *The Modification of Stuttering.* Englewood Cliffs, N.J.: Prentice-Hall, 1967.

BURDIN, G., The surgical treatment of stuttering, *Journal of Speech Disorders,* 5 (1940), 43–64.

CHERTOK, L., Theory of hypnosis since 1889. *International Journal of Psychiatry,* 3 (1967), 188–211.

CLARK, R., The status of speech correction and pathology in the U.S.S.R., *Cameo,* 26 (1959), 40–41.

COLUMBAT DE L'ISERE, M., *Du Begaiement et tous les Autres Vices de la Parole Traites par Nuvellea Methodes,* 2nd ed. Paris: 1831.

DE HIRSCH, K. and W. S. LANGFORD, Clinical note on stuttering and cluttering in young children, *Pediatrics,* 5 (1950), 934–40.

DENHARDT, R., *Das Stottern. Eine Psychose.* Leipsig: Keil's Machfolger, 1890.

DESPERT, J. L., A therapeutic approach to the problem of stuttering, *Nervous Child,* 2 (1942), 134–47.

DIXON, C. C., The effect of interjected non-propositional verbalization during oral reading on stuttering frequency, *Journal of Educational Research,* 51 (1957), 153–55.

DONATH, J., (Hypnosis in Stuttering Therapy) *Therapia. Gegeniv.* 73 (1932), 456–58.

EMERICK, L., Slow speech, *Life and Health,* 15 (1967), 17.

FALCK, F. J., Stuttering and hypnosis, *International Journal of Clinical and Experimental Hypnosis,* 12 (1964), 67–74.

FERNAU-HORN, H., *Die Sprechneurosen.* Stuttgart: Hippokrates-Verlag, 1969.

FITZ, O., *Schach dem Stottern.* Freiburg: Lambertus-Verlag, 1961.

FLANAGAN, B., I. GOLDIAMOND, and N. AZRIN, Operant stuttering: The control of stuttering behavior through response - contingent consequences, *Journal of Experimental Analysis of Behavior,* 1 (1958), 173–77.

FLETCHER, J. M., *The Problem of Stuttering.* New York: Longmans, Greene, 1928.

FRANK, J. D., *Persuasion and Healing.* New York: Schocken, 1961.

FREUND, H., Der induktiv vorgang im stottern und seine therapeutische verwertung, *Zeitschrift fur Neurologie und Psychiatrie,* 141 (1932), 180–92.

————, *Psychopathology and the Problems of Stuttering.* Springfield, Ill.: Charles C Thomas, 1966.

FROESCHELS, E., A technique for stutterers —"ventriloquism," *Journal of Speech and Hearing Disorders,* 15 (1950), 336–37.

————, *Selected Papers of Emil Froeschels.* Amsterdam: North Holland, 1964.

GARDNER, W., personal communication, 1960.

GENIESSE, H., Stuttering, *Science,* 82 (1935), 518.

GOLDIAMOND, I., Stuttering and fluency as manipulable operant response classes, in L. Krasner and L. P. Ullman (eds.), *Research in Behavior Modification: New Developments and Their Clinical Applications.* New York: Holt, Rinehart & Winston, 1964.

GORDON, J. E. (ed.), *Handbook of Hypnosis.* New York: Macmillan, 1966.

GREENE, J. S., Stuttering—what about it? *Proceedings of the American Speech Correction Association,* 1 (1931), 172–73.

GUTZMANN, H., *Das Stottern: Eine Monographie fur Aerzte, Pedagogen und Rehorden.* Frankfort: Rosenheim, 1898.

HALL, M., *On the Diseases and Derangements of the Nervous System.* London: Balliere, Tindall & Cassell, 1841.

HANICKE, O. and R. LEBEN (Contributions to Modern Views on the Treatment of Stuttering), *Deutsche Gesundheitswegen,* 19 (1964), 545–49.

HELTMAN, H. J., *First Aids for Stutterers.* Boston: Expression Co., 1943.

HILGARD, E. R., *Hypnotic Susceptibility.* New York: Harcourt, Brace & World, 1965.

HIRSCHBERG, J., (Stuttering), *Orvosi Hetilap.* (Hungary), 106 (1965), 780–84.

HOLLINGSWORTH, H. L., Chewing as a technique of relaxation, *Science,* 90 (1939), 385–87.

HULL, C. L., *Hypnotism and Suggestibility, an Experimental Approach.* New York: Appleton-Century-Crofts, 1933.

HUNT, J., *Stammering and Stuttering,* 1861. Reprinted by Hafner, New York, 1967.

IDEHARA, M., (Stuttering-curing Apparatus and its Method of Use), *Japanese Dental Association Journal,* 30 (1937), 640–42.

ITARD, J. M. G., Memoire sue le begaiement, *Journal Universe des Science Medicale, Paris,* 7 (1817), 129–44.

JOHNSON, W., *People in Quandaries.* New York: Harper & Row, 1946.

————, *Stuttering and What You Can Do About It.* Garden City, N.Y.: Doubleday, 1961.

JOHNSON, W., Some fundamental objectives in special education, *Journal of Exceptional Children,* 10 (1944), 10–11.

KASTEIN, S., The chewing method for treating stuttering, *Journal of Speech Disorders,* 12 (1947), 195–98.

KIMURA, S., Hypnosis in speech and language habilitation, *Proceedings of the International Congress for Psychosomatic Medicine and Hypnosis.* (Kyoto, Japan: Abstract, p. 75.)

KING, S. H., *Perceptions in Medical Practice.* New York: Russel Sage Foundation, 1962.

KINGDON-WARD, W., *Stammering: A Contribution to the Study of Its Problems and Treatment.* London: Hamilton, 1942.

KLINE, M. V., Hypnotherapy, in B. B. Wolman (ed.), *Handbook of Clinical Psychology.* New York: McGraw-Hill, 1965.

KLINGBEIL, G. M., The historical background of the modern speech clinic, *Journal of Speech Disorders,* 4 (1939), 115–32.

KNUDSEN, R., Behandling of talefejl: frankrig, *Nordisk Tidsskrift for Tale og stemme,* 10 (1946), 48–66.

KORZYBSKI, A., *Science and Sanity: An Introduction to Non-Aristotelian Systems and General Semantics,* 2nd ed. New York: Non-Aristotelian Library Publishing Co., 1941.

KUSSMAUL, A., Disturbances of speech, in

H. V. Ziemssen (ed.), *Cyclopedia of the Practice of Medicine,* 4th ed. Leipsig: Vogel, 1910.

KWAKAMI, R. (Practical results of the Idehara method of correction), *Dental Monthly* (Japan), 17 (1937), 439–41.

LIEBMANN, A., *Vorksungen uber Sprachstorungen.* Berlin: Colbentz, 1898.

LEVBARG, J. J., Hypnosis—treatment used with stutterers with marked mental disturbances, *Eye, Ear, Nose and Throat Monthly,* 20 (1941), 55–56, 60.

LUCHSINGER, R. and G. E. ARNOLD, *Voice-Speech-Language.* Belmont, Calif.: Wadsworth, 1965.

LUTHE, W. and J. H. SCHULTZ, *Autogenic Therapy.* New York: Grune and Stratton, 1968.

MACKAY, D. G., To speak with accent: Effects of nasal distortion on stuttering under delayed auditory feedback, *Perceptual Psychophysics,* 5 (1969), 183–88.

MADISON, L., The use of hypnosis in the differential diagnosis of a speech disorder, *International Journal of Clinical and Experimental Hypnosis,* 2 (1954), 140–44.

MATHUR, M. L., *Causes and Cure of Stammering.* Jodhpur, India: Mathur, 1960.

McCARTHY, C., Speaking clearly about stuttering, *Washington Post,* October 19, 1970, a–12.

McCORD, H., Hypnotherapy and stuttering, *Journal of Clinical and Experimental Hypnosis,* 3 (1955), 210–14.

McCORMAC, H., *A Treatise on the Cause and Cure of Hesitation of Speech or Stammering.* London: 1828.

MEARES, A., *Hypnography.* Springfield, Ill.: Charles C Thomas, 1957.

MERKEL, C. L., "Stottern, in C. Schmidt (ed.), *Encyclopedia der Gesammten Medizin,* 2nd ed. Leipsig: 1844.

MOCHIZUKI, S. (Subjective and Objective Attitude Toward Stuttering), *Voice and Language Medicine* (Japan), 6 (1965), 13–14.

MOORE, W. E., Hypnosis in a system of therapy for stutterers, *Journal of Speech Disorders,* 11 (1946), 117–22.

MUIRDEN, R., *Stammering.* Springfield, Ill.: Charles C Thomas, 1968.

NAO, C. (The Result of Hypnosis as a Stuttering Therapy), *Mental and Physical Medicine* (Japan), 4 (1964), 176–77.

NEWMAN, P. W., An explanation of the distraction effect in stuttering. Convention address, American Speech and Hearing Association, Denver, 1968.

PLATEN, M. (The New Method of Healing). Berlin: 1907.

PLATONOV, K., *The Word.* Moscow: Foreign Language Publishing House, 1959.

POTTER, S. O. L., *Speech and Its Defects.* Philadelphia: Blakiston, 1882.

RAZRAN, G., The observable unconscious and the inferable conscious in current Soviet psychophysiology: Interoceptive conditioning, semantic conditioning, and the orienting reflex, *Psychological Review,* 68 (1961), 81 147.

REICHEL, C. W., *Stop Stammering and Stuttering.* New York: Vantage Press, 1964.

RICHTER, P., *Das Stottern und Seine Heilung Durch Hypnotische Suggestion.* Dresden: Rudolph, 1928.

ROBBINS, S. D., *Stammering and Its Treatment.* Boston: Boston Stammerer's Institute, 1926.

————, The contribution of suggestion and of distraction to the treatment of stammering, *Proceedings of the American Speech and Hearing Association,* 2 (1932), 103–10.

ROBINSON, F. B., *Stuttering.* Englewood Cliffs, N.J.: Prentice-Hall, 1964.

ROSEN, H., *Hypnotherapy in Clinical Psychiatry.* New York: Julian, 1953.

ROTHE, K. C., Zur klarstellung einiger

fragen über stottern, *Hilfsschule,* 21 (1928), 437–39.

Rousey, C. L., Hypnosis in speech pathology and audiology, *Journal of Speech and Hearing Disorders,* 26 (1961), 258–62.

Salter, J. M., *Conditioned Reflex Therapy.* New York: Creative Age Press, 1949.

Sander, E. K., Talking plainly about stuttering, *Central States Speech Journal,* 21 (1970), 248–54.

Sarbin, T. R., Contributions to role-taking theory: I. Hypnotic behavior, *Psychological Review,* 57 (1950), 255–70.

Sato, I. et al. (The Speech Facilitating Apparatus and Its Resulting Cures), *Chiba Medical Magazine* (Japan), 30 (1954), 494–95.

Schilling, A., Die behandlung des stotterns, *Folia Phoniatrica,* 17 (1965), 365–458.

Schmalz, E., *Beiträge zur Gehoer und Stimmheilkunde,* Vol. I. Leipsig: 1846.

Schneck, J. M., *Hypnosis in Modern Medicine.* Springfield, Ill.: Charles C Thomas, 1959.

Schoolfield, L., The development of speech correction in America in the 19th century, *Quarterly Journal of Speech,* 24 (1938), 101–16.

Schulthess, R., *Das Stammeln und Stottern.* Zurich: Schulthess, 1830.

Schultz, J. H., *Das Autogene Training.* Stuttgart: Thieme, 1964.

Schultz, J. H. and W. Luthe, *Autogenic Training,* New York: Grune & Stratton, 1959.

Swift, W. B., Why visualization is the best method for stammering, *Proceedings of the American Speech Correction Association,* 1 (1931), 83–91.

Takeyama, K. (Hypnotic Therapy for Stuttering) *The Study of Hypnosis* (Japan), 7 (1963), 246–47.

Van Riper, C., Adventures in stuttering therapy, in J. Eisenson (ed.), *Stutter-*

ing: A Symposium. New York: Harper & Row, 1958.

————, *Speech Correction: Principles and Methods,* 5th ed. Englewood Cliffs, N.J.: Prentice-Hall, 1971.

————, The symptomatic treatment of stuttering, in L. E. Travis (ed.), *Handbook of Speech Pathology.* New York: Appleton-Century-Crofts, 1957.

————, The rhythm method, *Western Michigan University Journal of Speech Therapy,* 8 (1971), 12–13.

————, The role of reassurance in stuttering therapy, *Folia Phoniatrica,* 7 (1955), 217–22.

Vogel, V. H., Stuttering cured by hypnotism, *Scientific American,* 151 (1934), 311–13.

Watkins, J. G., *Hypnotherapy of War Neuroses.* New York: Ronald Press, 1949.

Wedberg, C., *The Stutterer Speaks.* Redlands, Calif.: Valley Fine Arts Press, 1937.

Williams, D. E., A point of view about stuttering, *Journal of Speech and Hearing Disorders,* 22 (1957), 390–97.

Williams, M. C., Twelve years of visual treatment of stuttering, *Proceedings of the American Speech Correction Association,* 1 (1931), 37–42.

Wilton, G., *How to Overcome Stuttering.* New York: Harper & Row, 1950.

Winn, B. (ed.), *Psychology in the Soviet Union.* Stanford, Calif.: Stanford University Press, 1957.

Wolberg, L. R., *Hypnoanalysis.* New York: Grune & Stratton, 1945.

Wolpe, J., *Psychotherapy by Reciprocal Inhibition.* Stanford, Calif.: Stanford University Press, 1958.

Wyneken, C., Ueber das stottern und dessen heilung, *Zeitschrift fur rationelle Medizin,* 31 (1868), 1–29.

Yearsley, W. A., *A Treatise on Stammering.* Accrington: privately published, 1909.

Relaxation Therapies

Workers with stutterers have long observed that the severity and frequency of stuttering decrease dramatically when the person is very relaxed. This seems to be due to several reasons. First of all, the physiological response to fear is tension, the individual responding to alarm by preparing his musculatures for action. If a person is very relaxed, one can be sure that he is not afraid, and if he is fearful, we can be certain that he is not completely relaxed. Training the stutterer to speak while under relaxation has always produced fluency because the relaxation meant that the fears which seem to precipitate so much of the difficulty were temporarily reduced or absent. Secondly, the concentration on all the complicated rituals necessary to create the relaxed state certainly take the stutterer's attention away from his speech. When one is concentrating on letting his arms and legs go limp, it is unlikely that he will be searching for stuttering-colored cues or assuming abnormal motor sets with his mouth. In short, relaxation is distractive. Thirdly, if the stutterer is completely relaxed, he cannot force or struggle since these activities demand tension. To ask the stutterer to be relaxed while speaking is to ask him to have no fear, to pay no attention to his speech, and not to struggle.

Nevertheless, through environmental controls and suggestion, it is possible to create the necessary conditions of safety which will permit a temporary state of relaxation sufficient to produce temporary fluency in many but not all stutterers. Such procedures have been used all over the world in the treatment of stuttering. Methods used to facilitate relaxation have varied all the way from exhortation, through complicated systems of muscle training, to hypnotic suggestion and drugs. There are innumerable permutations and combinations of these, each with its enthusiastic advocates and claims of cures. In a very early reference, Hoffman (1840) writes:

The patient must use no muscular effort in the throat, tongue or lips. Further he must avoid working other parts of the body such as the arms, feet, etc., since this makes the trouble worse and rarely offers more than temporary relief. . . . The greatest relaxation of the body must occur during speech.

Relaxation here is used primarily to prevent the stutterer from struggling, and the method is exhortation. We find such commands throughout the literature.

The use of general bodily relaxation to inhibit anxiety was the heart of Sandow's therapy as long ago as 1898. He protested against the tongue gymnastics and breath and vocal training so current in his time. "Away with these dangerous speech exercises," he wrote. "The one proper method for over-excitable nerves is rest; and this rest should alternate with gentle, natural and unforced movements." Sandow felt that smooth flowing speech depended upon a feeling of physical ease and well-being, i.e., the freedom from anxiety. He advised his stutterers to move slowly and restfully and to speak in the same fashion. "For example, lifting a hand to tip his hat should be done as though he had all the time in the world." Sandow anticipates some resistance from his cases:

The stammerer need have no fear of carrying this repose and relaxation to excess. The hearers will certainly not find the matter displeasing. And even were this not the case, the stammerer has to consider himself and not the hearer. Every speaker has his idiosyncracies, so why should the patient not have his? Especially as his happens to be the most natural in the world. The patient always has the right (and no reasonable person will gainsay it) to consider himself in the first place, and also himself in the second, third and fourth; and last of all to consider the hearer just a little. The stammerer should make the most abundant use of this privilege. And let me once more emphasize the fact that this restful and unhurried speech always strikes the hearer pleasantly.[1]

We have no doubt that many stutterers would be fluent *if* they could achieve such repose and calm and maintain it in the stress of normal living, but the *if* is gigantic. Certainly, in the therapy room or laboratory, if we can relax the stutterer, he will speak very well, for the fact that he is relaxed means that he is not under the stress that usually tends to trigger stuttering. A few stutterers doubtless can learn a more relaxed way of living and doubtless they should. If they can live limply and achieve some fluency thereby, more power to them! However, most adult stutterers find the world too full of past or present threats to remain relaxed and without anxiety when they leave the therapeutic harbor and sail out on the stormy sea.

Relaxation training has often been administered in large groups. The stutterers would lie on floor pads and cots as the therapist intoned his directions and suggestions in a soporific voice. Let us quote a bit from Gifford (1940) to know what the therapist might be saying in those pear-shaped, soothing tones:

[1] Quoted in Bluemel, 1913, p. 211.

Relaxation is refreshing. It rejuvenates your whole body and your attitude toward life as well. When you are in a condition of deep, complete rest, you seem to be floating down a smoothly flowing stream after a strenuous effort in battling upstream against the currents. Your body, your mind, your whole self, seem, without beginning or end, saturated with a feeling of unlimited and perfect peace. It is as though you were reaching some unfathomed inner center within you, a state of equilibrium in the very core of your being.

While you are thus resting, with eyes still closed, imagine a lovely orchard far out in the country where it is very still. See the trees full of blossoms and the cool green grass. You are lying on the soft grass and looking through the trees. All nature is resting in the sweet warmth of mid-day. There is no sound in all the orchard. It is very quiet. The clouds are slowly floating overhead. They drift, drift across the sky. The air is very lazy, too. It moves with a slow rhythmic motion. You can feel it on your face, pouring through your body as you breathe. In and out of your nose and throat it pours, constantly flowing. Feel your chest gently expand and contract. Unwilled, involuntary breathing goes on all day and all night. Nature goes on all day and all night. Nature takes care of it for you. *All you have to do is let your breath flow in this tranquil, natural way.*[2] (pp. 13–14)

Having thus induced the relaxed state by these and other almost hypnotic suggestions, the stutterers were then instructed to sigh gently and freely with soft vocalization, then to

[2] We are reminded here of Schilling's (1965) observation that when an initially peaceful background image was suggested "like lying in a smoothly moving boat on a calm lake" the imagined scene often shifted to unwanted stormy interruptions as the lake was disturbed by gunships or the boat being carried by a strong current into a wide strange ocean or suddenly sinking down to the bottom of that calm lake.

produce relaxed tones, and from this to begin speaking or chanting phrases and sentences. We have watched such a therapist sitting on a stool in the middle of a roomful of these recumbently relaxed stutterers, controlling them with her voice as an orchestra conductor manages his musicians. They would repeat after her such sentences as "I am happy." "I am calm." "I am relaxed." "I am serene." "I can speak easily." Then gradually they would arise slowly, with their arms dropping, and eyes shut, and intone other sentences of the ilk. They looked like Zombies, the living dead, but there in the room, they were fluent. We have also seen these same people in the hallway on their way home from the session talking excitedly to each other and stuttering violently. Nevertheless, we have known a few who profited from such therapy. One of them, Conrad Wedberg (1937), says this in his autobiography:

[Fluent speech can be produced] . . . in twenty minutes or less. I make this statement with assurance for I have never found a stutterer who could not speak fluently when totally relaxed. . . . Repeated practice in effortless, relaxed and smooth flowing speech will establish new auditory and kinesthetic perceptions of talking. You must actually hear and feel your voice gliding smoothly over all speech sounds, concentrating on no sounds in particular, but sensing the feeling of ease and passivity with every spoken word. Each successive experience will tend to relieve the tension and will gradually change the anticipation of blocking to a feeling of confidence in the smooth coordination of the speech organs. (p. 70)

For two decades (1920–1940), relaxation therapy was the dominant form of treatment in this country and England though often it was combined with other techniques. Robbins (1926) describes his procedures as follows:

In order, at a moment's notice, to relax completely like a cat, you must practice the relaxation exercises in the supplement every day until you have acquired the ability to relax any muscle in your body at will. Then practice relaxing two muscles at a time, three at a time, four at a time, and so on until you can relax every muscle together at a moment's notice. If you then practice this complete relaxation several times a day until normal speech has become a firmly fixed habit, you will be able to relax completely the instant you become afraid you are going to stammer and in this way will partly counteract the increased flow of blood to the brain which otherwise might make you stammer. (pp. 42–43)

Swift (1931), a very influential physician, advocated relaxation exercises as an adjunct to his visualization therapy. For 15 minutes, three times a day, his cases practiced extending their arms slowly over the head while inhaling, then lowering them slowly and evenly as they vocalized the vowel "ah" while varying its pitch. This was said to induce bodily relaxation while speaking. In the previous year, Elsie Fogerty (1930), director of one of the first training centers for therapists in England, had published her book *Stammering* which so stressed the role of relaxation that it, along with the texts by Boome and Richardson (1931) and Kingdon-Ward (1942), influenced British therapy for many years and indeed still continues to be widely used. A typical exercise illustrating the kind of relaxation therapy advocated by Fogerty (1930) may be illuminating:

Place the child lying down with head on a small cushion; gently stroke the eyes and chin till they relax and lie quiet at rest; very softly lift one hand and teach the child to relax it completly so that it drops softly the moment you let go; touch the knees softly till they fall softly apart and quite loose; go on until the whole body is lying as if it were floating on water with no strain of any kind. While you are doing this, talk gently to the child in a very soft voice, either telling him some little story or asking him to let everything go loose, or to think of some one pleasant colour like a deep-blue sky, or to pretend he is going to sleep. As soon as you see the whole body is really limp, stop talking for about one minute, then touch the side of the chest very lightly with four fingers and say very steadily, "breathe in, breathe out," in a very slow, sing-song voice, taking about eight seconds for each sentence, and gently pressing the chest while you say "breathe out" and lifting your hand away while you say "breathe in." Continue this for about two minutes, then help the child to sit up, first folding both arms round the raised knees and resting his head on his arms for about three seconds; then, with one hand on the ground jumping to his feet. A good time to do this exercise is in the evening after tea, or, if the child is young enough to be put to sleep, do the first part before he goes to sleep and the second part when he wakes up. (pp. 41–42)

Other similar exercises follow wherein relaxed body movements are accompanied by slow rhythmic breathing. Then speech is gradually inserted into the activities, using the stutterer's slow exhalations to whisper, then to phonate isolated vowels, then to intone phrases and sentences suggesting calmness. Accompanying hand movements are recommended. This is fine therapy—for the therapist. It produces fluency immediately; it has the smell of magical incantations; it is economical since large groups of stutterers may be treated in unison. But alas, it has one fatal flaw: the transfer to real-life situations leaves much to be desired.

In this country, books by Blanton and Blanton (1936), Gifford (1940), and Hahn (1941) also made strong cases for relaxation therapy, though the Blantons advocated deep relaxation in conjunction with psychotherapy to relieve the tension and to permit new speech habits to be formed. Hahn used relaxation along with many other methods. This use of relaxation as an adjunct to other therapy is also demonstrated by Wendell Johnson (1946) in his *People in Quandaries*. Though he maintains, as we do, that the best sort of relaxation is that which comes as a by-product of the well-being which comes from adequate adjustment to one's problems, he did devise a technique he called semantic relaxation in which the person gently strokes himself with his hands to heighten the awareness of the self. He differentiates between relaxation for rest and relaxation for work or "optimal tonicity," and the latter is what he seeks.

By using this technique for brief periods a few times a day, one tends to cultivate a more or less consistent state of optimal tonicity. . . . It counteracts our common tendency to make hard work of whatever we do, to frown and grimace unduly, to overreact, to carry on our daily activities with a greater degree of tension that is necessary. (p. 235)

Johnson makes clear that he feels little confidence in relaxation exercises specifically designed to produce fluent speech. He writes:

. . . so long as one is basically maladjusted it is not likely that any direct attempts at eliminating one's self-defensive

tensions will prove very successful. The relaxation that you achieve by deliberately relaxing is not quite as "genuine" as that which you achieve simply by living according to sound principles. (p. 230)

Perhaps the most influential book of all was *Progressive Relaxation* written by Edmund Jacobson in 1938. Through electromyographic studies he showed that when muscle tension was reduced almost to zero through an intensive course of relaxation training, anxiety and its so-related symptoms seemed to disappear. This scientific approach, coupled with rigorous and specific training procedures to induce relaxation, had something more than suggestive value.

Jacobson had his subjects define the tension by first contracting specific muscle groups (the toes, legs, arms, etc.) then relaxing them, and after each set of musculatures showed electromyographically that no residual tension was present, a new set of muscles was relaxed, hence the term *progressive* relaxation. Jacobson also gave us the concept of differential relaxation, showing that, after intensive training, one set of muscles could remain relaxed while others were active. Since Jacobson's protocols showed that three stutterers exhibited "marked improvement" as the result of his training, his methods were soon adopted with variations by most of the American therapists who used relaxation. Unfortunately, though Jacobson insisted that his subjects lie down and work to relax each of the muscle groups in a definite prescribed sequence and never to move onward until one group was *completely* relaxed, few of those who have followed his methods were as careful. (Thus Hahn [1941] let his stutterers sit up but darkened the therapy room, asking them first to close their eyes, commanded them to relax first the gross muscles, then the finer ones, and then begin to phonate and speak.) Moreover, Jacobson felt that several hundred training sessions were required before the near zero levels of muscular tonus needed to counteract "nervous hypertension" could be achieved. Few therapists who profess to follow Jacobson's methods have met his criteria of truly relaxed states.

Jacobson's progressive relaxation methods have been adopted by many of the advocates of behavior modification, notably Wolpe and his followers and we shall describe the application of relaxation to systematic desensitization in a later section. However, there are other forms of relaxation therapy which have had a profound influence on our European colleagues though they have been rarely used in the United States. We present them now.

Sleep therapy

The Russians have long used prolonged therapeutic sleep in the treatment of various ills, and at present they are reported[3] to have set up some 300 "sleep stations" in the U.S.S.R. where more than a half million persons, including some stutterers, have been treated. Sleep therapy in Russia is based upon Pavlov's concept of protective or restorative inhibition. In the Pavlovian view, neurosis is the result of overload, the person's nervous system having been overwhelmed by tasks beyond its power of integration. Sleep therapy therefore is designed to provide the needed protective inhibition so that

[3] "All Wired for A Trance," *Life Magazine*, 64 (March 11, 1968), pp. 81–82.

further breakdown will not occur, and also to help restore the person to normal functioning. Andreev (1960) describes the daily program:

The program for the day was built up in accordance with the form of therapeutic sleep used. The morning period of sleep began at 10 A.M. and continued until lunch, i.e., until 2 P.M., although the patients usually got up by themselves sooner; the patients went to bed a second time after lunch, at 3 P.M., and were allowed to sleep until supper, i.e., until 7 P.M., but most of them again awoke sooner. They retired for the night's sleep at 10 P.M. In the morning the patients were up from 8 A.M. to 9 A.M. (p. 46)

The duration of enrollment in one of these sleep centers varies but usually it lasts at least two or three weeks. Therapeutic sleep is induced through conditioning procedures, hypnosis (including the hypnotron, a device which drives the brain waves by imposed electrical stimuli from an apparatus attached to the scalp), and by drugs. Among the latter, both tranquilizers and narcotics are used.

We have found a few references which describe the application of therapeutic sleep therapy to stutterers. The first, by Knoblechova (1951), treated 20 stutterers with protracted sleep, reporting that five of them were "nearly completely healed" and that only two cases seemed unable to profit from the regime. In her doctoral thesis Pavlova-Zahalcova (1962) describes the utility of therapeutic sleep for stutterers, and Derazne (1966) summarizes the therapy as follows:

We recommend an increased amount of hours of sleep (not less than 11 or 12 hours a day) with consultation from a neurologist if the patient has insomnia. This method of removing stuttering is usually administered to children of 7–8 years and older. For children younger than 7–8 years we use medication such as bromium and calcium chloride which are taken internally 2–3 times a day in Pavlov doses, depending on the age. . . .

A few thousand children who received medication with prolonged sleep, while maintaining a strictly organized regime each day and who also paid attention to their speech difficulties in speech situations got rid of stuttering entirely after 2–3 months of rehabilitation. If in isolated cases we did not get the expected positive results, in the third month we stopped using the medication and then after 4–5 months again administered the medication but for a longer period—half a year or more. In these cases we obtained consistent results in the removal of stuttering. (p. 617)

It is interesting to note that as long ago as 1902, Lewis, the founder of a noted commercial institute for stutterers in Detroit, stated that "sleep is curative." He insisted that every stutterer in his institute should get more sleep than the average person and reported that prolonged sleep made successful treatment possible for especially refractory clients. To our knowledge the next person to advocate sleep therapy in this country was Bluemel (1913) who recommended that beginning stutterers be put to bed under medication for several days of prolonged sleep. Upon awakening, the child was to go through a transitional period in which first only whispered speech, then soft drawled speech, and then finally ordinary speech could be used.

Other methods for producing relaxation

Balneotherapy—the use of therapeutic bathing—has been an old therapy for many human ailments,

doubtless because of its relaxation and placebo effects. A long warm bath does seem to reduce muscular tensions and we find it being prescribed by several workers in the countries behind the Iron Curtain, notably Daskalov (1963). He writes:

In 1954 we introduced a new type of therapy, namely the balneo-sanatorium treatment of stutterers. Here we associated logopedic activities with the healing effects of the naturally favorable climate and the baths. Bulgaria is rich in mineral springs, usually located among splendid landscapes in the most favorable climatic conditions.

Daskalov also used protracted sleep along with drugs and many other types of therapeutic activities and agents, most of which seem to be designed to promote relaxation in the first stage of his treatment. Petkov and Iosifov (1960) describe a stuttering colony in Tyrnov:

We chose for the site of the colony the village of Vonesh located in beautiful mountainous country and being a good climatic health resort. It contains one of the best hydrogen sulfide springs in the country and its waters are beneficial for a number of ailments. . . . The children were divided into five age groups each containing ten members; one teacher and one nurse were attached to each group. The logopedic physician and the lay logopedist were responsible for the conduct of the entire program, and they daily visited the different groups and carried out individual sessions with children who suffered from severe stuttering.

The children stayed in the colony for 45 days; a special day curriculum was evolved for studies and for therapy.

On the first day of studies the medical logopedist and the lay logopedist carried out a thorough general physical, neurologic and logopedic investigation of all the children. This examination revealed etiologic factors responsible for the onset of the logoneuroses.

A wide range of treatment was given: in the early days and in the third week of stay in the colony sleep therapy was carried out (the children received luminal and bromide for three days); they received general tonic agents such as arsenic, iron, calcium, vitamins etc. Debilitated children received intramuscular injections of insulin (daily doses were gradually increased from four to 20 units). In addition to drug therapy the children received psychotherapy, gymnastic therapy and remedial exercises, and had air, sun and aqueous baths. A potent psychotherapeutic agent was the tape recorder on which speech was recorded at the beginning, middle and conclusion of therapy. Individual tape-recorded sequences were kept, enabling the development of speech by the stuttering child to be followed.

The program included systematic breathing and speech exercises, rhythmic vocal exercises with musical accompaniment, singing, games accompanying speech etc. A correctophone (auditory masker) was used in dealing with cases of severe stuttering.

A noteworthy feature was that the outcome of treatment depended considerably on training and discipline of the children. (p. 904)

Massage has also been employed in reducing the stutterer's tension states. We find it mentioned in the Russian literature and, as one might expect, in the Swedish as well. Ohlsson-Edlund (1965) describes the use of vibratory massage to produce relaxed, "harmonious" breathing for both silence and speech. Some of this was done manually but a foam-rubber vibrator was also used. Massage therapy is also mentioned by Daskalov (1962) and by Hirschberg (1965) as being used in stuttering therapy. In one of the European clinics that we visited we observed the use of another vibrating apparatus consisting of a steel ball (the size of a large orange) capping a metal arm which rose from an apparatus on the floor. The therapist placed the ball against the chest of the stutterer, set the vibration rate to coincide with his fundamental pitch, and then started it vibrating as he read prepared sentences. Its fast thumping did seem to prevent some of the laryngeal blocks he had been having but he became more fluent according to the therapist, because it relaxed him. We tried it out but it jarred our molars and certainly did not relax us.

Somewhat related is the painful physiotherapy technique called structural integration or *rolfing* from which some stutterers have seemed to benefit. By intensive manipulation of the fascia of the major muscle groups, the body is "realigned," or rebalanced, and all of the muscles freed from improper tensions.[4] Two stutterers who underwent the prescribed ten hours of rolfing reported to us that not only had they achieved relaxed and balanced tonicity of the whole body which made it impossible for them to stutter severely but also they experienced some profound emotional upheavals which were evidently cathartic. They reported a marked decline in the severity of their stuttering due to the looseness and relaxation of the general body musculatures. Some reduction in frequency was also experienced. Unfortunately we have been unable to achieve an adequate follow-up for either of these two individuals, but we would suspect that the relief

[4] A popular article by S. Keen describing rolfing will be found in *Psychology Today*, 4 (October 1970), 59–61.

would not be very permanent. However, we would not attribute all that relief to the simple cessation of punishment (the hitting-your-head-with-a - hammer - because - it - feels - so - good - when - you - stop effect). There is a sense of well-being that has a postural substrate as was shown by F. Mathias Alexander (1932) who developed a set of procedures for modifying the basic body postures to promote integration of the body image and the self. Alexander was the teacher of John Dewey and Aldous Huxley among others and a considerable part of his fascinating book *The Use of the Self* is devoted to the treatment of stuttering. He maintained that most of us come to misuse and abuse our bodies and develop improper habits of posture, locomotion, and action that create localized foci of tension which in turn lead to many human ills, and he offers a therapy to restore the person to his natural state of a relaxed, balanced tonicity.

We have covered most but not all of the various techniques used to teach the stutterer to be generally relaxed. There are others such as music therapy, the therapeutic dance, the surrounding of the stutterer by an environment of cool colors, the use of Fernau-Horn's breath training, autogenic formulae, various forms of Yoga, and meditation, and relaxing drugs. All have helped but none has solved the problem of stuttering.

Relaxation in behavior therapy

After some lapse of interest in relaxation for several decades, therapists have again rediscovered it, this time as it is used by Wolpe, Eysenck, and others who were seeking to devise a therapy for the neuroses based upon learning theory and especially upon classical conditioning. In their writings and research, various phobias which are viewed as conditioned anxiety reactions have received most of their concern. It is not surprising therefore that stuttering has also received some attention from those intrigued by the promise of behavioral therapy. The basic premise underlying this form of therapy, as Wolpe stated it in 1954, is that "if a response incompatible with anxiety can be made to occur in the presence of anxiety evoking stimuli it will weaken the bond between these stimuli and the anxiety responses (p. 208)." In clinical practice, the two most common competing responses used to inhibit the anxiety of stutterers have been assertive behavior and relaxation. Wolpe (1958) has described the successful treatment of one stutterer by deconditioning his anxiety through training in the use of assertive behavior when confronted by feared speaking situations. However, most of the workers who have attempted behavioral therapy with stutterers have employed relaxation and Wolpe indicates that he feels this is the appropriate method. He writes:

Stutterers seldom stutter all the time. Usually they can speak quite well when they are alone, or when they are with certain people. Close questioning reveals that the stutterer's problem occurs when he is anxious. The anxiety varies with the social situation, the number of persons present, who they are and how they behave. The greater the anxiety, usually, the worse the stuttering is. Once we find the cause of the anxiety we can treat it just as though it had revealed itself as a phobia. As we inhibit the anxiety through relaxation, the stuttering recedes. (p. 36)

Before we describe its use in the systematic-desensitization type of behavioral therapy, we wish to stress that relaxation can be a major focus of therapy even if no hierarchically arranged, anxiety evoking scenes are being imaged sequentially. We have already shown how therapists have often used various forms of relaxation in treating stutterers to ease their anxiety and to promote fluency. Let us now quote from an article by Damsté, Zwaan, and Schoenaker (1968) to demonstrate how relaxation was designedly programmed to decrease the situational and speech fears of some Dutch stutterers. (We ourselves attended such a group session in Utrecht and the account given describes exactly what we witnessed.)

Next to the training to stop at the right moment, relaxation is the most important therapeutic method. According to the principle of reciprocal inhibition, relaxation diminishes situational fears, but it also prevents motor disturbances in speaking, and primary and secondary accompanying movements. Relaxation in itself, however, does not suffice just as it is not sufficient to teach the stutterer how to breathe. We are fighting a chain of responses that starts with fear of a situation and runs via disturbances in tonus and breathing functions toward repetitions, blocks and accompanying movements. Subsequent feelings of guilt and anxiety for future situations close this vicious circle. Optimal use of relaxation is made if we follow the course of events that takes place when a disturbance occurs: breathing precedes speaking. Relaxation is learned by a method of self observation when resting and in movement in which the following stages can be distinguished:

(1) We usually start in the supine position with closed eyes. In this position the patient is taught full awareness of the presence of his body. In the beginning his attention is directed to the most simple observations, for instance to the sensations of the parts of the body that touch the floor. The movement of breathing is observed by the patient. Sensations in limbs can also be made the object of observation. Self-observation of this kind may lead to a better balanced muscle tonus of the whole body.

Little by little, movements are introduced. Still lying on the floor with closed eyes, movements of the arms, head and legs are experienced. At last, movements of breathing and speaking are experienced. In this uncomplicated situation, every stutterer we have met until now can speak fluently. Demands are minimal, the only points stressed being that the stutterer keeps on relaxing and observing the movements of his respiration. He waits until the breathing movement has reached its top; only then is he allowed to start speaking. Speaking consists of reproduction of simple sentences, and enumeration of series of words or numbers.

(2) Self observation now is no longer limited to the supine position, but extended to movements of the whole body leading to other postures. As long as the patient's attention remains directed upon himself, movements leading to sitting or standing positions do not interfere with his ability to speak fluently. In this situation the patient moves in full concentration on the movement, and with his eyes closed. He speaks to himself and the speaking refers to the movements and accompanying sensations. There is no contact with others and there are no demands regarding social behavior.

(3) Awareness of the environmental space is the next step, followed by awareness of the presence of other people around him. When the patient is a member of the group the other members are drawn more and more into the field of his attention. This is realized in circular or row like settings in which each member listens to the other's speech and in which the process of giving and receiving answers is going on.

Awareness of body or bodily movements and breathing function is our starting point. By a process of self observation a relaxation state is obtained in which every stutterer has a normal breathing function. What matters next is to retain this relaxation and breathing function improvement in situations in which self observation is not or hardly possible. Therefore a good mastering of the art of relaxation is a first require-ment, in order that the relaxation re-sponse becomes an automatized reaction to speaking situations in general. On the other hand, the group may contribute to a gradual mastering of situations as well. When all group participants are in the supine position, with eyes closed, relax-ation is relatively easy. Neither is it dif-ficult to repeat, together with the other members, the sentences prompted by the therapist. It is more difficult to repeat such a sentence alone or with the group listening. Personal communications and confidential questions rank still higher in the hierarchy of speaking difficulties. Delivering a speech before the group, or being cross-questioned by it, marks the ultimate possibility offered by the group. But the group gradually has become fa-miliar to each participant, and therefore we have not yet arrived at the difficult level of real life situations. (pp. 333–34)

Relaxation in systematic desensitization therapy

Relaxation as the dominant treat-ment of stuttering declined rapidly in the United States after 1945 pri-marily because of its failures. Most therapists could not teach it and most stutterers could not maintain it out-side the therapy room. However, in the last decade or two, due to the in-fluence of Wolpe's and Eysenck's behavior therapy for the neuroses as represented by "systematic-desensitiz-ation," a marked resurgence of in-terest in relaxation has been shown.

In essence, this therapy consists first of procedures to induce a rela-tively relaxed state in the stutterer by a modified version of Jacobson's

methods, or by suggestion, hypnosis or drugs.[5] Then, based upon a pre-liminary interview, a hierarchy of speaking situations graded in terms of their anxiety potential is presented, step by step, to the stutterer *while in the relaxed state* as he imagines him-self participating in the situation. Beginning with the lowest step on the hierarchy (the one least feared) and helped by the therapist to visualize it vividly, the stutterer is required to imagine it over and over again until his signalling (or more rarely some other more objective measure) indi-cates to the therapist that the anxiety has subsided. Then the stutterer is asked to imagine that situation on the hierarchy which had been ranked as slightly more anxiety provoking than the first. Then the densensitiz-ing process is repeated until all of the steps of the hierarchy have been worked through.

The following accounts may illus-trate the desensitizing process once the relaxation has been achieved: The first comes from Brutten and Shoemaker (1967):

When the hierarchy with which to be-gin therapy has been chosen, the thera-pist informs the patient that he will de-scribe a stimulus situation and on a pre-arranged signal the patient is to imagine being in that situation as vividly as he possibly can. The patient is also instructed that if he experiences any negative emo-tional response such as "fear, anxiety, uneasiness or disgust" he is to signal this. The therapist then describes the lowest ranked stimulus in the chosen hierarchy and snaps his finger or provides some other prearranged cue for the patient to begin imagining or experiencing the sit-uation. If the patient signals that he is ex-periencing some negative emotional reac-tion, the therapist immediately instructs

[5] A detailed description of the relaxation training used in systematic-desensitization will be found in Paul (1966).

him to stop imagining the situation, to return his attention to the therapy room, and to relax. . . . If the reaction is a mild one, the patient is given a short time to relax and the noxious stimulus is presented again. Generally, if the response is weak, with each repetition it becomes weaker until no response is reported by the patient. After several further repetitions, the next situation on the hierarchy is presented, and so on. (p. 115)

One of the problems which immediately confronts the therapist is the creation of an appropriate hierarchy and another is the ability to get the stutterer to relax deeply enough. Rosenthal (1968) describes some of his difficulties in this regard:

Hierarchy construction also proved a formidable task. In most phobic conditions, the eliciting cues such as crowds or snakes remain external, and can be graduated by number or proximity as the discrimination of intensity is achieved. In stammering, at least in the present case and some others in treatment by the writer, there seems to be an all-or-none effect such that if the dreaded blockage occurs, perception of producing the non-fluency can elicit additional anxiety and further blockage; thus, difficulty on a nominally easy item may trigger emotional arousal disproportionate to the external speaking situation the patient imagines. On the grounds that strong anxiety responses must be prevented from occurring, very gradual item-steps are suggested. Max's extreme anxiety-proneness made gentle graduation especially necessary.

Consequently, a 215-item hierarchy was constructed to embody a very wide range of speaking situations; nevertheless as many as 17 presentations were required to attain a criterion of two successive tension-free responses. In the main, fewer presentations were needed in the latter half of the hierarchy after progress had begun. The following items will illustrate the hierarchy: 1. Talking to yourself silently. 21. Stating your opinion to a child. 41. Chatting with a girl friend you know well, while dancing. 61. Complaining about a girl employee in a store to direct you to the men's rest-room. 101. Chatting with a pretty girl you have recently met at a dance. 121. Giving travel directions to a stranger. 141. Putting your thoughts into words in conversation with a wise-guy. 161. Reading out loud to a group. 181. Asking a clerk for fairly detailed information on the telephone; the connection is poor and you must speak loudly. 184. Telling non-sexy jokes to a large audience. 210. Telling a very pretty girl that you'd like to go to bed with her. 212. Talking over the telephone to a man high in authority. 215. Speaking forcefully to a big drunk who might hit you. It can be seen that later items combined speech with social situations that, originally, aroused fear because of Max's limited social skills. (p. 126)

We should state that this is the longest hierarchy we have ever known to be set up in desensitization therapy. Usually, the hierarchies consist of no more than ten items and when the evident anxiety on one of the items proves too difficult to extinguish, sub-items are devised and incorporated after taking the stutterer back to a previous level. But there are other difficulties too. In clinical practice, we seldom have access to galvanic skin recorders, palmar sweat prints, or electrical skin conductance apparatus and so we must rely upon observation to determine the amount of anxiety being felt since one cannot always trust the stutterer to be able to signal its occurrence or strength. Some therapists have asked the stutterer to verbalize his awareness of anxiety, or even to add to the therapist's presentation of the imaginary scene, using the amount of stuttering demonstrated as a measure both of the anxiety and of the depth of relaxation being experienced, a procedure which seems of dubious validity.

Some of the difficulties involved in systematic desensitization are described by Perkins (1967) as he considers the possible alternative responses to the therapists requests:

The first request would be for the subject to imagine an anxiety eliciting thought. He can think such a thought, or not; whatever his response, it may or may not arouse anxiety; his report of what he does experience may or may not be true, but true or not, this report will determine the presentation of the next request. When anxiety is reported, the next instruction would be to stop thinking and relax, and the cycle of alternatives would be repeated. When no anxiety is reported, the next step is to imagine another anxiety-laden thought, and so the cycle goes, piling uncertainty on top of uncertainty. (pp. 15–17)

Although, with the usual phobia, such as the fear of touching spiders, the use of imagining rather than contact with the real situation seems to be fairly effective, in the stutterer the amount of transfer from the imagined to the actual experience of speaking is often unimpressive.[6]

Accordingly some therapists combine imagining with some verbalized role playing at each step of the hierarchy, the stutterer actually speaking aloud as he imagines the scene or repeating after the therapist what the latter is saying. Others create testing situations outside the therapy room which parallel the imaginary scenes

[6] A summary of the literature and an experiment by Barlow, Leitenberg, Agras, and Wincze (1969) indicates that even with the phobias, imagined contacts with the feared situation in desensitization therapy were not entirely successful and that actual contacts when introduced hierarchically with relaxation facilitated transfer.

and use the stutterer's actual performance as the indication of the success of the desensitization. There are dangers inherent in this policy since often the testing may produce much stuttering even after the anxiety had been reduced in the imagined sessions and then the stutterer tends to reject the therapy. On the other hand, if no outside checking is done, the stutterer may climb every step of the hierarchy to the top and then, when he sallies forth into the real rather than the imaginary world, he may find again the anxiety arousal and the stuttering he has worked so hard to extinguish. (In part this is due to the presence in the real situation of other anxiety arousing cues which had not been desensitized in the therapy room.) Stuttering, alas, unfortunately presents a much more complicated stimulus picture than that of a harmless laboratory snake. Lazarus (1969), for example, tells of one of his cases, a woman stutterer who came to him full of assorted anxieties and other problems, and with whom he applied a broad spectrum of behavior therapy. He writes: "The young lady was transformed into a shapely, non-phobic, confident, self-sufficient, mature, feminine and delightful person who was soon married and who was also distinctly non-frigid, according to her husband; her stutter, however, remained as pronounced as ever." (p. 42.)

Another of the difficulties experienced by therapists in applying behavior therapy to stuttering is due to the probability that stuttering behavior perhaps consists not only of conditioned anxiety responses but also of instrumental acts of coping behaviors, reactions which have been created and maintained by their consequences as the operant therapists have so stoutly insisted. These instrumental behaviors by themselves can generate anxiety. For this reason most clinicians rarely confine themselves only to the relaxation used in systematic desensitization or to any of the other "reciprocal inhibition" techniques.

Moreover, one of the key questions concerning systematic-desensitization therapy is whether the alleged effectiveness of the technique is due to the relaxation state, or to the hierarchic dosage of anxiety evoking scenes, or to both, or to neither. The early studies as summarized by Rachman (1965) indicated "that relaxation alone or hypnosis alone does not reduce the phobia," and that "Desensitization administered in the absence of relaxation appears to be less effective than systematic-desensitization treatment (p. 101)." However in a later article, Rachman (1968) argues convincingly that *muscular* relaxation (as opposed to "mental calmness") is not a necessary part of the systematic desensitization process. He points out that most of the relaxation training advocated by Wolpe (who recommended about six sessions) and others is very perfunctory. Some of the reports tell of using as few as three sessions (Paul, 1966) or only one (Cooke, 1966). As Rachman (1968) comments, "In all these studies, successful results were obtained. These findings would seem to suggest one of two things. Either muscular relaxation *per se* is unnecessary or, it if is necessary, it can be achieved in one to three training sessions (p. 159)." In this connection we should remember that Jacobson's subjects often required up to 100 hours of intensive progressive relaxation before their electromyographic recordings indicated that a truly relaxed state had been achieved.

Our own interest here, of course, is to know if relaxation is a key ingredient in the reduction of fear. That this might not be true has been indicated by several experiments with snake phobias. Lang, Lazovik, and Reynolds (1965), for example, did a very interesting experiment in which a psychotherapeutic placebo group was used. The members of this group received training in general relaxation and also were hypnotized and an additional suggestion of deep relaxation was given during the imagination of nonfearful scenes associated with the items of the hierarchy. Despite the deep relaxation achieved, the members of the placebo group showed little fear reduction when later presented with the actual snake.

Moreover, several studies have indicated that successful desensitization to phobic stimuli can be achieved without any relaxation at all being used, and, indeed, even when the subjects were tensing their muscles as they went up the hierarchy (Nawas, Welsch, and Fishman, 1970; Wolpin and Raines, 1966). Lader (1967) and Matthews and Gelder (1969) also found that the electromyographic recordings taken at the very time that a subject verbally reported feeling relaxed and calm often showed pronounced bursts of EMG activity in the muscles. Finally, Miller (1970) showed that the usual programming of a progressive hierarchy of imagined visual scenes was unnecessary. In a desensitization experiment on snake phobias, he found that items presented in random order were just as effective as those programmed in sequence. He therefore rejects Wolpe's "assertion that anxiety to a low hierarchy item must be dissipated before one proceeds to the item next on the hierarchy."

Indeed we have recently witnessed

a strong attack on the basic concept that the reduction in fear which has been demonstrated to occur in systematic desensitization is due to counterconditioning or reciprocal inhibition. Breger and McGaugh (1965), and especially Lomont (1965), have assembled some impressive evidence indicating that simple extinction rather than reciprocal inhibition may explain what happens when a subject visualizes a threatening scene while relaxed. Exactly what takes place in systematic desensitization therapy still remains, as Lomont insists, an open question.

What then are the real reasons for the presumed effectiveness of relaxation in stuttering therapy? Rachman (1968) explains the possible utility of desensitization as being due to its facilitation of "calmness" or "decreasing arousal," both being verbal constructs. Muscle relaxation and "calmness" are not the same though the former may be able to generate the latter by suggestion. Bandura (1969) summarizes a great many studies in these words:

The various findings, taken as a whole, indicate that relaxation is a facilitative rather than a necessary condition for the elimination of avoidance behavior. Evidence that relaxation often hastens the extinction process does not verify that the benefits derive from the explicit manipulation of muscular activities . . . feelings of calmness induced by the procedure rather than muscular relaxation *per se* is the decisive factor at work. In this alternative explanation, relaxation instructions and presentation of pleasant scenes to the imagination reduce affective arousal which attenuates responsiveness to aversive stimuli. (p. 439)

Nawas et al. (1970) go even further, ˚saying that relaxation simply serves as a distractor. "The 'crowding

out' of the anxiety response by the more adaptive and repeated occurrence of the relaxation response renders the probability of occurrence of the latter higher than the probability of occurrence of the former (p. 54)." Our own explanation would include these items along with reciprocal inhibition but would also add some others. The state of relaxation, by definition, precludes much of the symptomatology of stuttering —the contortions, tremors, and struggle behaviors. It would alter or prevent preparatory sets to assume the abnormal postures that act as proprioceptive cues to recoil or avoidance. Under deep relaxation as under alcoholic intoxication, time pressure is decreased, cues representative of possible social penalty are poorly discriminated, and speech itself becomes slower and imprecisely monitored. Perhaps the speech servosystems return to a more normal state under relaxation with more reliance upon proprioceptive than upon possibly defective auditory controls. Were it possible for the stutterer to spend all his verbal life in a deeply relaxed trance, we would suspect he wouldn't stutter very often or very severely. Alas, we do not spend our lives half asleep and even if we did, there are stutterers, as Freund (1966) has reported, who even stutter in their dreams.

How effective is systematic desensitization therapy with stutterers?

The strong advocacy of relaxation in desensitization therapy for stutterers by Brutten and Shoemaker (1967) as an application of their two-factor theory does not seem to rest so much upon outcome studies as it does upon armchair theorization. At the time of this writing, the evidence for its effectiveness is far from satisfactory. All we have are some individual case reports, some unpublished long-term studies, and some general impressions. Controls are absent. Wolpe (1969) tells of a stutterer whom he trained to relax and to undergo a desensitization hierarchy focused about humiliation (*in addition to training in rhythmic syllable-timed speech!*) "After 9 desensitization sessions in the course of four months, his fear of these 'humiliation' situations steadily declined and his speech was judged to have improved 90–95 percent." Walton and Mather (1963) first trained a single stutterer in shadowing; found no significant change, then gave him systematic desensitization based on relaxation. Some improvement was shown but "He still considers himself lacking in sufficient confidence to take a teaching post. Talking before a group of people or reading out loud to them would in his estimation still be too stressful for him (p. 125)." Lanyon (1969) trained one mild stutterer in "Jacobson" relaxation in four sessions, then presented a hierarchy of 27 fear-evoking situations centered about speaking. After 24 weeks of this therapy, Lanyon reports that a 40 percent improvement in frequency of stuttering during reading and a 56 percent improvement in narration occurred together with significant change in attitudes. Perkins (1967) in an unpublished study gave systematic desensitization to two stutterers who had previously undergone training in rate control and he reported unsatisfactory results. Webster (1970) tells of treating three stutterers with typical relaxation desensitization. Using the frequency of stuttering during reading of passages before and after treatment, some improvement was shown, especially in the situations that had been used for visualization under relaxation, but other feared situations remained evocative of stuttering, and some situations such as making phone calls were resistant to desensitization. None of the stutterers were cured. (The results of his study are shown in Figure 2.1.) One long term study on systematic desensitization therapy with a substantial number of stutterers is also unpublished. It was done by Gray (1968). He reports that there was little significant reduction in the frequency of stuttering though the severity declined and so did the accompanying anxiety. Adams (1971) had 19 graduate students in speech pathology administer systematic desensitization therapy to 18 stutterers on a one-to-one basis, at least once a week for 10 weeks. Six of these dropped out of therapy. The average improvement in the others was 60 percent in a six-month period. Three failed to improve at all; 8 made some improvement; 5 were "dismissed as cured" (whatever that means). Finally, we have such an unsatisfactory commentary as that given by Brutten (1969):

. . . About thirty stutterers have received inhibition therapy. Clinical experience with these stutterers does not permit the proclamation that inhibition therapy has been universally effective; some of the stutterers have shown dramatic improvement and some have failed to evince more than a limited degree of behavior change. Nevertheless, I think it would be fair to say that inhibition therapy has produced more positive behavior change and taken less clinical time than any clinical methodology which I have previously employed. (pp. 8–82)

When we consider, as mentioned by some of these workers, that many stutterers who begin systematic de-

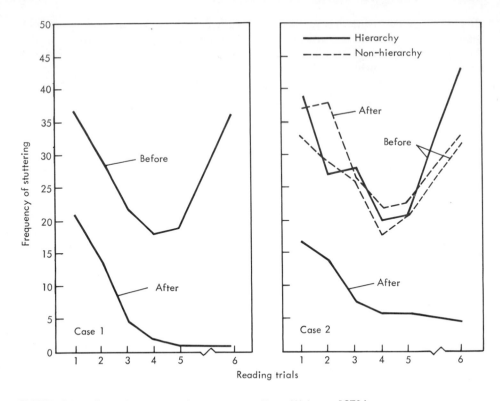

FIGURE 2.1 Effect of systematic desensitization. (From Webster, 1970.)

sensitization drop out early in the programs, the reported "cures" and percentages of improvement do not seem particularly impressive. Wolpe has stated that systematic desensitization therapy is appropriate primarily for phobic and neurotic anxiety, for those unpleasant emotional states that continue to be evoked by a stimulus configuration when that stimulus pattern is no longer followed by punishment. But are the fears of spiders or of open spaces, etc., comparable to the fears of stutterers? To us, the fears of stutterers seem to be realistically based on the expectation of the very real punishment of communicative breakdown, and social penalty, and self-derogation, and many other aversive consequences. They are no more unreasonable or inappropriate than the fear of trying to cross a Los Angeles freeway on foot at 6 P.M. If the stutterer can indeed relax, we can be pretty sure that the speaking situation in which he finds himself is not very threatening. Through relaxation and desensitization and suggestion we can create such nonthreatening situations in the therapy room and we can extinguish some of the unreasonable and exaggerated fraction of the fears which confirmed stutterers often evidence. However, so long as he continues to face the probability of frustration, struggle, abnormality, and penalty when he talks, the stutterer's hopes for finding permanent relief through any form of relaxation therapy will rarely be realized. It's biological insanity to stride out into a world full of knives with a blithe, relaxed, soft underbelly.

In saying this we do not wish to imply that we reject the basic principles of behavioral therapy. In the section of this book in which we describe our own therapy for stutterers they will be illustrated many times. We ourselves have found the use of relaxation in systematic desensitization to have some adjunctive value especially in helping the stutterer to confront a specific speaking situation such as applying for a job or meeting his parents when he returns home. We often have trained our stutterers to use assertive behaviors to inhibit their anxiety responses. We commonly use the hierarchic presentation of anxiety-evoking speaking situations and were using them long before we ever heard of behavioral therapy though we have always preferred *in vivo* desensitization to the imagining of potentially traumatic scenes. We suspect that we are biased, through personal and professional experiences, against the use of relaxation either as the sole vehicle of treatment or as the major counterconditioner in desensitization. We know, of course, that we can produce some temporary fluency by getting our stutterers to relax. Such a goal is easily attained by a hundred techniques but what we seek is a program that will enable the stutterer to be reasonably fluent for the rest of his life.

We also wish to state that though we find little utility in training the adult stutterer to attain a state of generalized body relaxation, this does not mean that we reject the evident need of stutterers to reduce their hypertensed musculatures during the stuttering act. Our own therapy is largely based upon the modification of the behaviors exhibited during the period of threat or blocking and we do everything we can to teach the stutterer that he should not struggle violently, that it is possible to work one's way into and out of a feared word without supercharging the articulators with hypertension. In the description of our own therapy program later in this book, it will be evident that we do not reject relaxation *in toto* for we use it in many ways. Our objection is to training the stutterer to try to remain limp in the presence of real alarm and to base his fluency upon such a demand. Leanderson and Levi (1967), for example, found that when stutterers entered a difficult speaking situation, their excretion of adrenaline increased over 300 percent. To ask a stutterer to stay relaxed with all that adrenalin pouring through his system is to make an outrageous demand. All stutterers have been told or have been taught or have tried to relax so that they could speak more fluently. Moreover, they find that when completely relaxed they do speak very well. Unfortunately, all the training in the world has not seemed to enable them to remain relaxed when the speaking situation become truly stressful. Again, they feel a loss of control of the self. If they only "had enough will-power" they could remain relaxed when stuttering is threatened or experienced. Instead, they get tense, stutter worse, and add guilt and impotence to their other burdens. We feel that much of the training in general body relaxation has done more harm than good.

Bibliography

ADAMS, M. R., The efficacy of reciprocal inhibition procedures in the treatment of stuttering, Unpublished paper, 1971.

AGRAS, W. S., An investigation of the decrement of anxiety responses during systematic desensitization, *Behaviour Research and Therapy*, 2 (1965), 267–270.

ALEXANDER, F. M., *The Use of the Self*. New York: Dutton, 1932.

ANDREEV, B. V., *Sleep Therapy in the Neuroses*. New York: Consultants Bureau, 1960.

BANDURA, A., *Principles of Behavior Modification*. New York: Holt, Rinehart & Winston, 1969.

BARLOW, R. H., H. LEITENBERG, W. S. AGRAS, and J. WINCZE, The transfer gap in systematic desensitization, *Behaviour Research and Therapy*, 7 (1969), 191–96.

BAUMLER, F., Mehrdimensionale stotterbehandlung von kindern und jugenlichen in sprachleilgruppen, *Zeitschrift fur Psychotherapie med. Psychol.*, 7 (1957), 99–104.

BLANTON, S. and M. G. BLANTON, *For Stutterers*. New York: Appleton-Century-Crofts, 1936.

BLUEMEL, C. S., *Stammering and Cognate Defects of Speech*. New York: Stechert: 1913.

BOOME, E. J. and M. D. RICHARDSON, *The Nature and Treatment of Stuttering*. New York: Dutton, 1931.

BRANKEL, O., Sinn and grenzen des autogenen trainings im rahmen der stotterbehandlung, *Folia Phoniatrica*, 10 (1958), 112–19.

BREGER, L. and J. L. McGAUGH, Critique and reformulation of "learning theory" approaches to psychotherapy and neurosis, *Psychological Bulletin*, 63 (1965), 338–58.

BRUTTEN, E. J., Stuttering: Reflections on a two-factor approach to behavior modification, in B. B. Gray and G. England (eds.), *Stuttering and the Conditioning Therapies*. Monterey, Calif.: Monterey Institute, 1969.

——— and D. J. SHOEMAKER, *The Modification of Stuttering*. Englewood Cliffs, N.J.: Prentice-Hall, 1967.

COOKE, G., The efficacy of two desensitization procedures: An analogue study, *Behaviour Research and Therapy*, 4 (1966), 17–24.

CROWDER, J. E. and D. W. THORTON, Effects of systematic desensitization, programmed fantasy and bibliotherapy on a specific fear, *Behaviour Research and Therapy*, 8 (1970), 33–41.

CURLEE, R. F. and W. H. PERKINS, Conversational rate control therapy for stuttering, *Journal of Speech and Hearing Disorders*, 34 (1969), 245–50.

DAMSTE, P. H., E. J. ZWAAN, and T. J. SCHOENAKER, Learning principles applied to the stuttering problem, *Folia Phoniatrica*, 20 (1968), 327–41.

DASKALOV, D. D. (Basic principles and methods for the prevention and treatment) *Zhurnal Nevropatologii i Psikhiatrii imeni S.S. Korsakova*, 62, (1962), 1047–52.

DAVIDSON, G. C., Systematic desensitization as a counterconditioning process, *Journal of Abnormal Psychology*, 73 (1968), 91–99.

DERAZNE, J., Speech pathology in the U.S.S.R., in R. W. Rieber and R. S. Brubaker (eds.), *Speech Pathology*. Amsterdam: North Holland, 1966.

DESPERT, J. L., A therapeutic approach to the problem of stuttering, *Nervous Child*, 2 (1942), 134–47.

EYSENCK, H. J., *Behaviour Therapy and the Neuroses*. New York: Pergamon Press, 1960.

FERNAU-HORN, H., *Die Sprechneurosen*. Stuttgart: Hippokrates-Verlag, 1960.

———, Hemmungszirkel und ablaufzirkel in der pathogenese und therapie des stotterns, *Med. Monatschrift*, 5 (1952), 323–27.

———, Prenzip der weitung und federund in der stimmtherapie, *H.N.O.*, 5 (1956), 365.

———, Über die beziehungen zwischen symptom und ursache beim stottern, *Arch. Ohr. Nas. Kehlkopfh.*, 169 (1956), 521–23.

FOGERTY, E., *Stammering*. New York: Dutton, 1930.

FREEMAN, G. L., Dr. Hollingsworth on chewing as a technique of relaxation, *Psychological Review*, 47 (1940), 491–93.

FREUND, H., *Psychopathology and Problems of Stuttering*. Springfield, Ill.: Charles C Thomas, 1966.

FROESCHELS, E., Pathology and therapy of stuttering, *Nervous Child*, 2 (1942), 146–61.

GIFFORD, M. F., *How to Overcome Stammering*. Englewood Cliffs, N.J.: Prentice-Hall, 1940.

GRAY, B. B., *Some Effects of Anxiety Deconditioning upon Stuttering Behavior*. Monterey, Calif.: Monterey Institute, 1968.

GROSSBERG, J. M., Behavior therapy: A review, *Psychological Bulletin*, 62 (1964), 73–85.

HIRSCHBERG, J. (*Stuttering*) *Orvosi Hetilap*, 106 (1965), 780–84.

HOGAN, R. A., The implosive technique, *Behaviour Research and Therapy*, 6 (1968), 423–32.

HOLLINGSWORTH, H. L., Chewing as a technique of relaxation, *Science*, 90 (1939), 385–87.

HAHN, E., A study of the relationship and effect of remedial treatment on the frequency of stuttering in oral reading, *Journal of Speech Disorders*, 6 (1941), 29–38.

————, *Stuttering: Significant Theories and Therapies*. Stanford, Calif.: Stanford University Press, 1943.

HOFFMAN, A., *Theoretisch-praktische anweisung zur radicalheilung stotternder*. Berlin: Schroeder, 1840.

JACOBSON, E., *Progressive Relaxation*. Chicago: University of Chicago Press, 1938.

JASPERS, K., *General Psychopathology*, 7th ed. Chicago: University of Chicago Press, 1963.

JOHNSON, W., *People in Quandaries*. New York: Harper & Row, 1946.

KASTEIN, S., Chewing method of treating stuttering, *Journal of Speech Disorders*, 12 (1947), 195–98.

KEEN, S., Sing the body electric. *Psychology Today*, 4 (October 1970), 36–61.

KINGDON-WARD, W., *Stammering: A Contribution to the Study of its Problems and Treatment*. London: Hamilton, 1942.

KNOBLECHOVA, J., Leconi koktavesti trevalia spankem, *Neurologii i Psikhiatrii Ceskoslovakia*, 14 (1951), 223–31.

KRAFT, T., A short note on forty patients treated by systematic desensitization, *Behaviour Research and Therapy*, 8 (1970), 219–20.

LADER, M. H., Palmar conductance measures in anxiety and phobic states, *Journal of Psychosomatic Research*, 11 (1967), 271–81.

———— and A. M. MATHEWS, A physiological model of phobic anxiety and desensitization, *Behaviour Research and Therapy*, 6 (1968), 411–22.

————, Comparison of methods of relaxation using physiological measures, *Behaviour Research and Therapy*, 8 (1970), 331–38.

LANG, P. J., A. D. LAZOVIK, and D. J. REYNOLDS, Desensitization suggestibility and pseudotherapy, *Journal of Abnormal Psychology*, 70 (1965), 395–402.

LANYON, R. I., Behavior change in stuttering through systematic desensitization, *Journal of Speech and Hearing Disorders*, 34 (1969), 253–59.

LAZARUS, A. A., Case history of a stutterer treated as an obsessive-compulsive disorder by broad-spectrum behavior therapy, in B. B. Gray and G. England (eds.), *Stuttering and the Conditioning Therapies*, Monterey, Calif.: Monterey Institute, 1969.

————, The elimination of children's phobias by deconditioning, *Medical Proceedings*, 5 (1959), 261.

LEANDERSON, R. and L. LEVI, A new approach to the experimental study of stuttering and stress, *Acta Otolaryngologie*, Supplement 224 (1967), 307–10.

LOMONT, J. F., Reciprocal inhibition or

extinction, *Behaviour Research and Therapy*, 3 (1965), 209–19.

_____ and J. E. EDWARDS, The role of relaxation in systematic desensitization, *Behaviour Research and Therapy*, 5 (1967), 11–25.

LUTHE, W. and J. H. SCHULTZ, *Autogenic Therapy*, Vol. III, *Applications in Psychotherapy*. New York: Gruen & Stratton, 1969.

McGLYNN, F. E. and R. H. MAPP, Systematic desensitization of snake avoidance following three types of suggestion, *Behaviour Research and Therapy*, 8 (1970), 197–201.

MATHEWS, A. M. and M. G. GELDER, Psychophysiological investigations of brief relaxation training, *Journal of Psychosomatic Research*, 13 (1969), 1–12.

MAXWELL, R. D. H. and J. W. PATERSON, Meprobomate in the treatment of stuttering, *British Medical Journal*, 1 (1964), 151.

MEYER, V. and J. M. M. MAIR, A new technique to control stammering: A preliminary report, *Behaviour Research and Therapy*, 1 (1963), 251–54.

MILLER, H. R., Control of aversive stimulus termination in systematic desensitization, *Behaviour Research and Therapy*, 8 (1970), 57–61.

NAWAS, M. M., W. V. WELSCH, and S. T. FISHMAN, The comparative effectiveness of pairing aversive imagery with relaxation, neutral tasks and muscular tension in reducing snake phobia, *Behaviour Research and Therapy*, 6 (1970), 63–68.

OHLSSON-EDLUND, E., Über vibrationsbehandlung von stottern und hypertonen zuständen bei cerebraler parese, *De Therapia Vocis et Loquellae*, 1 (1965), 421–24.

PAUL, G. L., *Insight Versus Desensitization in Psychotherapy*. Stanford, Calif.: Stanford University Press, 1966.

PAVLOVA-ZAHALCOVA, A., *Komplexe Schlaftherapie des Stotterns als Logopadische Rehabilitationmethode*, Doc-

toral thesis, Institute of Defectology, 1962.

PERKINS, W. H., *Modification of Stuttering by Rate Control*. Final Report, VRA, Research Grant #RD-2180-S. Washington, D.C.: Department of Health, Education and Welfare, 1967.

PETKOV, D. and I. IOSIFOV (*Our Experience in the Treatment of Stuttering in a Speech Rehabilitation Colony*) *Zhurnal Nevropatologii i Psikhatrii imeni S.S. Korsakova*, 60 (1960), 903–4.

RACHMAN, S., Studies in desensitization. I. The separate effects of relaxation and desensitization, *Behaviour Research and Therapy*, 3 (1965), 245–51.

_____, Systematic desensitization, *Psychological Bulletin*, 67 (1967), 93–103.

_____, Studies in desensitization. II. Flooding, *Behaviour Research and Therapy*, 4 (1966), 1–6.

_____, The role of muscular relaxation in desensitization therapy, *Behaviour Research and Therapy*, 6 (1968), 159–66.

RIEBER, R. W. and R. S. BRUBAKER, *Speech Pathology*. Amsterdam: North Holland, 1966.

RITTER, B., The group desensitization of children's snake phobias using vicarious and contact desensitization Procedures, *Behaviour Research and Therapy*, 6 (1968), 1–6.

ROLF, IDA, *Structural Integration*. Pamphlet available from Guild for Structural Integration, 1874 Fell St., San Francisco, Calif. 94117.

ROBBINS, S. D., *Stammering and Its Treatment*. Boston: Boston Stammerers Institute, 1926.

ROSENTHAL, R., Experimenter outcome orientation and the results of the psychological experiment, *Psychological Bulletin*, 61 (1964), 405–12.

ROSENTHAL, T. L., Severe stuttering and maladjustment treated by desensitiaztion and social influence, *Behaviour Research and Therapy*, 6 (1968), 125–30.

ROTHE, K. C., Zur klarstellung einiger fragen über stottern, *Hilfsschule,* 21 (1928), 437–39.

SANDOW, I., *Mechanik des Stotterns.* Nordhausen, Germany: Edler, 1898.

SCHILLING, A. (The Treatment of Stuttering), *Folia Phoniatrica,* 17 (1965), 365–458.

SCHULTZ, J. H., *Das Autogene Training.* Stuttgart: Thieme, 1956.

———— and W. LUTHE, *Autogenic Therapy.* I. *Autogenic Methods.* New York: Grune & Stratton, 1969.

STAMPFL, T. G. and D. S. LEVIS, Essentials of implosive therapy, *Journal of Abnormal Psychology,* 72 (1967), 496–503.

SWIFT, W. B., Why visualization is the best method for treating stutterers, *Proceedings of the American Speech Correction Association,* 1 (1931), 83–91.

THOMAS, K., Professor Dr. J. H. Schultz, the leader of German medical hypnotism, *British Journal of Medical Hypnosis,* 57 (1956), 153–60.

VALINS, S. and A. A. RAY, Effects of cognitive desensitization on avoidance behavior, *Journal of Personal and Social Psychology,* 7 (1967), 345–50.

VAN RIPER, C., Symptomatic therapy for stuttering, in L. E. Travis (ed.), *A Handbook of Speech Pathology.* New York: Appleton-Century-Crofts, 1957.

WALTON, D. and M. D. MATHER, The relevance of generalization technique to the treatment of stammering and phobic symptoms, *Behaviour Research and Therapy,* 1 (1963), 121–25.

WEBSTER, L. M., A clinical report on the measured effectiveness of certain desensitization techniques with stutterers, *Journal of Speech and Hearing Disorders,* 15 (1970), 369–76.

WEDBERG, C. F., *The Stutterer Speaks.* Magnolia, Mass.: Expression Co., 1937.

WOLPE, J., Behavior therapy of stuttering: Deconditioning the emotional factor, in B. B. Gray and G. England (eds.), *Stuttering and the Conditioning Therapies.* Monterey, Calif.: Monterey Institute, 1969.

————, For phobia: A hair of the hound, *Psychology Today,* 3 (June 1969), 34–37.

————, Reciprocal inhibition as the main basis of psychotherapeutic effects, *Archives of Neurology and Psychiatry,* 72 (1954), 205–26.

————, *Psychotherapy by Reciprocal Inhibition.* Stanford: Stanford University Press, 1958.

———— and A. A. LAZARUS, *Behavior Therapy Techniques: A Guide to the Treatment of Neuroses.* Oxford: Pergamon Press, 1966.

WOLPIN, M. and J. RAINES, Visual imagery, expected roles and extinction, *Behaviour Research and Therapy,* 4 (1966), 25–38.

Rhythmic, Timing,

and

Rate Control Therapies

One of the oldest and most universal of all the various forms of treatment used to help stutterers become fluent is that which is based upon the alteration or regulation of the rate of speech. There are a host of such methods and recently, after two or three decades when they fell completely from favor, we are witnessing their resurrection. Old theories and therapies for stuttering never die; they rise and fall but always appear again in slightly altered form. Each time they are greeted with enthusiasm; each time some new rationale for their existence is cited by their adherents and cures are claimed. Perhaps each new generation of stutterers and those who treat them must learn anew the old lesson that stuttering is a slippery disorder and refractory to change.

Metronomic or syllable-timed speech

Rate control, tempo-regulating, and time-beating methods have always been based upon some certain remarkable facts; most stutterers (not all of them) as soon as they begin to speak at an even-measured syllabic pace will suddenly become completely fluent; most stutterers (again not all of them), after demonstrating severe stuttering in *speaking* the words of a song, will be able to sing those same words without any stuttering at all; stutterers, when speaking in unison with some other speaker, usually again are completely fluent. These dramatic changes are so striking that any naive therapist who rediscovers them is almost certain to feel that he has found the magical method of Mo! If stuttering is basically a neurosis, as many claim, it must be a very strange one to have all its symptoms suddenly eliminated by the tick of a clock or metronome. If stuttering is simply a conditioned response to situational or linguistic cues, it is hard to see why extinction comes so instantly and so completely. There must be some underlying explanation for this "rhythm effect" which should throw new light on the nature of the disorder itself.[1] Although we anticipate ourselves, we hasten to say that the use of tempo-regulating methods, despite their ability to produce immediate fluency, have not solved the problem of stuttering. The rhythm effect is often transitory. Stutterers eventually refuse to talk in singsong. They and their listeners reject syllable-timed speech or the other variants as too artificial and abnormal. Little generalization occurs outside the therapy situation and relapse is almost universal. Any method which for at least a century and a half has failed so consistently to produce any real cure for stuttering and still manages to be used so widely must have something pretty vital in it. We think that vitality resides in the fact that it works. Yes, temporarily and unfortunately it works! This measured sort of speech can produce temporary fluency in the same way that singing can produce fluency in most stutterers. Listeners will not accept and most stutterers won't use syllable-timed speech. Those that do tend to relapse. It is very difficult to shape evenly tempoed utterance into the irregularly timed patterns of normal speech. Many have tried but few have succeeded. Indeed most of the lands of the earth doubtless contain

the dust of stutterers and their teachers who have valiantly tried to do so. If this were the answer to stuttering, the ancient problem and riddle would have been solved long ago.

Let us look at the ancient history of this method. As he strode up the mountain and walked the seashore, Demosthenes is said to have declaimed his orations to the beat of his steps and the recurring roar of the waves. Thewall (1812) tells us of the therapy advocated by Serre d'Alais: "His method comprised the separate forcible pronunciation of every syllable, aided by synchronous movements of the arms in severe cases. He afterwards acknowledged the uselessness of the system which had even failed to cure himself." Most writers have mentioned Columbat (1830) as the father of the rhythm method, and he was not averse to accepting credit for its discovery. He writes:

And in truth, one of the principal methods that I employ in combating stuttering is rhythm. . . . One must take pains to speak all the syllables metrically, beating time with the foot and pressing the thumb and forefinger together at every syllable, or after the second, third, fourth or sixth syllables. . . . The stutterer must give his entire attention to this regular regulation of the syllables and rely upon it.

To aid the imposition of the beat, Columbat invented a sort of metronome called the "mutonom" and won the Monthyon prize from the French Academy for his feat. The rhythm method caught on immediately and according to Bluemel (1913), "Rhythmic utterance has been the basis of perhaps 30 to 40 percent of all the various systems introduced since the time of Columbat. Rhythm was employed or recommended by Cull, Klencke, Katten-

---

[1] The author has attempted such an explanation in his book *The Nature of Stuttering* (1971) but is not very happy with it.

kamp, Guttman, Rosenthal, Lehwess, Krutzer, Günther, Shuldenham and a dozen other of the older teachers and writers."

An examination of how the rhythm method was taught a century ago may be illuminating. A Dr. Graves wrote the following in 1848:

I have recently discovered a method by which the most inveterate stutterer may be enabled to obtain utterance for his words with tolerable fluency. It is simply by compelling him to direct his attention to some object, so as to remove it from the effort he makes to speak. Thus, I direct him to hold a rule or a bit of stick in his right hand, and with it strike the forefinger of the left, in *regular time* with the words [apparently not the syllables] he is uttering; the eye must be fixed, and all the attention directed to the finger he is striking, and the time must be strictly kept. This method I have tried in several instances with complete success, and Dr. Neligan informs me that, since I first mentioned it to him, he has found it completely effectual in numerous cases. Although, of course, when thus employed, this plan can only be regarded as a means of affording temporary relief, I have no doubt, that if it were perseveringly followed out with young persons who stammer, both in reading and speaking, it would cure them permanently of the unpleasant affection. (quoted in Bluemel, 1913, p. 179)

Some modern advocates of syllable-timed or metronomic speech might envy the operant laboratory type of setting in which stutterers were treated by Klencke (1862). They lived in his home. Their lives were rigidly controlled; their diets prescribed; their speech constantly monitored. He manipulated his stutterers with a heavy hand, drilling them for hours in interminable breathing and vocal gymnastics, partly to engender good speech habits and partly because he felt that most

stutterers were undisciplined and erratic. He speaks of their dislike of the training and their passive opposition, boredom, and fatigue and says:

Every stutterer is strongly inclined to fall into a thoughtless mechanism, which, to a large degree, neutralizes the practice. The muscles should not alone be exercised, but also brought under the influence of the will and become susceptible to normal nervous excitation. In order to keep up this stage of the cure, he must practice combined exercises, during which he, with the strictest discipline and the closest attention, must conform to the quick or slow movements of my stick. . . . The greatest rigor and exactness are required to accomplish this. For this reason, I liken the drill to that of an orchestra, where a strict leader reproves every mistake in measure, tone and precision.

Once the stutterers have learned to breathe and to phonate "correctly" [sic!] they were introduced to rhythmic speech and contingent aversive consequences followed any failure to speak in unison with the beat. The training was thorough and painstaking. Klencke comments on some of the difficulties he encountered and how he solved them:

From the day the stutterer enters the third part of the cure he must not stutter, and must speak every word in strict accordance with the rules. My pupils generally watch one another, and rebuke every violation of the rules. I encourage this strife by sanctioning the small fines which the pupils voluntarily impose upon themselves. This plan has a most salutary effect in making them careful and bringing their minds into healthful action. . . .
Another important matter is to be observed in this measured talking. The stutterer gradually learns to speak measuredly and renew his breath in my presence

or when alone, but fails when a stranger is present. He becomes embarrassed and is ashamed of beating time which he tries to hide, and consequently falls into stuttering. . . . When required to beat time in my family circle, at table, or in the presence of other patients, [he] almost without exception, has a feeling of false shame and must be wrought upon by various means before [he] becomes willing and sufficiently bold to observe the rule. . . .

When he acquires calmness, self-control and precision, I permit him to beat the time more and more secretly, for example, with a finger in the other hand, then with a finger in the same hand, or on the thigh, then again with the hand in the pocket, etc., until finally, he has the tempo in his feeling and no longer needs the outward indication. Meanwhile the stuttering grows less and less, the will power increases with self-observation, as do also his courage with his boldness and his thought-logic with his feeling of emancipation.

Wyneken (1868) was himself one of these stutterers and we feel it is pertinent enough to quote verbatim a passage describing this treatment:

Now comes the most difficult task for the stammerer—resorting to rhythmical speech. He must pronounce every sentence as a polysyllabic word. He must speak slowly, and must accord all syllables a like duration. Where one would punctuate, he must carefully inhale.

When the pupil has observed metrical speech for several weeks in the Institute, and has become throughly accustomed to it, he is permitted—if no difficulties have occurred—to come gradually into contact with strangers. He is sent on errands (this usually furnishes a difficult task for the stammerer), and is at various times addressed suddenly and unexpectedly. If he successfully withstands these tests after he has employed rhythmic speech for several months, he is discharged as cured.

This is the formal procedure if progress has been continual and uninterrupted; but unfortunately this seldom occurs. Only a very few fortunate cases find themselves permanently rid of their stammering. The majority immediately relapse and for some time the impediment is often worse then it was originally. . . .

This relapse comes sooner or later. Usually it occurs while the student is still at the institution; sometimes it happens while he is packing his things to depart; occasionally it occurs after he has returned to his former occupation and environment. It is very seldom that the relapse does not occur at all. And now it is indeed a difficult task to reconquer doubt. I remained at the institution in question continuously for two and a half years, but in this time I never spoke as fluently again as at the end of the first six weeks. [Note: These first six weeks were observed as a period of silence.]

One of the chief reasons for the relapse lies in the employment of rhythmical speech which mode of utterance is exceedingly difficult to follow. It was never difficult for me to observe silence. I know many pupils who fulfilled the requirements in this regard to the very letter; but I have known only one who followed rhythmical speech afterwards in life. . . . To silence one can accustom himself, but to rhythmic speech never. (Bluemel (1913), pp. 174–75)

During the latter half of the nineteenth century there were other writers such as Hunt (1870) who objected to these practices: "Nothing can be more erroneous than to assume that rhythm, however skillfully employed, is sufficiently potent to remove a severe impediment," he wrote in an eloquent (though certainly optimistic) article entitled "A Death Blow to Tapping" appearing in the *Elocutionist,* January 1865, which carries this account of one stutterer's experience:

I have been trying for some time the practice of reading aloud very slowly, and beating time with my finger and thumb, tapping them sharply together at difficult consonants. From this I seem to derive benefit for a day or two; but being unexpectedly asked to read aloud in the presence of others, all my confidence deserted me. I was in a tremor from head to foot, and I cannot remember without humiliation what a terrible failure I made. The next day, *by myself* (having lost faith in my thumb!), I was worse. If anyone had been listening I should not have got out two words consecutively.

There were others who also declaimed against the use of what they called "this rhythmic trickery." Nevertheless, the immediate and dramatic effect of regularly timed speech is so powerful that this variety of therapy has probably been more universally used than any other single method. Often it has served as the key feature of a therapy that also contained many other techniques and some psychotherapy (Holgate and Andrews, 1966). Regularly timed utterance has been prescribed, as we have seen, throughout the years and it is doubtless practiced in every country today. It was the major technique employed by the owners of the commercial stammering schools and

institutes that victimized stutterers for a century and a half.

Thirty years ago, after its usage had markedly diminished for a decade or two, due to its failure to produce anything but temporary relief, the technique reappeared when Van Dantzig (1940) published an article in our own *Journal of Speech Disorders* entitled "Syllable-Tapping: A New Method for Helping Stammerers." In truth, she had devised a new gimmick although once again it was based on the old synchronization of regularly-timed syllables with body movements. We quote (from p. 130):

The *first stage* of the method of *syllable-tapping* consists of teaching the pupil to accompany the pronunciation of the successive syllables by noiseless taps of the fingers of one hand. This movement, which shows some analogy with a very elementary exercise for piano-playing, should be performed with the right or the left hand according to the preference and the handedness of the patient (but always with the same hand) and I prefer to have it started from the little finger and then continuing towards the thumb and *not* in the opposite direction. The motives that lead to this "one-way-traffic" will be stated below.

Example of syllable-tapping:

I'll	*try*	*to*	*speak*	*in*	*this*	*man-*	*ner*
little	ring	middle	index	little	little	ring	middle
finger	finger	finger	finger	finger	finger	finger	finger

The author claims that "syllable-tapping can be learned by every non-imbecile adult or child above the age of about eight years," and she recognizes the inherent suggestion in it:

Because from the very first lesson on, already the stammerer can be told that in any eventual difficult situation he may try to apply syllable-tapping in order to

overcome his difficulties; teaching this method has the effect of giving the patient an *amulet* against his disorder. The teacher need not be afraid of exploiting the suggestibility of the patient for this purpose. The stammerer's *anxiety* with respect to his own speech and to the occasions he has to speak in public or to important persons for instance will diminish by this quasi-magic *amulet effect* of syllable-tapping. (p. 130)

Also:

. . . syllable-tapping has to be combined with supplementary treatments, such as administering medicaments, relaxation, general rhythmical cures, persuasion and suggestion, psycho-analysis, or whatever other important modern method is judged the right one for each special case.

We find this method still being used in Holland. Droogleever Fortuyn (1965) says "When a school-age stutterer is asked to read aloud, pronouncing each syllable with the beat of his left palm striking the table top, he will not stutter."

Lennon (1962) in his book *Le Begaiement* says:

With the metronome set at a slow speed, the subject reads a passage aloud, saying a word to each stroke of the metronome. The speed may be increased gradually. Borel-Maisonny states that some stutterers have great difficulty synchronizing their speech with the metronome for they have no idea of the speed of their utterance since it changes constantly. It is necessary to train them in a regular rate and to make them advance only one step per syllable.

Although in the thirty years prior to 1960, the use of rhythmically timed speech nearly disappeared in the United States, some researchers soon corroborated its fluency enhancing capacity. Johnson and Rosen (1937) explored a series of conditions such as changes in rate, pitch, loudness, unison speaking with a model, and syllabic timing. All of these produced some decrease in stutterings during oral reading (only in part due to the adaptation effect) and the one which produced the greatest reduction was the imposition of a regular syllabic rhythm. Barber (1940) showed that timing

the rate of utterance with a metronome set at 92 beats per minute generated more fluency than when it was set at 184 beats per minute and also that the rhythm effect was demonstrated not only when auditory but also when visual and tactual stimuli were used to time the utterance.

However, it was not until the 1960s that syllable timed speech again caught the attention of researchers and therapists. Meyer and Mair (1963) developed a portable electronic pacer device, outwardly resembling a hearing aid and tried it out on five stutterers, asking them to speak in time with the beat until they were fluent and then to turn it off and to continue to speak in the same fashion as though the beat were still present. When the beat was set at 90 per minute, all achieved temporary fluency at first. When the beat was faster, or irregular but predictably patterned in time, or irregular and unpredictable, the reduction of stuttering was much less, and the last of these conditions had no effect. They noted that no transfer of the

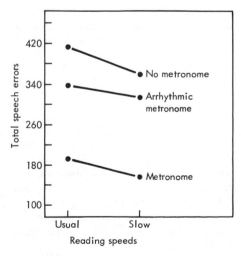

FIGURE 3.1 **Effects of metronomic speech.** (From Beech and Fransella, 1968).

improvement to unaided speech was shown, i.e., that there was no carry-over. Fransella and Beech (1965) showed that a rhythmic metronomic timer produced more fluency than an arhythmic one (see Figure 3.1). This was corroborated by Brady (1969). Fransella (1967) sought to determine whether the rhythmic effect was merely a distraction and asked stutterers additionally to copy numbers while reading to a metronomic beat and found that more errors occurred in this latter task. This might merely signify that the stutterers were distracted from their distraction but Fransella concluded that the rhythm effect was not due primarily to distraction, a conclusion which is not entirely convincing to us because of apparent errors in design.

Some application of these findings was soon in print. Andrews and Harris (1964) reported the results of intensive training in syllable-timed speech with 35 stutterers both adults and children. They were taught to use

a form of speech from which all the stress and syllable contrasts were removed. They were taught to speak syllable by syllable, stressing each syllable evenly and each to a regular even rhythm. This for us is syllable-timed speech. It is not particularly difficult but if stutterers are to become proficient at it they need considerable practice. Most of our subjects had up to 100 hours of practice, most of it intensively in the first 10 days. (p. 150)

Andrews and Harris found an immediate reduction in stuttering for "all cases for at least a few days," though a relapse "in a major or minor degree has occurred in most of the subjects."

Holgate and Andrews (1966) reduplicated the study in Australia but added psychotherapy and longer training. Again they found relapse and recurrence of stuttering and stated, "The treatment of stutterers with syllable timed speech results in immediate but short-term improvement, so that substantial relapse occurs within twelve to twenty-four months." Brandon and Harris (1967) supplemented syllable-timed speech training with psychotherapy and desensitization to outside situations. They report some long-term improvement (about 60 percent) in about two-thirds of their cases but no details are given. Horan (1968) in a preliminary report states that the disfluency rate for all her subjects, irrespective of their severity, fell below two percent when paced by an electronic metronome set at two beats per second. Wohl (1968), in a study which is almost impossible to evaluate, found that 14 out of 146 stutterers, "acquired fluency," 55 showed little or no improvement, and the rest showed "great or considerable improvement." Brady (1968) combined metronomic speech with desensitization and reports that three of the six stutterers treated "have acquired fluency within the normal range (unaided by the metronome)." Alford and Ingham (1969) used tokens (buttons which when collected could be exchanged for some reward) to reinforce normal speech in small groups (N-4 and 5) of young stutterers. No change occurred until syllable-timed speech was instituted; then a marked decrease in stuttering (though not to zero) occurred but stuttering increased again at time of follow-up. We also note that a visual pacer, the Perceptoscope, and also a metronome were used by Goldiamond (1965) in his operant studies for controlling stuttering. Still another variant timing procedure was employed by Curlee and Perkins (1969) who used a delayed feedback device set at 250 msec. delay. The stutterer "was instructed to slow down his speaking rate by prolonging syllables so that his utterances coincide with the delayed feedback." This speaking in cadence with the delayed echo usually results not only in an abnormally slow "speaking rate of 30 to 35 words per minute" but in our experience, it also produces a rhythmic, evenly cadenced type of utterance. Columbat's metronome was a simpler instrument. Meyer and Cromley (1969), in a preliminary study which is also hard to judge, found that 17 of 48 stutterers were unable to master rhythmic speech and that most of these were those who showed "hard blockings." Bilateral metronomic aids were less well tolerated than monaural. Half of their 48 stutterers received metronome-aided and half unaided syllabic timed speech training for a period of twelve weeks. Three from each of these two groups "achieved complete fluency" and all subjects improved.

In a series of papers, Andrews and Ingham (1971), Ingham and Andrews (1971), and Ingham, Andrews, and Winkler (1972) the authors describe further attempts to apply the techniques of rhythmic, syllable-timed speech to several groups of Australian stutterers. To exert greater control, these stutterers were hospitalized and placed under a token economy so that necessities (such as food and drink) and luxuries such as cigarettes had to be purchased by the tokens. These were earned by showing *progress* in eliminating stutterings or increasing the rate of syllables spoken per minute after the stutterers had been taught to speak the syllables with a regular cadence. They talked conversationally with

each other for about twelve hours a day for two or three weeks. During the initial stages of treatment the frequency of stuttered syllables and the rate of speaking were measured seven times a day, with tokens awarded for achieving certain criteria of stuttering reduction. Tokens could also be taken away if regression occurred. Booster sessions averaging eight hours a month for nine months were also given. Under this incredibly intensive therapy program, and seeking to progress from rhythmic to normal speech:

"Nearly half of the stutterers did not stutter when assessed on the Iowa Job Task nine months later, but only a quarter of them spoke at normal rates of speed. The others, handicapped either by the patterned syllable timed speech or by their residual stuttering were limited in their rate of speaking." Those who showed the best results were those whose initial stuttering was mild. Andrews and Ingham conclude "that syllable timed speech is not a preferred method of treatment." They also mention the reluctance that many of the stutterers showed toward using syllable-timed speech outside the hospital.

This to date forms the far from impressive research upon which the current commercial promotion of metronomically-aided training for stutterers is based. It clearly shows the tendency toward relapse; it indicates that stutterers and listeners find this kind of speech unpleasant; the methods used for assessment of outcome are very inadequate; the contamination produced by other forms of adjunct therapy is apparent; the transition into normal speech from the unnatural regular tempo produced by the metronomes or by instruction seems to be very difficult to stabilize. From all we have read, and from all we have seen and personally experienced, we would conclude that, at least in its present form, the use of this kind of speech training for the confirmed stutterer is inadvisable.[2] The stutterer's fund of hope is too small to be wasted.

The suggestive effect of rhythmic speech

Nevertheless, we feel that it is important to try to understand why this tempo-regulating therapy has any effect at all—since it does improve the fluency for many stutterers temporarily. Consider just the effect of suggestion alone. When *each* syllable or word is spoken in regular rhythm a powerful suggestion is brought into being. Since most stutterers speak the great majority of their words and syllables without stuttering, the fluent items gain a stimulus value under the rhythmic patterning that they ordinarily do not possess. The stutterer hears and feels himself being fluent on these utterances and since their only commonality is the regular beat, the latter becomes easily invested with an almost magical efficacy. There is little time to scan for feared words or sounds when the mandate of the inexorable beat predominates. All words, all syllables are the same; the fear is homogenized out of them when they are uttered metronomically. No one sound sticks its head up long enough to be feared. The cumulative effect of all this self-suggestion, indirect though

2 Because of these reasons we regret the full page advertisements in *Asha*, the professional journal of the American Speech and Hearing Association, describing the behind-the-ear-miniaturized metronome (Figure 3.2) hailing its use as "A New Behavioral Approach to Stuttering" and claiming that "clinical reports are very encouraging."

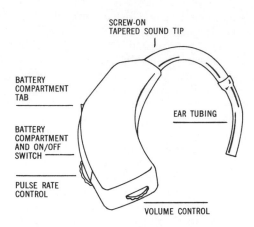

SCREW-ON TAPERED SOUND TIP

BATTERY COMPARTMENT TAB

EAR TUBING

BATTERY COMPARTMENT AND ON/OFF SWITCH

PULSE RATE CONTROL

VOLUME CONTROL

FIGURE 3.2 The pacemaster electronic metronome. (Reproduced by permission of Associated Auditory Instruments, Upper Darby, Pennsylvania.)

it is, can be tremendously powerful. The technique is simple; it is easily performed, it usually produces immediate, if temporary, fluency and so seems to possess almost magical properties; by concentrating on the timing the stutterer is distracted from the phonemic and situational cues that precipitate his fears.

Rhythm as reassurance

It might seem as though there could be little psychotherapy in this singsong speech or syllable tapping or other forms of rhythmic utterance. Yet if we can accept reassurance as belonging to the family of psychotherapies we find some of it in these activities as they are taught. There does seem to be something reassuring about being caught up in a regular rhythm and we should remember the mother's rocking and lullabies, the witch doctor's dance, the effects of massage, the rhythmic nature of incantations and hypnotic suggestion. As one who was subjected to treatment that emphasized the use of body swaying, rhythmic chanted speech usually as a member of a large group performing simultaneously, the author can attest to the conviction that there is something tremendously reassuring in these rhythmic vocalizations. (Sometimes he felt as an autistic child might feel, rocking back and forth interminably singing his perseverative little tune.) Caught up in the hypnotic hours of vocalized rhythm practice, for the time being he felt safe and secure. In a world full of traumatic change and sudden hurt, there is something to be said for regularity, for continuity. While doubtless there are other factors (such as the facilitation of timed utterance involved), we should not be unaware of the anxiety reduction which accompanies such rhythmic rituals.

Rhythmic speech as a distraction

Bloodstein (1969) makes a statement concerning the distractive value of syllabic-timed speech which probably represents the beliefs of many sophisticated therapists:

Almost any circumstance that momentarily reinforces the stutterer's awareness of himself as a stutterer or focuses his attention on cues representative of stuttering is likely to bring on more stuttering. Conversely, any condition under which his attention to such cues is weakened by competing stimuli may bring about a temporary elimination of speech difficulty. (p. 198)

Under such distractors, Bloodstein lists singing, speaking in a singsong, or in a monotone, or "in time to rhythmical movements such as those of a metronome."

In a separate section we have considered the dynamics of distraction in stuttering and here we wish to say

again that only so long as the novelty persists and the stutterer must direct his attention to the precise timing of each syllable, do the phonemic and word fears fail to raise their ugly heads. Once the new way of talking becomes habituated, the distraction effect is lost and the fears return as strong as ever, the resulting disillusionment often precipitating more severe stuttering than had previously been evidenced. On this we can give personal testimony. Upon returning home from one of the stuttering institutes where hope had first been created, then lost in despair, we remember thinking that above the portals of each of these institutions there should be inscribed the same words that Dante placed above the gates of hell: "All hope abandon ye, who enter here." Some of us are more suggestible than others. In some of us, the stuttering behaviors have been less strongly reinforced. Some of us may be better integrated than others or less vulnerable to stress. And so some of us may improve when speaking for a time in this abnormal way.

Other explanations for the rhythm effect

Although we recognize that distraction may account for some of the temporary fluency which is produced by syllable-timed speech, we do not think it to be the only factor. Indeed we feel that its primary influence is due to its facilitation of the timing of the basic synergies of respiration, phonation, and articulation which appear to be disrupted in stuttering, and the timing involved in the co-articulation of the syllable and the motor patterns of the word. Since we have discussed this matter elsewhere (Van Riper, 1971a), we shall not elaborate further except to say again that the very predictability of the accessory signals provided by the metronome or finger movement or other external or internal stimuli tends to drive the temporal patterning of nervous impulses required for integration.

In a very interesting article by Allan (1970) the point is made that

. . . a disturbance of the precise temporal relations that normally exist between voluntary presetting of the phonatory musculature and continuous reflex adjustment of the tonus of this musculature may be involved in stammering—particularly the fact that stammering may be suppressed during singing or recitation of rhythmically accented verse, and the fact that the disorder may be ameliorated by practicing syllable-timed speech.

A similar point of view has been expressed by Moravek and Lagova (1968). They say, "We regard the prephonational or initial tonus as the key to the problem of stuttering." From this point of view, the metronomic or other signals make possible the appropriate presetting of the laryngeal structures via the gamma loops involved and so long as they serve this timing function, the motor patterns of the syllable are integrated. Unfortunately, these signals tend to lose their value as an accessory timer when they lose their novelty or stimulus value, and, also, though they are useful timing mechanisms when predictable (as occurs in measured, regular syllabic utterance), they are less successful when ordinary speech is attempted since ordinary speech is irregular and constantly variable.

Other timing methods

Stutterers themselves have invented a host of behaviors which they use to time the moment of speech attempt—head jerks, sudden abdominal contractions, jaw openings, preparatory vocalizations such as a prolonged vowel, a sudden shift in pitch or loudness, the stamping of a foot, the twitch of a finger, a hand gesture, a nod. Any therapist will recognize these as being present in the symptom pictures of severe stutterers and as contributing greatly to the abnormality of the disorder. What is not recognized too often is that most of these behaviors are the automatized residues of timing devices once used to facilitate utterance on feared words. At first these behavioral timers do facilitate utterance just as the beat of a metronome does until habituation reduces its stimulus and signaling value. As we might expect, therefore, many who have had to treat stuttering have incorporated such timing devices into their therapy. Accessory timing signals need not be externally imposed; they can be given by the stutterer himself. They also resolve the approach-avoidance conflicts, the ambivalence which results from the urge to speak and the fear of demonstrating abnormality or suffering frustration. They terminate postponement behaviors which have run too long. They help the stutterer to get started.

The use of these self-timers or starters has had a long history. Serre d'Alais (1829) recommended that the stutterer accompany his speech attempts by vigorous gestures. We see no point in describing all of the various timing activities given to stutterers and so will content ourselves with Bluemel's (1913) account:

A few of the specific gestures prescribed by teachers of stammerers are: nodding the head, throwing the head back with a jerk, snapping the fingers, pulling at a coat button, pressing the thumb against the chin or larynx, waving the hand, raising a handkerchief to the mouth, tapping the foot. . . . (p. 178)

These methods were far from being universally accepted even by the contemporaries of those who advocated them. Alexander Melville Bell in 1853 protested that "such cures were worse than the malady" and the anonymous author ("A Minute Philosopher") of "The Irrationale of Speech" (1859) says of them, "As long as the fresh trick which had been taught compelled the patient to speak slowly and with attention to his words, so long was he benefited; as soon as he began to speak freely and with ease, all of his old bad habits returned along with the new one (p. 8)."

Nevertheless, we find similar practices used today. Travis (1931) and Bryngelson (1952) devised a simultaneous talking and writing exercise in which stutterers timed their utterance with the dominant stroke of the first letter of the words being spoken. Hours were spent daily in such practice as the present author well remembers, and although at times his pen froze on the paper with the fixation of his mouth, usually the words were spoken without stuttering. Transfer to ordinary speaking situations was not satisfactory. At one of the stammering schools we attended long ago, the basic method for initiating utterance was to describe a figure eight in the air with the forefinger, trying to make the speech attempt exactly at the intersection. It was a fine method for the therapist. If we stuttered, he told us we had failed to say the word exactly at that imagined point; if we said it normally, he assured us that we had, and no proof of either was possible. Many of us developed figure eight movements with our eyes when blocking. Metraux (1965) tells us of witnessing some stuttering therapy in France in which the stutterers had to draw a wavy line on a paper, the waves of which "were automatically coordinated with the syllables and terminated with each phrase (p. 21)." Froeschels, whose breath-chewing therapy dominated German and Austrian stuttering therapy for years, inadvertently designed another set of timers. By speaking while chewing the breath, the utterances became timed with the strong jaw movements and thus produced some fluency. In this connection it is interesting that Denhardt (1890) suggested that the stutterer make "great mouth movements" when he talked and also to put an *h* sound before words beginning with vowels.

It would also be possible to regard the use of voluntary stuttering (Bryngelson, 1952) or "the bounce" (Johnson, 1946) as timing mechanisms. Bryngelson recommended that the stutterer should deliberately keep repeating the first syllable of a feared word until he felt he had absolute voluntary control over it and only then to speak the word. The possibility that this would be used to time the speech attempt is obvious and in fact, using this procedure, it became apparent that many of our cases fell into set patterns of repetition, usually producing a stereotyped set of three syllables before attempting the word. The repetitions were regular and the final attempt was in rhythm with them. Despite our instructions to vary the tempo, most stutterers did not seem to be able to resist the timing facilitation produced by the regularity.

Zaliouk (1954) in Israel tells of teaching children who stutter to jump or walk on floor tiles as they pronounced syllables or words and also, in conjunction with gross movements, he used pencil facilitation "in which the child would draw straight vertical lines in different colours." As he spoke he used phonetic gestures to accompany the speech attempt.

Breathing rituals

Another set of techniques designed to treat stuttering involves the use of specific instructions concerning how to breathe at the moment of speech attempt. The obvious breathing abnormalities shown by stutterers, their gasps, holding of the breath, discordance in thoracic and abdominal respiration, and their attempts to speak while holding the breath or at the very end of exhalation, all these seemed to demand correction. Accordingly, the early history of stuttering therapy [3] is replete with a hundred differing kinds of training intended to teach the stutterer how to breathe—despite the also obvious fact that he breathes normally in silence and also during the large fraction of his speech in which he is fluent. The many hours spent by stutterers in following these instructions probably did little harm though a few persons, like this author, suffered from hyperventilation and occasionally became dizzy and fainted. It was also apparent that when these prescribed rituals of breathing were applied to speaking the stutterers did become more fluent at least temporarily. What occurred of course is that the prescribed manner of breathing served both as a distraction and as a timing device. When one was intent upon a slow deliberate inhalation, or a deep inhalation, with the abdomen distended or the thorax expanded (according to the particular

system being taught), or when one tried to make sure that the speech attempt was timed exactly with the felt outflow of the breath through the lips (or nose!), one became pretty oblivious to the cues in the situation or in the word which had previously been associated with stuttering. So concerned were we with performing the intricate ritual, we could not assume the old trigger postures or rehearse covertly the patterning of the stuttering that ordinarily we would have done. Again, the tricks worked. But again, as soon as they became habituated, they no longer were able to distract or to perform their timing function and so the stuttering returned. One of the worst consequences of this training was that we felt very guilty when it did. We felt that we had not been vigilant enough; we had not done what we were supposed to do; and our teachers were not reluctant to turn their scorn upon us for our failures.

We see no utility in providing any detailed account of this sad breath training that characterized our last century and part of this one.[4] Instead we present some evidence to indicate that the same methods will survive today. A common older technique was to stop when a feared word approached, to inhale-exhale once or several times before beginning to vocalize on inhalation, then to speak the word on the final exhalation.[5] We find something very similar in an article by Rethi (1965): "It is explained to the patient that normal speech is only produced while the subject is breathing out. The spasm in-

---

[3] One of the earliest prescriptions for breath training was offered by Avicenna, an Arabian physician and philosopher. He suggested that the stutterer always take a deep breath before beginning to speak. The same advice has been given to many stutterers ever since—often leading to abnormal involuntary gasping.

[4] A detailed description of them will be found in Bluemel (1913), Chapter 2.

[5] Wyllie (1894) tells of a stutterer who used "drawback phonation," doing his vocalization on the inhalation. "Practicing this method voluntarily at first, he soon found that it became habitual and involuntary."

duced by stammering can only thus occur during exhalation. If vocalization is begun during inhalation, then the stammering could not take place even if the subject wanted to stutter. . . . The vowels are formed during inhalation and continued into exhalation (p. 270)." Fernau-Horn (1952) also trains her subjects to attack feared words by beginning with a vowel and using a brief inspiratory catch. Hanakawa (1965) in Japan writes, ". . . he must be trained to control his breathing whatever may happen. It is good for this training to practice to strain the abdomen and to breathe out gradually, raising the diaphragm." Facchini and Gozzi (1965) in Italy recommend a variety of forms of breathing while vocalizing vowels. DeParrel (1965), a French therapist, provides a series of breathing exercises "since controlled respiration is the cornerstone of remedial treatment." Damsté (1970) gives this glimpse of therapy in the Netherlands:

On the second day, the tension-control session is spent with a further survey of the sensations involved in the process of breathing. The therapist says a sentence, and we say it after him, everyone in his own time, and at the moment that is appropriate for him. For example, "I feel the movement of my breath." (The group repeats the sentence.) "I notice the air entering through my nose." (The group repeats.) "I feel my trunk expanding a little." (Repeat.) "I pay attention to the peak of inspiration." (Repeat.) "I make the transition from inspiration to expiration a fluent one." (Repeat.) "When my phrase is finished, I let the remaining air run off, sshhh." (Repeat.) "Then I wait for the next inspiratory phase to occur, and I let it flow in without any tension." (Repeat.) "Thus I continuously increase my self-reliance." (Repeat.) All of us in the group feel satisfied after this session because we have penetrated further into

one of the roots of the stuttering problem. We stretch and yawn uninhibitedly before we get up. (p. 87)

Various forms of breath training have been used abroad. Trojan and Weihs (1963) in Austria describe a training in relaxed breathing and vocalization leading to the rhythmical chanting of syllables accompanied by movements and gestures. And in our own country, although the former emphasis on breath training as shown in the writings of Hahn (1950) and Gifford (1940) has just about disappeared, we still find Reichel (1964) advocating diphragmatic breathing while whirling the hands and directing the breath nasally. In our opinion, most of these techniques are at best mere vehicles of suggestion, self-discipline, or distraction. Perhaps some of them, such as Rethi's inhalatory prefix to vocalization may help the stutterer momentarily to unlock a laryngeal closure. We are pretty sure that the breath pulse plays an important role in timing the necessary synergies of respiration, voice, and articulation in producing a sound or syllable and that some of the minor effectiveness of this breath training may be explained in this way. Yet there are dangers in the deliberate control of the breath for speaking. The automaticity may be further impaired or the behaviors taught may turn into gross abnormalities. We feel that most of the gasps and breathing abnormalities shown by stutterers are the habituated residues of techniques they devised themselves to time the speech attempt.

Vocalized timing rituals

The well known difficulty that many stutterers show in getting started, in initiating phonation, has led them and their therapists to explore ways other than breathing to begin their speech attempts. Some of these we have mentioned earlier in our chapter on suggestion but one of them, Arnott's system, involved the use of a prefixed vowel to time the utterance and so it is pertinent here. Dr. Neil Arnott was a physician and physicist and he believed that the core of the stutterer's problem lay in his inability to produce phonation due to the jamming of the vocal cords. To help him, Arnott suggested the use of a starter vowel after any pause and the elimination of as many pauses as possible. Hunt (1861) tells us:

Dr. Arnott advises us to begin pronouncing or droning any simple sound, as the *e* of the English word *berry* whereby the glottis is opened, and the pronunciation of the following sounds is rendered easy. The words should be joined together, as if each phrase formed but one long word, nearly as they are joined in singing; if this be done, the glottis never closes, and there is, of course no stutter. (p. 86)

In one of the stuttering schools we attended we were taught to preface the beginning of our sentence with an upwardly inflected schwa vowel. While at first we achieved some surprising fluency in this drunken-sounding speech because the initial *ah* did act as a distractor and timing signal, soon that *ah* began to become longer and longer, and soon we were repeating it clonically, then tremors crept into these repetitions and finally we were unable to even produce the *ah*. A few stutterers, however, left the institute within a few weeks without much stuttering though still speaking in this abnormal way and our instructor claimed that they had been cured. Potter (1882) gives an example of "Arnott's old trick." The sentence

is "Would you willingly aid in securing unanimous consent?" It would be spoken, according to Potter in this way: "Oooould-eeeooo-oooillingly-aid-ins-ec-uring-eeoonanimous-econsent?" The way we had to slur was even worse than this and once, when going down town on an errand, we had to ask a policeman "Uhwhereuhisuh-theuhbusuhstation?" and he took us to the police station instead whereupon we hastily returned to our old form of stuttering to make ourselves intelligible enough to validate our sanity.

Other practitioners soon adopted Arnott's method (though he failed to include it in a revised edition of his physics book) and, as usual, they made modifications. Some of them scoffed at the vowel he used as a timing prefix and insisted that the *ah* should be used instead. Others, noting that the nasal channel formed an alternative channel for the lip- and tongue-blocked mouth, taught their stutterers to start their feared words with an *n* sound instead, thus bypassing the blockade.[6] Many used a vocalized sigh to initiate all utterance, thus combining relaxation with suggestion and timing. Such a procedure was advocated in this country by Gifford (1940) and by Hahn (1950). If anyone would assume that this trick is no longer used, we suggest they listen incredulously to the recordings of the expensive set of cassette therapy lessons copyrighted by Lee (1970) and intended for stutterers to do at home. One of the major evils of this technique is that the accessory vowel often becomes an in-

[6] In Japan, Kotoji Satsuta (1937) "invented" the technique of having the stutterer preface the first sound of each word on which he expected to stutter by inserting the *n* sound prior to the speech attempt. It has been called the Satsuta method.

tegral part of the stuttering pattern and the abnormality is thereby increased. We worked with an Indian from Oklahoma once, who had been taught to start all feared words with an *uh* sound. He had no other abnormality, no other repetitions, prolongations, tremors, or anything else but he had yards of repeated *uhs*. We remember that at our first interview we asked him where he came from and he answered, "Uh . . uh . . uh . . uuuuh . . uh . uhuhuh . . . uh . . uuuuuuh . . . uhuhuhuhPa-ris." [7] He had a starter that didn't start.

At that, he might have developed a worse one. In our chapter on suggestion we described how Scripture (1923) trained his stutterers to use the "octave twist," a technique which stutterers were to use when they anticipated stuttering. It was not too complicated, the stutterers simply having to raise or lower their voices a full octave as they attacked the feared word. Some bizarre vocal symptoms usually result from this practice. We have had seven stutterers who discovered this sudden shift of pitch by themselves, usually employing it to terminate an overlong prolongation or series of syllables. Despite the fact that they were terribly distressed by the audience reactions to the behavior, we found the behavior very difficult to extinguish. It had been reinforced too often by being followed by the utterance of the word they had feared. There are other techniques of this ilk but we feel we have given enough examples.

From singing to speaking

The well known observation that stutterers generally have little diffi-

culty when singing has also led to various methods for treating the disorder. Witt (1925) and Nadoleczny (1926) found that less than ten percent of their stutterers had any trouble during singing. Fletcher (1928), Johnson and Rosen (1937), and Klemm (1958) also found fluency in the stutterer's singing. Accordingly, we find in the literature numerous references to the use of singing in therapy. The stutterers were first trained in choral singing, then in choral speech, and then in melodic utterance with exaggerated inflections, and finally in normal speaking with attention to melodic patterning and accentuation. We find here some excellent examples of the shaping of responses, even though the early therapists knew nothing about conditioning. Another program used a series of substeps in which singing was shifted to singsong then to chanting, then to speaking in a monotone and finally to normal speech. All of these methods were used in the commercial schools for stutterers and were advocated by various authors during the last half of the nineteenth century. That they still are being used in one form or another is evidenced in the modern literature. Stoneley (1955) writes that his stutterers were able to speak more easily by singing their messages. "Indeed, where simple monosyllables had previously been insuperable barriers, whole phrases were sung easily, and thence it was but a simple matter of gentle persuasion to steer the child from the notes to spoken words." He goes on to say that there was nothing new in his method, that King George VI of England had profited from it but that "the cure takes time and requires ability."

Rau (1953), Prevbrayenskaya (1953), Petkov and Iosifov (1960) and other Russian and Bulgarian au-

---

[7] There is indeed a Paris, Oklahoma.

thors describe the kind of unison sing-ing-speaking training given to their stutterers, often associated with the rhythmic steps of folk dancing or gymnastics. Nekrasova (1953) for ex-ample suggests intoning speech, be-ginning with simple materials and proceeding to more complex ones, chanting very loudly. Rozenthal (1968) in Poland has developed a lo-gorhythmic form of therapy based on the Jacques-Delacrose system which combines musical and body rhythms with speech. In her therapy, autosug-gestive formulae are also employed: "1. Je respire tranquillement. 2. Je regarde mon interlocuteur dans les yeux, je l'écoute et puis je parle. 3. Je prononce les sons nettement" and so on up to the final item, number 20: "Je gagne la liberté." Our only venture into this form of therapy (Van Riper, 1958) resulted in the Dance of the Wild Cucumber which is best left undescribed and unappreci-ated.

In Germany, Moll (1939) wrote an article entitled "From Singing to Speaking" in which he recommended that stutterers be provided with a hi-erarchy of transitional utterances of the same sentences, first sung with a pronounced melody, and then modi-fied into nonsinging speech. He stressed the importance of having this singing end on the stutterer's habitual pitch level if the transition were to be accomplished. More currently, Os-kar Fitz (1961), whose group therapy methods have been very influential in Germany, has this to say:

The basic enemy in stuttering is the use of a wrong technique in speaking. If we can eliminate all the stutterer's in-appropriate behaviors and assumptions, then only the correct movements remain. In playing a musical instrument, the per-former must always be in the right place at the right time. In speaking, all move-ments occur in space and time and they must be timed instantaneously. Unfortu-nately in the stutterer this timing is han-dled very inadequately. . . . In the art song (Kunstgesang) the vowel has to co-incide exactly at the time of the musical beat and the rhythm of the verse parallels the words recited. For this reason, the rhythmical, ordered speech (of the art song) helps the stutterer significantly and his everyday speaking also becomes lively, rhythmical and melodic. The tone is based on the vowel, not on the conso-nant. The characteristics of the consonant depend upon the vowel and are influ-enced by them. (p. 266)

Fitz claims that 92 percent of all stut-terers can be fluent when using this art song.

Another European author, Svend Smith, of Denmark, should be men-tioned in this section on rhythmic therapy. His therapy is complex and sophisticated and he rejects the use of many of the methods we have been describing: "The use of unnatural tricks in treating stuttering is certain-ly not advisable. The stutterer him-self has used these tricks for some time. Do not give him any more (Smith, 1955)." Svend Smith, how-ever, does use an interesting rhythmic therapy, designed to integrate the synergies of utterance and at the same time to free the stutterer from his in-hibitions. In his "accent therapy," for example, the therapist may beat a drum in various strange rhythms, al-most African in nature, and leads the stutterer in chanting nonsense sylla-bles in time with the beat. We have seen Svend Smith demonstrate these procedures and the performance is impressive. The participants do tend to lose their vocal inhibitions; they become aware of the potential flexi-bility in tone production and articula-tory movements which they have always possessed but never have experienced. As Smith says, "This conduct has in itself a psycho-therapeutic effect." Goraj (1963) gives this description: "He (Smith) has developed a kind of chant, using loose up and down jaw movements which the patients use to pronounce one vowel sound after another. To motivate and relax at the same time, he uses a deep drum which he beats in rhythms that are like real speech; he calls them 'life rhythms.' He does not repeat a pattern so that it becomes mechanical but varies it continually." Schilling (1965) whose account of current European stuttering therapy is probably the most comprehensive, offers this further information: "Svend Smith starts with general relaxation, lying supine, with the stutterer placing his hand on the upper abdomen to sense the abdominal exhalation and the short pause (rest) which follows it. Then the stutterer groans on exhalation; then the rhythmic beats are given (the stutterer now standing) and the stutterer groans (vocalizes) and moves his articulators freely and easily but with the accent on the vowel, the tempo increasing, and then shifting to continuous speech."

Unison speech

Still another remarkable feature of stuttering, that chameleon of speech disorders, is that it tends to disappear whenever the person speaks in unison with others or when echoing them. Kussmaul (1877) observed that for the stutterer "the impediment disappears as soon as someone pronounces the word for him," but it was probably Liebmann (1898) who developed the use of unison speaking as a major part of his therapy, one which is still practiced today by a few workers. Schilling (1965) describes the Liebmann method as follows (our translation):

The method itself is simple. After a short period of instruction, the therapist starts immediately to speak short, simple sentences with the stutterer. He ignores any hesitations and continues speaking. The stutterer is therefore forced to pay attention to the therapist's words and his speech becomes fluent. If the therapist would wait for the stutterer to catch up, the latter would have time to focus his attention again on his speech and so the latter would remain disturbed. In the second phase, simultaneous repeating of certain sentences is emphasized. Gradually the therapist lowers his voice intensity so that it becomes weaker and weaker and finally he speaks in pantomime as the stutterer continues to speak fluently and entirely alone. Then short anecdotes provide the stimulus material. . . .

Schilling reports that five of the 150 therapists who answered his questionnaire still followed Liebmann's methods.

In this country several researchers have investigated the unison effect, among them Johnson and Rosen (1937), Barber (1939) and Pattie and Knight (1944). One of the more interesting of Barber's findings was that the stutterers spoke fluently even when the model speaker was reading different material. This to us indicates that it may have been the timing effect of the stimulus pulses provided by the model which enhanced the fluency. Other possible explanations, of course, may include distraction, lack of propositionality, or masking. Pattie and Knight said that the chorus reading served as an accessory pacemaker. At any rate, speaking in unison with the stutterer has been a technique used in many differing therapies. We even find Andrews and Harris (1964) using the "concurrent reading" of prose as one of the steps they used to teach syllable-timed speaking, and it is included in the tape-recorded therapy program of Peins, Lee, and McGough (1970). Stecher (1964) describes a therapy session in Germany in which a group of stutterers would begin by speaking in unison, and then, in rotation, one member after another would drop out until finally only one stutterer was speaking the sentences being recited. This too is an ancient timing method, often used in the old commercial schools to convince the stutterers that they could be fluent.

Shadowing

This technique is closely related to unison speech since the stutterer is asked to echo what the model speaker is saying as soon as he can, and with a minimum of delay. It is echo speech, not unison speech or choral speech, but when done correctly and skillfully there is little time lapse. Cherry (1957) explains it in this way:

A tape recording is made of a reading from a passage of prose and played through headphones to a listener; the listener is instructed to repeat what he hears concurrently, in a subdued or whispered voice. He is then listening and speaking at the same time, but this is found to be an extremely simple task. His spoken repetition tends to be in irregular detached phrases and, with most people and most texts, is given in a singularly emotionless voice as though intoning. It seems as though he is unable to copy the emotional content of the words he hears and, since he is following so close upon the heels of these words, he is unable to see far enough ahead to create his own

emotional content. He mouths the words like an automaton and extracts little semantic content, if any. (p. 279)

There are several studies which demonstrate that shadowing can produce at least some temporary fluency. Cherry and Sayers (1956) found that when stutterers "shadowed" the speech of a model speaker almost complete "suppression" of stuttering occurred. In a further study, Cherry, Sayers, and Marland trained five stutterers in shadowing over a period of from two to four weeks and state that "striking improvement" took place. A case report of improvement in which shadowing was combined with systematic desensitization is given by Walton and Mather (1963). Kelham and McHale (1966) report impressive success when three different therapists administered shadowing training primarily to child stutterers using a hierarchy of speaking situations which gradually increased in difficulty. Jones (1969) gives a less favorable report. Fifty adult stutterers were given training in shadowing practice over a period of eight weeks. He writes, "The results have not been completely analyzed but it is already clear that, although a few patients improved dramatically, the overall success of the therapy is unlikely to be greater than when more traditional methods are employed over the same period." More favorable results, however, seem to be found when shadowing is used with child stutterers, Kondas (1967) reporting a seventy percent "success rate" based on a two- to five-year follow-up. We too have found unison speech and echo speaking of value in reinforcing the normal speech of very young stutterers who were showing struggle but no avoidance reactions, but with adults these methods, by themselves, produced no permanent transfer of the fluency into other speaking situations.

Rate control therapy

Another hoary old method for producing temporary fluency has recently been exhumed from the grave where it belongs. It consists of training the stutterer to speak very slowly, usually by prolonging the vowel sounds or by pausing longer than usual after each phrase. At first, the stutterer speaks only one word about every two seconds or about 30 words a minute as he reads or recites memorized material. Then, as the stuttering disappears, the rate is gradually increased until hopefully it approximates the normal tempo of utterance. Who first discovered that this odd way of talking does indeed reduce or eliminate stuttering is unknown but Denhardt in Germany and Chervin in France were using it more than a hundred years ago. That at one time it found wide acceptance is illustrated by this quotation from Bluemel (1913):

Slow speaking is advocated by most teachers of stammerers. This slow speaking usually involves lengthening the vowels and protracting the ordinary pauses. Kingsley's oft quoted advice was to "Read and speak slow." Another English writer declares that "The stammerer, if he wishes to be cured, *must,* on all occasions, speak slowly and deliberately, dwelling on the *vowels,* so as to give time for forming the laryngeal sounds. . . ." In an English stammering school, slow speaking is carried to the point where the pupils utter only one word on a breath at the beginning of treatment. (pp. 121–22)

In this quotation by Bluemel we made mention of the two major methods for slowing down the speech rate—increasing the length of the pauses and elongating the vowels. Many of the old drill books are full of reading passages with diagonal lines marking the place where the stutterer must insert a lengthy pause and many of the old pedagogical therapies stressed this sort of phrasing practice along with slow deliberate speech. The treatment of stuttering in a book by Bender and Kleinfeld (1938) was primarily based upon rate control and we find an account of its use in an article by Bender (1944) who tells of a stutterer, aged forty, whom he treated.

The psychologist explained to him that only he could help himself. That he might well adopt the attitude that his stuttering could not be cured in any miraculous way. But by relearning to speak through conscious management of the speech process, he could at least control the symptoms of stuttering. Training was given him each morning, before he reported for work in *rate-control.* . . . These principles were applied to the oral reading of sounds, then syllables, and then words, and finally phrases and sentences. Once the technique was mastered in oral reading, the same principles were applied to improvised speaking. He was asked to talk about pictures that were flashed to him. After this step was mastered, he was requested to talk impromptu about a scale of subjects that required ever-increasing attention to the subject matter, always using the rate that allowed him to speak smoothly. The final step was to apply rate-control over the telephone and before a formal audience. (pp. 223–24)

Except to say that the technique was used widely in the past by the old therapists, we will mercifully skip mentioning the many dead advocates of rate control and turn to our livelier contemporaries. Thus we find Wilton (1950) exhorting the stutterer: "Slow-

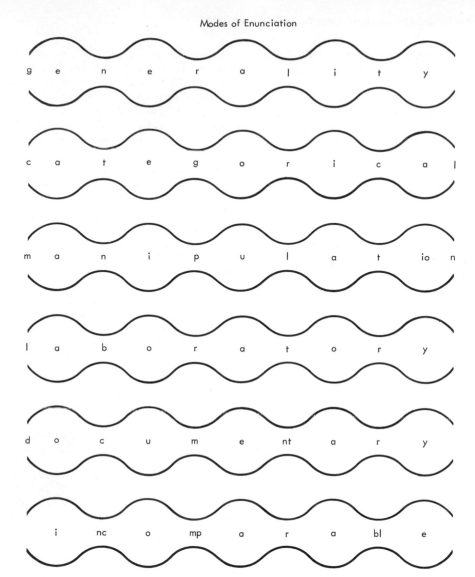

In this exercise the volume of sound is supposed to increase with the distance between the lines.

FIGURE 3.3 Programmed reading material to produce rhythmic speech. (From Bluemel, 1913.)

ness—slow, slow, slow. This must be your watchword. This is the word for you to make thoroughly your own, to go to bed with you at night, to keep with you through all the night (p. 4)." Despite such a bedfellow, the alteration of one's habitual rate of speaking is very difficult to maintain and most of the old therapists made their stutterers read and speak slowly many hours of each day. Strong penalties were administered (including "a substantial thrashing") when they forgot to use the method. Indeed most stutterers seem very reluctant to adopt this extremely slow pace. To aid them, Bocks (1967) currently has his stutterers learn to read slowly by making it difficult for them to read faster: "The book or paper is held upside down, and starting from the bottom, the page is read from right to left (p. 99)."

Several modern investigators have accomplished the same purpose in more elaborate ways. Among them is Goldiamond (1965). If we desire to understand the kind of speech he got his stutterers to use, and if we ignore for the moment his operant rationale for doing so, we find once again that they were trained to speak slowly and to prolong their vowels. Goldiamond used various ways of achieving this result. One was to use a metronome; another employed a visual pacer, the perceptoscope, which exposed the reading materials on a screen at a pace controlled by the experimenter; a third involved the use of the delayed feedback apparatus, and a fourth consisted of direct instructions to speak slowly and to use prolonged speech. That the rate of speaking was initially extremely slow is demonstrated by his figure of 34 words per minute or approximately one word every two seconds. Though DAF was used in a negative reinforcement manner, the stutterer being able to escape the DAF if he did not stutter, there is no doubt that it aided Goldiamond's instructions to the stutterer that he should use prolonged speech, since the elongation of vowels is one of the effects often shown by normal speakers exposed to delayed feedback. That this author was quite aware that he was in fact teaching the stutterers to speak in a novel and abnormal way may be indicated by his statement: "The fact that this pattern had unusual components, such as prolongation, does not

necessarily contraindicate its use, since procedures exist which can eliminate such undesirable features." These procedures turn out to be the same old ones of gradually shortening the vowel prolongations (by progressively shortening the delay time) and the gradual speeding up of the rate (via the pacer's acceleration). Yates (1969) makes this pertinent comment: "Why should Goldiamond wish to spend long periods in training the stutterer in the acquisition and shaping of a *new* form of speech until it approximates normal speech, when we already know empirically that all stutterers are capable of perfectly fluent speech, *albeit under special conditions?* (pp. 165–66, italics added)"

We now turn to the "conversational rate control" therapy as advocated by Curlee and Perkins (1969). The stutterer begins conversing with the therapist by speaking under a DAF delay of 259 msec. with "the unit set of the maximum loudness acceptable to [each] client. He is instructed to slow down his speaking rate by prolonging syllables so that his utterances coincide with the delayed feedback. In addition, he is instructed in the use of short, syntactically appropriate phrases." Under such a regime, the stutterers timed each new word with the echo of the immediately preceding word at a rate of about 30 to 35 words per minute and when they no longer showed any stuttering, the delay time was reduced in 50 msec. steps until no stuttering occurred at zero delay. "Once the client has met the no-stuttering criterion at 0 msec. speaking rate and delay, he is instructed to use a slow enough articulatory rate and short enough phrases to maintain freedom from instances and expectation of stuttering, and is removed from the DAF equipment." Even in the clinic, Curlee and Perkins found it necessary to institute a time-out punishment program [8] for failure to use the new rate control techniques for stuttering and also devised a rather elaborate transfer program so that the gains made in the laboratory would not be lost. They describe the transfer training as consisting of two steps:

First, the treatment sessions are moved to a different room in the clinic. Then another individual, who is a stranger to the client, is introduced into the treatment sessions, and his participation is gradually increased. Following the inclusion of several more strangers into the treatment sessions, the client is seen with members of his family and/or friends, and with other stutterers at the same stage of treatment in a group situation. Finally, the clinician goes with the client into some selected social situations normally encountered by the client. In this manner, the client is gradually weaned from a stereotyped treatment session.

Step 2. This step is programmed individually for each client in the following manner. Given a list of 40 general speaking situations and any supplementary information obtained in earlier sessions, the client is asked to rank order all the speaking situations from most to least difficult. As a homework assignment, he is instructed to apply the techniques he has learned in treatment in an outside situation, starting with the least difficult. When he reports that he has been able to maintain the same level of fluency in that outside situation as in treatment, the next situation in the hierarchy is assigned. These procedures continue until the client has extended his use of the treatment techniques from the least to the most difficult situations successfully, at which point treatment is terminated. (p. 248)

Other workers, notably Ryan (1971) and Andrews and Ingham (1971), have used more or less the same DAF and instructional techniques in creat-

ing slow but fluent speech though they used positive reinforcement rather than punishment.

It is difficult to evaluate these newer applications of slow prolonged speech but we remain highly skeptical of the permanence of the improvement claimed. In our chapter on the outcome of therapy, we will examine these and other claims in terms of the rigorous criteria which must be applied to all forms of treatment—and especially to therapies such as those that employ the ancient techniques of rate control and prolonged vowels. Moreover, there may be real dangers in training a stutterer to prolong his vowels in the effort to slow down. Some of the severest stutterers we have ever known were those whose major abnormality consisted of interminably long vowel sounds. Indeed, we are always highly concerned when a beginning stutterer stops repeating syllables easily and begins to elongate his vowels and then combines these with an upward inflection. Such fire-siren behaviors can be extremely traumatic to both the stutterer and his listeners. We personally would be loathe to run this risk, especially with young children. Most of the older ones will probably not be permanently hurt; they will just stop using retarded speech and vowel prolongations and return eventually to their old forms of stuttering after the novelty fades. They will lose some of the hope that is so tragically in short supply. They will have little faith in modern speech pathology. The old workers in our vineyard unfortunately did not have the benefit of our modern technology. They had no perceptoscopes or DAF apparatus. Sadly deprived of the magic of the machine, they simply did the same things that some of us are still doing today. They trained the

---

[8] This will be described in our chapter on the punishment and reinforcement therapies.

stutterer first to speak very slowly and to prolong his vowels and then gradually to change this odd way of talking into normal speech. They rewarded the stutterer when he did and punished him when he didn't. Once again, if this were the route to fluency, the age old problem would long ago have been solved.

Bibliography

ALFORD, J. and R. J. INGHAM, The application of a token reinforcement system to the treatment of stuttering in children, *Journal of the Australian College of Speech Therapists,* 19 (1969), 53–57.

ALLAN, C. M., Treatment of non-fluent speech resulting from neurological disease—treatment of dysarthria, *British Journal of Disorders of Communication,* 5 (1970), 3–5.

ANDREWS, G. and M. HARRIS, *The Syndrome of Stuttering.* London: Heinemann, 1964.

ANDREWS, G. and R. J. INGHAM, The effects of alterations in auditory feedback with special reference to synchronous auditory feedback, Unpublished paper, 1971.

ARNOTT, N., *Elements of Physics and Natural Philosophy,* 7th ed. Vol. 2. New York: Appleton-Century-Crofts, 1877.

BARBER, V., Studies in the psychology of stuttering: XV. Chorus reading as a distraction in stuttering, *Journal of Speech Disorders,* 4 (1939), 371–83.

————, Studies in the psychology of stuttering: XVI. Rhythm as a distraction in stuttering, *Journal of Speech Disorders,* 5 (1940), 29–42.

BEECH, H. R., Stuttering and stammering, *Psychology Today,* 1 (1967), 48–51.

———— and F. FRANSELLA, Explanations of the "rhythm effect" in stuttering, In B. B. Gray and G. England, *Stuttering and the Conditioning Therapies.* Monterey: Monterey Institute, 1969.

————, *Research and Experiment in Stuttering.* London: Pergamon Press, 1968.

BELL, A. M., *Observations on Defects of Speech, the Cure of Stammering and the Principles of Elocution.* London: Hamilton-Adams, 1853.

BENDER, J. F., Do you know someone who stutters? *Scientific Monthly,* 59 (1944), 221–24.

———— and V. M. KLEINFELD, *Principles and Practices of Speech Correction.* New York: Pitman, 1938.

BLACK, M., Speech correction in the U.S.S.R., *Journal of Speech and Hearing Disorders,* 25 (1960), 2–7.

BLOODSTEIN, O., *A Handbook on Stuttering.* Chicago: National Easter Seal Society for Crippled Children and Adults, 1969.

BLUEMEL, C. S., *Stammering and Cognate Defects of Speech,* Vol. 2. New York: Stechert, 1913.

BOCKS, U. D., *Freedom From Your Stammer.* London: Modern Publications, 1967.

BRADY, J. P., A behavioral approach to the treatment of stuttering, *American Journal of Psychiatry,* 125 (1968), 843–47.

————, Studies on the metronome effect on stuttering, *Behaviour Research and Therapy,* 7 (1969), 197–204.

BRANDON, S. and M. HARRIS, Stammering —an experimental treatment programme using syllable-timed speech, *British Journal of Disorders of Communication,* 2 (1967), 64–68.

BRYNGELSON, B., Suggestions in the theory and treatment of dysphemia, and its symptom, stuttering, *The Speech Teacher,* 1 (1952), 131–36.

CHERRY, E. C., *On Human Communication.* Cambridge, Mass.: M.I.T. Press, 1957.

————, and B. M. SAYERS, Experiments upon the total inhibition of stammering by external control and some clinical results, *Journal of Psychosomatic Research,* 1 (1956), 233–46.

_____ and P. MARLAND, Experiments in the complete suppression of stuttering, *Nature,* 176 (1955), 874–75.

COLUMBAT, (DE L'ISERE), M., *Du begaiement et les autres vices de la parole.* Paris: Masut, 1830.

CURLEE, R. F. and W. H. PERKINS, Conversational rate control therapy for stuttering, *Journal of Speech and Hearing Disorders,* 34 (1969), 246–50.

DAMSTE, P. H., A behavioral analysis of a stuttering therapy, In Speech Foundation of America, *Conditioning in Stuttering Therapy.* Memphis: Fraser, 1970.

DANTZIG, B. V., Syllable tapping: A new method for helping stammerers, *Journal of Speech Disorders,* 5 (1940), 127–31.

DEPARREL, S., *Speech Disorders.* Oxford: Pergamon Press, 1965.

DENHARDT, R., *Das Stottern Eine Psychose.* Leipsig: Keils Nachfolger, 1890.

DROOGLEEVER-FORTUYN, H. J. W., Stuttering, *Geneesk Gide,* 43, (1965), 83–85.

FACCHINI, G. M. and M. I. GOZZI, Concetti di trattamento della bulbrezie in eta prescholare, *Societa Italiana Di Fonetica, Foniatria E Audiologia,* 14 (1965), 118–24.

FAWCUS, M., Intensive treatment and group therapy programme for the child and adult stammerer, *British Journal of Disorders of Communication,* 5 (1970), 59–65.

FERNAU-HORN, H., (Circle of Inhibition and Expiration in the Pathogenesis and Therapy of Stuttering,) *Medizinische Monatsschrift,* 6 (1952), 323–27.

FITZ, O., *Schach dem Stottern.* Freiburg: Lambertus-Verlag, 1961.

FLETCHER, J. M., *The Problem of Stuttering.* New York: Longmans, 1928.

FRANSELLA, F., Rhythm as a Distractor in the Modification of Stuttering, *Behaviour Research and Therapy,* 5 (1967), 253–55.

_____ and H. R. BEECH, An experimental analysis of the effect of rhythm on the speech of stutterers, *Behaviour Research and Therapy,* 3 (1965), 195–201.

FROESCHELS, E., Therapy, in E. F. Hahn, *Stuttering: Significant Theories and Therapies.* Stanford, Calif.: Stanford University Press, 1943.

GIFFORD, M., *Correcting Nervous Speech Disorders.* Englewood Cliffs.: Prentice-Hall, 1940.

GOLDIAMOND, I., Stuttering and fluency as manipulable operant response classes, in L. Krasner and L. P. Ullman (eds.), *Research in Behavior Modification.* New York: Holt, Rinehart & Winston, 1965.

GORAJ, J. T., A report on three European speech facilities, *Asha,* 5 (1963), 860–64.

GUNDERMAN, H. and M. WEUFFEN, Über den nutzen von stottererkursen, *Z. Laryngol. Rhinol. Otol.,* 44 (1965), 517–21.

HAHN, E., *Stuttering: Significant Theories and Therapies.* Stanford, Calif.: Stanford University Press, 1950.

HANAKAWA, C., (Correction of Stuttering), *Voice and Language Medicine* (Japan), 6 (1965), 15–16.

HOLGATE, D., Comments on the electronic metronome in the treatment of stuttering, *Journal of the Australian College of Speech Therapists,* 17 (1967), 67–68.

_____ and G. ANDREWS, The use of syllable-timed speech and group psychotherapy in the treatment of adult stutterers, *Journal of the Australian College of Speech Therapists,* 16 (1966), 36–40.

HORAN, M. C., An improved device for inducing rhythmic speech in stutterers, *Australian Psychologist,* 3 (1968), 19–25.

HUNT, J., *Stammering and Stuttering: Their Nature and Treatment.* Originally published 1861. Reprint New York: Hafner, 1967.

INGHAM, R. J. and G. ANDREWS, Stuttering: The quality of fluency after treatment, *Journal of Communication Disorders*, 4 (1971), 279–88.

———— and R. WINKLER, A comparison of the effectiveness of four treatment techniques, *Journal of Communication Disorders*, 5 (1972), 91–117.

JOHNSON, W., *People in Quandaries*. New York: Harper & Row, 1946.

———— and L. Rosen, studies in the psychology of stuttering: VII. Effect of certain changes in speech pattern upon frequency of stuttering, *Journal of Speech Disorders*, 2 (1937), 105–9.

JONES, H. G., Behavior therapy and stuttering: The need for a multifarious approach to a multiplex problem, in B. B. Gray and G. England (eds.), *Stuttering and the Conditioning Therapies*. Monterey, Calif.: Monterey Institute, 1969.

KELHAM, R. and A. McHALE, The application of learning theory to the treatment of stammering, *British Journal of Disorders of Communication*, 1 (1966), 114–18.

KLEMM, M., Zur geschiche des Berliner sprachheilwesens, *Die Sprachheilarbeit*, 3 (1958), 50–57.

KLENCKE, H., Die Heilung des Stotterns. Leipsig: 1862. Translated in *The Voice*, Volume I. May, 1885.

KNUDSEN, R., (Stuttering Therapy in France), *Nordisk Tidskrifft for Tale og Stemme*, 10 (1948), 7–18.

KONDAS, O., The treatment of stammering in children by the shadow method, *Behavior Research and Therapy*, 5 (1967), 325–29.

KUSSMAUL, A., "Die Stoerungen der Sprach," In H. V. Ziemssen (ed.) [Cyclopedia of the Practice of Medicine,] Volume IV, 1877.

LEE, B., *Stuttering Therapy Cassette Tapes*. Holmdel, N.J.: Listen and Respond Tapes, 1970.

LENNON, E. J., *Le Begaiement: Therapeutiques Modernes*. Paris: Doin et Cie, 1962.

LIEBMANN, A., *Vorslesungen über Sprachstörungen*. Berlin: Coblentz, 1898.

LUCHSINGER, R. and G. E. ARNOLD, *Voice-Speech-Language*. Belmont, Calif.: Wadsworth, 1965.

MARLAND, R. M., Shadowing—a contribution to the treatment of stammering, *Folia Phoniatrica*, 9 (1957), 242–45.

MASON, N. H., *A Practical Guide and Introduction for the Natural System for the Cure of Stammering and All Defects of Speech*. London: Potter, 1905.

MATSUDA, A., (Therapy for Stuttering), *Japanese Medical News*, Issue 1671 (1965), 101.

METRAUX, R., Special report: Observations on stuttering therapy in France, *The Voice, Journal of the California Speech and Hearing Association*, 14 (1965), 20–22.

MEYER, V. and J. CROMLEY, A preliminary report on the treatment of stammer by the use of rhythmic stimulation, In B. B. Gray and G. England, *The Conditioning Therapies*. Monterey, Calif.: Monterey Institute, 1969.

MEYER, V. and J. M. M. MAIR, A new technique to control stammering: A preliminary report, *Behavior Research and Therapy*, 1 (1963), 251–54.

Minute Philosopher, The irrationale of speech, *Fraser's Magazine*, London, July 1859.

MOLL, A., Vom singen zum sprechen, (From Singing to Speaking), *Z. padag. Psychol.* 40 (1939), 47–56.

MORAVEK, M. and J. LANGOVA (The Patolphysiology of the Stuttering Attack), *Cas. Lek. Cesk.*, 107 (1968), 536–38.

NADOLECZNY, M., Stottern, in M. Flaundler, and A. Schlossman (eds.), *Handbuch der Kinderheilkunde*. Leipsig: Fogel, 1926.

NEKRASOVA, Y. B., Elocution training of young stutterers, *Proceedings of the Institute of Defectology*, Moscow: 1953.

PATTIE, F. A., and B. B. KNIGHT, Why

does the speech of stutterers improve in chorus reading? *Journal of Abnormal and Social Psychology,* 39 (1944), 362–67.

PEINS, M., B. J. LEE, and W. E. MCGOUGH, A tape recorded therapy method for stutterers: A case study, *Journal of Speech and Hearing Disorders,* 35 (1970), 188–93.

PETKOV, S. and I. IOSIFOV, Our experience in the treatment of stuttering in a speech rehabilitation colony, *Zhurnal Nevropatologii i Psikhiatrii imeni S. S. Korsakova,* 60 (1969), 903–4.

POTTER, S. O. L., *Speech and Its Defects.* Philadelphia: Blakiston, 1882.

PREVBRAYENSKAYA, V. D. (Work with Preschool Stuttering Children), *Experiences in Logopedic Practice.* Moscow: Institute of Defectology, 1953.

RAU, E. F., Experience in logopedic work with young stuttering children, *Proceedings Institute of Defectology.* Moscow: 1953.

REICHEL, C. W., *Stop Stammering and Stuttering.* New York: Vantage Press, 1964.

RETHI, A., Uber die heilung des stotterns und der dysphonia spastica mittels inspiratorish-experatorischer stimmbildung, *Monatschrift fur Ohrenheilkunden,* 99 (1965), 240–46.

ROZENTHAL, A., Logorhythmique comme un des moyens d'autopsychotherapie chex les enfants bégues, *Journal Francaise ORL,* 17 (1968), 205–7.

ROSENTHAL, M., Stottern. *Weiner Medicinalische Wochenschrift,* 1861.

RYAN, B. P., Operant procedures applied to stuttering therapy for children, *Journal of Speech and Hearing Disorders,* 36 (1971), 264–80.

SATSUTA, K. (Notes on Speech Therapy), *Otorhinology Journal of Japan,* 10 (1937), 284–86.

SCHILLING, A., Die behandlung des stotterns, *Folia Phoniatrica,* 17 (1965), 365–458.

SCRIPTURE, E. W., *Stuttering, Lisping and Corrections of the Speech of the Deaf.* New York: Macmillan, 1923.

SERGEANT, R. L., Concurrent repetition of a continuous flow of words, *Journal of Speech and Hearing Research,* 4 (1961), 373–80.

SMITH, SVEND (The Pedagogic Treatment of Stuttering), *Nordisk Larebog for Talepedagoger.* Copenhagen: Rosenkilde og Baggers Forlag, 1955.

————, The treatment of stuttering: Therapeutic exercises, *Report of the Conference on Speech Therapy,* London: Tavistock (1948), pp. 81–82.

STECHER, S., Speech therapy techniques in Germany, *Asha* (1964), 157–59.

STONELEY, H., Music as speech corrective, *Music and Letters,* 36 (1955), 39–40.

THEWALL, J., *Illustration of English Rhythmus.* London: Taylor, 1812.

TRAVIS, L. E., *Speech Pathology.* New York: Appleton-Century-Crofts, 1931.

TROJAN, F. and H. WEIHS, Studien sur stottertherapie, *Folia Phoniatrica,* 15 (1963), 42–67.

VAN DANTZIG, M., Syllable-tapping: A new method for treating stutterers, *Journal of Speech Disorders,* 5 (1940), 127–32.

VAN RIPER, C., Experiments in stuttering therapy, in J. Eisenson (ed.), *Stuttering: A Symposium.* New York: Harper & Row, 1958.

————, The rhythm method, *Western Michigan University Journal of Speech Therapy,* 8 (1971a), 1–2.

————, *The Nature of Stuttering.* Englewood Cliffs, N.J.: Prentice-Hall, 1971b.

WILTON, C., *How to Overcome Stammering.* New York: Harper & Row, 1950.

WALTON, D. and M. A. BLACK, The application of learning theory to the treatment of stammering, *Journal of Psychosomatic Research,* 3 (1958), 170–79.

———— and Mather, M. D. The relevance of generalization techniques to the treatment of stammering and phobic symptoms, *Behaviour Research and Therapy,* 1 (1963), 121–25.

WITT, M. H., Statistische erhebungen uber den einfluss des singens und flusterns auf das stottern, *Vox*, 11 (1925), 41–49.

WOHL, M., Reciprocal inhibition—a process of continuous diagnosis, in *British Journal of Disorders of Communication* Supplement: Speech Pathology Diagnosis: Theory and Practice. London: Livingstone, 1967.

———, The electronic metronome—an ‘evaluative study, *British Journal of Disorders of Communications,* 3 (1968), 89–98.

———, The treatment of non-fluent utterance: A behavioural approach, *British Journal of Disorders of Communication,* 5 (1970), 66–70.

WYKE, B., Neurological mechanisms in stammering: An hypothesis, *British Journal of Disorders of Communication,* 5 (1970), 6–15.

WYLLIE, J., *The Disorders of Speech.* Edinburgh: Oliver and Boyd, 1894.

WYNEKEN, C., Ueber das stottern und dessen heilung, *Zeitschrift für rationelle Medicin,* 31 (1868), 1–29.

YATES, A. J., The relationship between theory and therapy in the clinical treatment of stuttering, in B. B. Gray and G. England (eds.), *Stuttering and the Conditioning Therapies.* Monterey, Calif.: Monterey Institute, 1969.

ZALIOUK, A., A new therapy for stuttering, "Une Methode de Traitement de la Dysphemie (begaiement) Chez Enfants et Adultes," *Encephale,* 43, (1954), 337–346.

Punishment

and

Reinforcement Therapies

Anyone who reviews the literature dealing with the treatment of stuttering cannot fail to note the prominence of punishment. Over and over again, in forms that range from a blow to the head to a contingent blast of white noise, punishments of all sorts have been applied to stutterers of every land. The rationales for using punishment have also been many. Stuttering has been viewed as a verbal perversion, as evidence of the devil incarnate, as deviant behavior, and commonly as a bad habit to be broken as swiftly as possible by administering painful consequences. Stutterers have also been rewarded for not stuttering with social approvals and other rewards being granted for exhibitions of fluency. Numerous experiments have shown that positive reinforcement, negative reinforcement, and punishment can produce remarkable changes

in the frequency of stuttering. In this chapter we present an account of the practices that are based upon punishment and reinforcement and try to explain why they were used and why they produce some transient relief.

The suggestive effects of punishment

Disabilities and illnesses of all kinds have often been viewed as God's retribution for sin and evil. Many a stutterer has found a kinship with Job of the Old Testament who so eloquently kept asking his Lord what he had done to deserve such misery. Most of us have collected enough sins of omission or commission to store up some fund of guilt. If the stutterer believes that his stuttering is the penance he must pay for his real or fancied sins, then any other punishment he gets may serve as its surrogate. Anxiety has often been relieved by doing penance, by flagellation, by the suffering that heals. These guilt feelings are often expressed in deep psychotherapy and they are more common than one might expect. But we also find them being verbalized occasionally in the course of speech therapy as well. Sheehan (1970) has also pointed out how guilt in the stutterer arises from false role behavior and the creation of listener distress. When aversive consequences are applied to stuttering, some of that guilt may subside in certain stutterers. Some of our own cases have almost begged to be punished and we have had to restrain them from punishing themselves. Most stutterers do not present this picture but there are some who do.

Corporal punishment

Many of the punishments which have been administered to the stutterer have not been as corporal as that advocated by a Dr. Frank, mentioned by Hunt (1861), "who strongly recommends a good flogging," but we have been told by several adults that they had been cured of their stuttering after a parental whipping. Here is a case from our own files:

Jack was nine years old and a very severe stutterer with facial contortions and gasping behavior. He had begun to stutter just prior to school entrance, according to the mother's report. A very fearful child, he was prone to night terrors, enuresis, and tics. We worked with the boy and his mother very intensively for three months but without any success. Indeed the boy's stuttering began to increase in severity. After they failed to show up for therapy three consecutive times, we phoned the mother and she informed us that the boy had stopped stuttering, that he was completely cured, and that it was his father who had done

it. "As you know, my husband is a butcher and one night he brought home from work a basket of fish that had spoiled. He was going to use them for fertilizer in the garden. As he came in the gate, Jack ran up to him excitedly and he was stuttering bad, even worse than usual, and my husband, he was tired and irritated and couldn't stand it. So he dumped the whole basket of rotten fish over the kid's head and yelled at him, 'Don't you never do no stuttering like that to me again!' "

The mother insisted that Jack did stop stuttering from then on, that she hadn't heard a bit of it since, and that he was talking a lot. We went to the home to check and found that it was true. He was completely fluent. His teacher reported the same thing had happened in school. We followed up this case for five years and made a recheck at ten years and are convinced that the boy did not stutter again.

We also have other evidence that punishment may lead to the remission of stuttering. Glasner (1947) reports that 48 out of 101 preschool stuttering children had stopped stuttering and that many of them had been subjected not only to active correction by their parents but also had been punished for stuttering in one way or another. Since about four out of five children who begin to stutter show spontaneous recovery anyway (Andrews and Harris, 1964; Sheehan and Martyn, 1967) perhaps we should not be certain that the disorder's disappearance in Glasner's cases was due only to the punishing correction. Nevertheless, we are fairly certain that some persons (primarily children, not adults) have been freed from stuttering by the application of aversive stimuli.

We have known personally a few other children whose parents literally beat the stuttering out of them and have had more than a few such reports from "recovered stutterers." An American Indian told us that he had been cured of stuttering by having to speak through a knothole in a board which was banged by his father's club every time he stuttered or hesitated. Some of the operant conditioning people might highly approve of this scheduling of contingencies but we feel that the knothole was probably as important as the bang with the club. Some hocus pocus, some magic, some mumbo jumbo, some mystery seems to be needed to permit punishment to yield some permanence to the healing effect and not merely to suppress temporarily an unwanted behavior. A consideration of some folk remedies for stuttering may be of interest in this connection.

Folk remedies for stuttering

A fascinating account of primitive medicine by King (1962) helps us understand the healing power of suggestion and magic. He writes: "Even in a society dominated by the scientific method, magic is not as far away as we might like to think or hope. It is a background to which we are all heir and which we may be tempted to use in situations that are high in ambiguity and fraught with great threat. We may use it in disguised form, clothe it in up-to-date language, but it still exists." He speaks of the importance of swallowing unpleasant substances, of being injected by needles, of having the body cut and violated in creating the necessary condition for the healing that comes from hope and suggestion. The history of the treatment of stuttering is certainly illustrative. Stutterers have had their tongues slit and burned. Leeches have been placed upon their lips. They have been forced to swallow an incredible variety of vile substances including

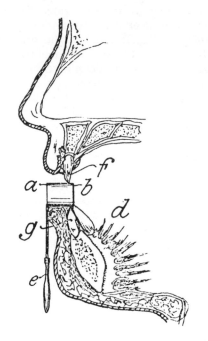

FIGURE 4.1   Knoch device to prevent dental or lip closure. (British Patent 16,045 [1906].)

goat feces. They have been purged, a Dr. Langenbeck in 1830 giving his stutterers heavy doses of that profound cathartic, croton oil. Perhaps this treatment did produce some alleviation of stuttering, since if the stutterers forced or struggled, they would produce a double emission of unpleasantness, or else they would be too weak to talk with any tension whatsoever.

It is easy to smile tolerantly at such ancient and quaint practices of long ago and far away but suddenly we find the same treatment being applied today. Witness Emerick's (1968) account:

Mrs. Ford said that it seemed as if the child had always stuttered. She did remember, however, that when Sherrie was about four years old, a relative had suggested a remedy for the stuttering problem. The "cure" consisted of a bottle of mineral oil and an eyedropper to be used as follows: whenever Sherrie blocked, Mrs. Ford was to squirt an eyedropper full of oil down the child's throat. I wonder if Skinner would term that an aversive stimulus. Sherrie's problem had grown steadily worse despite the lube job and the stuttering behavior was more ubiquitous than it had ever been. (p. 33)

Folk remedies for stuttering are found in widely differing cultures. Aron (1958) tells of the chewing of garlic by Bantu stutterers; the older Finns gave their stutterers a concoction called "Hirven Sarven Tippola" and the prescription is still available. We have a bottle of the vile stuff and uncorking it for two minutes empties the building pronto. In Japan, Umeda (1963) provides us with a comprehensive list of folk remedies, most of which can be considered very punishing. To overcome stuttering some stutterers were forced to pour ice-cold water over themselves outdoors at midnight in winter in a biting wind to build up the strong mind needed. Acupuncturation and moxacautery were applied, acupuncturation being the process whereby sharp long needles are inserted into the body while moxacauterization is produced by burning grass fibers (moxa) on the skin.[1] Stutterers were forced to drink decoctions of persimmon stones; to swallow raw eggs or to eat charred shrikers' or frogs' tongues.

[1] With regard to acupuncture, we came across this account in an old book by Hall (1869):
Some twenty years ago the New York world was struck with dumb amazement at the instantaneous remedy for stammering, which was thrusting a knitting needle through the tongue. But it cured only until the tongue got well, because, while the tongue was sore from the barbarous operation, of the extra energy expended in the instinctive effort to refrain from any other but a careful movement of the tongue.

If these strike the reader as being strange and far away, we suggest the reading of Pedrey's Letter to the editor, appearing in the 1950 Journal of Speech Disorders, wherein a stutterer tells how he had to eat the meat of a black tomcat at midnight, drink the urine of a virgin mare, eat a snake under a half moon, and undergo a terrible beating in an abandoned church—all in the vain hope that these rituals might cure his stuttering.

While we are not sure that the use of impletol blocking should be considered in this section on punishment therapies, perhaps some of the stutterers who have undergone it would agree that it belongs there. We find it being used primarily in the Iron Curtain countries. Daskalov (1962) describes it as follows:

Its technic is as follows. Daily for 10 to 12 days we subcutaneously inject at each of certain points in the Zakharin-Head zones of the speech organs (Figure 4.2)

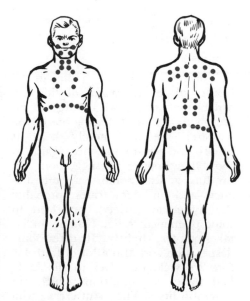

FIGURE 4.2 Injection points for Implemetol blocks. (From Daskalov, 1962).

0.5–1 ml. of a sterile solution of impletol (2% solution of procaine; 1.42% caffeine in physiologic saline; we use the preparation known as "iovoplex") using a total of 15 ml. per blocking session. The treatment course is repeated if necessary. The technic of subcutaneous injection of the solution is similar to that used for the Mantoux test, with observation each time for the appearance of a tiny papule-like infiltrate.

The therapeutic mechanism in this case is due to anesthesia of the cutaneous zones of the speech organs; reflexly the therapeutic influence spreads to the affected points in the cerebral centres of speech. Sometimes, immediately after the therapeutic block patients perceive facilitation of speech, diminution of rigidity of neck muscles and thoracic muscles and general restfulness. In addition to a clear favorable influence on the impaired speech function one also notes a favorable influence on other manifestations of the neurosis, especially on neuroautonomic disturbances. (p. 1050)

Platonov (1959) however declared that this method has been completely abandoned in Russia. "They were effective only in terms of their suggestive effect (p. 361)."

Surgery

There is a long, sad chapter in the history of the treatment of this disorder that deals with surgical attempts to cut the stuttering out of the stutterer. We shall merely sketch it briefly and we do so, once again, to show how powerful suggestion can produce at least some temporary fluency, and, in a few cases (probably the hysterical variety), can lead to some permanent relief. No one undertakes surgery lightly. It takes some desperation and also a lot of faith before we yield ourselves to the knife and these are conditions which aid suggestibility. The stutterers who sought surgical relief only did so after persuading themselves through intense self-suggestion that these drastic measures would do the job. We are not surprised therefore to find in the literature some accounts of cures and improvement produced by energy.

Galen (131–201 A.D.) is said to have recommended the cauterization of the tongue and the cutting of its nerves for the relief of stuttering. Five hundred years later, according to Klingbeil (1939), Aetius of Amica advised that a stutterer should have his frenum clipped, but it was not until January 7, 1841, that Dieffenbach, a German physician sliced through the root of a stutterer's tongue and started a wave of similar operations that spread throughout the world. And it all happened by chance. Here is Dieffenbach's (1841) own account:

Some time ago the stuttering defect arrested my attention, and I grew as anxious to find a radical and rapid remedy for it as the many stutterers who, believing themselves already free of their defects, slipped back again into the same errors, while others, were tutored in vain by skilled teachers. Suddenly I fell upon the idea that by completely severing the root of the tongue, perhaps a cure could be brought about from the altered nerve control, the relaxed vocal chords, etc. The success has justified most splendidly this new operation. The possibility of curing stuttering by cutting through the tongue muscles came to me one time when a squinting person came to me for an operation, and I listened to him explain his case in stuttering speech. He had a convulsive squinting of both eyes. (Strabism concomitans with nystagmus.) After that I found—since my attention turned in that direction—stuttering accompanied by squinting in several other persons. The latter defect was almost always convulsive squinting that differed greatly: now stronger, now weaker. Stuttering and stammering was the same way.

On the basis of such dubious reasoning Dieffenbach made a horizontal slice at the root of the tongue and took out a triangular wedge of tissue. He felt that this would weaken or prevent the stutterers muscular spasm. And it did. The stutterer spoke without his old spasms. Within two months Dieffenbach had performed nineteen such operations and shortly afterward stutterers were being butchered all over the world, though variations in technique were also tried, some surgeons preferring merely to cut the hyoglossus, the geniohyoid, and stylohyoid muscles instead. Fortunately, the enthusiasm died out in a few years when it became apparent that the initial relief was only temporary and when some stutterers died from the resulting abscesses. On April 29, 1841, Amussat, a French surgeon, "operated on a stuttering patient severing the genio-hy-glossi muscles. On May 17 the patient died," according to Klingbeil (1939). At least he never stuttered again! Appelt (1911) gives the requiem:

In 1851, however, Romberg was able to state that the surgical treatment of the affliction had been "rightly given up." Thus the blood-stained campaign ended with complete defeat, bringing disappointment to all who had hoped for relief, and some amount of censure on those who had conducted it. (p. 29)

It might be interesting to speculate on the reasons for the temporary fluency achieved by such surgery. The operant conditioners would say that struggle behaviors involving the hurt and tender tongue (hard contacts, forcing, and tremors) would get contingent punishment immediately after each instance of such struggle and so these behaviors would be extinguished. Perhaps certain workers would say that the relief stemmed from the penance paid in suffering for ancient guilts. Perhaps it just hurt too much

to talk and so he talked as little as possible thereby decreasing the frequency of stuttering. Perhaps, by having to compensate motorically, old tactual and kinesthetic cues associated with stuttering were avoided. Perhaps he had to speak more slowly and in a relaxed way. There are many possible reasons but we would certainly not omit the one we feel most reasonable—the influence of suggestion. As Appelt (1911) commented, "Any slight improvement which might take place is not due to the operation; rather it is due to autosuggestion on the part of the stammerer who, buoyed up by hope of relief at the surgeon's skillful hands, momentarily experiences that relief (p. 31)."

Although no further major surgery on the tongue of the Dieffenbach sort was performed thereafter, there are many accounts of other interventions. Braid and other English surgeons excised the tonsils and adenoids and we have had many reports from our own stutterers of such practices today and even of some temporary cures thereby produced. In the Japanese literature we find Kitagawa (1936) telling of a 22-year-old man who had begun to stutter at the age of eight. Kitagawa performed a tonsillectomy on this man, accompanied by strong suggestion that this would eliminate his stuttering. Three days after the operation his speech became remarkably fluent. Takasu (1945) cut the frenum of a stutterer (frenectomy or frenulotomy) and reported a reduction in stuttering. In Austria, Imre is reported by Hirschberg (1965) to have found spontaneous improvement after the surgical removal of tonsils resulted in normal respiration. In summary, Luchsinger and Arnold (1965) make a statement with which we would heartily agree: "Frenulotomy as a cure for stuttering is of as much value as the clipping of toenails would be for a hemiplegic walking disorder."

Nevertheless we may not be certain that the story ends here. Not too long ago we had clinical reports of stutterers who had gained remarkable fluency as the result of lobectomy and lobotomy operations and, at the time of this writing, we received a letter from a stutterer asking us if we felt a craniotomy advisable. He had heard of the dramatic cessation of stuttering reported by R. K. Jones (1966) on four epileptic stutterers subsequent to the removal of cortical tissue focal to the seizures.

Use of electrical shocks

Long before anyone had heard of operant conditioning, therapists were administering electrical shocks to stutterers, as the English surgical journal, *Lancet,* reported sardonically in May of 1841:

An unfortunate lad has lately been most cruelly victimized by one of the stammering operators. It is needless to say he stammers worse than ever. The most ingenious operation that has yet been proposed for relieving this infirmity, but which is likely to be claimed by numerous candidates for operative distinction, is the following: It consisted of the removal of extremity of the cocyx by means of a half-dozen elegant little instruments invented for the express purpose, and the insertion of a needle with a large eye at the extremity into the structure of the bone. The needle is so constructed as to admit of being attached to the conduction wire of a pocket galvanic battery, of about the size of and similar to an ordinary hunting-watch. When the patient wishes to speak, he attaches the wire to the end of the needle, and immediately the galvanic current being transmitted by the vertebral column issues through the fauces and keeps the velum palati distended like a sail, and the uvula floating upon its stream like a pennant,

while the voice is perfectly regulated. The eminent members of the profession who were present at the first operation performed on this principle, were completely electrified (sic!) at its wonderful success. It is proposed to petition Parliament for a patent for this truly philanthropic discovery.

We should remember in this context that the physicians of that time were very interested in the use of galvanic, static, or faradic electricity and that they applied it to a variety of ailments—usually those that we now call psychosomatic—and to increase muscle tone as in paralysis or hysterical flaccidity. Some of them did enough experimentation to prove that continued application of the inductive current to the head, larynx, or tongue muscles was completely ineffective but even today we find a few therapists exploiting the suggestive hocus pocus of electrical application.

The history of electric shock in treating stutterers unfortunately does not seem to have died with the last century. Old forms of treatment never die. Although the application of faradic electrical stimulation has long passed its heyday with most disorders, a surprising number of our own patients have reported receiving it and evidently the practice is still current in Europe for Luchsinger and Arnold (1965) feel impelled to make this strong comment:

In the treatment of stuttering, however, any local *electrotherapy is without value* because this disorder is never associated with organic paralytic lesions of the peripheral speaking musculature. Speech movements in stuttering usually proceed with excessive force. Why then further increase the augmented neuromuscular tonus by application of electricity? The possibility of a suggestive effect from electricity is similarly questionable, for suggestive effects fade away in stutterers as rapidly as they are enthusiastically accepted. Electrotherapy for stuttering may be justifiably compared to the application of the ill-reputed oral gadgets sold by imposters. (p. 762)

During the world wars, electroconvulsive therapy was used very widely in army hospitals in the treatment of "combat fatigue," and it was also applied to jolt the stutterer out of his symptoms. A detailed account of its use (together with warm baths and music!) can be found in the reference by Owen and Stemmermann (1947). Although we fortunately escaped the experience personally, we have known several stutterers who underwent the trauma repeatedly. They said that some temporary remission from their stuttering occurred but only while they were still feeling the aftereffects of the trauma. Poor bedevilled stutterers—God's guinea pigs!

Punishment in modern therapy

Thus far we have been mainly describing the punishment of stuttering as a disorder. We have seen punishment being used, as it was formerly for sin and insanity, as an attempt to "whip the stuttering out of him." Aikins (1929) even had an article entitled "Casting Out A Stuttering Devil," and most of the early punishing practices were probably based on a somewhat similar belief. Drastic measures were presumed necessary to eliminate a reprehensible verbal perversion.

The modern use of punishment is based upon the Law of Effect which states that the probable occurrence of behavior is governed by its consequences. When those consequences are unpleasant, the behavior will decrease; when they are pleasant, they will increase. The crucial difference between the older and modern use of punishment lies in specification of instrumental behaviors and the concept of contingency. Modern therapists do not punish the *person* for having a stuttering disorder. They use punishment as a specific consequence for certain stuttering behaviors or for specific stuttered words.

Punishment in modern therapy for stuttering is more widespread than many would believe and it is not confined solely to the advocates of operant conditioning as this passage from Shames (1968) demonstrates:

Others who object to the suggestion that punishment should be used in the clinic may not like to think of themselves as purveyors of punishment, even though it may be for the stutterer's ultimate good and well-being. It may be, however, that some of these same clinicians are already punishing their clients in other ways. For example, they may confront the stutterer with his behavior, either verbally or by having him look in a mirror. They may raise semantic questions about the way he talks about his stuttering. They may literally force their clients to talk in feared situations, under the threat of being dismissed from the clinic. They may ask the stutterer to repeat a stuttered word, thereby delaying his message and his social reinforcement. They may do all these things under the banner of therapy, without calling them punishment. Do these tactics become less acceptable if they are called punishment? The important question is whether these tactics are effective in treating stuttering. In this light, the laboratory data suggest that they might be more effective if they were administered on a consistent schedule as a consequence of some predesignated behavior of the client's. (pp. 26–27)

We ourselves (Van Riper, 1958) have at times employed a large variety of penalties in our clinical work, primarily making them contingent up-

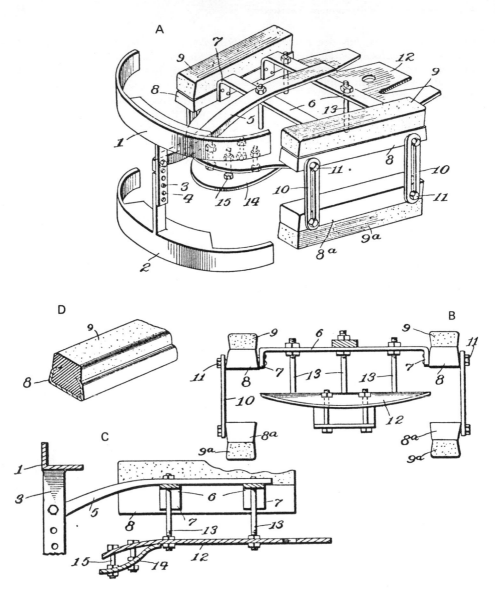

FIGURE 4.3   Beattie and Peake's stammer-cure device to minimize articulation. (British Patent, U.S. Patent 1,030,964 [1912].)

on specific instrumental behaviors so that these would be suppressed enough to enable us to substitute more appropriate ones. We have especially used the escape from unpleasantness as a negative reinforcer and motivator. We have used the threat of contingent punishment as an alerting device. In our technique of cancellation is found what later workers termed the "time-out" kind of aversive consequence. And we have found these uses of punishment to be effective. However, we have come to feel that consistent and severe punishment has no justifiable role in stuttering therapy. We use it as an alerter and insight-gaining procedure not as a systematic deconditioner. As Azrin (1959, 1960) and many others have shown, the initial suppression of the punished response simply does not usually last. Moreover, contingent punishment often creates other side effects which can interfere with effective therapy. When we use it, we use it sparingly and judiciously, not as the basic heart of therapy. Nevertheless we sympathize with Sheehan (1968) who says:

Life is too full of punishment to make it necessary or advisable to administer more of it in the clinic. Therapists who use punishment are probably incompetent to use anything else, or they have a neurotic need to assume the role of the punisher as a reassurance against their own fear of being in the role of the one punished. We have never encountered stutterers whose case histories lacked an abundance of punishment. They have been punished too much, not too little. And, if punishment were in any way effective, every stutterer would have been cured in childhood. (p. 132)

Sheehan's vehemence probably refers more to the use of severe punishments such as electric shocks or loud blasts of noise than to the sort of disapproval or milder penalties which characterize many therapeutic encounters. It is the deliberate and consistent use of punishment as the major tool of treatment which he so eloquently attacks. There are other tools which are even more effective.

Punishment in the operant conditioning therapies

Nevertheless, some modern American therapists have attempted to suppress stuttering by punishment, hoping thereby to extinguish it and most of them have done it in the name of operant conditioning. They have perhaps been unduly impressed by certain researchers which have indicated that the frequency of stuttering can be reduced by contingent punishment or its relief.

Various types of programs have been utilized in applying operant principles to stuttering. One of the common patterns follows the design of Goldiamond's (1965) research in which a novel way of speaking (usually speaking at a very slow rate or with vowel prolongation) is created by delayed auditory feedback or simply by instructions. As the stutterer becomes able to meet a designated criterion of fluency in his oral reading, the DAF is then faded out and the rate at which the reading materials are exposed is increased in gradual steps. As this occurs, the new way of speaking is alleged to gradually approach normal speech. Then attempts are made to transfer the fluency thus obtained into other speaking situations.

Goldiamond felt that he was punishing stuttering by using the delayed auditory feedback since, according to the special kind of definition which the operant conditioners use, any stimulus which causes a decrease in the behavior to which it is contingently applied must be punishing.[2] DAF (delayed auditory feedback) does interfere with the fluency of some nor-

[2] There are many psychologists who take issue with this definition, and it does create problems. For example Cooper, Cady, and Robbins (1970) followed each moment of stuttering by saying "right" or "wrong" or "tree." The neutral word "tree" caused as much reduction in stuttering as did the word "wrong." So did the word "right!" According to the operant definition, both "right!" and "tree" were punishers—and this just doesn't make sense.

mal speakers, and bursts of it, applied contingently to stuttering behaviors, might seem to be therefore aversive. However, we have some substantial research, reviewed by Soderberg (1969) and Van Riper (1971) which indicates that DAF *facilitates* fluency in many stutterers. If indeed DAF is punishing, which in our opinion is highly doubtful, it certainly is a mild form of punishment at best.

Another type of "punishment" was used by Curlee and Perkins (1969) in the conversational rate-control therapy we described in an earlier chapter. While it is relatively easy to get stutterers to speak very slowly by prolonging their vowel sounds for a short period, it is much harder to get them to use this kind of careful speech and phrasing very long. To insure compliance, the stutterers were punished for failure to use rate control by making complete cessation of speech contingent upon that failure, using the "time-out" procedure described by Haroldson, Martin, and Starr (1968). Curlee and Perkins described the process:

In our therapy program, treatment sessions consist of the clinician and the client conversing in a "blackout" room that is lighted by a single lamp. The client is instructed that he is to stop talking as soon as the light goes out. Whenever the client stutters, or his speech becomes "sticky," his rate "too fast," or his phrases "too long" (as defined by the clinician), the clinician turns the light off, and the two sit in silence and darkness for 30 sec, after which the clinician turns the light on and the client resumes speaking. These procedures continue until the no-stuttering criterion is met. The lights out interval is then reduced to 25 sec until the no-stuttering criterion is again met. In this manner, the lights out interval is reduced in 5-sec steps until a 5-sec lights out interval is obtained. Whenever

a client stutters more than 2 times in any 5-minute period (the stuttering criterion), the contingency is returned to the immediately preceding treatment procedures until the no-stuttering criterion is met again. (p. 247)

We also have some studies in which some very aversive stimuli were used contingently as punishment. Flanagan, Goldiamond, and Azrin (1958) had three stutterers read orally for 30 minutes until adaptation had occurred and a base rate of disfluencies seemed fairly stable. Then they turned on a very loud traumatic tone (105 decibels) and left it on continuously except that, whenever a disfluency occurred, the tone was turned off for five seconds. Under this condition of negative reinforcement the frequency of stuttering increased. Next the same stutterers were blasted by the 105-decibel tone every time they stuttered. This resulted in a decrease of disfluencies (not necessarily stutterings) for all three subjects and one became completely free from hesitancies there in the laboratory. Brady (1968) was perhaps kinder. When one of his stutterers violated one of the retraining rules (speeding up, becoming tense, or struggling with a blocked word) the experimenter zapped him with the blinding flash of a photographer's 400 candlepower gun. We no longer whip our stutterers; we deafen them or blind them.

In another book (Van Riper, 1971) we reviewed some of the other ways, less drastic ones, in which stutterers have been punished for stuttering. Again using three stutterers at the University of Minnesota, Martin and Siegel (1966b) studied the effects of administering contingent shock for different types of stuttering behavior (nose-wrinkling, tongue-protrusion, etc.) and found that these specific

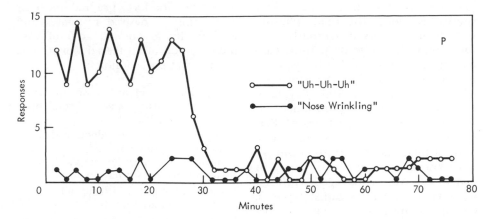

FIGURE 4.4 Effects of contingent punishment upon two stuttering behaviors. (From Martin and Siegel, 1966b.)

stuttering behaviors decreased but returned to baseline as soon as the contingent shock was removed (Figure 4.4). However, at the same time, an increase in prolongations occurred. In another experiment (Martin and Siegel, 1966a) with two male stutterers, these authors simultaneously "punished" stuttering by the words "not good" and rewarded fluency by the word "good." Both of these contingencies increased the fluency, and when they were no longer used, more stuttering occurred. A nylon strap used as a discriminative stimulus was shown to have some effectiveness. Brady (1967) shocked his subjects contingently for each moment of stuttering while reading a 1,000-word passage and found that there was less stuttering in this condition than when no shock was employed. Quist and Martin (1967) used the word "wrong" as a consequence for any repetition and prolongation in one stutterer and for "uh" or prolonged "n" sounds in two others after baselines had been established. They reported reductions in frequency of stuttering under these contingencies. The responses returned

to base rates when the contingencies were removed.

Gross and Holland (1965) showed a decrease in stuttering when shock was made contingent on stuttering, but they found too that shocking the *listener* for each stuttered moment produced a similar reduction in stuttering. Haroldson, Martin and Starr (1968) used a "time out" or silence period as a punishing consequence for stuttering and found a marked decrease in four stutterers, but Adams (1970), reviewing the same data, concluded that the instability of the base rates make their findings very doubtful.

In an attempt to replicate Flanagan, Goldiamond, and Azrin's research, Biggs and Sheehan (1969) used a 108-decibel-high frequency tone as an aversive stimulus in three conditions: presented contingently with a moment of stuttering, presented randomly, and stopping it when stuttering occurred. Since they found that stuttering decreased under all three conditions they attributed the decrease mainly to distraction.

Unfortunately, some speech therapists we have known have used these researches [3] to justify their administration of not only dangerously loud tones or white noise or painful electric shocks but also of verbally shaming or even slapping the stutterers when they stuttered. And they have used this contingent punishment as the major part of their therapy! Fortunately most of these persons lose most of their clients very soon but we have known some tragic instances in which captive, school-aged children were victimized by a sadistic public school therapist in the name of behavioral science.

Other types of operant conditioning programs

Lest we be accused of concentrating too much on punishing or aversive stimuli, we hastily outline an operant program designed by Ryan (1964) in which escape from punishment rather than contingent punishment was used. Indeed, it demonstrated very clearly how some of the techniques such as cancellation that we ourselves have advocated (Van Riper, 1971) can be implemented by operant conditioning. Negative reinforcement (the relief from the punishing task of having to read aloud for a long time) was the core of a program which consisted of eight steps arranged sequentially so that they

would provide for a gradual and easy acquisition of desired responses and lead finally to an end goal of easy prolongation of all feared words. The eight steps were as follows:

1. experimenter identification in which the experimenter gave a signal after each stuttered word;
2. experimenter-subject identification, in which the subjects and the experimenter concurrently signalled when they observed a stuttered word;
3. cancellation [1], in which the subjects reiterated stuttered words;
4. cancellation [2], in which the subjects reiterated stuttered words in a prolonged manner;
5. cancellation [3], in which the subjects reiterated stuttered words with a prolongation of the initial sound of the reiteration;
6. late pullout, in which the subjects interrupted stuttering behavior on a word with a prolongation of the initial sound of the word;
7. early pullout, in which the subjects interrupted stuttering behavior within a time limit; and
8. prolongation, in which the subjects prolonged the initial sound of words where stuttering behavior was anticipated.[4]

Reinforcement was provided immediately after each correct response. The nature of the correct response was different in each step but always specified in advance. As we have said, a long task of oral reading was used as the aversive stimulus situation in a negative reinforcement paradigm using continuous reinforcement. Whenever the subjects emitted the designated correct response, a clock, operated manually as a counter, signalled the subjects with a click indicating a reduction in the length of time they

---

[3] Siegel and Martin discontinued the use of contingent electric shock for stuttering after their first experiments because as Siegel (1970) says, "As compared to other methods, the shock did not prove to be a very powerful suppressor of disfluency." In one experiment Martin and Siegel (1969) found that the contingent presentation of "an ordinary doorbell buzzer" had a comparable suppression effect on the disfluencies of normal speakers and also that the same reduction could be procured by merely asking the subjects to read more carefully and without repeating.

[4] These definitions of cancellation and pullout are different from ours. See chapter 12.

had to read. (The click became a positive conditioned reinforcer during the program.)

Ryan set up criteria of performance for each step, and then used the negative reinforcement procedures to bring the stutterer's response up to criterion for each step in the sequence before going on to the next step, thereby shaping the stutterer's speech toward complete fluency. In other explorations, Ryan and his students have experimented with varying the number and sequence of steps, differentially reinforcing shorter and shorter prolongations, and other approaches to the problem of transfer and maintenance.

A description of another operant program is provided by Shames (1968). Both punishment and positive reinforcement in the form of the therapist's verbal disapproval or approval were used to shape the stuttering behavior so that it approximated fluency. A step by step outline of the procedure runs as follows:

In step 1, the stutterer is asked to pause after every stuttered word and to repeat the word, after which he is reinforced by the clinician. Saying a stuttered word again, even if it is stuttered the second time too, is considered a correct response provided the stutterer repeats the word before going on to the next word. To separate the word-repetition that is a stuttering behavior from the word-repetition that is part of the program, a correct response is defined as a stuttered word, followed by a pause, followed by an additional utterance of the word.

Step 2 is a refinement of step 1. The stutterer receives reinforcement if he repeats a stuttered word and also prolongs the first sound of the word, for example, "m-m-m-man (pause) mmman."

In step 3, the stutterer is reinforced when he stops himself while stuttering on a word and prolongs the first sound of the word being stuttered, for example, "m-m-

(pause) mmman." The prolongation of the initial sound of the word following the whole word repetition is also considered a correct response, for example, "not, not (pause), nnnot."

In step 4, the stutterer is reinforced when he prolongs the first sound of a stuttered word, for example, "mmman." This response is not differentiated from a stuttering prolongation, and both types of response are reinforced. The program may be extended by differentially reinforcing progressively shorter prolongation durations, thus more closely approximating normal speech.

In order to progress from one step to the next in this program the client must successfully complete the required task of each step on 90% of the words stuttered. When the 90% criterion is reached, the stutterer proceeds to the next step. Once the stutterer had progressed to the next step, he is no longer reinforced for the response required for an earlier step. The client and the clinician agree upon the theme of the discussion before the session begins. This helps prevent long silent periods and reduces the probability of emotionally loaded themes. (pp. 29–30)

Still another type of operant program is outlined by Shames, Egolf, and Rhodes (1969) who used operant conditioning procedures not only to shape the stuttering behavior toward fluent utterance but also to reinforce those interview statements by the stutterer which appeared to be beneficial to therapeutic progress. Therapist disapproval was made contingent upon those statements which seemed incompatible with recovery. Thus the therapist would give verbal approval *in the same way* to such a statement as this: "I stutter when I am around my family or people who know me well," but would withold approval or provide a negative reaction if the stutterer said, "The sound won't come out." This sort of conditioning of verbal responses not only decreased the number of negative statements but also decreased the amount of stuttering.

A later report by Ryan (1970) gives a careful play-by-play account of an operant program with a 14-year-old boy named Stan who "demonstrated a baseline rate of 4 stuttered words per minute in reading and 24 stuttered words per minute in monologue. No baseline measure was taken in conversation because we believed that the monologue sample was enough. His stuttering was composed mostly of part word repetitions, whole word repetitions, and exhalations of air preceding words. All of these behaviors occurred at a high rate (p. 64)." Ryan carefully describes his procedures in conditioning the identification of the stuttering behaviors, the establishment of their modification through cancellation and prolongation and the build-up of fluency, all of these carried out sequentially in oral reading, monologue, and conversation. Finally the conditioning procedures for effecting a transfer into normal communication are presented. Ryan used only positive reinforcement in this training, giving the boy approvals or "points" for the behaviors he wished to strengthen at each stage of the sequence. His report is well worth reading by all who seek to help the stutterer.

Another operant program is that described by Andrews (1971):

The token system is extremely simple. Tokens are earned for each ten per cent reduction in the severity of stuttering. The baseline is the average of the three best preceding sessions. "Rating sessions" in which tokens can be earned consist of 45 minute group discussions in which all speech is rated for errors. These sessions are held throughout the day. Food, liquor, and cigarettes and other luxuries can only be purchased by tokens. Australian currency is declared valueless during the programme. The patients sub-scribe the funds and administer the details of the programme themselves. Group morale ensures that rule breaking is negligible." (p. 9)

Andrews and Ingham (1971) have explored the use of this token economy with syllable timed speech, psychotherapy, negative practice, delayed auditory feedback, and amplified simultaneous feedback. The program is an intensive one, the stutterers spending up to 12 hours each day in a hospital for several weeks trying constantly to speak with less stuttering and to increase the rate of their speech. Tokens are sometimes taken away for regression to former fluency levels, but most of the reinforcement is positive. Success varied with the type of therapy administered, with negative practice, psychotherapy, and syllable tapping yielding the poorest outcomes, and feedback training the best results.

Clinical difficulties in using operant conditioning

The operant conditioning approach to stuttering has great appeal to many therapists. First of all, it has the smell of science about it. It seems to be highly objective since the therapist can count stuttered words and graph them to provide an immediate measure of success or failure. It employs the reinforcement principles of learning and unlearning. Secondly, as viewed by the naive therapist, the operant approach appears to be a rather simple procedure. The clinician, he erroneously believes, needs only to give positive reinforcements for fluency and to punish the stuttering, and lo, the disorder will disappear. Thirdly (and to many this is very attractive), by using an operant conditioning type of therapy, the clinician can disregard all the antecedents of stuttering since he concentrates only on changing its consequences. He thereby escapes any need for competence in psychotherapy or other related clinical skills. All the miserable complexities which characterize the stutterer as a person may be bypassed. And finally, as in all new approaches to this ancient disorder, there are the enthusiastic anecdotal (though rarely published) reports of cures.

This rather naive view of operant conditioning methods of course is not shared by those who have really tried to create a successful therapeutic operant program. There are many problems to be solved: problems in identifying the behavior to be given contingent reinforcement, problems in selecting the appropriate reinforcement or punishment and applying it at the right instant in time. There are decisions to be made concerning criteria of successful performance; judgments are required concerning the devising of steps in the shaping process and knowing when to shift from one step to the next or when to regress to an earlier one. And above all, the therapist must find ways for effecting transfer outside the laboratory. At the present time, stuttering therapy based upon operant conditioning principles must be regarded as still in the experimental stage as most of those who are exploring it would agree. Whether it will fulfill the optimistic hopes of its advocates or reveal itself as another path to the same old cul de sac is still to be determined. Nevertheless it is an approach which must be seriously considered.

Since this form of therapy is still in the experimental stage, it is difficult to describe because of its many variations. Nevertheless, there are commonalities which can be mentioned. One of the first things which operant therapists do is to identify the stuttering behavior which is to be elimi-

nated. This problem of definition is crucial, since unless the behavior can be specified with some exactness, the contingent stimuli such as punishment or time out from positive reinforcement cannot be applied in any consistent fashion. Usually the first step taken is either to have the stutterer signal each moment of stuttering (Goldiamond, 1965) or to have the therapist do the defining, or through preliminary training to achieve some specified percentage of agreement between therapist and stutterer as to what constitutes the behavior to be extinguished or reinforced.

There are some real problems in this specification of what is to be considered a "moment of stuttering" or a "stuttered word." Some experimenters have used so broad a definition (disfluencies or repetitions) that it is probable that many nonstuttering behaviors were punished. We also know of no research in which contingencies were applied to several abortive speech attempts on the same word. Hesitations and interjections which reflect formulative difficulties may get the same contingent aversive no-no as do those which all would agree were stutterings. Shall we turn on the shock if the stutterer pauses or if he repeats whole words or phrases or uses an *ah* or an *um,* or shall we reserve it for lip protrusion and headjerk? Should we turn up the volume of the blast of noise more for a long severe prolongation than for a very brief one? All we are saying is that many difficult decisions must be made in the presumably simple process of identification.

Next, it is necessary to get a stable baseline level or base rate of emitted stuttering. The stutterer reads, or speaks in a monologue, or converses until a fairly steady rate of emitted stutterings is shown. This often does not occur until after adaptation has taken place. Unfortunately some of the research indicates that even then the baselines are neither very stable or valid (Starkweather, 1971; Adams, 1970). Goldiamond (1965), for example, gives no objective criteria for his baselines, but his "standardized procedure" required three daily sessions in the base-rate condition. Other workers have been even less rigorous, some getting their baselines in ten minutes. Martin (1968) solved the problem in this way. He postponed his contingent reinforcement or punishment until the stutterer's base rate "was considered stable when the number of responses emitted by the subject during three consecutive two-minute periods did not vary by more than a given amount," the amount varying with the amount of stuttering emitted, and a sample of at least 30 minutes of oral reading being required. In view of the marked variability shown by most stutterers, this seems hardly sufficient. Moreover, few of the workers using operant procedures procure new baselines when they change the kind of speaking situation from oral reading to monologue or to conversational speech although conversation is often more variable in stuttering frequency. Nevertheless, some attempt is made to get a stable level of stuttering rate before the positive or negative reinforcement or punishment contingencies are introduced.

Another problem concerns the kind of reinforcement or punishment to be used. Most experimenters have employed such punishing stimuli as a loud blast of sound (tones or white noise at levels of 100 decibels or more) or a strong electric shock, or the introduction of an interval of delayed auditory feedback, or such verbal reprimands as the words "no" or "wrong" or "not good." Others have given the stutterer money and then have taken away pennies or nickels when he stuttered. Still others have used "time-outs" from concurrent gratification or other positive reinforcement as the penalty. Clinically, therapists have used such practices as having the stutterer get ducked every time he stuttered in the swimming pool, or taking away, for the moment, the ice cream cone or bottle of beer on a hot day or stopping the tape recorder when a long passage had to be read, or by breaking the connection of a telephone circuit and thus interrupting communication. Positive reinforcements have ranged all the way from verbal approval to contingent licks of an ice cream cone or the right to give the clinician a severe electric shock. We also find reports of the use of neutral stimuli such as lights, buzzers, or wrist bands and rings which had been previously associated with the punishment or reward. The clinician who wishes to do operant conditioning therapy with stutterers must make the right selection of these contingencies or invent ones more appropriate.

There are many problems involved in the selection and administration of aversive stimuli. For instance, adaptation to the aversiveness may occur. Individual sensitivity to electric shock is difficult to determine. How valuable is the penny that is taken away? How truly hurtful is the word "no" when delivered over and over again through earphones? Finally, if we wish to get transfer outside the laboratory or clinic, should we not use a kind of punishment which others or the stutterer himself can conveniently administer?

Our next task is to make sure that the punishment for stuttering or the reinforcement for fluency is given at the right time, i.e., contingently. This is not easily done and random delivery of aversive stimuli for example, according to some of the research, often seems to increase disfluency. It is very difficult for the experimenter to press the key that gives the electric shock, or turns on the noise, or to apply any punishment at exactly the right instant. In our clinical practice, we have often found that our stutterers were either unwilling or unable to apply unpleasant stimuli to themselves so that they would be truly contingent upon stuttering. On their longer struggling blocks they seem too involved in the stuttering to be able to press the key, while on the shorter ones they tended to disregard it. Often our stutterers have given themselves the blast of noise during the expectancy period prior to uttering a feared word or too long after the word has been uttered. Clinicians too have often found themselves punishing not the stuttered word but the fluent one that followed it. Webster's (1958) research showed how difficult it is even in the laboratory to time aversive stimuli so that they are truly contingent. Again when stuttering occurs in volleys, it is difficult to apply the prescribed aversive stimuli in any consistent way when this occurs. These difficulties probably are not crucial since the majority of the punishments are probably given close enough to the stuttering behavior (and often enough) to achieve what is desired but they do indicate that the *clinical* application of operant conditioning procedures to stuttering seldom approximates the scientific ideal.

Reinforcement for fluency

Because of some of these problems some clinicians have used positive or negative reinforcements for fluency rather than punishment for stutter-

ing. They evidently find it hard to punish or their stutterers simply refuse to undergo any therapy which adds to their miseries. But here again we find problems. Shall we reward the fluent utterance of each word, or demand a fluent phrase, or a sentence, or five seconds or five minutes of speaking in which no stuttering occurs before we give the reinforcement? In clinical practices, many arguments arise when the stutterer thinks that he had spoken fluently and yet failed to get the positive reinforcement he had been led to expect. Again, should we reinforce only the feared words which were spoken fluently or all words? If the former, how can we be sure?

Also, we face the problem of what kinds of positive and negative reinforcement can be used clinically rather than experimentally. Unlike rats or pigeons we cannot starve our human subjects. Other deprivations that might be available for our use are often very difficult to assess. Some therapists have paid their subjects money for fluent utterances. Some have used tokens which could be used for privileges or escapes from unpleasantness. Some therapists have used escape from continuous shock or high level noise when a designated period of fluent speech occurred. Some have confined themselves merely to saying "good" or "fine." What reinforcements should be used in operant therapy? "Those that work" is the usual answer but there are real problems in this area.

Satiation always plagues the therapist who uses positive reinforcement. How many M and M candies are too much sweetening for any mouth? How really important is the therapist's approval? Rickard and Mundy (1965), for example, found no effect at all when the therapist's verbal approval was given contingently for fluency in their operant therapy with a 9-year-old stutterer. Only when they used ice cream and other such reinforcements did his stuttering begin to subside, and, as their report of the follow-up demonstrated, the progress made was not sustained. Leach (1969) used money as a reinforcer for fluent utterances with a 12-year-old boy. After 42 sessions, the boy was stuttering at a rate of less than one word a minute during oral reading and some transfer to speaking situations outside the clinic was reported, but two months after the end of treatment he had relapsed. Russell, Clark, and van Sommers (1968) had three stutterers do machine reading of exposed words, phrases, and sentences in which fluent utterance was reinforced by lights, buzzers, and exposures of a new reading material. Their experiments demonstrated "some reduction" in the frequency of stuttering. As we mentioned earlier Martin and Siegel (1966b) also studied the effects of punishing stuttering with the phrase "not good" while rewarding a specified period of fluency with the word "good" with two stutterers doing oral reading, finding that this program also caused some reduction in stuttering. Ryan (1964) employed negative reinforcement through the use of a long period of required oral reading. The required reading time could be decreased and demonstrated on a clocking device for successful performance, in this case for progress in modifying the form of stuttering. How can these be applied in actual therapy? Or outside the clinic? Maintenance of gains is hard to accomplish.

The next problem involves scheduling. How often should the reinforcements or punishments be given? Usually most workers begin with a schedule in which each stuttered word is

punished or each period of fluency is reinforced since this sort of 100 percent schedule seems to bring the response under stimulus control more swiftly. However, as is well known, such consistent contingent reinforcement results in rapid extinction. The learning which occurs under such a schedule soon weakens when the punishment or reinforcement is removed. Consequently, partial or intermittent reinforcement schedules are usually employed to insure that the desired behavior will have a longer life. A clinician therefore must select the appropriate kind of partial reinforcement schedule (fixed or variable ratios or fixed or variable intervals) and this too is not always easily accomplished. Some operant therapists use a schedule of consistent punishment or reinforcement only until the rate of emitted desired response meets a specified criterion, i.e., until the stuttering is down to one stuttered word for every two minutes of talking time. If the criterion is set too low, the stutterer may never be able to meet it; if it is too high, the response may not have been strengthened or weakened enough to do any good.

All of these difficulties in applying the operant conditioning approach are not insurmountable and those who have had a solid grounding in behavioral science are able to cope with most of them. Our critical presentation has been offered primarily because these things should be understood and because some clinicians who profess to be using operant conditioning fail to understand them.

How effective is operant conditioning?

Clinicians who have hoped that operant conditioning would easily solve the problem of carryover of any fluency acquired in the therapy room to the outside world are likely to be disappointed. The problem of transfer has bedevilled the operant experimenters. Ryan (1964), for example, reported very little generalization of conditioned fluency in oral reading to spontaneous speaking and all workers have found similar difficulty. Some of the measures which have been taken to solve the problem have involved the use of tokens or other objects which had been paired often enough with the original response contingent stimuli until they showed some control over the speaking behavior. That they have not been entirely successful is illustrated by the following account of Wetzler (1967), one of Goldiamond's research assistants:

Mr. E. had stuttered since he was a child in Australia, and had had no speech therapy. When he came to the clinic he was 34 years of age, living in the United States, and a relatively successful engineer with N.A.S.A. Through operant conditioning he rather quickly learned a fluent manner of speaking, but reported that he tended to "forget" to use this way of speaking. He was, therefore, conditioned to use his fluent speech when he saw a poker chip which had, embossed upon it, an eagle in flight. The following week he returned to the clinic and reported tremendous success with the procedure. He did, however, state that on two occasions it had caused him some problems. One was when he was going down the hall at work with some equipment in his arms. As he passed a friend he found that he could not get his hands in his pocket to touch the chip and was unable to speak. The other time was when he was visiting friends and had the chip on the table in front of him. The three-year-old child of his friends picked the chip up and carried it out of the room thinking it was a plaything. Again he was without speech until he regained the chip. After this was reported, it was decided to make his fluency stimulated by

his speaking voice, and not by the poker chip.

Goldiamond reported verbally at a seminar in Carmel, California that a portable delayed auditory feedback apparatus which could be carried by the stutterer into the speaking situations of his daily life did facilitate transfer of the fluency acquired in the laboratory but no published account is available. Others have experimented with the gradual introduction of listeners into the conditioning sessions and the use of booster sessions (Ryan, 1968). Interestingly Andrews and Ingham (1971) using the intensive token reinforcement system with syllable-timed speech found that booster sessions did not improve the result obtained in the initial two week training period.

It is difficult at this time to evaluate the effectiveness of operant therapy with stutterers. The few reported long term follow-up reports have not been particularly impressive and most of the research studies show that though stuttering behaviors can be reduced in frequency by the scheduling of appropriate contingencies, the stuttering usually returns to former levels when these are discontinued. We are also very suspicious of any procedure which deliberately employs rate control or the prolongation of vowels to establish fluency. As we have seen, these methods have been used for hundreds of years (though not as systematically or precisely), and they have seldom had much permanent effectiveness. Even the temporary reduction of stuttering which these methods may produce may not reflect true extinction of learned behaviors. Most of these studies measure the reduction of stuttering in terms of frequency alone or more rarely in terms of rate. The former measure by itself without any consideration of the kind of stuttering shown may yield spurious impressions of progress if the stutterer shows fewer but more abnormal forms of stuttering or if he has recourse to avoidances, postponement pauses and the like to keep from being punished or to earn rewards. As Ingham and Andrews (1971) writes, "One severe block in one thousand syllables is rated as 0.1 syllables stuttered, yet it would be evident to any listener that the subject still stutters. It might not be quite as evident, however, if the single stutter was a mild repetition of a sound or syllable which was not effortfully produced nor a hindrance to the normal speech tempo. Thus it becomes important to make this distinction in the quality of fluency that results from a treatment (p. 281)." That different forms of stuttering (or frequency and rate of speaking) do not always covary together was shown by the experiment of Martin and Siegel (1966a). Again, some authors (Ryan, 1971) measure progress in terms of stuttered words per minute. This gives no real estimate of the amount of stuttering. A stutterer might be able to avoid or postpone most of his feared words, under the contingencies of approval or to obtain points that would bring toys, and thus show a marked reduction in overt stuttering. In conversing, he might say only the word "yes" in a minute, and if he said it fluently, he would show zero stuttering.[5]

Measures of rate of speaking (either in terms of words per minute or preferably in terms of syllables per minute of continuous discourse) would have the advantage of summating the durations of the individual stutterings and the studies of Andrews

and Ingham referred to earlier use this measure as well as frequency counts. Nevertheless, there are stutterers who respond to the threat or experience of blocking by a sudden burst of speed and others who when they expect to stutter on a word say the preceding ones very slowly. Moreover, it is possible to have a very severe grotesque moment of stuttering that may be very short in duration.

As we have said, if these are serious problems for the operant conditioner, we do not feel that they are insurmountable. If appropriate measures of frequency and speaking rate could be combined with some measure of the tension resulting from struggle, or the anticipation of stuttering, valid estimates of improvement could probably be obtained.

It is also important, however, to consider the claim that the reduction in stuttering produced by positive and negative reinforcement or punishment are due to these contingencies. An alternative explanation may lie in the possibility that stutterers, when faced by the possibility of being rewarded for fluent speech or punshed for stuttering, may use some of their old strategies for preventing it. As we have said, they may resort to the use of avoidance and postponement, but additionally, they may employ slow, paced speech, or drawl, or speak softly with different pitch or intensity levels or use any of the other kinds of different talking that have formerly enabled them to be temporarily fluent. Or they may assume the jovial or aggressive attitudes that often act as counterconditioners to speech anxiety. Toomey and Sidman (1970) for example showed that noncontingent shocking of their four stutterers altered not only the frequency of stuttering but also the pitch, volume, and rate. One subject read with longer pauses than usual, and more quiet-

---

[5]This criticism, however, does not apply to Ryan's work since he used a stopwatch to measure not just elapsed time, but minutes of actual talking time. Others have not been so careful.

ly. If these variations occur during noncontingent shock, surely those which resulted in a decrease of stuttering would tend to be adopted if that stuttering were punished contingently.

Furthermore, the *sudden* drop in frequency of stuttering that is evidenced by many of the operant studies at the moment the punishing contingency is administered makes it difficult to believe that only conditioning was involved. Few responses that are thoroughly conditioned extinguish so swiftly. Wingate (1959) showed experimentally that simply calling the stutterer's attention to his stuttering was sufficient to produce a significant decrease in blocking. He writes, "Analysis of the data suggests that these results were due to the stutterer's assuming a set not to stutter, that is, to avoid speaking nonfluently; there was no evidence that learning had occurred (p. 334)." We suspect that some of the improvement shown by stutterers who are punished for stuttering or rewarded for fluency may be better explained in this way, especially for the milder stutterers (and we must remember that, according to Soderberg, 1962), most college stutterers, the main source of experimental subjects, are classified as "mild" on the Iowa Scale of Severity. Our experience has been that mild stutterers can *temporarily* eliminate many of their minor repetitions when they really try to do so.

Some of the decrease in frequency shown in the operant studies may be the result of the suggestion and placebo effect inherent in any new form of treatment. Besides this, as the Biggs and Sheehan (1969) replication of the Flanagan, Goldiamond, and Azrin research has shown, the reduction obtained by pairing aversive stimuli with stuttering may be due to distraction rather than to actual deconditioning.

As we said in our section on distraction, when the stutterer realizes that he may get a blast of sound or an electric shock or even a frown or the word "wrong" every time he stutters, he will concentrate on the anticipation of these aversive stimuli and his usual preparatory sets and rehearsals of abnormality may be wiped out temporarily, thereby producing more fluency. If distractors could permanently distract, then we would have found the solution to stuttering but unfortunately they seem to lose effectiveness as time passes and the novelty fades. Avoidance reactions are notably resistant to extinction and the instrumental behaviors used by stutterers to cope with the threat or experience of being blocked have had a long history of vivid positive reinforcements based upon communicative progress. Booster sessions seem to be the hallmark of operant conditioning therapy so far as maintenance of gains is concerned and we are not surprised to find that they are needed. Certainly the published accounts of successful carry-over from the clinic or laboratory into real life have been conspicuously sparse, and, even in the laboratory, operant procedures rarely seem to extinguish stuttering completely.

In this presentation we have tried to inform the reader of the kinds of therapy based on punishment and reinforcement and their limitations. If we have been critical it is because we seek the truth fiercely. And surely we have not been as harsh as Wingate (1970) was in his assessment of operant based therapy:

"Demonstrations" of the learned character of stuttering have found their most vigorous expression ever in the recent frenetic rush to the Skinner box. The enthralling images of pigeons pecking colored buttons and playing ping-pong have landed the stutterer-as-subject on a baseline, exposed to apparatus through which mathematically arranged effects "control" his behavior. The medium for this control, of course, is punishment, an agent of amazing versatility which for a long time has assumed various roles in the service of explaining stuttering. On the current scene it has appeared as ridiculous, in the form of a 105 dB tone; as confounded, in the role of DAF; and as innocuous in such guises as brief periods of enforced silence, or impersonal utterances of "huh-uh." These "noxious consequences" are delivered with sterile detachment in the best scientific fashion, and the subject is then released. The procedure is hallowed; there would not be the excitement and satisfaction of the confirmation of expected principles if, for example, the subject were asked to report whether he caught on to the scheme. Besides, such tactics would violate the paradigm: the "consequences" must function here in the same blind mechanistic manner in which they are "known" to operate in all organisms, so it is important to pretend that the subject had no idea of what was going on. It would be even more unthinkable to see what would happen if one were to simply substitute for a contingency schedule some mundane procedure such as requesting the subject to make a special effort not to stutter. That too is just not in the scheme of things.

If one looks a bit beyond the terminology, the apparatus, and the charts there is ample reason to wonder whether there is anything in any of the proliferated and redundant operant studies which cannot be accounted for more reasonably and sensibly as due to some cognitive function—perhaps even something as plebian as knowledge-of-results. (p. 7)

It is likely that the real contribution of the operant conditioning studies will lie in their demand that clinical work with stutterers be less impulsive and more systematic. Some terribly unreasonable things have been done to stutterers in the name of therapy. By challenging the intuitive therapists to specify the behaviors they wish to change, by insisting that criterion goals be set, by demanding that progress be measurable, the operant conditioners cannot fail to produce a better treatment for stuttering. We suspect that the present programs are only primitive precursors of better things to come.[6] All therapy involves some learning and unlearning and all therapists use punishment and reinforcement in one form or another. At the present time it would seem wise to withhold final judgment and to hope that future developments will be more encouraging. If they are, we suspect that punishment will have a less prominent place in them than now exists and that operant procedures will be used, not as now to decrease the frequency of stuttering but instead as ways to modify its component behaviors of avoidance and escape. To hope that we can erase stuttering completely and forever by simply rewarding fluency or punishing stuttering seems unrealistic. The disorder, in the adult especially, is far too complex to yield easily to such measures. At the present time at least, we have no firm evidence that operant conditioning provides the ultimate answer to this ancient problem.

Bibliography

ADAMS, M. R., Some comments on "Time-out" as punishment for stuttering, *Journal of Speech and Hearing Research,* 13 (1970), 218–20.

AIKINS, H. A., Casting out a stuttering devil, *Journal of Abnormal and Social Psychology,* 18 (1929), 175–92.

ANDREWS, G., Editorial: Token rein-

6 Another critical presentation of the methods, values and weaknesses of the classical and operant conditioning approaches may be found in *Conditioning in Stuttering Therapy.* Speech Foundation of America, Publication 7, 152 Lombardy Road, Memphis, Tennessee: Fraser, 1968.

forcement systems, *Australian and New Zealand Journal of Psychiatry,* 5 (1971), 135–36.

———— and M. HARRIS, *The Syndrome of Stuttering.* London: Heinemann, 1964.

ANDREWS, G. and R. J. INGHAM, Stuttering: Considerations in the evaulation of treatment, *British Journal of Disorders of Communication,* 6 (1971), 129–38.

———— and K. R. MITCHELL, An approach to indentifying fluency due to pattern change from that due to reinforcement, Unpublished paper, 1971.

APPELT, A., *Stammering and Its Permanent Cure.* London: Methuen, 1911.

ARON, M., *An Investigation of the Nature and Incidence of Stuttering in a Bantu Group of School-Going Children.* Ph.D. Dissertation, University of Witwatersrand, Johannesburg, South Africa, 1958.

AZRIN, N. H., Punishment and recovery during fixed ratio performance, *Journal of the Experimental Analysis of Behavior,* 2 (1959), 301–5

————, Effects of punishment intensity during variable-interval performance, *Journal of the Experimental Analysis of Behavior,* 3 (1960), 123–42.

BIGGS, B. E. and J. G. SHEEHAN, Punishment or distraction. Operant stuttering revisited, *Journal of Abnormal Psychology,* 74 (1969), 256–62.

BLOODTEIN, O. N., Stuttering as an anticipatory struggle reaction, in J. Eisenson (ed.), *Stuttering: A Symposium.* New York: Harper & Row, 1958.

BRADY, J. P., A behavioral approach to the treatment of stuttering, *American Journal of Psychiatry,* 125 (1968), 843–47.

BRADY, W., *The Effect of Electric Shock on the Frequency of Stuttering.* Master's thesis, Pennsylvania State College, 1967.

BROOKSHIRE, R. H., Speech pathology and the experimental analysis of behavior, *Journal of Speech and Hearing Disorders,* 32 (1967), 215–27.

———— and R. R. MARTIN, The differential effects of three verbal punishers on the disfluencies of normal speakers, *Journal of Speech and Hearing Research,* 10 (1967), 496–550.

BRUTTEN, G. J. and D. J. SHOEMAKER, *The Modification of Stuttering.* Englewood Cliffs, N.J.: Prentice-Hall, 1967.

COOPER, E. B., B. B. CADY, and C. J. ROBBINS, The effect of the verbal stimulus words *wrong, right* and *tree* on the disfluency rates of stutterers and nonstutterers, *Journal of Speech and Hearing Research,* 13 (1970), 239–44.

CURLEE, R. F. and W. H. PERKINS, The effect of punishment of expectancy to stutter on the frequencies of subsequent expectancies and stuttering, *Journal of Speech and Hearing Research,* 11 (1968), 787–95.

————, Conversational rate control therapy for stuttering, *Journal of Speech and Hearing Disorders,* 34 (1969), 245–50.

DASKALOV, D., Basic principles and methods of prevention and treatment of stuttering, *Neuropatologii e Psikhiatrii imeni S.S. Korskakova,* 62 (1962), 1047–52.

DIEFFENBACH, J. F., *Heilung des Stotterns durch eine neue Chirugische Operation.* Berlin: Forstner, 1841.

EMERICK, L., A cure for Ankytaa, *Today's Speech* (November 1967).

————, A clinical failure: Sherrie, in Speech Foundation of America, *Stuttering: Successes and Failures in Therapy.* Memphis: Fraser, 1968.

FLANAGAN, B., I. GOLDIAMOND, and N. AZRIN, Operant stuttering: The control of stuttering through response-contingent consequences, *Journal of the Experimental Analysis of Behavior,* 1 (1958), 173–77.

GLASNER, P. J., Nature and treatment of stuttering, *American Journal of Diseases of Children,* 74 (1947), 218–25.

GOLDIAMOND, I., Stuttering and fluency as

manipulable operant response classes, in L. Krasner and L. P. Ullmann (eds.), *Research in Behavior Modification*. New York: Holt, Rinehart & Winston, 1965.

GRAY, B. B. and G. ENGLAND (eds.), *Stuttering and the Conditioning Therapies*. Monterey, California: Monterey Institute for Speech and Hearing, 1969.

GROSS, M. S. and H. L. HOLLAND, The effects of response contingent electroshock upon stuttering, *Asha*, 7 (1965), 376.

HALL, W. W., *The Guide Board*. New York: Fisk, 1869.

HAROLDSON, S. K., R. R. MARTIN, and C. D. STARR, Time-out as a punishment for stuttering, *Journal of Speech and Hearing Research*, 11 (1968), 560–66.

HIRSCHBERG, J. (Stuttering), *Orvosi Hetilap* (Hungary), 106 (1965), 780–84.

HUNT, J., *Stammering and Stuttering*. 1861. Reprinted by Hafner (New York), 1967.

INGHAM, R. J. and G. ANDREWS, Stuttering: The quality of fluency after treatment, *Journal of Communication Disorders*, 4 (1971), 279–88.

JONES, R. K., Observations on stammering after localized cerebral injury, *Journal of Neurology and Neurosurgery*, 39 (1966), 192–95.

KING, S. H., *Perceptions in Medical Practice*. New York: Russell Sage Foundation, 1962.

KITAGAWA, S. (Example of Successful Therapy for Stuttering), *Japanese Journal of Otorhinology*, 42 (1936), 741–42.

KLINGBEIL, G. M., The historical background of the modern speech clinic, *Journal of Speech Disorders*, 4 (1939), 115–32.

LEACH, E., Stuttering: Clinical application of response-contingent procedures, in B. B. Gray and G. England (eds.), *Stuttering and the Conditioning Therapies*. Monterey, Calif.: Monterey Institute, 1969.

LUCHSINGER, R. and G. E. ARNOLD, *Speech-Voice-Language*. Belmont, Calif.: Wadsworth, 1965.

MARTIN, R., The experimental manipulation of stuttering behavior, in A. W. Sloane and B. D. MacAuley (eds.), *Operant Procedures in Remedial Speech and Language Training*. Boston: Houghton Mifflin, 1968.

———— and G. M. Siegel, The effects of response contingent shock on stuttering, *Journal of Speech and Hearing Research*, 9 (1966a), 340–52.

————, The effects of simultaneously punishing stuttering and rewarding fluency, *Journal of Speech and Hearing Research*, 9 (1966b), 466–75.

————, The effects of a neutral stimulus (buzzer) on motor responses and disfluencies in normal speakers, *Journal of Speech and Hearing Research*, 12 (1969), 179–84.

OWEN, T. V. and N. G. Stemmermann, Electric convulsive therapy in stammering, *American Journal of Psychiatry*, 104 (1947), 410–13.

PEDREY, C., Letter to the editor, *Journal of Speech and Hearing Disorders*, 15 (1950), 266–69.

PLATONOV, K., *The Word*. Moscow: Foreign Language Publishing House, 1959.

QUIST, R. W. and R. R. MARTIN, The effect of response contingent verbal punishment on stuttering, *Journal of Speech and Hearing Research*, 10 (1967), 795–800.

RICKARD, H. C. and M. B. MUNDY, Direct manipulation of stuttering behavior: An experimental-clinical approach, in L. P. Ullman and L. Krasner (eds.), *Case Studies in Behavior Modification*, New York: Holt, Rinehart & Winston, 1965.

RUSSELL, J. C., A. W. CLARK, and P. VAN SOMMERS, Treatment of stammering by reinforcement of fluent speech, *Behavior Research and Therapy*, 6 (1968), 447–54.

RYAN, B. P., Operant procedures applied to stuttering therapy for children, *Journal of Speech and Hearing Disorders*, 36 (1971), 264–80.

————, An illustration of operant conditioning therapy for stuttering, in Speech Foundation of America, *Conditioning in Stuttering Therapy*, Publication 7, Memphis: Fraser, 1970.

————, *The Construction and Evaluation of a Program for Modifying Stuttering*. Ph.D. Dissertation, University of Pittsburgh, 1964.

SHAMES, G., Operant conditioning and stuttering, in Speech Foundation of America, *Conditioning in Stuttering Therapy*. Publication 7, Memphis: Fraser, 1968.

————, Verbal reinforcement during therapy interviews with stutterers, in B. Gray and G. England (eds.), *Stuttering and the Conditioning Therapies,* Monterey, Calif.: Monterey Institute, 1969.

———— and Sherrick, C., A discussion of nonfluency and stuttering as operant behavior, *Journal of Speech and Hearing Disorders,* 28 (1963), 3–18.

SHAMES, G., D. H. EGOLF, and R. C. RHODES, Experimental programs in stuttering therapy, *Journal of Speech and Hearing Disorders,* 34 (1969), 30–47.

SHEEHAN, J. G., Reflections on the behavioral modification of stuttering, in Speech Foundation of America, *Conditioning in Stuttering Therapy*. Publication 7, Memphis: Fraser, 1968.

————, *Stuttering: Research and Therapy*. New York: Harper & Row, 1970.

———— and M. M. Martyn, Spontaneous Recovery from Stuttering, *Journal of Speech and Hearing Research,* 10 (1966), 396–400.

SIEGEL, G. M., Punishment, stuttering and disfluency, *Journal of Speech and Hearing Research,* 13 (1970), 677–714.

SODERBERG, G. A., Delayed auditory feedback and stuttering, *Journal of Speech and Hearing Disorders,* 33 (1968), 260–67.

————, What is average stuttering? *Journal of Speech and Hearing Disorders,* 47 (1962), 85–86.

————, Delayed auditory feedback and the speech of stutterers: A review of studies, *Journal of Speech and Hearing Disorders,* 34 (1969), 20–29.

STARKWEATHER, C. W., The case against base rate comparisons in stuttering experimentation, *Journal of Communication Disorders,* 4 (1971), 247–58.

TAKASU, T. (A Cured Case of Tongue Adhesion Coupled with Stuttering), *Japanese Journal of Otorhinology,* 43 (1945), 382–85.

TOOMEY, G. L. and M. SIDMAN, An experimental analogue of the anxiety-stuttering relationship, *Journal of Speech and Hearing Research,* 13 (1970), 122–29.

TRAVIS, L. E., The unspeakable feelings of stutterers, in L. E. Travis (ed.), *Handbook of Speech Pathology.* New York: Appleton-Century-Crofts, 1957.

UMEDA, K., (Study and Therapy of Stuttering), Tokyo: Gakwin, 1963.

VAN RIPER, C., Experiments in stuttering therapy, in J. Eisenson (ed.), *Stuttering: A Symposium.* New York: Harper & Row, 1958.

————, *Speech Correction: Principles and Methods.* Englewood Cliffs, N.J.: Prentice-Hall, 1971.

————, *The Nature of Stuttering.* Englewood Cliffs, N.J.: Prentice-Hall, 1971.

————, The use of DAF in stuttering therapy, *British Journal of Disorders of Communication,* 5 (1970), 40–45.

WEBSTER, L. M., *A Cinematic Analysis of the Effects of Contingent Stimulation on Stuttering and Associated Behaviors,* Ph.D. Dissertation, Southern Illinois University, 1968.

WETZLER, P., personal communication, 1967.

WINGATE, M. E., Calling attention to stuttering, *Journal of Speech and Hearing Research,* 2 (1959), 326–35.

————, Stuttering 1970—where we stand, *Journal of Speech and Hearing Research,* 13 (1970), 5–8.

Servotherapy

Any comprehensive account of the various methods used to treat stuttering must include those which alter the stutterer's perception of his own speech. Although many of these were devised as a result of the discovery of delayed auditory feedback and its ability to disrupt the speech of normal speakers, there are others which have existed for many decades. The current interest in these methods stems in part from the great influence that cybernetic theory has had in almost every phase of modern living. Since we live in a world of computers and automatic controls it is not surprising to find that stuttering theory and stuttering therapy have also felt the impact of cybernetic concepts. Therapy sometimes precedes theory; sometimes it follows it; but always it is influenced by the views held about the nature of the disorder being treated.

Stuttering as a perceptual defect or disturbance

Since we have presented the theory and research concerning the view that stuttering results from disturbed auditory feedback elsewhere (Van Riper, 1971), we shall content ourselves here with only a brief summary. Essentially, the position is that stutterers possess a defective monitoring system for producing sequential speech and that the trouble seems to be due to distorted auditory feedback. Motor speech, being largely controlled automatically rather than voluntarily, requires a reliable flow of information from the output if it is to be integrated. This feedback returns through multiple bilateral channels (air, bone, tissue, tactile, kinesthetic, etc.) and is processed at many levels in the central nervous system—a situation which certainly permits distortion of the signals. Since speech demands an incredibly precise synchronization of simultaneous and successive bilateral motor responses, such distortion could produce asynchrony and lead to stuttering.

Some representative points of view

One of the earliest formulations of a tentative explanation in terms of information theory was presented by Cherry and Sayers (1956). They offer the assumption that ". . . the production of speech involves a closed-cycle feedback action, by which means a speaker continually monitors and checks his own voice production," and go on to say that stammering represents a type of relaxation oscillation caused by instability of the feedback loop. Mysak (1960, 1966) views stuttering as a disturbance of verbal automaticity in tonal flow due to disruption in any one of a series of internal or external servo-loop circuits. Along with others, Butler and Stanley (1966) suggest that the locus of the malfunctioning may be in the middle ear and that this interrupts the automatic programming of the motor output. Stromsta (1962) hypothesized that discrepancies in arrival times of bone-conducted and air-conducted sidetone may be different in stutterers than in normal speakers. Wolf and Wolf (1959) explain stuttering rather naively and inadequately as being due to a "dead-time lag" between the auditory input and motor output of speech.

More sophisticated, though far from being corroborated, is the theory of Tomatis (1963) who attributed the disruption of the stutterer's speech in terms of a delay created by the use of the nondominant ear for the self-perception of speech, an intracerebral delay interval which acts much in the same way as that involved in DAF. Gruber (1965) feels that too much information (overload) in the auditory as compared with the tactual and kinesthetic feedback circuits may produce fluency breaks. Sklar (1969), an engineer, sees stuttering therapy as needing to stabilize an oscillating servosystem and suggests that the best way of doing this is by reducing the auditory feedback. Webster and Lubker (1968) offer an auditory interference theory of stuttering. While accepting that this interference may be produced by various distortions in the feedback signals, they say, ". . . the nature of the interaction between air- and bone-conducted auditory feedback in the ear of the stutterer assumes increased importance. If interaction between air- and bone-conducted feedback components produces momentary phase or frequency-induced distortion it is possible that the resultant signal can be a sufficient stimulus to produce interference. Martin (1970), like the other theorists mentioned, also attributes stuttering to disruption of the auditory feedback system, but blames the criterion function of the comparator for the difficulty. "The perceiver is viewed as setting a decision criterion. When the intensity of the input exceeds the value of the criterion, the perceiver decides that the signal was present." He feels that stutterers, for many reasons, including speech anxiety, set too stringent a criterion and so incoming signals are misevaluated. "In the case of a moment of stuttering it is my hypothesis that the criterion becomes excessively conservative and the decision time in the comparator is slightly delayed. In this way, speech becomes distorted in a manner similar to the distortion in the speech of normals under DAF (p. 254)."

Most of this theorizing has come from some important research and observations which point to the auditory processing system as the possible culprit in stuttering. We have many studies, for example, which show that stuttering-like phenomena are produced by delayed auditory feedback in some normal speaking persons; others that indicate that the congenitally deaf rarely stutter; others that show that stutterers stutter less when their and finally that, under DAF, many stutterers suddenly become very fluent. Moreover, less stuttering seems to occur when whispering, and very little when pantomiming. When using an electrolarynx, stutterers achieve remarkable fluency. Adequate reviews of all this research are provided by Soderberg (1958) and Van Riper (1971). However, Wingate (1970) points out, and we agree, that neither the research nor the theory can be said to be adequate at the present time so far as producing an adequate explanation for stuttering. Nevertheless, this interest has led to certain therapeutic procedures and these will now be presented.

The use of masking noise

The earliest account of therapeutic deafening of stutterers that we have been able to find is one reported by Froeschels (1962) who states that R. Imhofer of Prague in 1927 recommended deafening as a method for treating various "speech and voice troubles." Denes (1931) mentioned the increased fluency shown by stutterers in the presence of noise. Kern (1932) had stutterers read aloud while a very loud Barany drum was being beaten but he seemed to regard the increased fluency produced thereby as being due to distraction. Freund (1932) in his listing of techniques which seemed to decrease stuttering, included pantomime, whispered utterance and low murmuring as ways of reducing the stutterer's morbid self-listening and fears of being heard. At the University of Iowa, Shane (1955) rediscovered the same phenomena. She fed 25 dB (decibels) and 90 dB of white noise into the earphones of 25 stutterers. The weaker voice had no effect but the 90 dB noise produced complete cessation of stuttering in eight of her subjects. Like Freund, she felt that the deafening freed the stutterer from the anxiety and embarrassment of having to hear himself stutter. Interpreting her finding in semantic terms, Shane felt that the noise prevented the stutterer from making the erroneous self-evaluations which the Iowa school believed to be the precipitants of stuttering.

One of the first researches to relate the masking effect of servotheory was performed by Cherry and Sayers (1956). When they had their stutterers simply plug their ears, no reduction in disfluency took place but, when they used a very loud masking noise sufficient to overcome bone-conducted self-hearing, practically all of the stuttering disappeared. By eliminating first the high frequency and then the low frequency components of the masking noise, they concluded that the latter procedure was most effective. Maraist and Hutton (1957), using various intensities of masking noise, found that the severity and frequency of stuttering decreased above 59 dB. Subsequent researches by Ham and Steer (1967), Stromsta (1958), May and Hackwood (1968), Murray (1969), and Burke (1969) have all showed the effectiveness of various kinds of masking in reducing stuttering.

The use of portable maskers

In actual therapy, as opposed to experimentation or demonstration, the use of masking had to wait for the development of devices which could be made small enough to be carried by the stutterer and used outside the laboratory. The first of these seems to have been invented by Derazne, (1966) a Russian. He writes:

Careful clinical observations of the behavior of stutterers indicated that stuttering was greatly reduced or completely absent in conditions where there was a considerably high noise level. Apparently this phenomenon occurs because of some kind of deafening or distraction process. In 1939 we constructed a special electric apparatus that had special earphones. By putting the phone to the stutterer's ears and switching on the machine, the continuous sound masked the patient's own voice. The intensity of the sound of this apparatus, which we called Derazne Correctophone (D.C.) can be loud or soft depending on the need. This can be regulated by a screw which is found at the back of the apparatus. In the U.S.S.R. these apparatuses are operated by electric current on 127 or 220 volts. They are also used with batteries. (p. 615)

According to our informants, the first portable masking devices required a knapsack to hold the heavy batteries but present ones are much smaller with an output of 60 dB and a low buzzer frequency of 50 Hz. However, Derazne came to the conclusion that if stutterers could be given daily practice under masking for a few months, the stuttering generally disappeared, and so the larger units were installed

in the clinics where the training was done.

Derazne's report of success runs as follows:

In looking over extended results in the treatment of stutterers (8 to 10 years), we confirmed the fact that it was possible for us to remove stuttering in the majority of our cases. In a small number of cases we noticed recurrences but this happened as a result of a repeated breakdown of the higher nervous function or of a repeated experience of fear, trauma, infectious disease, etc. Those stutterers who had suffered relapses were again treated with the D.C. but for a shorter period of time (2 or 3 weeks) and consequently resumed normal speech. Our methods did not give positive results in stuttering which was of an organic nature. (p. 616)

Along with the correctophone, Derazne also employed training in smooth exhalation, increasing the rate of speech, and prolonged sleep.

The use of the correctophone masker has been reported by many writers in the Iron Curtain countries. Most of these view it as an adjunct to other comprehensive therapy. Petkov and Iosifov (1960) in Bulgaria indicate that it is used only for cases of severe stuttering. Neimark (1968) used a 100 Hz. portable correctophone in treating 25 stutterers, primarily adults, using it in an audience situation.

From the first sessions we tried to train the patients to master difficult speech in front of an audience. . . . The group method was more valuable in a psychotherapeutic sense as well; the instantaneous normalization of speech in the reader which occurred when the earphones were put on produced a remarkable impression upon the listeners, i.e., those patients who were waiting their turn to read with muffling (masking). (p. 334)

Neimark notes that after some training, the stutterers improved even when the noise level was not sufficient to mask the voice. "Sometimes it was only necessary to put on the earphones for improvement to occur." He also reports that repeated daily sessions for a month or more were necessary before any carry-over took place. No cures were reported. Neimark feels that "muffling" should not be used in treating children and that it has no value with "organic stuttering."

Razdol'skii (1965), whose therapy is based upon reading and speaking alone without a listener and gradually introducing listeners, used the correctophone for those who did not improve under this regime. Using the apparatus,

The patients were advised to practice reading and speaking aloud for 1 to 2 hours every day with rests, observing the principle of gradual progressing from easy forms of speech to those more difficult. The results after one or two months were these: most of the adults who had previously stuttered only slightly when alone were completely freed from their disability, while the solo speech of the rest was greatly improved. This improvement in self-talk when alone, however, was not reflected in their speech in the presence of other people, and this of course vexed them. Later we treated these patients successfully by conditioned reflex methods. (pp. 1718–20)

The most detailed account of long term therapy employing a portable masker is that by Trotter and Lesch (1967). Dr. Trotter, himself a stutterer, reports using such an aid for two and a half years and his subjective experiences are illuminating. He says:

When I was wearing the aid and felt that I was going to stutter, or was in the middle of a block, I would turn the aid on from a switch in my trouser pocket and instantly receive a 90 to 100 dB low-frequency masking noise in my ears. The aid was used in all types of speaking situations but principally while giving lectures, attending university committee meetings, and using the telephone. These are the situations in which I have the most difficulty. I used the aid at least once a week during the time that the university was in session. I wore it about 360 days, of the approximately 800 days that this report covers, for about 15 minutes a day. I rarely wore it in the evenings, on weekends, during vacation periods, or between school semesters, since at these times my stuttering was so minimal that I did not feel the need to wear the aid.

I have stuttered since I was six years old. I received formal therapy at the University of Iowa from 1949 to 1951. Ordinarily I am a mild stutterer. By *mild* I mean that during a 50-minute lecture I will have, on the average, 47 blocks of less than 1 second duration, 16 blocks of 1 to 3 seconds duration, 12 blocks between 4 and 5 seconds in length, and 4 blocks greater than 5 seconds. When I use the stutter-aid in this same situation I have less than one-fourth this number of stutterings, and only an occasional one of these would be longer than one second in length. Although there is a reduction in both the frequency and duration of my stuttering, it has never been entirely eliminated.

One situation in which my stuttering has been almost entirely eliminated is in reading before my class, while using the aid. If I read a 200-word passage without the stutter-aid most students will note severe stuttering incidents. With the aid most of them do not identify a single instance of stuttering. Frequency of stuttering is similar with and without the aid at meetings of the Board of Graduate Studies of Marquette University. When I use the aid there is, however, a reduction in the duration of my long blocks.

If I use the aid during the first 25 minutes of a 50-minute lecture there is considerable "carry-over" during the last 25 minutes. Several times I have tape-recorded 50-minute lectures in which I wore the aid during the first 25 minutes and not during the last 25 minutes. When I counted the stutterings during the second half of the lecture, I noted that I stuttered about 15 times. Other tape recordings show that I will usually stutter about 40 times during the second half of a lecture if I do not wear the aid during the first half. This "carry-over" does not last, however, and by the next day my stuttering will be at its usual level of about 80 blocks per 50-minute lecture. There is no permanent "carry-over". (pp. 271–72)

Despite the favorable reports of Derazne and others, the use of masking noise in the treatment of stuttering has not gained complete acceptance in Russia or Bulgaria, Hungary, and Czechoslovakia, many of their workers feeling that its major effects are due to distraction and fail to eliminate the source of the problem. Thus Zinkin (1968) writes:

It has been noted that weakening auditory reception by providing noise as interference decreases stuttering. But it is quite evident that such a method can in no way serve as a cure for this defect. Whatever the external interference, one's own speech continues to be heard through the bone and muscle conductors. To remove the defect it is necessary to remove its cause, i.e., to normalize inductive relations and restore the auto-regulation of speech movements. This is why speech exercises cannot lead to positive results. The stutterer has a normally-formed verbal stereotype and only the moment of its initiation is disrupted. Nor can the goal be achieved by the training of breathing, since the disruption of the regulation of aerodynamic conditions is itself a consequence of a pathological change in inductive relations. (p. 432)

Moravek and Langova (1965) in Czechoslovakia also explored the use of masking. They point out that much

of the stutterer's problem lies in the initiation of utterance, in the preparation for phonation. Since masking can only affect phonation after it has already taken place, these authors feel that it does nothing about the cause or core of the difficulty. They write, "We conclude that the causes of stuttering are to be sought in mechanisms other than the sense of hearing itself."

Masking in the Western world

It was not until 1963 that Parker and Christopherson, two British psychiatrists, designed a portable electronic masker to aid them in their psychotherapy with stutterers whose blockings were so severe that they could not verbalize sufficiently to be helped. These authors reported that the masker was very effective. Van Riper (1965) also designed one which could be carried in the hand and which fed the noise into an ear mold. In 24 or 25 stutterers, a marked reduction in severity of stuttering and a slight decrease in frequency was achieved in spontaneous speaking under stress when the noise was turned on *only at the moment of stuttering*. Murray (1969) showed that continuous masking produced more fluency and less severe stuttering than either random or stuttering-contingent masking. Klein (1967) was granted a United States patent for a random noise generator (Figure 5.1) with a contact microphone which could be fitted against the mastoid process or the laryngeal region. The ear pieces which transmitted the masking noise were hollow, thus permitting the person to hear other conversation but not his own voice since the masker only came on when actuated by the voice. Another portable masking device has been described by Donovan (1971).

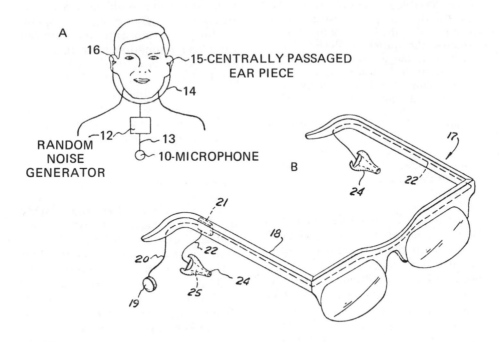

FIGURE 5.1   Klein auditory masker. (U.S. Patent 3, 349, 179[1967].)

It combines an electronic metronome which produces a square wave 180 Hz. tone "resembling a croak" fed into the ear piece of a hearing aid and controlled by the subject. Donovan writes:

We have found that the speech improvement due to auditory masking and paced masking and paced speech can also be obtained by using an interrupted or periodic masking tone. Here the masking tone is interrupted at regular intervals except that the actual sound is longer in duration and can be varied to suit the patient. (p. 87)

Another report of extended use of masking noise is provided by Perkins and Curlee (1969). Three adult stutterers, who had previously been receiving rate control therapy but had been unable to transfer the fluency gained in the clinic to outside situations, agreed for several days to use one masking device which produced a pulsing signal of variable rate and intensity and another device which produced white noise. Both types of units eliminated or decreased stuttering but the pulse device was preferred over the white noise unit. The subjective reports of the stutterers may be of interest:

One subject, the aviator, thought that the aid was effective because it forced him to concentrate on the content of what he was saying rather than on how he would speak the words on which he expected to stutter. Another subject, the engineer, thought that the aid was effective because it induced a feeling of psychological isolation. He said he knew he was speaking in a social situation, but that the masking sound made him feel as if he were speaking alone—a condition under which he would normally not stutter.

All the subjects felt that if they could learn to manage their speech without the aid, they would much prefer not to use one and would not get one unless they were convinced that further improvement in their speech was not likely. In that event, all felt that they would want such an aid if it were available, despite having several objections to it. All objected to the mechanical inconvenience of it and to the induced hearing loss in social conversation. All tended to fear that they would use it as a crutch. None liked the idea of the ear plugs as an advertisement of disability, regardless of whether the suspected difficulty was hearing loss or stuttering. All felt, however, that the instrument would be valuable to them even if they used it only to maintain easy speech in otherwise difficult, but important, speaking situations. (p. 362)

Clinical use of masking

All of the researches have shown conclusively that masking does reduce the frequency and severity of stuttering though there is no real certainty concerning the reason for this effect. The clinician needs to know why he does what he does and it is unfortunate that in this case he cannot be sure. Is it merely a distraction—whatever that means? Sutton and Chase (1961) demonstrated that administering the masking noise during the silent intervals of speech produced a similar decrease in stuttering, a finding which was first criticized by Webster and Lubker (1968) and then later corroborated by Webster and Dorman (1970). The latter authors, however, point out that this finding may not spoil their auditory interference explanation since middle ear muscle reflexes may be set off by the anticipation of noise as well as its presence. There are other bits of evidence in-

dicating that something more than a shift of attention is involved. Distractions usually wear out swiftly; Trotter found his masker to be effective for some years. Trotter and Lesch write:

Some speech pathologists have asked me if I thought the stutter-aid was another distraction device that would eventually become useless. I do not think so. In the two and one half years that I have worn the aid, I estimate that I have turned the aid on between 5,000 to 6,000 times. My stuttering blocks are shorter or absent as a result.

The major effect of masking is found at lower frequencies of masking;[1] if it is only a distractor, why should we find this difference? The masking is also most effective at intensities sufficient to overcome bone-conduction; why again should this be so? On the other hand, we have a study by Barr and Carmel (1969) which used a high-frequency narrow-band noise, one which would not mask out the stutterer's voice. This too decreased stuttering. These authors suggest, however, that their findings might still be explained in terms of interaural phase differences or differential auditory adaptation in stutterers. We are certain that some distractive effects are present as they are in all therapy but not so sure that they constitute the essential influence in promoting fluency.

It has been stated by Wingate (1970) that masking is effective perhaps because it causes the stutterer to speak more loudly (the Lombard effect); or makes him speak more slowly or drawl out his words or in other ways alters

---

[1] Bohr (1963) and May and Hackwood (1968) found no difference between masking levels above and below 500 Hz. as producing increased fluency. Some difficulties in their experimental designs may explain this finding.

his usual manner of initiating phonation. However, Cherry and Sayers (1956) and Shrum (1962) found that masking still increased fluency when stutterers spoke quietly. The other factors have not been investigated to our knowledge.

Other clinical uses of masking

We have employed the masking effect for some years in our own therapy, but in other ways than those presented in the studies mentioned previously. We soon found that when we used it solely to create speech entirely free from stuttering, little transfer of that fluency to other speaking situations took place. Our stutterers also became dependent upon the masker; they made no effort to overcome their fears or to modify their struggle and avoidance behaviors. Without the masker, they were helpless. What was more common, as we have seen in the Perkins and Curlee (1969) article, the stutterers resented having to use it. The continuous loud noise gave them headaches; the earmolds reduced their hearing even when the sound was switched off; others treated them as though they were deaf; or they tended to talk too loudly and at too high pitch levels (as they discovered when the noise was terminated). In short, we found most of the objections that arise when hearing aids or glasses are first fitted.

But there was something more. No matter how long the stutterers used the masker, they did not adapt to it. Indeed it grew more unpleasant with extended use and eventually they just refused to wear it or to turn it on. "I'm still a stutterer," one of them said. "This trick gadget hasn't changed me a bit. If I don't use it or if it would break I'd be just as bad as ever—maybe worse." We were inclined

to view this resistance as neurotic protest until we wore the masker ourselves for two days, turning it on every time we talked. It was a cumulatively unpleasant experience. Perhaps under the strict controls of a Russian hospital clinic, stutterers could be forced to wear it long enough to stabilize the precarious fluency the masker produced but it became very obvious that few of our own cases would do so. As a permanent prosthesis, it was simply not tolerable.

Intermittent masking

Our next endeavor was to reduce the distress by training the stutterer to use the masking noise intermittently rather than continuously. We first trained our cases to turn on the noise at the precise moment they began to fear they might stutter. If the noise was just a distraction, this procedure should have maximized the effect. We found, however, that the reduction in stuttering was not nearly as substantial as when continuous masking was used though some decrease did occur. First of all, a surprising number of stutterings were not anticipated; the stutterer found himself blocking before he could turn on the device.[2] Moreover, since expectancy of stuttering is not an all or none affair but appears in a gradation of calculated probability, most of our cases only turned it on when they were *certain* that they would stutter. This led to the evoking of many more stutterings than when continuous masking was employed. Again, it was difficult for the stutterers to press the switch when the fear flared suddenly just at the moment of

---

[2] In this clinical experimentation, the masker was used only in spontaneous speech since we had found that preliminary practice with individual words or in oral reading was unnecessary.

speech attempt. For these and other reasons we discarded the use of masking contingent upon expectancy.

Contingent masking

We then investigated the utility of making the masking contingent upon the perception of stuttering itself. This technique was more effective since it exerted some operant control over the behavior and also served as an alerting device. Primarily this procedure reduced the severity of stuttering although some moderate decrease in frequency was also apparent. The moment the masking came on, the compulsive repetitions would cease or the tonic fixations would end and the word would be spoken. The technique seemed to facilitate "pull outs," and we have continued to use it as an aid in teaching the stutterer how to work out of his repetitions and prolongations voluntarily.

Difficulties with masking

Nevertheless, we found difficulties. Some stutterers used the masker as an accessory timing device to initiate the moment of speech attempt rather than to make it contingent upon the perception of fixation or tremor or repetitive recoil. Those whose symptom picture was characterized by postponement behaviors ("ah's," "um's," etc.) would not turn on the noise until they had postponed long enough to "satisfy their fear," as one of our cases phrased it. They turned it on only at the moment of genuine speech attempt but not at the moment of felt stuttering. Had this resulted in a decrease in the postponement time, we would have felt better about it, but instead the number and duration of postponement behaviors increased and the therapeutic loss was greater than

the gain. These "postponing stutterers" seemed unable to make the noise contingent upon actual overt stuttering.

Another difficulty concerned the timing of the masker synchronously with the onset of stuttering. The stutterers tended to press the switch too soon or too late. Ideally the masking should be sensed at the very first sign of fixation or oscillation but this timing was difficult to achieve. Even when the therapist turned on the noise, his reaction time often delayed the contingent sound so that it came on, for example, after too long a duration of tremor or some time after the stuttering was terminated and a subsequent fluent word was being spoken. Despite intensive training some stutterers never seemed to be able to turn on the masker at the onset of stuttering. Those who were able to time the noise contingently did seem to profit from the technique greatly. Their stuttering would terminate almost as soon as it began and the resultant decrease in overall abnormality was impressive. Very severe stutterers became very mild stutterers. Some of them reported that even without the masker they could end their "blocking" merely by making a tiny finger movement similar to that which they had used in turning on the noise device. This bothered us since we didn't want any finger-stuttering and we knew that these timing movements could grow when they were followed by the powerful reinforcement of utterance. In two of our cases this did happen. First they would only have to crook their finger once and the "word came out"; then they would have to press it twice or three or four times. One of them developed a tremorous finger twitching even during expectancy. These were exceptions however. After reviewing our clinical experiences with continuous, expectancy-contingent and stuttering-contingent masking, we decided some other approach was necessary. Even though all of these procedures did reduce stuttering, often dramatically, we felt their difficulties and disadvantages outweighed their effectiveness.

Masking as an aid to proprioceptive feedback

Accordingly, we sought to use masking as a teaching and training technique to help the stutterer learn to monitor his speech primarily by proprioceptive, tactile, and kinesthetic feedback. Although we did not know the cause of stuttering nor the neurological factors which may be vital in its precipitation, there are, as we have said before, some strong indications that some malfunction of the auditory system may be involved. Once again we call attention only to the rarity of stuttering in the congenitally deaf, to the production of "artificial stuttering" in the normal speaker by delayed auditory feedback, to the production of phonatory blockage in normal speakers by sidetone distortion, and to the absence of stuttering in laryngectomees (who had previously stuttered) when they learn esophageal speech.

All of these findings point, in one way or another, to the possibility that, if we can bypass or attenuate self-hearing and emphasize somosthesia in the monitoring of ongoing speech, we may be able to help the stutterer speak more fluently. Or, even if no perceptual auditory problem exists, the morbid attention directed to the way the stutterer thinks he sounds to others seems sufficient to justify more concentration on some other feedback than the auditory one. We want to get the stutterer to stop cocking his ear for trouble. We want him to do what normal speakers do, monitor his speech by somosthetic cues primarily. Normal speakers can speak well even in a boiler factory. They have learned to control their speech by "feel", not by "sound." Even when they become deaf, they do not stutter and their articulation remains adequate for a surprisingly long time. They have learned to use their ears to hear their own unfolding thoughts and the messages of others. They seem to monitor their speech primarily by taction and proprioception. We feel that most stutterers ignore what their mouths are doing, perhaps because they do not want to know. We feel they need more information in their somosthetic feedback circuits.

Our present use of masking is therefore designed to aid the stutterer to monitor his speech by nonauditory feedback. We do not use it primarily to give him some temporary fluency (though in some special circumstances we may). What we do is to fade out the noise in gradual steps in a reverse hierarchy, beginning with noise loud enough so that he cannot hear himself at all and finishing with the masker turned off. Throughout the process we ask the stutterer to focus his attention on the feel of his articulatory and respiratory movements, primarily the former, and to keep speaking in the same way. Often the jaw movement seems to serve as the primary integrator, the prime mover, of the motor sequence and to this we ask the stutterer to attend by scanning his proprioception and his taction and his kinesthesia as the masking noise diminishes. In addition to fading out the noise gradually, we also have him practice turning off the masker for increasing lengths of time while continuing to monitor his speech by the way it feels.

With training, the stutterer becomes able to do this on all of his speech, not only on the words he fears but on all the words. We try to get him to achieve a generalized scanning set for this type of feedback information, to stop listening to himself and to feel what he is doing motorically. Once he has learned to monitor his speech in this way, very little stuttering remains. The portable masker is soon employed merely as an aid in recapturing the kind of somosthetic scanning set used by normal speakers and it need not be used very often. Our stutterers learn that they do not need the masker, that they can feel their mouths move without it but it is a valuable aid in training.

We have experimented with the programming of this kind of masking at different times during the course of our stuttering therapy. As we shall see later in this text, we find that it is most effective when deferred to the later stages of treatment, in that stage which we have termed stabilization. We do this for several important reasons. First, we delay masking because we need enough stuttering to work with. We need time to reduce and extinguish his fears. Unless we have stuttering behaviors to manipulate, we cannot break them up or weaken their strength. We need stuttering so that we can use it in our accompanying psychotherapy. We do not want to *suppress* the avoidance and coping responses which have been so powerfully reinforced. Were we to neglect them or merely repress them, they would lie latent as strong as ever. We do not seek temporary fluency. That is easily procured by a hundred methods. Instead we try to change the stutterer as a person as well as a speaker. We want him to come to grips with his problem in its totality. In our therapy there is an important place for

masking but it does not come early in the treatment.

Delayed auditory feedback (DAF) [3]

When a normal speaker's speech is returned to his ears a fraction of a second after the time it normally would arrive, certain changes in his speech tend to occur. His verbal output tends to be slowed down (Black, 1951); repetitions of syllables and prolongations of sounds which resemble stuttering are observed (Lee, 1951); the speech becomes slurred and certain sounds are distorted or omitted (Ham and Steer, 1967). This "artificial stutter" and articulation errors were viewed by Fairbanks and Guttman (1958) as the primary behaviors produced by the delay while the other accompanying behaviors such as an increase in the pitch of the voice or an increase in vocal intensity, together with pauses, palmar sweating, and flushing, were seen as reactions to the experience.

It should be mentioned immediately that there exists a wide individual variability in all these reactions to DAF, whether primary or secondary (Beaumont and Foss, 1957). Some normal speaking individuals seem to be relatively unaffected by DAF. Yates (1965) offers the explanation that those normal speakers who show little speech disruption under the delay are probably those who depend very little upon auditory feedback for its motor control and who probably monitor their speech primarily by proprioception, taction, or kinesthesia. Other persons are very vulnerable. Some

[3] Portions of this section were included in Van Riper, C., "The Use of DAF in Stuttering Therapy," *British Journal of Disorders of Communication*, 5 (1970), 40–45. Permission for its use here has been granted.

show a proclivity toward syllable repetitions while still others prolong their vowels. Some react with marked pitch changes or increases in loudness; a few even demonstrate difficulty in word finding (Meyer-Epler and Luchsinger, 1955). Males also seem to be more vulnerable to DAF than females according to Bachrach (1964).

Chase and his coworkers (1961) reported that older children and adults are more affected than the younger ones but other recent research by MacKay (1968) and Buxton (1969) does not substantiate this. Children had more trouble than adults but the DAF times for maximal disruption were much longer. Adaptation to DAF can be achieved, despite some of the earlier research (Atkinson, 1953), but usually only after prolonged exposure (Goldiamond, 1965; Winchester, Gibbons, and Krebs, 1959). Some lingering effects in terms of disrupted speech has been reported by Black (1951) and others but these seem to be transitory.

The question has been posed as to whether or not the repetitions and prolongations shown under DAF are similar to or identical with stuttering behaviors. Neelley's (1961) research seemed to indicate that they were not; however, Yates (1963b) and others have criticized the design of his study and especially his conclusions. We ourselves would define them as stuttering behaviors. Some of the difficulty is doubtless a semantic one. If our own definition of stuttering in terms of temporally disrupted sounds and syllables (Van Riper, 1971) is accepted, then DAF can produce stuttering. It does not create stuttering as a disorder but it can break up the integrated motor sequences of sounds, syllables and words. Rawnsley and Harris (1954) and Agnello and Kagan (1966) showed that the sonograms of DAF

"stuttering" in normal speakers resembled the fluency disruptions of stutterers. Certainly, many normal speakers say that the DAF experience makes them stutter.

The effect of DAF on stuttering

A rather surprising finding is that certain stutterers, especially the more severe ones, speak much better under DAF than under normal feedback conditions (Soderberg, 1969). Chase (1958) had reported earlier that normal children who were usually more hesitant and repetitive spoke better under DAF than those who were relatively fluent. In Germany, Nessel (1958) found that certain stutterers became much more fluent under DAF but termed it a distraction effect. Lotzman (1961) who studied 60 stutterers, and used a variety of delay times, also showed that it made stutterers fluent. Bohr (1963), in South Africa, Zerneri (1966) in Italy, and a number of workers in the United States have demonstrated that many stutterers speak much more fluently under DAF. Soderberg (1969) has reviewed these and other studies and comes to the following conclusions:

(1) Under DAF the stutterers' rate of speech is generally prolonged and the frequency of stuttering is reduced; (2) the effect of DAF on the fluency of stutterers seems to persist after the delay has been eliminated from the feedback, and oral reading rate subsequently can be shaped to a more normal pattern; (3) DAF may be a more effective means of reducing stuttering than is auditory masking. (p. 28)

The following account was written by a very severe stutterer shortly after she had failed to show any improvement under masking and then became very fluent under DAF:

I am in a state of emotion I can't describe. I heard—no I didn't, I *felt* myself talking so freely I couldn't believe it was my own mouth. I almost felt like crying with hope at last. I could see feared words coming in the book you gave me to read and it was a shock and a surprise to find them coming out as smooth as a dream. That echo pulls me onward. It won't let me stick. It drives me.

A very interesting study was done by Cohen and Edwards (1965). They attempted to interfere with the stutterer's presumed reliance on normal auditory feedback by randomly programming delayed feedback with synchronous feedback. They found that, though the stuttering did not disappear under this constantly changing scheduling, it varied in its form. The severe secondary reactions of struggle and avoidance were replaced by simple repetitions and prolongations and training for 15 sessions over a three-week period showed persisting effects for as long as six months. Another interesting finding was by Bohr (1963) who noted that former stutterers were not markedly affected by DAF. MacKay (1968) showed that normal speakers could overcome the DAF disruption by voluntarily drawling or prolonging the duration of syllables, a technique which has been used in stuttering therapy for years. MacKay (1969) also discovered, as we have reported earlier, that when normal speakers used very nasalized speech, they become relatively fluent under DAF, a finding which is paralleled by the fluency of stutterers when using a dialect or other strange manner of speaking.

Finally we should make clear that DAF does not always produce an immediate decrease in stuttering, especially when only one delay time is being used. Thus Logue (1962) and Ham and Steer (1967) showed no significant differences between a small group of stutterers and their controls. We have found, however, with extended practice and directions to "try to beat the machine" *by attending to proprioception* that most stutterers become very fluent in oral reading under DAF.

Therapeutic use of DAF

Suggested uses of the delayed feedback apparatus in therapy have been sparse. Since Chase (1958), had found that syllabic repetitions could be facilitated by DAF, Soderberg (1969) used DAF to help the stutterer to learn to stutter with short, easy repetitions and prolongations rather than with their old abnormal struggle. Delayed auditory feedback does seem to prevent the usual forcing and struggle so characteristic of many stutterers. It also seems to create conditions which help the stutterer to move onward in the speech sequencing or at least to facilitate some change in his stereotyped behaviors.

Adamzyck (1963) contrived a city-wide telephone hook-up in Lublin, Poland, so that stutterers could call a certain phone number and practice speaking under DAF while being observed by their clinicians. The stutterers were trained "to synchronize the syllables to be pronounced with the syllables of the echo." This specific application uses the echo as a timing signal and the improvement reported by Adamzyck may be due in part to this. If so, he might as well have hooked up a metronome to the telephone. We should mention some support for this possibility. Novak and Petrik (1965) showed that when high pass or low pass filters were introduced into the DAF circuit, it still was able to reduce stuttering. Even when the echo was so distorted it resembled meaningless noise, it still maintained its effectiveness.

In applying operant conditioning to stuttering, Goldiamond (1965) viewed DAF (as most normal speakers might) as an unpleasant experience and his research showed that when DAF was made contingent upon stuttering, the stuttering decreased, i.e., that it was punishing. Then he turned off a continuously administered delay (for 10 seconds) whenever a stuttered word appeared. This at first resulted in an increase of stuttering but, surprisingly, under the same "negative reinforcement" scheduling, the stutterers began to talk more slowly, prolonging their syllables, and became very fluent. Goldiamond, evidently had considered the possibility that DAF alone, and quite apart from its alleged punishment role, might be fluency-enhancing for he applied continuous DAF to one stutterer for a short time and found no improvement. That this attempt to control for DAF ability to decrease stuttering was insufficient was pointed out by Webster and Lubker (1968) who demonstrated that stutterers with enough exposure can learn to withstand DAF disruption and gain fluency from its effect alone and without its operant contingencies. They write:

In our laboratory 4 of 14 stutterers did not show immediate improvement in fluency when they first experienced continuous DAF. These were subjects whose stuttering seemed to be comprised of strong anticipatory struggle responses. We discovered that while they were on DAF, they could follow instructions to drop out the struggle responses and could then successfully emit words they initiated. They found that if speech was initiated without struggle, DAF permitted fluency. The 14 subjects used to date in our laboratory have shown marked improvements in fluency while under continuous DAF. (p. 759)

Our own cases have reacted in much the same fashion when helped to disregard their self-hearing and to concentrate on proprioceptive, tactile, and kinesthetic cues.

Another attempt to apply DAF in the treatment of stuttering was made by Curlee and Perkins (1969). Using it in what they called Conversational Rate Control Therapy, and with accompanying instructions to prolong the syllables and to speak slowly in short simple sentences, they were able eventually to get fluent speech from their stutterers at the rate of from 30-35 words per minute in conversation. The DAF initially was set at 250-msec. delay and the stutterer was to try to say his syllables so that they would coincide with the delayed feedback (a procedure that results in a regular rhythmic utterance of words). Then the delay was progressively decreased in 50-msec. steps until simultaneous feedback was attained. Finally time-out procedures were used to punish the stuttering which remained, and transfer of the fluency to outside situations was attempted. Curlee and Perkins report some favorable results:

Clients have estimated that their stuttering has decreased 75% to 95% in those situations not easily available to the clinician. In addition, both clients and clinicians have reported that the severity of individual instances of stuttering also has decreased noticeably in and out of the clinical laboratory. (p. 249)

Ryan (1968) applied the Goldiamond procedures described earlier in this section to six stutterers over a nine-month period using concurrent programs of oral reading, monologue and conversation under DAF. His basic conclusions are as follows:

Comparisons of performances under DAF in the three modes of reading, speaking, and conversation revealed that these situations were independently affected by the DAF procedure. Reading in a fluent, prolonged manner under DAF did not generalize to speaking without DAF. The highest frequency of reoccurrence of dysfluencies under DAF occurred in conversation, followed by monologue and then reading. Although it is possible to dramatically reduce the frequency of stuttering in monologue and conversation concurrently with reading using DAF, it would appear that the increased re-occurrence of dysfluencies makes this a questionable procedure. The use of base periods following each break probably is not necessary and only detracts from the ongoing program. It increases the possibility of dysfluency.

In France, Tomatis (1963) designed an "electronic ear" device to counteract the influence of transcerebral delay times. These he felt were present in stutterers because they monitored their speech through auditory information coming through the nondominant ear. Although both cerebral hemispheres process auditory information, Tomatis came to believe, through various experiments, that there was a "directing ear" for side-tone perception and that 90 percent of stutterers had hearing losses in that ear. This forced them to use the nondominant ear for perception and introduced a transcerebral delay time of approximately 0.2 seconds, a delay which usually disrupts speech in the adult male. Tomatis' finding that a unilateral hypoacousia existed in stutterers was not corroborated by Moravek and Langova (1964) or by Aimard, Plaintier, and Wittling (1965) nor did the latter workers find any evidence of central lateral dominance for auditory perception. Backe (1965) in Norway found that there was less stuttering when the DAF was applied only to the preferred ear. Asp (1965) however found some evidence that Toma-

tis may have been correct in his concept of the dominant ear. At any rate, the electronic ear is a gating circuit with two channels, each of which can be modified to change the shape of the envelope. It is basically used to retrain the stutterer to use his natural "directing ear," and so to prevent the operation of transcerebral delay. We have only anecdotal accounts of its success.

Our experience with DAF therapy

Our own attempts to determine the utility of DAF in stuttering therapy have only been exploratory and we can give only tentative impressions as to its success. Nevertheless, it is out of such observations that new clinical practices and researches have their origin. Early in therapy, we have found that we can use the DAF to help the stutterer recognize that other people can be made to stutter too and that their responses to broken words are very similar to the stutterer's reactions to his own moments of disruption. Letting the stutterer turn on the delay that precipitates a breakdown in the fluency of a normal speaker (or the therapist perhaps) seems to relieve some of his frustration.

Next, we use it, much as Soderberg did, to show the stutterer that his stuttering behavior is modifiable. By using a variety of delay times and intensities and randomized schedules of delay and normal feedback, most of our stutterers have changed the way they characteristically stuttered—or else they became remarkably fluent. By recording these new easier forms of stuttering and asking the stutterers to duplicate them when they are heard or seen on videotape, the variability becomes very vivid to them and they then recognize that they can markedly alter their stuttering behaviors. Moreover, since the stutterings on DAF are seldom very long, are more easy, more repetitive, much simpler, and with very few contortions or avoidance or struggle behaviors, our stutterers realize that their stuttering is not only modifiable but that it can be reduced in severity.

Some of the commercial DAF instruments unfortunately are not adequate for effective clinical use since they provide too limited delay intervals or fail to have sufficient gain. Like Lotzmann (1961) we have found that certain delay times are critical both for producing a maximal amount of disruption or, with a different setting, a maximal amount of fluency, depending on what we desire at the moment. The researches of MacKay and Buxton mentioned earlier demonstrated that for maximal disruption, children require much longer delay times than the approximately one-fifth of a second usually employed. For maximal

disruption females also seem to require longer delays than males according to Mahaffey and Stromsta (1965) MacKay (1968), and Buxton (1969) which is interesting in view of the sex-ratio of stuttering.

Much research has shown that individuals of any age or sex group may differ markedly in their vulnerability to different delay times. The same may also be said about the intensity of the delayed signal which is fed back to the speaker's ears. Accordingly, one of the first things we do diagnostically is to vary both the delay and the gain so as to determine the settings for optimal fluency or optimal disruption. Each individual seems to have his own crucial settings for therapeutic use. If we need to give our stutterers the feeling of fluency under stress, we use the critical setting of delay and gain which yields that fluency. If, on the other hand, we need to train the person to resist disruption through

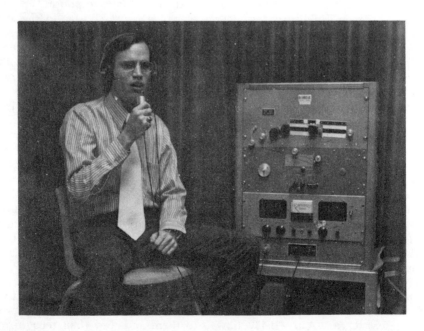

FIGURE 5.2   A stutterer using delayed auditory feedback.

adaptation and desensitization techniques, we use that delay or gain which tends to create blockages or repetitions.

Although some but not all of the research has indicated that little adaptation to DAF occurs, we have found it possible through systematic desensitization training to teach the stutterer to "beat the machine." We do this systematically in three ways: (1) by inserting brief moments of delay, while the stutterer is being fluent and gradually increasing the frequency and duration of the delay dosages (yet always trying to remain below the threshold of breakdown), the stutterer can be trained to speak very well despite the DAF stress; (2) by beginning with continuous DAF using the delay time which is most conducive to fluency, and then gradually changing the delay interval until it approximates the delay time which produces the maximal disruption; (3) by starting the person out under the delay time which usually produces the most disruption but initially setting the volume control so low that the delay is barely sensed. Then through progressive steps in which the gain is increased up to the threshold of breakdown but not above it, the stutterer can be trained to resist the DAF even at the critical levels. Combinations of these three desensitization methods can also be employed.

As we have mentioned, different individuals respond differently to the stress of DAF. Therefore, in our diagnostic sessions, we also seek to determine how a given stutterer characteristically tries to cope with the disturbance when he is first exposed to the delay. There are several common reactions. If he does not become completely fluent as many surprisingly do, he may show a slow down in the rate of his utterance. Or he may stop and

try again, or use the burst of speed which so often results in articulatory distortions and omissions. Or the loudness or pitch of his voice will markedly increase as the stutterer seeks through bone and tissue conduction to overcome the effects of sidetone delay. He may prolong the vowels and continuant sounds or he may repeat syllables compulsively. Word-finding difficulties, disturbances in formulation may occur. There are many ways that people use to cope with the disruption of delayed feedback. The stutterer, like the normal speaker, finds a strong urge to do what he can to bring his utterance back under the automatic control of his servosystem.

Most of the above mentioned coping mechanisms, we feel, are unwise and should not be reinforced in the stutterer. There is a better strategy—to ignore the disrupting auditory signals and instead to concentrate upon the proprioceptive and tactile feedback and to use this information for the monitoring of speech. At first it is difficult for the subject to do this, especially when the return flow of speech is amplified so greatly. Nevertheless, through the desensitization training we have outlined, the stutterer finds it possible to learn to rely on his proprioceptive and tactile cues and so to resist the delay successfully. In training the stutterer, we have found it essential to weaken and prevent the other types of coping reactions and to insist upon, and to reinforce, somesthetic monitoring.

Often in facilitating this kind of control, we precede the DAF training by using powerful masking noise or pantomimic speech, or the electrolarynx for a period before we turn on the delay. One way to check whether the person is using proprioceptive controls rather than other coping devices is to record the speech with and without the delay and to see if the rate and loudness and prosodic patterning of the speech is similar under both conditions. When some exaggeration of articulatory movements is seen, the overarticulation apparently signifies an early form of proprioceptive

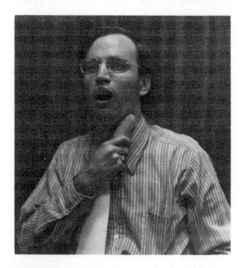

FIGURE 5.3 A · stutterer using the electrolarynx.

monitoring. As the stutterer learns to "beat the machine" through proprioception, his speech becomes not only more fluent but much more precise. The movements, especially of the jaw and lips, are more marked. They are stronger even when unexaggerated.

The stutterer should aim eventually to be able to talk no differently under delay than he does when no delay is present. He should not be using the "DAF voice." Through training in selective attention, a marked carry-over in fluency to ordinary speaking occurs. Some of our stutterers almost became addicted to the DAF apparatus. We have seen them using it intensively before phoning a girl to ask for a date and so on. Nevertheless, we say we do not encourage this depen-

dence. By fading out the delay in gradual steps, it is possible to teach the stutterer to monitor his speech primarily by somosthesia even when he is not hooked up to the apparatus.

All therapists have long desired better ways of getting carry-over from the laboratory or clinic into real life speaking situations. It is our impression that this proprioceptive-tactile-kinesthetic monitoring transfers very easily, probably because normal speakers seem to rely primarily upon it rather than upon self hearing for their temporal programming of motoric speech.

It is also possible that a stutterer who could free himself from his morbid concern with how he sounds could also escape being controlled by the unfortunate learning experiences to which he has been subjected, most of which involve auditory or visual cues in the conditioning. If he has some basic coordinative difficulty, more somosthetic controls should help. Or, if there exists some perceptual problem due to blockage of phonation or other asynchrony produced by distorted sidetone, then training in somosthetic monitoring might be able to bypass these possible precipitants. Finally, if the stuttering has a neurotic origin, the new concentration on the awareness of the self and the responsibility for its control could have some value. We hold no brief for any of these speculative reasons for employing DAF in therapy. It is enough for us that we find it to be a highly effective clinical tool.

Let us also mention a few other uses of delayed auditory feedback. If we employ very long delay times, a segment of stuttering behavior can be recycled and, during the long delay, the stutterer can attempt to cancel or modify the behavior thus vivifying the contrasts involved. We have also explored using DAF in conjunction with videotaping in this way. As the stutterer watches himself stuttering and modifying the behavior in a cancellation process, we ask him to duplicate what he is seeing but to improve upon it. By replaying the videotaped DAF stuttering and its cancellation several times, the stutterer learns very swiftly to adopt new and more fluent ways of stuttering in ordinary communication. We have also required the stutterer (primarily one with clonic or repetitive stuttering behaviors) to fake one of his repetitive blocks and to keep it from becoming uncontrollable, inhibiting the recycling at the therapist's signal. DAF therapy permits stutterers to have successful experiences in controlling the uncontrollable.

One of the interesting discoveries in recent research is that by MacKay (1968) mentioned earlier who found that a person's vulnerability to DAF correlated negatively with his maximum speech rate, i.e., those stutterers whose *maximum* speech rates were slow tended to show more stutterings under DAF than those subjects who could at times speak very swiftly. We have been doing some exploring to see if it is possible to train stutterers to speak at much faster rates of speech (not in conversation but only in the training sessions) to see if increasing the maximum rate of utterance might not only reduce the amount of stuttering on DAF but elsewhere. In this connection it is said that the American TV entertainer, Gary Moore, claimed that once he had learned to speak incredibly fast, his stuttering at ordinary rates disappeared. Most stutterers however find it very difficult to maintain fast rates of speech for any length of time even when alone. Ingham and Andrews (1972) in a series of experiments dealing with the effectiveness of various forms of therapy used both amplified synchronous auditory feedback and delayed feedback finding that both conditions decreased the frequency of stuttering in a small number of subjects, though the DAF produced a marked slowing of speech rate. They make a strong point that any treatment resulting in abnormally slow speech will not be an effective one. "Stutter-free speech that is still tied to a rate of under 100 words per minute is not fluent speech." They stress that the reduction in the frequency of stuttering should be paralleled by a corresponding increase in rate.

These observations and experiences indicate that the use of delayed auditory feedback as a clinical tool holds some promise. Portable units resembling a hearing aid, some models of which we have tested, have not as yet proved themselves sufficiently flexible or powerful or durable enough for general clinical use but they will come.

Bibliography

ADAMCZYK, B. (Use of instruments for the production of artificial feedback in the treatment of stuttering), *Folia Phoniatrica*, 11 (1959), 216–18.

————, (Correction of Speech in Stutterers by Means of a Telephone with the Use of an Artificial Echo), *Otolaryngologia Polska*, 17 (1963), 482–84.

AGNELLO, J. G. and M. A. BUXTON, Effects of resonance and time of stutterers and nonstutterers speech under delayed auditory feedback, National Institute of Mental Health, 1968, H.E.W. Project No. 11067–01.

AGNELLO, J. C. and H. C. KAGAN, *Delayed Auditory Feedback and Its Effect on the Manner of Speech Production.* National Institute of Mental Health, 1966, H.E.W. Grant No. 11067–01.

AIMARD, P., A. PLANTIER,, and M. WIT-
TLING, Le begaiement, çontribution
a l'etude de l'audition et de l'integration phonetique, *Rev. Laryngol.*
(Bordeauz), 87 (1965), 254–56.

ANDREWS, G. and R. J. INGHAM, The effect
of alterations in auditory feedback
with special reference to synchronous
auditory feedback, unpublished paper, 1971.

ASP, C. W., An investigation of the locali-
zation of interaural stimulation by
clicks and the reading times of stutterers and non-stutterers under monaural sidestone conditions, *De Therapia vocis et Loquelae,* 2 (1965), 353–
55.

ATKINSON, C. J., Adaptation to delayed
sidetone, *Journal of Speech and
Hearing Disorders,* 18 (1953), 386–91.

BACHRACH, D. L., Sex differences in reactions to delayed auditory feedback,
Perceptual and Motor Skills, 19
(1964), 81–82.

BACKE, L., Delayed feedback og stamming,
*Nordisk Tidsskrift for Tale og
Stemme,* 25 (1965), 54.

BARR, D. F. and N. R. CARMEL, Stuttering
inhibition with high-frequency narrow-band masking noise, *Journal of
Auditory Research,* 9 (1969), 40–44.

BEAUMONT, J. and B. Foss, Individual differences in reacting to delayed auditory feedback, *British Journal of Psychology,* 48 (1957), 85–89.

BEREDAY, G. Z. F., W. W. BRICKMAN, and
G. H. READ (eds.), *The Changing
Soviet School.* Boston: Houghton-
Mifflin, 1960.

BLACK, J., The effect of sidetone delay
upon vocal rate and intensity, *Journal of Speech Disorders,* 16 (1951),
50–56.

BOHR, J. W. F., The effects of electronic
and other external control methods
on stuttering: A review of some research techniques and suggestions for
further research, *Journal of South
African Logopedic Society,* 10 (1963),
4–13.

BURKE, B. D., Reduced auditory feedback
and stuttering, *Behaviour Research
and Therapy,* 7 (1969), 303–8.

BUTLER, R. R. Jr. and P. E. STANLEY, The
stuttering problem considered from
an automatic control point of view,
Folia Phoniatrica, 18 (1966), 33–44.

BUXTON, L. F., An investigation of sex and
age differences in speech behavior
under delayed auditory feedback, *Dissertation Abstracts,* 29 (1969), 904.

CHASE, R. A., Effect of delayed auditory
feedback on the repetition of speech
sounds, *Journal of Speech and Hearing Disorders,* 23 (1958), 583–90.

CHERRY, E. C. and B. M. SAYERS, Experiments on the total inhibition of stammering by external control, and some
clinical results, *Journal of Psychosomatic Research,* 1 (1956), 233–46.

————, S. SUTTON, D. FIRST, and J.
ZUBIN, A developmental study of
changes in behavior under delayed
auditory feedback, *Journal of Genetic
Psychology,* 99 (1961), 101–12.

CHERRY, E., B. M. SAYERS, and P. MAR-
LAND, Some experiments on the total
suppression of stammering; and a report on some clinical trials, *Bulletin
of the British Psychological Society,*
30 (1956), 43–44.

COHEN, J. G. and A. E. EDWARDS, The ex-
traexperimental effects of Random
sidetones, *Proceedings of Annual
Convention of American Psychological Association,* 6 (1965), 211–12.

CURLEE, R. F. and W. H. PERKINS, Conversational rate control therapy for stuttering, *Journal of Speech and Hearing Disorders,* 34 (1969), 245–50.

DENES, L., Diagnostik und therapie der
functionellen stimmund sprachstörungen mit ausschaltung des gehoers,
*Proceedings IVth Congress Interna-
tional Association of Logopedics and
Phoniatrics,* Berlin, 1931.

DERAZNE, J., Speech pathology in the
U.S.S.R., in R. W. Rieber and R. S.
Brubaker (eds.), *Speech Pathology.*
Amsterdam: North Holland, 1966.

DONOVAN, G. E., A new device for the
treatment of stuttering, *British Jour-*

nal of Disorders of Communication, 6
(1971), 86–88.

FAIRBANKS, G. and N. GUTTMAN, Effects of
delayed auditory feedback upon
articulation, Journal of Speech and
Hearing Research, 1 (1958), 12–22.

FREUND, H., Der induktive vorgang im
stottern und seine therapeutische
verwertung, Zeitschrift fur Neurologie
und Psychiatrie, 141 (1932), 180–92.

————, Psychopathology and the Problems of Stuttering, Springfield, Ill.:
Charles C Thomas, 1966.

FROESCHELS, E., A survey of European
literature in speech and voice pathology, Asha, 4 (1962), 172–81.

GOLDIAMOND, I., Stuttering and fluency
as manipulatable operant response
classes, in L. Krasner and L. P. Ullman (eds.), Research in Behavior
Modification. New York: Holt, Rinehart & Winston, 1965.

————, C. J. ATKINSON, and R. C.
BILGER, Stabilization of behavior and
prolonged exposure to delayed auditory feedback, Science, 137 (1962),
437–38.

GRUBER, L., Sensory feedback and stuttering, Journal of Speech and Hearing
Disorders, 30 (1965), 378–80.

HAM, R. and M. D. STEER, Certain effects
of alterations in auditory feedback,
Folia Phoniatrica, 19 (1967), 53–62.

HANLEY, C. N., W. R. TIFFANY, and J. M.
BRUNGARD, Skin resistance changes
accompanying the side-tone test for
auditory malingering, Journal of
Speech and Hearing Research, 1
(1958), 286–93.

IMHOFER, R. (Pathogenisis of Stammering: Neurosis of Expectation), Med.
Klin., 23 (1927), 628–31.

INGHAM, R. J. and G. ANDREWS, The
quality of fluency after treatment,
Journal of Communicative Disorders,
5 (1972), 91–117.

KERN, A., Der einfluss des hoerens auf
das stottern, Archiv. Psychiatrie
Nervenkr., 97 (1932), 429–49.

KLEIN, M. E., Anti-stuttering device and

methods, United States Patent No.
3,349,179, Oct. 24, 1967.

LANGOVA, J. and M. MORAVEK (Experimental study on stuttering and
stammering), Casopis Lekaru Ceskych,
101 (1962), 297–300.

————, Some results of experimental
examinations among stutterers and
clutterers, Folia Phoniatrica, 16
(1964), 290–96.

LEE, B. S., Artificial stutterer, Journal of
Speech and Hearing Disorders, 16
(1951), 53–55.

LOGUE, L., The effects of temporal alterations in auditory feedback upon the
speech output of stutterers and nonstutterers, Unpublished Masters Thesis, Purdue University, 1962.

LOTZMANN, G. (On the use of varied delay times in stammerers), Folia
Phoniatrica, 13 (1961), 276–310.

MACKAY, D. G., Metamorphosis of a
critical interval: Age-linked changes
in the delay in auditory feedback
that produces maximal disruption of
speech, Journal of the Acoustical Society of America, 19 (1968), 811–21.

————, To speak with an accent: Effects of nasal distortion on stuttering
under delayed auditory feedback,
Perceptual Psychophysics, 5 (1969),
183–88.

MAHAFFEY, R. B. and C. STROMSTA, The
effects of auditory feedback as a
function of frequency, intensity,
time and sex, De Therapia vocis et
Loquelae, 2 (1965), 233–35.

MARAIST, J. A. and C. HUTTON, Effects
of auditory masking upon the speech
of stutterers, Journal of Speech Disorders, 22 (1957), 385.

MARLAND, P., Shadowing — a contribution
to the treatment of stuttering, Folia
Phoniatrica, 9 (1957), 242–45.

MARTIN, J. E., The signal detection hypothesis and perceptual defect theory
of stuttering, Journal of Speech and
Hearing Disorders, 35 (1970), 252–55.

MAY, A. E. and A. HACKWOOD, Some effects of masking and eliminating low
frequency feedback on the speech of

stutterers, *Behaviour Research and Therapy*, 6 (1968), 219–23.

MEYER-EPLER, W. and R. LUCHSINGER, Beobachtungen bei der verzögerten ruckkupplung der sprache, *Folia Phoniatrica*, 7 (1955), 87–99.

MORAVEK, M. and J. LANGOVA, Hearing and auditory feedback in stutterers, *Proceedings Congress of Otolaryngology*, Prague, 1964.

————, Some electrophysiological findings among stutterers and clutterers, *Folia Phoniatrica*, 14 (1962), 305–16.

————, Patofyziologie zachvatu kohtavsti, *Casopia Lekaru Ceskych*, 107 (1968), 536–38.

————, Sensorische rückkoppelung beim stottern, *De Therapia Vocis et Loquellae*, 1 (1965), 429–32.

MURRAY, F. P., An investigation of variably induced white noise upon moments of stuttering, *Journal of Communication Disorders*, 2 (1969), 109–14.

MYSAK, E. D., Servo theory and stuttering, *Journal of Speech and Hearing Disorders*, 25 (1960), 188–95.

————, *Speech Pathology and Feedback Theory*. Springfield, Ill.: Charles C Thomas, 1966.

NEELLEY, J. N., A study of the speech behavior of stutterers and nonstutterers under normal and delayed auditory feedback, *Journal of Speech and Hearing Disorders Monograph Supplement*, 7 (1961), 63–82.

———— and R. J. TIMMONS, Adaptation and consistency in the disfluent speech behavior of young stutterers and nonstutterers, *Journal of Speech and Hearing Research*, 10 (1967), 250–56.

NEIMARK, E. Z., The treatment of the stuttering neurosis on the basis of the physiological interpretation of its mechanisms, in Robert E. West (ed.), *Russian Translations in Speech and Hearing*. Washington, D.C.: American Speech and Hearing Association, 1968, pp. 333–35.

NESSEL, E., Die verzogerts sprachruckklop-

plung (Lee-effect) bei der stotterern, *Folia Phoniatrica*, 10 (1958), 199–04.

NOVAK, A. and M. PETRICK, The influence of frequency-modified Lee effects on the speech of stutterers, *De Therapia Vocis et Loquellae*, 1 (1965), 425–27.

PARKER, C. S. and F. CHRISTOPHERSON, Electronic aid in treatment of stammer, *Medical Electronics and Biological Engineering*, 1 (1963), 121–25.

PERKINS, W. H. and R. F. CURLEE, Clinical impressions of portable masking unit Effects in stuttering, *Journal of Speech and Hearing Disorders*, 34 (1969), 360–62.

PETKOV, D. and I. IOSIFOV, Our experiences in treatment of stuttering in a speech rehabilitation colony, *Zhurnal Nevropatologii i Psikhistrii imeni S. S. Korsakova*, 40 (1960), 903–4.

RAWNSLEY, A. I. and J. D. HARRIS, Comparative analysis of normal speech and speech with delayed sidetone by means of sound spectrograms, U.S.N. Submarine Research Laboratory Reports, 13 (1954), No. 248.

RAZDOL'SKII, V. A., State of speech of stammerers when alone, *Zhurnal Nevropatologii i Psikhiatrii imeni S. S. Korsakova*, 65 (1965), 1717–20.

RYAN, B. P., The use of DAF in the establishment of fluent reading and speaking in six stutterers, Convention Paper, American Speech and Hearing Association, Denver, 1968.

SHANE, M. L. S., Effect on stuttering of alteration in auditory feedback, in W. Johnson (ed.), *Stuttering in Children and Adults*. Minneapolis: University of Minnesota Press, 1955.

SHRUM, W. F., A comparison of the effects of masking noise and increased vocal intensity on the frequency of stuttering, *Asha*, 4 (1962), 408.

SKLAR, B., A feedback model of the stuttering problem—an engineer's view, *Journal of Speech and Hearing Disorders*, 34 (1969), 226–30.

SMITH, K., *Delayed Sensory Feedback*. Philadelphia: Saunders, 1962.

SMITH, K. U., M. MYSZIEWSKI, M. MERGEN,

and J. JOEHLER, Computer systems control of delayed auditory feedback, *Perceptual Motor Skills,* 17 (1963), 343–54.

SODERBERG, G. A., Delayed auditory feedback and stuttering, *Journal of Speech and Hearing Disorders,* 33 (1968), 260–66.

————, Delayed auditory feedback and the speech of stutterers, *Journal of Speech and Hearing Disorders,* 34 (1969), 20–29.

STROMSTA, C., The effects of altering the fundamental frequency of masking on the speech performance of stutterers, *Technical Report,* National Institutes of Health, Project B-1331, 1958.

————, A spectographic study of dysfluencies labeled as stuttering by parents, *De Therapia Vocis et Loquellae,* 1 (1965), 317–20.

————, Delays associated with certain sidetone pathways, *Journal of Acoustical Society of America,* 34 (1962), 392–96.

————, Experimental Blockage of Phonation by Distorted Sidetone, *Journal of Speech and Hearing Research,* 2 (1959), 286–301.

SUTTON, S. and R. CHASE, White noise and stuttering, *Journal of Speech and Hearing Research,* 4 (1961), 72.

TIFFANY, W. R. and C. HANLEY, Adaptation to delayed sidetone, *Journal of Speech and Hearing Disorders,* 21 (1956), 164–72.

TOMATIS, A., *L'Oreille et le Language.* Paris: Editions du Senil, 1963.

————, Recherches sue la pathologie du begaiement, *Journal Francaise O.R.L.,* 3 (1954), 382–87.

TROTTER, W. D., and M. M. LESCH, Personal experiences with a stutter-aid, *Journal of Speech and Hearing Disorders,* 32 (1967), 270–72.

VAN RIPER, C., Clinical use of intermittent masking noise in stuttering therapy, *Asha,* 7 (1965), 381.

————, *The Nature of Stuttering.* Englewood Cliffs, N.J.: Prentice-Hall, 1971.

————, The use of DAF in stuttering Therapy, *British Journal of Disorders of Communication,* 5 (1970), 40–45.

WEBSTER, R. L. and M. F. DORMAN, Decrease in stuttering frequency as a function of continuous and contingent forms of auditory masking, *Journal of Speech and Hearing Research,* 13 (1970), 82–86.

WEBSTER, R. L., and B. B. LUBKER, Masking of auditory feedback in stutterer's speech, *Journal of Speech and Hearing Research,* 11 (1968), 219–23.

WINCHESTER, R. A. and E. W. GIBBONS, Relative effectiveness of three modes of delayed side tone presentation, *Acta Otolaryngology,* 65 (1957), 275–79.

———— and D. F. KREBS, Adaptation to sustained delayed sidetone, *Journal of Speech and Hearing Disorders,* 24 (1959), 25–28.

WINGATE, M. E., Effect on stuttering of changes in audition, *Journal of Speech and Hearing Research,* 13 (1970), 861–73.

WOLF, A. A. and E. G. WOLF, Feedback processes in the theory of certain speech disorders, *Speech Pathology and Therapy,* 2 (1959), 48–55.

YATES, A. J., Delayed auditory feedback and shadowing, *Quarterly Journal of Experimental Psychology,* 17 (1965), 125–31.

————, Delayed auditory feedback, *Psychological Bulletin,* 60 (1963a), 213–32.

————, Recent empirical and theoretical approaches to the experimental manipulation of speech in normal subjects and stammerers, *Behavior and Research Therapy,* 1 (1963b), 95–119.

ZERNERI, L., Tentatives d'application de la voix retardeé (delayed speech feedback) dans la therapie du begaiement, *Journal Francaise O.R.L.,* 15 (1966), 415–18.

ZINKIN, N. I., *Mechanisms of Speech.* The Hague: Mouton, 1968.

Psychotherapies, Drugs,

and

Group Therapies

CHAPTER 6

Psychotherapy

Many of the forms of treatment which we have described in preceding chapters of this text might have been included in the present one on psychotherapy. The following quotation by Watkins (1965) is illustrative: ". . . one form of psychotherapy, suggestion, has probably been used to treat more cases of illness than all the other therapeutic agents put together, throughout the entire history of mankind (p. 457)." The term psychotherapy seems to resemble a very large, circus tent-like structure housing a very large and motley collection of rationales and techniques (including also a few freaks). The precise definition of what we mean by psychotherapy is very difficult to achieve, but its aims are fairly universal: to

relieve distressing anxiety and its related symptoms, to develop self-esteem and social adequacy, and to increase the person's ability to tolerate stress. Some speech pathologists have felt that they should not and must not do any form of psychotherapy with stutterers. It is our view that they are deluded because they have no choice in the matter. They will do some psychotherapy whether they wish to or not.

Psychotherapy in one form or another is an ancient art but it has had only a short history. Long before the Christian era, the priests and oracles of Greece counseled their patients as they reclined on the stone couches of the temples, thus anticipating the couch procedure of classical psychoanalysis and, as we have seen in our chapter on the punishment therapies,

140

during the Middle Ages various kinds of shock treatment were used on those whose bizarre behavior seemed to be the sign of demonic possession.[1]

Many of the older writers on stuttering such as Moses Mendelsohn, Schulthess, Merkel, Wyneken and Sandow (most of them stutterers themselves), showed remarkable insights into the psychopathology of stuttering and built some supportive psychotherapy into their treatment. Nevertheless, psychotherapy as we know it today began in the 1890s with the work of Freud.

Is formal psychotherapy needed?

We have said that some psychotherapy is inherent in almost any kind of stuttering therapy. Here we consider whether or not it should serve as the sole or dominant focus of treatment. As one might expect in a disorder characterized by anxiety, by symptoms which often look symbolic, by apparent compulsivity and certainly by socially unacceptable behaviors, there are those who insist that stuttering is clearly a neurosis and that psychotherapy must therefore be the only appropriate way to treat it. For example, Glauber (1958) declares ". . . it is impossible for stutterers, as for other patients with phobias, on their own consciously and regularly to resist phobias through will power.

[1] A stutterer who came to us from Arabia for treatment told us that in his religion, God was in you when you were highly aware of yourself and in control but that, when you were not, Al Kohol, the devil incarnate inhabited your skin. He said that epileptics, persons with cerebral palsy, and stutterers were viewed by the uneducated as being posessed by the devil and accordingly were severely penalized and rejected. "Women would take their children and flee in mortal terror when they heard me stutter."

They can be resolved by means of psychoanalysis alone (p. 110)." In opposition to such an opinion, we find Froeschels (1951) writing, "The days of cathartic psychoanalysis are over. One does not believe any longer that remembering alone of formerly repressed thoughts and emotions may result in a cure or even an improvement." He insists that speech therapy should certainly be tried first and that if psychotherapy is done with certain rare cases, it should be used either in combination with speech therapy or should follow it. Barbara, Goldart, and Oram (1961) do not agree. They say:

Stuttering is to be considered not as an isolated disorder of the speech mechanism, but as the outward expression of a more basic character disorganization. Any effective treatment must also be directed toward helping the individual to understand his particular neurotic difficulties, with their neurotic solutions, and to arrive at some resolution of the underlying conflicts. (p. 46)

Those who are so certain that formal psychotherapy is the only appropriate method for treating stuttering are those who believe very strongly that stutterers as a group differ from normal speakers in their personality structure and traits—in short, that they are neurotics. The many researches that have been performed to test this assumption have been critically scrutinized by Goodstein (1958), Sheehan (1958), and Van Riper (1971b), and all three of these reviewers came to the same conclusion—that the research does not support the belief that stutterers differ from normal speakers in basic personality structure and that they do differ from those who have been classified as neurotics. If this is true, then do stutterers really need psychotherapy? Sheehan (1970) states his position vividly:

To say that stutterers need psychotherapy or can profit from it is like saying that people need psychotherapy or can profit from it. As Wendell Johnson reminded us, stutterers are people. If we are to recommend psychotherapy routinely for stuttering, we may as well tap each person we meet on the street and recommend psychotherapy. (p. 132)

We are not prepared to go as far as Sheehan in this crucial matter. Most of the researchers used tests designed to ferret out the indications of what we would term primary neuroses of the classical sort and even for them these instruments are far from being entirely satisfactory. We feel there are neurotic features shown by many confirmed stutterers that arise *as the result* of the stuttering and its consequent communicative frustration and social rejection. We believe that there can be secondary as well as primary neuroses and that the kind usually displayed by stutterers is a secondary neurosis though we also find a few cases in which both primary and secondary forms are present.

Freund (1966) points out that there exists a group of neurotic disorders among which are included writer's cramp, stage fright, some forms of sexual impotence, and other similar problems that differ essentially from the classical forms of neurosis.

All these forms of expectancy neurotic disturbances have as a common characteristic that they are based upon actual "primary" traumatic experiences of failure in the performance of a learned skill or simple motor or sensory act, often though not necessarily, in socially embarrassing situations. The anticipation of their dreaded recurrence leads, then via inhibition, etc., to the establishment of a vicious spiral. In opposition to the pho-

bias, the dread here is not of a symbolic nature but based upon actual experience. (p. 37)

Earlier we have met similar concepts in the Rand and Kern types of neurosis posited by Schultz (1964) and by Fernau-Horn (1969). Freund's description of the distinctions between the neurotic features of stuttering and those of other recognized neuroses is illuminating. Moreover, he shows that many current concepts of stuttering may well be included under this rubric.

Today some of the leading American students of stuttering seem close to the concept of "expectancy neurosis," though under different names and using different frames of reference. Johnson (1956) who refuses to call stuttering a "neurosis" defines it as an "anticipatory apprehensive hypertonic avoidance reaction;" Bloodstein (1958) calls it an "anticipatory struggle reaction;" Van Riper (1955) and Sheehan (1954) view it under the heading of an "approach-avoidance" conflict, which naturally presupposes the anticipation of the approaching "difficulty." (pp. 49–50)

Perhaps again the problem is merely one of nomenclature and definition. The confirmed stutterer does show excessive anxiety even though it is primarily speech anxiety, and not the generalized free-floating anxiety often characteristic of most so-called neuroses. He shows inappropriate motor behaviors in his attack upon his feared words. He displays many situational and word fears and avoidance reactions. His attitudes toward social interaction often seem morbid. Whether we call them neurotic or not these features of the disorder require some help from the therapist if they are to be changed or ameliorated. And if the therapist tries to do something about them, he may be said to be doing some kind of psychotherapy. The term psychotherapy, once rigidly confined to classical psychoanalysis, has become elastic enough to cover a host of procedures ranging all the way from exhortation and advice to reciprocal inhibition. Most of them, as we shall see, have been applied to stuttering.

What type of psychotherapy should be used with stutterers?

This, of course, is a meaningless question to some practitioners who are so blinded by theoretical bias that they fail to recognize the variability in individuals who stutter and the limitations of their own points of view and practices. The field of psychotherapy is presently in great flux. Classical psychoanalysis has been for some years under direct attack. Both its theory and effectiveness have been challenged from many sectors. Rogerian counseling is similarly threatened by the behavior therapists who regard it as merely an inefficient and unsystematized shaping process involving differential reinforcement by the counselor of certain classes of the client's verbal behaviors. Again, deviation from and modifications of orthodox Freudian theory have led to so many innovations in practice that it is impossible even to talk about psychoanalysis without specifying a name and theoretical position. What kind of psychotherapy would be recommended for the stutterer: Sullivan's, Horney's, Adler's, Jung's, Alexander's, Roger's, Wolpe's, Frankl's, Perl's, Ellis's, Salter's, whose? We can not discuss psychotherapy without describing the kind of therapeutic strategies employed. Are they active–passive, individual–group, supportive–reconstructive, nondirective–directive, reality therapy, logotherapy, gestalt

therapy, release therapy? The list seems endless. When a speech therapist has to refer a stutterer to someone else for psychotherapy, he should know something about the kind of approach that will be employed as well as something about the nature of the stutterer's emotional problems which make that referral necessary. And certainly he should know something about the psychotherapist.

It is probable that any individual stutterer might profit to some degree from any of the myriad kinds of psychotherapeutic methods now available, but it is unlikely that he would profit equally from each approach. For example, although our review of the research has indicated that the majority of stutterers do not show the patterns of behavior characteristic of severe psychopathology, we always find a few of them who do. We once had referred to us as a stutterer a girl of 20 who initiated almost every speech attempt after a pause with a hypertensed eye-closing, mouth shutting, hand and foot clenching, and a simultaneous constriction (so she reported) of the vagina and anus. In the throes of her hard blocking she would sometimes even squat. We were able to interest a famous analyst in this person and three years later, all the bizarre behavior had disappeared and she spoke fairly fluently albeit with an excessive amount of unforced syllabic repetitions. We doubt very much that any treatment other than long-term deep psychotherapy might have helped this person. When one fishes for whales, it is not wise to use a fly-rod.

What we are saying is that the kind of emotional problems presented by the stutterer should dictate the kind of psychotherapy that he should have. Most of the adult stutterers seen in college and university speech clinics do not seem to show the kinds of behaviors illustrated by the girl in the case just described. They are intelligent, fairly verbal despite their blockings, and within the normal range on most of our personality tests. But there are others who show profound disturbances and deep emotional conflicts. In these persons, the stuttering is woven into the basic fabric of their personalities and life styles.[2] In our experience, the supportive and counseling forms of psychotherapy do not seem to be able to help these people. The so-called reconstructive kinds of psychotherapy sometimes can. Among them is psychoanalysis.

Psychoanalysis

Most speech therapists have an elementary understanding of the Freudian principles which underlie psychoanalysis and we see no necessity for summarizing them here. Fortunately in the literature there are also enough accounts of its application to stuttering to help us know what our stutterers will experience if we refer them for such treatment. It will be expensive; it will be long-term, perhaps three years or longer. The stutterers in analysis will explore their past and present through free association, dream interpretation, and the analysis of their behaviors and resistances both overt and covert. They will undergo catharsis, transference, aberection, and many other unnerving experiences. Hopefully new insights, which help them to understand why they feel and behave as they do in terms of their past, will also enable them to live more adaptively in the present.

In traditional Freudian psychoanalysis, the therapist does not reveal himself as a person but rather serves

2 We hate to use this kind of language but have no other which seems adequate.

as a therapeutic mirror in which the patient can perceive him as his own parental or other significant figure and, by so doing, discover and relive the early traumatic experiences which are the sources of his present difficulties. The analyst listens to the flood of verbalized memories and feelings. Occasionally the analyst may interpret to the patient the meanings of his transference feelings or resistances or projections, always seeking to bring repressed material up into consciousness, where it can be reexperienced. The aim is to have the patient understand in terms of his past *why* he now feels and behaves as he does. With these new insights he is enabled to react more appropriately.

Most orthodox psychoanalysts seem to consider stuttering to be a pregenital conversion neurosis based upon oral or anal fixations. Some of these such as Coriat (1931) and Stein (1949) emphasize the oral component. Stein writes:

The stammerer unconsciously wishes to remain a suckling. The patient, owing to anxiety, unconsciously reverts to the suckling stage and so replaces consonants with clicks. He can release these but fails to release or join them to the vowel. (p. 118)

Coriat, who insists that stutterers should not smoke nor chew gum because these may foster the already morbid oral pleasure, says:

When a stammerer attempts to talk, the mouth movements are the persistence into maturity of the original sucking and biting lip-nipple activities of infancy. In this connection it is also significant that the labials (p. b, m) which are usually the most difficult sounds for stammerers to enunciate, are also among the earliest sounds made by children. The physiological lip movements utilized to produce these sounds are the same movements employed in nursing at the mother's breast or in sucking at the rubber nipple of the nursing bottle. The stammerer, therefore, in the course of his development, has not successfully overcome this early nursing phase, but remains fixed at this infantile stage of oral tendency which inflexibly binds the individual to the sucking and biting period of infantile oral erotic gratification.

Other analysts emphasize the anal-erotic or anal-sadistic features of the neurosis. Thus Brun (1923) claims that the repressed pleasure from an anal infantile fixation is transformed into coprolalia according to the following scheme: (1) dirty talk is forbidden; (2) one is not quite sure that a nasty word might not escape all the same. There is no solution except to be entirely silent. Since speaking must be maintained, it must be also checked. The repression thus only partially succeeds and so stammering results. Fenichel (1933) offers a more sophisticated presentation based on anal sadism:

The anal-sadistic significance of the symptom of stuttering is also in keeping with the typically anal-sadistic personality make-up of the stutterer. The momentous regression (or arrest of development) is not limited (to the stuttering).

In a later passage, Fenichel (1945) does not sound very optimistic about psychoanalytic therapy for stutterers:

Concerning psychoanalytic therapy for stutterers, the main difficulty is that the function of speech is disturbed, and talking is the very instrument of psychoanalysis. But this is not the only difficulty that has to be overcome. Having gone through a pathogenic regression to the anal-sadistic level, stutterers in general present the same difficulties in analysis as do compulsion neurotics. The prognosis for such analyses, therefore, is in general the same as in compulsion neuroses. When stam-

mering represents a rather simple "inhibited state" the prognosis is much more favorable, and quick cures have been reported. The deeply pregenital types of stuttering are as difficult to influence as are other pregenital neuroses. However, it is a favorable fact that the symptom of stuttering itself can often be eliminated before the underlying pregenital elements are thoroughly worked through in analysis. In general psychoanalytic treatment should be advised, and a trial analysis undertaken with the same caution as in a compulsion neurosis. (p. 317)

Glauber (1953, 1958, 1968), a more modern proponent of the psychoanalytic treatment of stuttering finds both oral and anal elements in the neurosis and attributes them to mother-child relationships and dependency needs. The hesitancy in stuttering is seen as the symptomatic resolution of the wish to speak and not to speak. A statement of Glauber's (1943) position is as follows:

The profound craving for oral dependence on mother—subjectively felt as Omnipotence—is regarded by the ego as a threat to its integration or very life. It regards it as an oral aggression upon itself and reacts by wishes to retaliate in kind. Besides, it is itself identified with aggression. When this psychic ambivalence is viewed from the standpoint of its somatic expression, we see that speech and respiration, which "take in" the environment, express this oral dependence and oral aggression. (p. 177)

Glauber feels that psychoanalytic therapy cannot be used with all persons who stutter since some do not meet the essential requirements. They may be too young; they may lack sufficient motivation; they may remain too passive; they may continually sabotage by "acting out" outside the therapy room; they may refuse to relinquish the secondary gains which the symptoms confer. For some of these stutterers Glauber recommends an analytically oriented psychotherapy. This differs from analysis proper in that there is more direct ego support, the therapy relationship is utilized rather than analyzed, and the goals of therapy are more limited.

The psychoanalytic literature dealing with stuttering is fairly large but only a small portion of it deals with therapy. Perhaps the most accessible and insightful examples of the sort of emotional material produced by stutterers undergoing analysis are those found in the chapter entitled "The Unspeakable Feelings of Stutterers" by L. E. Travis in his *Handbook of Speech Pathology* (1957).[3] We provide one brief excerpt:

Suddenly I see my father and I hate him. He's responsible for me having no husband, no home, and no children. Now I see my hairline structure (pubic hair) and it doesn't disgust me anymore. I'm riding nude on a bare-back horse and the horse becomes my father and I hate him and I hate you too, terribly, sitting there coldly trying to figure me out in a professional way. I lie here on the defensive. I've been belching him up for years, my hate for him. I don't need to stutter him up any more. Through lip service I was supposed to love him but I didn't. I was lying. It was sinful to hate your father. It was a commandment to love thy father and thy mother. This lie I stuttered. (p. 938)

How successful is psychoanalysis with stutterers? One of Freud's early patients, Frau Emmy, had a good many problems and one of them was a sort of stuttering, a disorder which had begun in adulthood. Although Freud was able to help her solve

[3] A friend of ours, a psychoanalyst, commented that the chapter was mislabeled, that it should be worded "The Unspeakable Feelings of Everyone."

them, we have several reports indicating that he didn't feel that psychoanalysis was an appropriate method for treating stutterers.[4] Nevertheless we have accounts of successful psychoanalytic therapy with some individual stutterers, most of whom were either children (who might have overcome it anyway) or persons whose stuttering began in adulthood or at least much later than its usual onset (perhaps indicating a possible hysterical origin). We know of no outcome studies which involved any controls.

Even in the treatment of the traditional neuroses, psychoanalysis has been under strong attack. The efficacy of its therapy has been especially challenged by behavioral modifiers such as Wolpe and Eysenck. Eysenck's review (1952) showed that the results of psychoanalysis were not much better than those methods which used simple reassurance, suggestion or persuasion and Wolpe (1961) cites a number of follow-up studies that demonstrate the relative ineffectiveness of psychoanalysis. Although the author of the present text has himself undergone orthodox psychoanalytic treatment, and has profited from the experience in many ways, he is far from being convinced that it alone is an effective way of attacking the problem of stuttering.

Other analytic therapies. Freud constantly revised his theories and practices during the course of his long career to such an extent that he could be said to be less Freudian than many of his orthodox followers. Sev-

[4] According to Glauber (1958) Freud allegedly told Esti Freud that "the psychoanalytic method offered neither insight nor help in this disorder," and Froeschels (1951) says, "I quote in this connection Freud himself who in a private talk admitted that he has given up treating stutterers for he has not succeeded in a single case."

eral of his students, notably Adler, Rank, and Jung, created their own psychoanalytic systems, each of which has had considerable influence on modern psychotherapy. Adler stressed the drive toward power and status as being more important than sexual drives. His concepts of the inferiority complex, the ego ideal and the patient's life style have been especially important. Many Adlerian psychotherapists have been interested in stuttering and perhaps the most influential of these was Appelt (1929) whose book *Stammering and Its Permanent Cure* served as a basic text for some years.

Jung also made many contributions, some very mystical such as his concepts of the collective unconscious mind, and inherited archetypes from mankind's primordial past, but he also emphasized the need to build a unique, integrated individuality. Jung and Adler both freed the patient from the psychoanalytic couch, feeling that direct confrontation with the therapist was more helpful. Rank's major effects on modern psychotherapy can be seen in his emphasis upon the present rather than the past and in the importance he placed upon the client's will and responsibility for becoming whole and well. All these men influenced later psychotherapists who had to deal with stuttering.

One variant psychoanalytic approach was formulated by Karen Horney (1939) and it has had considerable influence on the psychotherapy of stuttering. Horney felt that though early childhood experiences determined the unique character of the personality type and could predispose the person to neurosis, the essential conflicts which had to be resolved were due to cultural influences involving such human relationships as those due to the constant competition for power and status, the need for independence in a world which constantly controls our activities, and the need for love in an environment which is often hostile. She believed that neurotic anxiety is the result of the "basic hostility" generated in the early relationships between parent and child and thereafter projected upon others. She felt that much of our alienation from others and from ourselves is due to this anxiety and hostility. Horney makes much of the "tyranny of the shoulds," showing how driven we are to achieve impossibly ideal selves in the hope that this achievement will free us from negative emotion.

Horney has had a strong influence on the kind of psychotherapy used with stutterers as illustrated especially in the prolific works of Dominick Barbara (1954, 1957, 1962). His psychotherapy, though it employs dream analysis, and free association, also employs direct questioning in the "spontaneous give-and-take of ideas, feelings and beliefs . . . in an atmosphere where satisfactory exchange can take place (1962, p. 264)." The therapist is less passive than in orthodox psychoanalysis. He observes and listens carefully, but also participates actively in exploring not only the past but also the present conflicts and feelings. Barbara feels that the function of psychotherapy is to reveal and attack the various blockages other than those of speech which characterize the stutterer. The stutterer is helped to confront not only the stuttering blocks but his preference for helplessness, his inability to relate to the therapist and others, his reluctance to reveal or express emotion, his refusal to surrender his ideal image of himself as a sort of Demosthenes, the perfect orator, in chains. All these and many other blockages prevent the stutterer from achieving independence and self-esteem. These feelings and concepts must be brought to light, understood, and accepted before the stutterer will change. Yet once this has occurred, according to Barbara, the stutterer will come to accept himself as he really is, discard his neurosis, and all his various blockages including those of stuttering.

Barbara, who is himself a psychiatrist and a stutterer, is under no illusions about the difficulties to be faced by the stutterer in psychotherapy. His first book, *Stuttering: A Psychodynamic Approach to Its Understanding and Treatment* (1954) should be read by every prospective therapist for it vividly and authentically describes the covert features of the disorder and helps us understand the stutterer's resistances. Summing up, he states:

> Treatment in the adult or confirmed stutterer is a difficult, tedious, and serious undertaking. . . . Its main goal is to help the stutterer unravel himself and free himself from his neurotic web, so that he can avail himself of constructive forces and energies necessary for healthy growth and self-realization. (p. 265)

Another variation from traditional psychoanalysis can be found in the position of Harry Stack Sullivan (1953), and this too has markedly influenced the kind of psychotherapy used with stutterers. Sullivan's theory views neurotic behavior as stemming from disturbed interpersonal relationships, first arising in childhood when the basic needs for physical satisfaction and security have been thwarted by the parents. Anxiety is created when the child feels that he cannot meet the parental expectations. He internalizes the negative evaluations of others and rejects himself. When he does so, he finds it difficult not to reject others and the barriers of alien-

ation thus erected in turn create more anxiety. Sullivan shows how this alienation from self and others continues and developes as the individual grows older, until in maturity we find a person who cannot give or receive love, a person who craves security and self-esteem but who cannot establish the close relationships with others which might help him get them. Stuttering may be viewed as one of the defenses erected by the person to protect himself against establishing relationships which might once again hurt him. Using questioning, free association and discussion of the history of interpersonal relationships, Sullivan sought to remove the barriers between the self and others, to help his clients learn how to express emotion, to give and receive love openly, and to use real life situations in developing a less self-defeating way of living in a world full of social relationships, in short, to like and respect himself and his companions.

The most lucid application of the Sullivan approach to stuttering is that found in the book by Murphy and Fitzsimons, *Stuttering and Personality Dynamics* (1960). These authors view stuttering as learned behavior, originating in defective interpersonal relationships and persisting "as a consequence of old and contemporary interpersonal discomforts." "Stuttering can be defined as 'what a person is.' . . . Stuttering gives us an idea of what a person thinks of himself, how he feels about himself, and how he thinks others regard him (p. 145)." Though Murphy and Fitzsimons use projective play and client-centered counseling and do not closely follow his methods of psychotherapy, their excellent book reflects very vividly the concepts of Sullivan. Speech therapy is played down; psychotherapy is emphasized. They feel that the primary

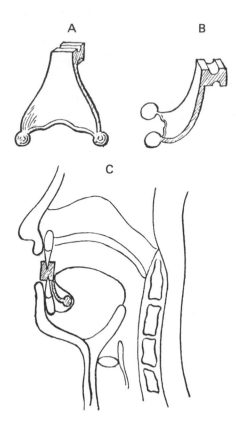

FIGURE 6.1   The Housstein device to prevent tongue fixations. (German Patent 255, 645 [1913]).

psychotherapeutic goal is the "modification or reduction of the demands of an overwhelming conscience." Depending on the demands made by each individual client, the speech pathologist must help him:

1. to release and to gain more understanding of the repressing forces of conscience which are plaguing him (by seeing the unreality and the non-productivity of its demands);

2. to reexperience and reassess his introjected objects to perceive his parents, siblings, and teachers as they are, to perceive himself as he really is;

3. to accept others and himself as they actually are with all their strengths and weaknesses;

4. to learn socially acceptable and developmental modes of satisfying the demands of the conscience;

5. to increase his awareness or consciousness of his world in every way;

6. to chart and to activate his own behavior rather than be driven by the twisted and archaic introjections of childhood.[5] (p. 112)

Another modern writer who shows the Sullivanian influence is Eugene Cooper (1968). His IPC (interpersonal communications) approach to therapy is based on the concept that through the therapist's control and manipulation of the psychotherapeutic interaction as evidenced in speech, the stutterer undergoes a learning experience in improved interpersonal relationships which eventually will solve his problems.

Other psychotherapies based on psychoanalysis

There are many psychotherapies that, in one way or another, use some of the techniques of psychoanalysis in modified forms. Most of them involve some kind of abreaction or acting out. Among those that have been applied to stuttering are the *psychodrama* and the *kinetic discharge therapies*.

Moreno (1956) developed a psychotherapy called psychodrama in which various hypothetical situations are arranged on stage, and a cast selected to play the various roles while inventing the action and the verbal interchanges on the spot. The person being treated plays his own role and directs the others in their parts. When

5 From A. T. Murphy and R. M. Fitzsimons, *Stuttering and Personality Dynamics*, Copyright © 1960. The Ronald Press Company, New York.

successful, much emotion is displayed, acted out, and cathartic effects are very evident. By being actor, director, and spectator in the psychodrama, the person also achieves real insights concerning his interpersonal relationships and the hidden feelings which have been revealed. Lemert and Van Riper (1944), Honig (1947), and Murphy and Fitzsimons (1960) provide examples of how psychodrama has been used with stutterers.

Trojan (1965) describes a "new psychotherapeutic method" for treating stuttering called the kinetic discharge therapy. Basically an acting out of imaginary scenes with the significant people who have played a part in the stutterer's life, he is asked to imagine such a person very vividly in a situation which would or did arouse fear, hate, sexual desire, or other strong feelings, then to act out motorically and without inhibition the emotions which are generated. The whole body must be brought into play and the behavior is accompanied by appropriate cries or verbalizations. After structuring the behavior desired, the therapist absents himself or remains behind the stutterer as he performs. A profound catharsis is said to occur with marked feelings of relief and these too are verbalized. Trojan claims that this therapy is much swifter than psychoanalysis and free from the morbid brooding and sexual emphasis which traditional Freudian therapy encourages.

Finally, we find in the literature a good many case reports by psychiatrists, rather than avowed psychoanalysts, that describe their psychotherapeutic work with stutterers. Most of these are based upon psychiatric interviewing techniques that rely more upon direct questioning and exploration than on free association and dream analysis or other major features of the Freudian method. These reports are often illuminating and help us see the changes in attitudes and adjustment which might result from such treatment. Two that could be called representative of the rest are those by Bergman (1968) and by Miller (1962). An excerpt from Bergman's report illustrates their anecdotal flavor:

In these early interviews, Jeffery began to tell me some of his fantasies. In the fifth hour he told me that he liked to sit by the lake and daydream about being a king in an earlier civilization. He imagined himself to have worked very hard so as to become president and then dictator of the United States so that he had command of the vast resources of material and technology necessary to make a time machine. Once he had the time machine, he would travel back to some ancient kingdom where he would so impress the people with a few modern inventions that they would make him king. Then, at last, he could stop working and have hundreds of wives and just lie back and enjoy himself. He said that he felt guilty about not taking his parents along on this adventure, but he did not want them there because even though he would be king they still could boss him around. He also thought of taking along some of his classmates for companionship, but was afraid that he would have to compete with them, and that they might mess everything up. He had decided that he would take Bruce, because his brother would be kind of an equal but easy to dominate. (p. 19)

The counseling approach

The most common type of psychotherapy used with stutterers in this country seems to be that devised by Carl Rogers. His books, *Counseling and Psychotherapy* (1942) and *Client-Centered Therapy* (1951), provided one of the first real challenges to psychoanalysis. The fact that the case he presented in his first book to il-lustrate his nondirective, client-centered therapy was a stutterer (though with many other problems) probably accounts for its influence in the field of speech pathology. The book also provided a breakthrough in demonstrating that psychotherapy was no longer a special prerogative of the psychiatric branch of the medical profession. Roger's theory is that the client possesses the basic potential for healing himself. This potential can be realized provided that he has the opportunity to explore himself in the presence of a permissive therapist who can understand, accept and reflect the feelings he expresses. Counseling psychotherapy made it possible for trained psychologists and speech pathologists to help many clients who otherwise would have had to be referred to psychiatrists. Though the strategies and techniques of client-centered therapy are far from simple, they appear to be, and this in itself encouraged many speech therapists to explore and use this kind of psychotherapy with stutterers.

Examination of the *process* of Rogerian psychotherapy shows that certain happenings usually follow in sequence as the client seeks to heal himself in the favorable climate provided by the empathetic and nonjudgmental therapist. First, the verbal interchanges concern the patient's complaints and the definition of the psychotherapeutic situation, the counselor encouraging free expression of all feelings, and the patient testing to see if indeed the counselor is as truly accepting as he seems to be. Then comes a period in which significant emotional material is verbalized, the counselor serving as a clarifier and, subtly, reinforcing the positive emotional responses. Next comes, in our experience, a period of self-evalua-

tion and self-acceptance which generates certain decisions for resolving the problems. And finally, the client begins to report that he has taken positive actions, has experienced good feelings about himself and others, and is happy about the changes that have occurred. In short, as Rogers might say, the client has become a person. We do not, of course, wish to imply that this sequence is straight line. The course of therapy oscillates, halts, regresses, moves forward again. And sometimes, unable to bear the therapist's insistence that the patient must set the goals and accept the responsibility for his self-healing, the client may flee the self-confrontation and be lost. Client-centered therapy demands much of the counselor.

Besides the case Rogers used in his first book, we have many other accounts in the literature which illustrate client-centered therapy with stutterers. The book by Hejna, *Interviews with a Stutterer* (1963); the taped recording entitled *The Case of Jim* (Seeman, 1957), the text by Murphy and Fitzsimons (1960), and the article by Schultz (1947) describe the psychotherapeutic process. Additionally, if students would wish to see Rogers doing some actual therapy with a client, the film "Three Approaches to Psychotherapy" [6] contrasts the approach of Rogers with that of Perls and Ellis.

Psychotherapy based upon learning theory

The psychoanalytic and counseling approaches to psychotherapy which we have been describing have been based largely upon explorations of the dynamics of behavior. They seek to

[6] This film is available from Psychological Films, 205 Twentieth St., Santa Ana, California 92706.

help the client understand why he behaves and feels as he does in terms of the past and present. In recent years, as we have seen earlier in this text, a new emphasis on *what* the patient does and how his overt and covert behaviors are maintained and reinforced has appeared in psychotherapy. Applying the "laws of learning" (and they are still far from being completely understood), the behavioral psychotherapist seeks to create a therapeutic environment in which anxiety and maladaptive behaviors are counteracted and extinguished, and healthy attitudes and adaptive behaviors are strengthened. Psychotherapy then is viewed as a process of conditioning and deconditioning.

This approach is the direct result of the attempt to apply to maladaptive behavior the principles of learning theory described variously by Pavlov, Thorndike, Hull, and Skinner. The psychotherapist provides settings and experiences in which learning may occur and carefully controls reinforcement so that the desired change in the client can be effected. Both classical and operant conditioning procedures are employed, the first being focussed on the anxiety and other feelings, the latter on the inappropriate habits of behaving. Wolpe, Eyesenck, and Salter apply the classical conditioning procedures of desensitization and counterconditioning in extinguishing anxiety and its associated responses. Ullmann and Krasner (1965), among others, have demonstrated the use of positive and negative reinforcement in applying operant conditioning to the kinds of behavior often termed neurotic. Both the classical and operant conditioning approaches have influenced not only the speech therapy but the psychotherapy of stuttering as we shall see.

In addition, stuttering therapy has been affected greatly by the various forms of the two-factor theory of Herbert Mowrer (1950, 1960, 1967) as represented by Brutten and Shoemaker (1966) and by the approach-avoidance conflict theory formulated by Dollard and Miller (1950) as represented by Sheehan (1970).

If we accept the behavioral therapists' revised definition of psychotherapy which holds that "neurotic behavior consists of persistent habits of learned (conditioned) behavior acquired in anxiety generating situations and that therapy depends upon the unlearning of this behavior (Wolpe, 1962)," then much of what we have always done in stuttering therapy could be viewed as psychotherapy. Certainly, we have long used relaxation, assertive behaviors and other kinds of counterconditioning agents to promote fluency. Since we have discussed rather thoroughly the use of relaxation in systematic desensitization earlier in this text, we turn now to the assertive behavior recommended by Salter (1949), and by Wolpe and Lazarus (1966) as also allegedly being able to reduce inhibition or to eliminate anxiety.

Assertive behaviors in anxiety reduction

The ancient history of psychotherapy is full of mand statements. "Go out and sin no more!" "Be not afraid!" "Take the bull by the horns!" "Excelsior!" The stutterer Demosthenes followed Satirus' admonitions and, shouting as he assertively climbed the mountain with leaden plates on his chest or yelled against the sound of the surf, drove himself into fame as the best orator of Greece. Anxiety is constrictive, inhibitory, and, as Sal-

ter (1949) has shown, assertive outgoing behavior seems to reduce fear.
We find this point of view reflected
in the old southern mountain legend
of the hoop snake that takes its tail
in its mouth and chases you if you
fearfully run away, but rolls away itself if you chase it. This principle of
the reciprocal inhibition of anxiety
through the use of assertive responses
has been used by psychotherapists of
all persuasions and for all sorts of
neuroses.

The utilization of assertive behaviors in stuttering therapy is as ancient
as suggestion and time beating.
Freund (1966) tells of its being used
in the early years of the nineteenth
century:

An expressive technique, which in some
way is the opposite from what we have
described as calming and relaxing procedures, was introduced by Serre d'Alais,
a famous French ophthamologist and himself a stutterer, as far back as 1829. He
showed that by using a loud and rapid
mode of speech accompanied by exaggerated gesturing and facial expressions,
both denoting strong inner convictions
and intensifying in retrograde self-reliance and determination, the spell of inhibition, as it were, can be broken. The
stutterer here assumes the role and de-
meanor of those self-assured and authoritarian persons whom he usually mostly
dreads and in front of whom he experiences his most humiliating defeats. (pp.
165–66)

Freund also tells us that Voisin
(1794–1872), a French psychiatrist,
believed that stuttering was due to a
weakness of the coordinating mechanism for speech and recommended
talking in a loud, forceful, and angry
voice. Hunt (1861) observed that "It
is well known that when stammerers
are roused by indignation, a sense of
wrong, etc., they are frequently re-

leased from their infirmity, or at least
the latter is considerably diminished."
Yearsley (1909) has this exhortation
for the stutterer:

Court every possible opportunity of
conversing with strangers and superiors,
especially in public places and shops
where the attention of a number of listeners is concentrated upon you. Do not
fear any man's censure. Let him know
that you possess (to use a slang expression) some "gift of gab." Drag him into
argument. Debate with him. Tongue
thrash him "hip and thigh." (p. 178)

Hatfield (1910) also echoes the
thought: "Stoutly assert your divine
right to hold up your head and look
the world in the face; step boldly to
the front." In this, we see the suggestion of the "good eye contact" so
often recommended by therapists today, in itself an assertive behavior.

This emphasis upon assertiveness
in entering feared situations is also
one of the common practices to be
found in American speech therapy
today. For example, Wendell Johnson
(1961) had this to say to his stutterers:

Would you talk to more people? Then
go ahead. Talk to as many as you can
bring yourself to approach. Would you recite in your classes? Then make the best
beginning you can muster. Would you
go out with girls—and do you have a particular girl in mind? Ask her for a date,
if not immediately, then as soon as you
can talk yourself into it. (p. 199)

Also those therapies based upon the
conflict hypothesis of Dollard and Miller (1950), especially that advocated
by Sheehan (1958, 1970), emphasize
assertiveness. At each of Sheehan's five
levels of conflict, he stresses the need
to increase the strength of the approach tendencies by assertive behav-

ior. Thus at the word and situation levels the stutterer is urged to seek our feared words and situations, to enter them deliberately and aggressively while, at the conflict level of emotional expression, he is urged to break through "the inhibitory dam" and to demonstrate assertively how he feels both in words and actions.

The use of assertive behaviors is found also in the works of Bryngelson (1966) and Frankl (1960, 1965). Frankl developed a logotherapy treatment based upon what he termed "paradoxical intention" and applied it to a number of obsessive, compulsive, and phobic problems, including stuttering. If we may oversimplify Frankl's position, we might say that his phobic patients are trained to seek out what they fear, to assertively wish for what they dread. Thus an insomniac is urged to try to stay awake, the heart patient to try voluntarily to produce fibrillation, the stutterer to try hard to stutter on purpose. In short, they endeavor to talk themselves into desiring the experience they fear. All those of us who have done any research with stutterers will recall how often our subjects could not stutter for us when they and we desired them to do so. In Frankl's words,

Paradoxical intention is based on the fact that a certain amount of pathogenesis in phobias and obsessive-compulsive neuroses is due to the increase of anxieties and compulsions caused by the effort to avoid them. Paradoxical intention consists in a reversal of the patient's attitude toward his symptom, and enables him to detach himself from his neurosis. (1960, p. 534)

Bryngelson (1966) has long advocated in his "psycho-talk therapy" that the stutterer should assertively expose his sensitivities, verbalize them

first to himself before a mirror and then before a group, and then to advertise them aggressively in his daily activities. He views voluntary stuttering, not only as a means of gaining cortical control of a poorly integrated speech mechanism, but also as a means for overcoming the neurotic defenses produced by anxiety.

We find in the limited literature that provides accounts of self-recovery from stuttering, numerous examples in which deliberately assertive behavior seemed to play a major factor in the recovery. One of these is an old account given by Quidde (1926) who tells how, after various attempts at therapy had failed, he went to a strange environment and started talking to everyone available. He asked directions on the street, he attended a dancing school so he could talk to young ladies. He inserted himself into every conversation. The result was "miraculous." His fears disappeared and his speech became fluent. The researches by Shearer and Williams (1965), Wingate (1964) and Sheehan and Martyn (1966) provide similar evidence. Our own collection of recovered stutterers, in which they attempted to account for their acquisition of fluency, also demonstrates that in the majority of instances, the stutterers who "cured themselves" found ways of replacing avoidance with assertive behavior.

Finally in this connection we provide a quotation from a 1970 newspaper clipping concerning the stuttering therapy administered by a traveling "research psychologist" who cured stammerers with anger in only twelve days. One of his cases is speaking:

"For three-hour sessions, twice a day, we were instructed to sit straight in hard plywood chairs," Magee said. "We couldn't smoke. He made us as angry at him as he could. He used insults and egotistical behavior. But he did it with a point in mind," the former stammerer said. "You cannot be apathetic about something and hate it at the same time. Daily he strove to build animosity and to fill us with feelings of fear, hate, or respect. He quoted the writings of the world's greatest authors and minds and filled us with his own ideas. I felt ready to kill. But I did not have a stammer after half a day." (Dunlop, 1970)

The article mentioned that speech therapists at the demonstration expressed scepticism!

Feeding and sexual responses and counterconditioners

The psychosomatic literature on obesity includes many references to excessive eating as being due to the need to allay anxiety and some experimental evidence that this has some basis in fact is found in the research by Mary Cover Jones (1924), Lazarus (1969) and others. We find few direct applications of food being used as a counterconditioner in stuttering except for that mentioned by Van Riper (1968) but it is interesting that chewing, one of the components of feeding, has been used for years in treating stutterers. For completely different reasons each of the following authors, Froeschels (1942), Robbins (1932), Hollingsworth (1939) and Despert (1942), recommended the use of chewing as an important therapeutic technique. Froeschels used breath chewing to convince the stutterer of the normalcy of his speaking mechanism; Robbins employed it to help the stutterer shift from the consonant into the vowel; Hollingsworth found that chewing produced relaxation; and Despert recommended it as a means for safely reliving old conflicts first developed in a family feed-

ing situation. And we might also remember Demosthenes pebbles here. Perhaps the active principle in all this chewing is merely the anxiety reduction or relief which occurs when we have been fed.

Sexual satisfaction has also been mentioned in the literature as being able to inhibit anxiety. We have often seen marked progress in therapy to occur when the stutterer does establish a satisfactory relationship with some member of the opposite sex. However, the only direct application of which we know comes from the case report of a stutterer who came to us from Arabia. He reported that a standard treatment for stuttering, which he had undergone, was to wait until the boy was 16, then to take him to a house of prostitution, where he had to keep talking throughout the intercourse. He said that he had known others who were said to have been cured that way but all that happened to him was that he became impotent and remained so for some time afterward. Counterconditioning works best when the anxiety is weak.

Respiratory responses as counterconditioners

As long ago as 1929, Lovenhart, Lorenz, and Waters found that psychotics showed a temporary remission of symptoms following the inhalation of progressive amounts of carbon dioxide. This went unnoticed until Meduna (1950) used carbon dioxide inhalations with a motley group of 100 assorted anxiety-neurotics, including some stutterers, and reported that 68 of them improved enough after 20 to 150 treatment sessions to be termed cured. He provided no data on follow-ups. In Meduna's CO_2 therapy, the patient takes about 20 to 30 inhalations of a mixture of 30 percent

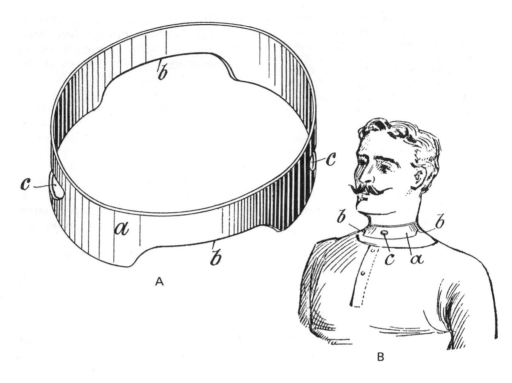

A

B

FIGURE 6.2 Samual neck band to stimulate muscles of the throat. (British Patent 10,256 [1913].)

carbon dioxide and 70 percent oxygen until he becomes unconscious for two or three seconds. This treatment is given three times a day for from four to five or six months. Smith (1953) reported that about a third of 33 stutterers so treated showed remarkable improvement, a third showed some improvement, and a third showed none. Kent (1961b) reviewed much of the research and queried the American medical members of the Carbon Dioxide Association about their use of this form of treatment. Her conclusion was that the "question of the efficacy of this treatment for stuttering has not been answered adequately either through research or through the experiences of clinicians." A different form of carbon dioxide therapy is reported in Wolpe and Lazarus (1966) who used it not to produce unconsciousness but hyperventilation and relaxation and they claim that "one or two inhalations may remove pervasive anxiety for weeks." Three of our own stutterers who had previously undergone CO_2 treatment told us that they had benefitted temporarily and attributed the change to the profound relief experienced when they again could breathe good air.

Humor as antagonistic to anxiety

Stutterers have often found that humor can be used to relieve some of their anxiety and momentarily increase their fluency. Van Riper (1971) has mentioned this as among the antiexpectancy devices commonly used and there are occasional accounts throughout the literature of "laughing stutterers." Bryngelson (1935) has strongly recommended that stutterers learn to joke about their disorder, not only to disarm their listeners, but to attain less morbid attitudes toward the problem. Luper and Mulder (1964) have this to say:

We agree with others who feel it helps the stutterer to be able to tell jokes about his stuttering. As he becomes better able to laugh at himself, he prevents adverse audience reactions by not becoming completely embarrassed when his stuttering does have a comical side. (p. 165)

Used too often, however, such behaviors become conspicuously fraudulent. Stuttering is no laughing matter!

Semantic and rational psychotherapies

One of the oldest ideas about stuttering is that it is due to disordered thinking. A common admonition heard by all stutterers is that they should think about what they are saying before they say it, a prescription which doubtless stems from the speech hesitancies shown by all of us when we are having difficulties in formulating. Hippocrates insisted that stutterers thought faster than they could speak. This view has been echoed by many others since that time. Some workers however have felt that it was not the excessive rapidity of thought but rather its disorganization which was the core of the disorder. Beasley (1897) was only one of a large number of early stuttering therapists who demanded the organization of thought. Speaking of the stutterer he writes, "Let him learn again the art of speaking, and having learned, think before he speaks, and say his

thoughts calmly, with self-respect, as a man who does not talk at random (p. 51)." Scripture (1931) insisted that stutterers need training in proper thinking. He notes how often they seem unable to "go directly to the point" of what they desire to say; how often they frequently break off a sentence midstream and get tangled in revisions. Perhaps however it was Bluemel, a psychiatrist, who in his book *The Riddle of Stuttering* (1957) developed "thinking therapy" most thoroughly. Using modelling as the basic approach, and intensive exercises in the silent, pantomimic, whispered, and finally overt formulation of sentences spoken in answer to questions, Bluemel sought to reorganize the disordered thinking which he felt was at the bottom of the problem.[7] We find some of the same sort of training being advocated for clutterers by many writers, notably Weiss (1964). We should make clear, however, that Bluemel as a psychiatrist also considered stuttering to have many of the features of a secondary neurosis and his thinking therapy was also seen by him as being a useful means for calming his patients and relieving much of their anxiety.

Semantic psychotherapy. Although we have already presented the semantic interaction therapy of Wendell Johnson, Williams and others of the Iowa School in our section devoted to the suggestion and persuasion therapists, it should also be included in the psychotherapies. Johnson's book *People in Quandaries* (1946) is

---

[7] Having known Dr. Bluemel fairly well, it is our impression that his own stuttering had a very strong cluttering component. This might account for his emphasis on the need to organize the thinking processes. One of his colleagues once said to us that Bluemel's book should really have been entitled *The Riddle of Cluttering*.

in fact a book on psychotherapy, not only for stuttering but for other problems usually considered neurotic. Johnson felt that the stutterer must come to examine the language he uses when he is concerned about stuttering and, by revising that language, to eliminate the misperceptions and mis-evaluations in which the problem is anchored. Through group and individual discussions, and an almost Socratic type of questioning by the therapist, the stutterer is helped to examine and test his erroneous assumptions that there is anything really wrong with him as a person or that there is anything really wrong with his speech except the maladaptive ways with which he reacts to his misperceptions. Bloodstein (1969) indicates the directive nature of this psychotherapy as follows. The stutterer

. . . is trained to set aside, at least temporarily, such words as "stuttering" in order to talk descriptively about his problem, with the expectation that, as he becomes more and more vividly aware that there is nothing to prevent him from going on except the things which he himself does when he talks, he will gradually become better able to talk without doing these things. On the basis of this sort of semantic reorientation, then, Johnson proceeds to place major emphasis on a great deal of actual speaking by the stutterer—with attention to "going ahead and talking" on the assumption that ~there are no basic physical or emotional reasons for not doing so. (p. 249)

Nevertheless, as Kent (1961a) points out, one of the chief goals of this therapy is to modify the stutterer's belief system about his speech and his speech disorder so as to reduce his anxiety and avoidance reactions.

Perhaps the most succinct exposition of Johnson's semantic or interaction therapy is to be found in his book *Stuttering and What You Can Do About It* (1961) where he condenses the recommended treatment into four mandates: (1) Pay much more attention to your normal speech than to what you think of as your stuttering. Cultivate increasingly the feelings and attitudes and ways of thinking that go with normal speech. Be warmly accepting of yourself as a person. (2) Pay enough attention to the things you do that interfere with your normal speech, the things you do that you call your stuttering, to understand that they are unnecessary and then change and eliminate them. (3) Do more talking. (4) Work at "being a normal speaker."

Rational psychotherapy. The present interest shown by speech therapists in *rational psychotherapy* as advocated by Ellis and Harper (1961) reflects the influence of the older semantic therapy. According to Ellis, rational psychotherapy is based on the assumption that human beings become emotionally disturbed through acquiring irrational and illogical thoughts, philosophies, or attitudes. To Ellis, "Neurosis essentially consists of stupid behavior by a non-stupid person." "A neurotic is a potentially capable individual who in some way or on some level of functioning does not realize that he is, or how he is, defeating his own ends." Ellis is concerned primarily with the self-talk of neurotics, with the unrealistic and irrational sentences with which they brainwash themselves and so maintain their anxieties and inappropriate behavior. What the therapist does in *rational therapy* is to analyze the fear and anger and guilt feelings of the client and to reveal their origins in the distorted thoughts of the present rather than in past trauma. He helps the client to reverbalize, to think straight, and to test his new straightened thinking in actual experiences.

The treatment is highly directive and the therapist is aggressive as the following quotation shows:

Rational psychotherapy makes a concerted attack on the disturbed individual's irrational positions in two ways: (1) the therapist serves as a frank counter-propagandist who directly contradicts and denies the self-defeating propaganda and superstitions which the client has originally learned and which he is now self-propagandistically perpetuating. (2) The therapist encourages, persuades, cajoles, and at times commands the client to partake of some kind of activity which itself will act as a forceful counterpropagandist agency against the nonsense he believes. (Ellis, 1958, pp. 44–45.)

While to date we have no published reports of the success of rational psychotherapy with stutterers, we are personally finding more and more clients who have experienced it before they come to us, and many speech therapists have told us that they have found it very useful. It is our impression that rational psychotherapy, like semantic psychotherapy, may be effective with a certain kind of stutterer, one who despite his mild stuttering is highly verbal and fonder of intellectualizing than performing speech therapy assignments. Our experiences in applying either of these kinds of psychotherapies to very severe, hard-blocking stutterers have not been very successful. Perhaps their mantles do not fit our own therapeutic lamps and contours.

Reality therapy

As advocated by Glasser (1965), this psychotherapy seems to appeal most to those avoidance-prone, timid stutterers who feel lost and helpless, those who have withdrawn from others and live miserably within the walls of their avoidance prison, the ones of

very low self-esteem. In this form of psychotherapy there is no digging up the dead cats of the past, no unearthing of what Glasser calls "psychological garbage," for this only degrades the person. Instead, the psychotherapist actively involves himself with the client, insists that the latter test reality, fulfill his needs, accept the responsibility for all his behavior, and seek to do what is right and not to do what is wrong. Confrontation and no excuses! It too is highly directive and supportive.

Gestalt therapy

At times it seems as though new psychotherapies sprout like weeds. In this text we have not and could not cover all of them. Those we have presented are ones which have been applied to stutterers with whom we come in contact or ones which we have employed ourselves. The final one in our series, Gestalt therapy, is fairly recent but two of our present cases seem to have profited greatly from it and so we provide a brief description. The therapy seems only remotely based upon Gestalt psychology and perhaps reflects existential concepts more than any other. Essentially, it is an action therapy, the clients performing a series of experiments in self-awareness, recognition of conflicts, remembering, concentrating, verbalizing, and then reporting their reactions. Emphasis is placed upon manipulating the self through contact, insight, and action. The person learns to change anxiety into excitement and to use the energies so released for constructive purposes. The best source is *Gestalt Therapy* by Perls, Hefferline, and Goodman (1951).

In a lifetime devoted to the treatment of stuttering, the author of the present text has referred to psycho-

therapists of different persuasions prospective patients who seemed to have
emotional problems too profound for
his own limited competence or available time. He has collaborated closely
with some of these professionals and
has done speech therapy with their clients after the psychotherapy had been
terminated. In only two instances did
the psychotherapy completely free
the person from stuttering and these
were individuals whose stuttering was
monosymptomatic and began in adulthood very suddenly. All the others
with whom we came into therapeutic
contact later seemed to be stuttering
about as frequently though not as
severely as they had done prior to entering psychotherapy, and this was
true despite the variations in rationale
or practice. Nevertheless, it is our impression (and that is all it could be)
that these highly disturbed stutterers
had profited substantially from the
psychotherapy. They seemed less morbid about their speech problem; their
anxieties had lessened; they seemed
to possess more sustained motivation.
It was interesting that although their
social fears had markedly decreased
and they were talking more in more
situations, their phonemic and word
fears had not changed. To summarize,
though they stuttered about as frequently as they did before their psychotherapy, they were not as unhappy
or as miserable. We felt that our referrals had been wise.

Drug therapy

Drugs of various kinds have been
used to relieve anxiety for as long as
mankind can remember. We need only mention the opium poppy of the
Orient; the wines and nepenthe of
the Greeks, Romans, and Omar Khay-
yam; the cocoa leaves of the Incas;

the Rauwolfia roots of India; or the
peyote and psychedelic mushrooms of
the Mexican Indians to see that this
is so. Francis Bacon was not the first or
last person to prescribe hot wine for
the congealed tongues of stutterers.
The dulling of anxiety, the changed
perceptions, the buffering effects
which drugs can confer have always
made them attractive to those who
live in fear and deprivation. Modern
psychopharmacology has provided
hundreds of new medications, each
with highly advertised claims of effectiveness, and the literature shows
clearly that the pink pill of hope has
been swallowed by thousands of stutterers seeking relief from their troubles.

Though, as Dews (1962) insists,
"the terms may have outlived their
usefulness," most of the drugs employed in the treatment of stuttering
have been classified as stimulants, sedatives, or tranquilizers. Their differing effects have been variously attributed to the altering of the biochemis-
try of different parts of the nervous
system—the cortex, the thalamus, the
hypothalamus, the reticular formation, the sympathetic or parasympa-
thetic systems. Unfortunately, there
are few drugs which have single specific effects or clearly defined sites of
action. As with other drugs, alcohol
can serve both as a stimulant or a depressant; much depends on the dosage
and the time interval after ingestion.
Individual differences in drug tolerance are always found. Some so-called
sedatives can produce almost manic
states in certain people at certain
times. Placebos can often produce the
same symptomatic relief as the drugs
themselves. In short, psychopharmacology is in its infancy.

With these observations in mind,
one must examine the literature with
some care. First of all, we find many

reports of successful drug therapy with stutterers—reports that are completely inadequate. Drugs are administered but no dosages or length of time are reported; no placebos are used or, if they are, the giver (who was also the evaluator) knows which was being given or the subject may also know that one *might* be given. If improvement is claimed, no objective measure of the gain is employed. Often far too few subjects are tested. A few studies attempt objective measurements of stuttering severity, counting the frequency of stutterings in a repeated reading passage or getting reading times or judgments by an expert listening panel. While these procedures themselves leave much to be desired (see Van Riper, 1971, chapter 9) in providing valid and reliable measures of severity, most of the literature expresses the results of drug administration in terms of "speech improvement." Rarely do we find an account of "cures" and even when we do, we never know whether these are laboratory cures or if carry-over to outside situations has been obtained. Rarely do we find any careful follow-up studies after a lapse of time. Often, the improvement cited is in terms of subjectively estimated attitude change: "On the drug, the stutterers seemed more cheerful and relaxed as compared with when they were on the placebo."

Placebos must be used carefully. As Uhr and Miller (1960) point out, placebos should ideally have the same side effects as the drugs themselves, and certainly the basic criteria underlying the double-blind procedure must be followed. For example, on the one hand, we find such studies as Gutzmann (1954) reporting that "Beginning in 1949, we have prescribed glutamic acid so far in 130 cases with different clinical symptoms and have

usually obtained good results." In contrast, Leanderson and Levi (1968), using a careful double-blind procedure and objective measures of improvement found that placebos had the same effects as did the drug opipramol.

The scheduling of the drug administration is also of vital importance, yet often we find either no account of when the drugs were given or for how long, or we discover that critical evaluation of the drug is not even possible. Thus Corneliu (1968) first gave tranquilizers, then shifted to stimulants, then to relaxation training, to orthophonic exercises. He reports that in 90 percent of his cases, "positive improvement was shown." Daskalov (1968) also provides only impressions although drugs formed an integral part of his therapy with 815 Bulgarian stutterers. He used some of them for "protection" against stress, others as a tonic, and finally still others as a stimulant. Although he reports very favorable results from his complex therapy, we are completely unable to assess the value of the drugs used therein. The determination of the efficacy of drugs demands very precise procedures, and careful replication is essential.

In the light of these observations, we almost hesitate to review the literature. We do so only in the hope that better studies may be done and also to provide possible promising directions for future research. It should be recognized however that drugs are currently being used fairly widely in the treatment of stuttering. In this country, mild sedatives and tranquilizers are frequently prescribed by physicians, if not by speech pathologists, and in other countries the use of drugs is even more widespread. Thus Luchsinger and Arnold (1965) indicate that the use of sedatives, atropine,

prostigmin and the rauwolfia tranquilizers is very common in Europe.
Yannatos (1960) in Greece found hy-
droxygine (Atarax), when used along
with speech therapy, facilitated treatment but did not produce any cures
when used alone. Lennon (1962) in
his book *Le Begaiement* says that
drugs produce improvement but not
complete recovery and are best used
as adjuncts to other forms of therapy.
Daskalov (1962) in Bulgaria states
that he uses: "sedatives and soporific
medications, neuroleptic and ataractic
drugs, drugs regulating the neuroautonomic mechanisms, muscular relax-
ants, spasmolytic drugs . . . and ton-
ics such as vitamins B_1, B_6, and C,
arsenic, phosphorous, iron and calcium.". These drugs, however, are
used along with other therapeutic
methods. Kochergina (1965) in Russia uses cholinolytic drugs for stuttering patients with breathing abnormalities, elatine (a curare-like alkaloid)
which is a powerful relaxant of muscle tonus for those who are very tense,
and a series of tranquilizers (meprobramate, trioxazine, and librium) for
patients with high anxiety. This writer also used combinations of drugs. In
Japan, we find Imazeki (1960) using
Astyn (a tranquilizer), and Fujita et
al. (1964) employing Insidiom, Tran-
copal, and Scopolamin, but the results they report are not impressive.

Though the literature is full of clinical observations and inadequately
controlled experiments, we have
found only a few studies which even
approximately fulfill the proper evaluative procedures using a double-
blind controls and some objective
measures of improvement. The first of
these, by Mitchell (1955), which employed Serpasil and the reversal of
groups on the drug and placebo for
16 stutterers showed no significant

changes in rated severity or frequency
of stuttering that could be attributed
to the drug though "introspective reports" by the subjects who were receiving speech therapy at the time
indicated that under the drug condition they had less anxiety, shorter
blockings, and better control. Kent
and Williams (1959) divided 15 stutterers into placebo and drug groups
(crudely matched in terms of severity,
previous therapy, MMPI scores, etc.)
and, using double-blind procedures,
administered meprobramate (Mil-
town). As in the Mitchell study, all
subjects were receiving speech therapy concurrently with the drug or
placebo and this may possibly have
contaminated the results. They found
no significant differences between the
two groups during a 99-day period.

Perhaps the most careful study was
performed by Aron (1965), in South
Africa, using 46 stutterers and a combination of two drugs—trifluoperazine
(Stelazine), a tranquilizer, and amylobarbitone, a barbiturate sedative. Placebo and drugs were reversed each
three weeks of a 15-week period for
each subject and careful measures of
stuttering severity were employed frequently and systematically. No speech
therapy was given during the period.
Aron reports that 80 percent of her
subjects showed improved speech
while under the drugs as compared
with the placebo but no one was
cured. The improvement seemed to
be due not to lessened frequency of
stuttering but to decreased severity.
The judged severity for stuttering
showed a significant drug effect. According to Aron, "it was postulated
that reduction of anxiety and tension,
brought about by the drug, had greater influence on the severity of the stuttering than on the frequency with
which it occurs."

A fourth study was performed by Goldman and Guth (1965) using two drugs (but not in combination)—Thioridazine (Mellaril) and Chlordiazepoxide (Librium). Four conditions were scheduled: (1) no drug, (2) placebo, (3) Mellaril, (4) Librium. Subjects were evaluated in terms of frequency of stuttering while reading and being interviewed, in terms of reading time, and as judged by experts from films of their performance. No statistically significant differences were found in terms of frequency or reading times but six of the far too few eight subjects were rated by the judges of their films as having milder stuttering when taking Mellaril. Seven of the eight stutterers reported feeling better when taking this drug. Librium produced no significant results. As in the Aron study, speech therapy had been discontinued during the experiment. The authors are very cautious, probably because of their small sample of subjects, concluding that "the fact that the stutterers reported feeling some improvement under Mellaril might warrant consideration of the use of this drug as an adjunctive aid to traditional speech therapy."

One very well controlled study by Sack (1968) explored a different drug, sodium dilantin, usually prescribed for epileptics. Although in many ways, the design of this research may serve as a model, Sack found no significant differences in the severity of stuttering between the placebo and the sodium dilantin. The two available reviews of the literature on drugs and stuttering, by Burr and Mullendorf (1960) and by Kent (1963), generally conclude that tranquilizers have no important effect upon stuttering. In view of the somewhat more positive findings of Aron and Goldman and Guth, which were published

later than these reviews, it is possible that sedative or depressant drugs, used alone or in combination with a tranquilizer, may prove more promising.

Less valid studies

We now include a brief review of studies which unfortunately fail to fulfill even minimal criteria for adequate assessment but which may provide some leads for future investigators. Hogewind (1940) used bellergal and phenobarbital, reporting that "on the whole, the results were satisfactory, sometimes very good." Schaubel and Street (1949) tried prostigmin for three months on ten stutterers finding some decrease in stuttering severity. Penson (1952) and Hale (1951) found some improvement resulting from the administration of vitamins (Thiamin hydrochloride), about as much as Palasek and Curtis (1960) discovered when they gave nothing but a placebo. With regard to the latter finding, Anton Schilling (1963b) also showed that placebos had about the same effect as tranquilizers when both were compared to the no drug condition.

In Italy, Serra (1960) gave large doses of iodine with inconclusive results. At the University of Iowa, Love (1955) compared the effects of the stimulant amphetamine with the sedative phenobarbital, finding no significant differences. Fish and Bowling (1965), in an admittedly uncontrolled study, found that amphetamines helped some stutterers while tranquilizers helped others.

Bibik (1966) states that preschool stutterers given benactyzine, a tranquilizer, showed remarkable improvement. Four out of five "lost" their stuttering in six weeks. Hanicke and Leben (1964) administered meprobromate to 20 young stutterers. Class teachers reported improvement in 13 of them but also pronounced side effects such as sleepiness and lack of energy occurred. When older children were given the drug, only one of 15 showed any improvement. Cozzo and Gabrielli (1965) gave haloperidol and triperidol to 48 stutterers. Of this number, 16 showed marked and 17 slight improvement. No lasting effects following termination of the drugs were found.

Influenced by the theories of Seeman (1959), tranquilizers such as Librium, Valium, and Seduzen have been used by many Czechoslovakian workers. Seeman believes that strong negative emotions influence the cortex (perhaps by cancelling its usual inhibitory role on the lower brain centers) so that pronounced autonomic activity occurs. He therefore suggests the use of various drugs such as sedatives, hypnotics, and tranquilizers to reduce the negative emotionality and thus to prevent stuttering. Sedlackova (1970) concluded that these drugs act on the thalamus to improve coordination of proprioceptive-exterioceptive impulses, and on the limbic system to reduce the intensity of "logophobias" and generalized anxiety. Stimulants were also used experimentally by these workers to combat negative emotion but with less favorable results, since thinking became chaotic and impaired.

Maxwell and Patterson (1958) stated that meprobramate was effective during speech therapy, though their study indicates that when the placebo was substituted for the drug, the stutterers still continued to improve. DiCarlo, Katz, and Batkin (1959) randomly assigned their 30 stutterers to placebo, meprobramate, and no drug groups, using only frequency counts in oral reading of a passage as the measure of severity. They report a "substantial reduction" in stuttering for the drug group but the differences were not statistically significant. Holliday (1959) also used random assignment of 20 stutterers to meprobramate and no-drug control groups for three weeks of treatment using ratings of frequency, duration, and a checklist of overt stuttering behaviors, finding that the meprobromate subjects were rated as less tense than the controls. We also have individual case reports of the successful use of Serpasil in Tuttle (1952) and Meffret (1956). Hommerich and Korzendorfer (1966) concluded that placebos were just as effective as Librium. One recent study by Wells and Malcolm (1972) should also be mentioned. They used a controlled, double-blind procedure for investigating the effectiveness of a combination of haloperidol and orphenadrene, the latter being included to avoid tremors and other side effects. Of the 12 patients taking the medication, 10 showed "considerable improvement" while 2 were somewhat worse. Assessment was made on the basis of tape recordings. Speech therapy continued throughout the treatment. There are some basic errors in design of this study that make us skeptical of the favorable results reported especially in the areas of assessment and follow-up. Replication is certainly needed.

Perhaps, in summary, the words of Bachrach and Quigley (1966) should be emphasized:

It must be realized that the final general assessment and recognition of the psychotherapeutic value of any drug must rest not only upon its widespread use but most critically on the basis of carefully controlled evaluation. General experience has shown that original claims nearly always prove to be overly optimistic, and only gradually, as the evidence of controlled studies accumulates, will the therapeutic value of the drug be assessed. (p. 542)

In the light of the preceding review of the research and also as the result of our own experimental administration of many of these drugs, we find little justification for their use as the sole method of therapy. Perhaps, for certain individuals, certain drugs can be used profitably as an adjunct to treatment procedures but to date at least pharmacology has not solved the stutterer's problem. Pollard and Bakker (1960) provided a sane commentary to conclude this section:

In some carefully planned programs the giving of drugs has been an integral part of the total therapy, but the capsule of love without understanding can become the bitter pill of rejection. We are well aware of the placebo response and of the various diligent manipulations of double-blind studies, of large samples, and of controls, but we are critical and suspicious of evaluations that do not even begin to cope with the uniqueness of human beings. (pp. 203–4)

Group Therapy

Until about thirty years ago, group psychotherapy was generally rejected as having little scientific value and as being sociologically and psychologically unsound. During and after World War II, however, the large numbers of soldiers in need of psychotherapy required such procedures and soon a similar need for treating patients in mental hospitals or child guidance clinics gave great impetus to the movement. It was soon found that group therapy had advantages of its own: (1) The client comes to realize that his problems are not unique, that he is not alone, that others share his difficulties. (2) The group situation is in itself a facsimile of social interaction, the area in which most of their interpersonal difficulties reside. (3) Through group tolerance, understanding and support, powerful forces are brought to bear that promote healing. (4) It is economical of the therapist's time and energies. (5) The group provides a safe place in which to attempt new ways of behaving. (6) The individual members of the group not only learn from each other new approaches to the solutions of their problems; they also assume the role of therapists for other members and finally for themselves.

There are also some difficulties and disadvantages: (1) Often the composition of the group may be too heterogeneous to facilitate interaction or may contain exploiters and saboteurs. (2) At times unhealthy attitudes may become contagious. (3) Some members who most need to participate may remain on the fringes of the group and stay uninvolved. (4) The group may become a safe harbor and refuge and prevent the person from making the adjustment to reality of which he is capable. (5) Certain members may be overwhelmed by group pressures for premature disclosure of events and feelings and either leave the group or become shattered. (6) Group therapy requires a very skilled and competent leader and there aren't many of them.

In the treatment of stuttering, group therapy has been used for many years and all over the world. Though much of this group treatment has been focused on the facilitation of fluency rather than improving interpersonal adequacy, there is no doubt that it always contains some potentially potent psychotherapy. One of the first advocates of group therapy for stutterers was James Sonnet Greene who operated a clinic for stutterers at the National Hospital for Speech Disorders in New York City. In 1942, he wrote that "group therapy is the most important factor in the treatment of the stutterer" and five years later (Greene, 1947) he suggested that the stutterer be exposed to several different groups and therapists, proceeding from smaller "low pressure groups" to larger more challenging ones as he became able to withstand the pressures. Repeatedly he insisted that the goal of this therapy was to "treat the person as a whole" and not the symptom. He also founded a social-therapeutic group of stutterers called the Ephatha Club which survived for several years. Slavson (1947) whose book, *The Practice of Group Psychotherapy,* was perhaps the first to have important impact in the field of psychotherapy due to his systematic presentation of principles and methods. In its section dealing with the problem of stuttering, the goals of group therapy with these "speech sufferers" are (1) to break down the stutterer's old unadaptive emotional reactions and to build new healthy ones; (2) to decrease the patient's specific fears and anxieties; (3) to create better social adjustment strategies; and (4) to develop a more mature, adequate, and integrated personality. Slavson felt that both individual and group therapy were usually necessary.

One worker who for a time had a marked influence in promoting group therapy in speech pathology was Ollie Backus. Beginning with an early article (Backus and Dunn, 1947) she applied the theoretical approaches of Lewin, Horney, and Sullivan to build a unique combination of group psychotherapy and speech therapy based upon conversational patterns. Moreover she felt it unnecessary to have homogeneous groups of individuals with the same kind of speech disorder. Indeed she felt that groups con-

sisting of members with dissimilar speech disorders offered special advantages and in any event the basic purpose of all therapy was to create the optimal "atmosphere" and conditions which would permit the person to heal himself.[8] Several different kinds of group interaction have been described by Van Riper (1958) in an account of his 20 years of exploratory therapy with stutterers. A partial description of the therapy program for 1955–1956 may illustrate just one of the variations:

This year, the final year of our five-year emphasis on psychotherapy, we decided to go hog-wild in permissiveness and nonstructuring of the therapy. No assignments were required; no self-therapy reports fill these files. The student therapists played a minor part, being more observers and conversationalists than their predecessors had been. The therapist himself assumed little leadership of the group, letting it go where it would. At times he played the scapegoat and whipping-post roles more than any other. Occasionally, if they permitted him to do so, he reflected a feeling or two, or protected one of the group from the savage attacks of others. He was used by the group also as a sort of encyclopedia of therapy, providing information as requested but only when requested. The stutterers early were given a list and explanation of all the techniques we or others had used to help stutterers, and from there on it was a free-choice affair, as unstructured as play therapy with children. Often during the semester we were struck with the similarity to play therapy. These stutterers played with their stuttering, with the various techniques used to reduce it, with their clinicians and this therapist, as freely as children at a mud table. (p. 379–80)

[8] This all too brief description does not do justice to the theoretical complexity of the Backus approach. For further reading, see Backus (1952, 1957), and Backus and Beasley (1951).

As we had expected, this particular kind of group therapy featuring the therapist's abrogation of any responsibility for leadership was not very effective and Sheehan (1970) reports a similar experience (p. 298). Nevertheless, he writes:

Since stuttering is an interpersonal self-presentation disorder and occurs in a social context, group therapy is a natural choice for adults. In combination with varying degrees of subgroup and individual therapy, we have worked out a fairly unique structure unifying stuttering therapy with major aspects of psychotherapy. Stutterers can do things for each other in groups that no individual therapist can accomplish. Social isolation, at least in the lonesome sense of feeling like a probable freak—or an improbable one—is a core feeling in stuttering. Against this background, the discovery that you are not alone, that your experiences are shared and shareable with others like you, can be in itself enormously therapeutic. Particularly is this true if the group is used as a springboard to action. (p. 297)

There have been several other descriptions of group therapy with stutterers having a psychotherapeutic flavor. Oscar Fitz (1961) in Germany had long advocated group therapy with the stutterers "placed before a large circle of listeners in order to convince them of their own ability to speak (p. 265)." Jessler (1962) evidently uses similar methods. Hooper (1964) describes a play-by-play account of a group therapy program of combined speech therapy and pychsotherapy in Australia, concluding:

I have tried to stress that a group is a therapeutic unit through which a person may experience social relationships and be stimulated and encouraged in his battle—because it is a battle—to learn to talk easily when and where he likes. (p. 14)

Stromsta (1965) presents an interesting account of a group therapy program based upon sociometric procedures, the stutterers revising their self-concepts in terms of the group's consensus. Leith and Uhlemann (1970) and Ingham and Andrews (1971) have explored the use of conditioning principles including token rewards in group treatment of stutterers.

In the studies we have been reporting, the group therapy often was bimodal in aims and activity, some of it being concerned with speech therapy and some of it with psychotherapy (if, indeed, they can be so separated). A group of workers however have relegated the speech therapeutic component to a very minor role or have ignored it completely. Brody and Harrison (1954) were among the first to apply psychoanalytic principles to group therapy with stutterers. They found it extremely difficult as this quotation indicates:

From the very beginning this group of strangers formed a cohesive band that seemed to look upon the psychotherapist as an outsider who could not possibly understand their problem. The presenting picture was that of a long-suffering, persecuted minority group. Their concept of how stuttering could be overcome by the individual was striking in its uniformity. They expressed the opinion that the symptom should be dealt with violently. They felt if they were strong, they could force themselves to stop stuttering by means of "cutting it out" and "ripping it away." They said they were unable to accomplish this only because they "lacked the strength," had "no guts," or were "too inferior." The psychotherapist tried to encourage the group, but this seemed to cause the men to become more resentful. The psychotherapist found himself fighting to extend a ray of hope to the group. He offered his interpretation that each of these individuals was prejudiced against himself, and perhaps, if as individuals each could accept and be proud of himself including his stuttering, that would be his first step toward overcoming it. The group reacted as a unit, saying that this substantiated their feeling that the psychotherapist could not understand them at all. (p. 155)

(Reading this, the present author permits himself a wry grin.)

Barbara, Goldart, and Oram (1961) describe the dynamics of group psychoanalysis (based on the Horney approach) with stutterers, presenting the rationale, application, and resistances. They write:

In the group process it is essential not to deal specifically with the stuttering manifestation, but to understand what the stutterer is trying to express when he speaks, and especially at the time he stutters. The therapist must intercept and decode the messages the stutterer sends by the way he presents himself in speaking, his hidden meanings, feeling tones, anxieties, inhibitions, hesitations, and especially his own word jargon. (p. 55)

A similar position, that stuttering represents a defense against facing infantile, narcissistic needs, was adduced by Sadoff and Siegel (1965) in a pilot study with six adult stutterers receiving group psychotherapy. In the same year, Miele (1962), a stutterer, provided a general survey of the principles of group psychotherapy with stutterers and mentions one of his problems:

The therapist who stutters will at first be quickly accepted as "one of us." The patients soon realize that the therapist's goal is to examine the attitudes and feelings unrelated to speech and the staggering realization gradually emerges that the therapist believes that each patient suffers not only from stuttering but from a more basic emotional disturbance. This is a crucial stage in the group. At this point the resistance takes the form of

"fluency based logic." Mental health is equated with fluency and the therapist is confronted with the question of how he "can set himself up as an authority on mental health" if he still stutters. (p. 237)

Self-therapy groups

Stutterers have on occasions banded together to form groups to take care of the need for belonging which most stutterers feel. Some of these are quasi-therapy groups; others are primarily social. Some have been instigated and supported by therapists (Damste, Zwaan, and Schoenaker, 1968) to promote stabilization of the gains made in intensive therapy. Others such as the famous *Plus Club* of Sweden were initiated and operated by the stutterers themselves. Mogren and Leanderson (1965) describe the formation and working of this organization in detail and we quote from the summary of their article:

In order to bridge the gap between therapy and situations met in reality a few adult stutterers on their own initiative worked together. In joint training they tried to apply techniques they had learned earlier as patients with various speech therapists. In their efforts to transfer speech practice from artificial to real situations of speech the focus of interest shifted from problems of speech technique to psychological questions. The speech exercises were replaced by analytical discourses. This caused a relaxation of the ambitions of the participants to suppress the stuttering but stimulated their desire to vindicate their personal integrity as stutterers. In a period of ten years the group developed into a national liaison organization and debate society for stutterers and therapists. (p. 440)

A comparable organization in the United States is the National Council for Adult Stutterers which began with the following plea by Heffron (1966):

I would like to form a group of stutterers—or join one that already exists—in which the members want to help themselves and to help other stutterers. Such a group would be dedicated to making the public aware of the problem of stuttering, to soliciting the public's help and understanding, and to reaching all those stutterers who have never sought help for themselves. It would seek to make stutterers proud—not that they stutter, for only a fool can take pride in affliction—but that they are doing something to help themselves.

Ideally, there would be a national organization with the competence, authority, personnel, and funding to develop and direct a nationwide campaign. Associated with this organization would be state and local groups, bringing into local focus the broad appeals of the national body. Some day this may be.

My immediate concern, however, is to establish a local group where I live (Washington, D.C.) and to urge others throughout the country to consider similar plans for themselves. I will meet for the first time with a small group of stutterers who—I hope—will form with me the nucleus of an organization dedicated to the goals I have outlined. I will propose that the following means of achieving these goals be considered:

a. Prepare and deliver talks to local business groups such as the Lions, the Rotarians, and the Civitans, to church, PTA, and fraternal groups.

b. Contact local newspapers, radio, and television stations; be prepared to offer full cooperation in the preparation of news items, dramatic presentations, and personal interviews.

c. Solicit the aid of the public and private schools—especially at the college level—in making known to stutterers within their systems the goals of our organization.

d. Publish a newsletter keeping all area stutterers informed and encouraging their cooperation and participation.

e. Solicit financial support for research into the problem of stuttering.

f. Make known to the public the fine work of the many local people, schools, and organizations concerned with stuttering.

As a stutterer, I feel nothing but revulsion at the thought of publicly displaying my misfortune. But as an adult of some enlightened self-interest, I feel that the value of doing something about my own problem and of extending my selfish energies to help others would be beyond measure. I'm willing to try it, I want to find others who will join me, and I want the advice and aid of all interested parties. (pp. 168–69)

Most of the self-initiated groups of stutterers, unlike those of most deviants, have had only an emphemeral existence, usually breaking up in a few months or years and this has been our experience too. Lemert (1970) says:

. . . stutterers—unlike the blind, the deaf, the physically handicapped, narcotics addicts, criminals and other deviants—do not form groups of their own, nor do they develop a subculture. Furthermore, they neither organize nor support therapy groups comparable to Alcoholics Anonymous. Stutterers have no opportunities to make use of socially acquired techniques and subcultural ideologies for dealing with the rejection and social degradation they experience in society. (pp. 181–82)

Nevertheless, both the Plus Club and the National Council of Adult Stutterers have been flourishing for some years and the latter has shown an impressive spin-off in creating other stuttering groups.[9] Much depends upon the leaders chosen by these

[9] The address of the Plus Club is Postbox 755, 101 30 Stockholm, Sweden; and that of the National Council of Adult Stutterers is the Speech and Hearing Clinic, Catholic University of America, Washington, D.C. Both organizations publish a little journal.

groups and the functions they perform. Certainly in at least some minor measures they provide some supportive psychotherapy for their members.

Bibliography

ANDREWS, G. and M. HARRIS, *The Syndrome of Stuttering*. London: Heineman, 1964.

ALEXANDER, F. M., *The Use of the Self*. New York: Dutton, 1932.

APPELT, A., *Stammering and Its Permanent Cure*. London: Methune, 1929.

ARON, M. L., The effects of the combination of trifluoperazine and amylobarbitone on adult stutterers, *Medical Proceedings* (South Africa), 11 (1965), 227–33.

ARNOTT, N., *Elements of Physics and Natural Philosophy*. Edinburgh: 1828.

BACH, G. R., *Intensive Group Psychotherapy*. New York: Ronald Press, 1954.

BACHRACH, A. J. and W. A. QUIGLEY, Direct methods of treatment, in I. A. Berg and L. A. Pennington (eds.), *An Introduction to Clinical Psychology*, 3rd ed. New York: Ronald Press, 1966, pp. 482–560.

BACKUS, O. L., Group structure in speech therapy, in L. E. Travis (ed.), *Handbook of Speech Pathology*. New York: Appleton-Century-Crofts, 1957.

———, The use of group structure in speech therapy, *Journal of Speech and Hearing Disorders*, 17 (1952), 116–22.

——— and J. BEASLEY, *Speech Therapy with Children*. Boston: Houghton-Mifflin, 1951.

BACKUS, O. L. and H. M. DUNN, Intensive group structures in speech rehabilitation, *Journal of Speech Disorders*, 12 (1947), 39–60.

BARBARA, D. A., *Stuttering: A Psychodynamic Approach to Its Understanding and Treatment*. New York: Julian, 1954.

———, Some aspects of stuttering in light of adlerian psychology, *Journal of Individual Psychology*, 13 (1957), 188–93.

——— (ed.), *The Psychotherapy of Stuttering*. Springfield, Ill.: Charles C Thomas, 1962.

———, N. GOLDART, and C. ORAM, Group psychoanalysis with adult stutterers, *American Journal of Psychoanalysis*, 21 (1961), 40–57.

BEASLEY, B., *Stammering: Its Treatment*, 17th ed. Birmingham: Hudson, 1897.

BERGMAN, R., A case of stuttering, *Journal of American Academy of Child Psychiatry*, 7 (1968), 13–30.

BIBIK, V. A., Experience with the use of tranquilizers in the treatment of stuttering, *Zhurnal Nevropathologii i Psikhiatrie, imeni S. S. Korsakova*, 68 (1966), 1089–90.

BLOODSTEIN, O., *A Handbook on Stuttering for Professional Workers*. Chicago: National Society for Crippled Children and Adults, 1969.

———, Stuttering as an anticipatory struggle reaction, in J. Eisenson (ed.), *Stuttering: A Symposium*. New York: Harper & Row, 1958.

BLUEMEL, C. S., *The Riddle of Stuttering*. Danville, Ill.: Interstate, 1957.

BRILL, A. A., Speech disturbances in nervous and mental diseases, *Quarterly Journal of Speech Education*, 9 (1923), 129–35.

BRODY, M. W., and S. I. HARRISON, Group psychotherapy with male stutterers, *International Journal of Group Psychotherapy*, 4 (1954), 154–62.

BRUN, R., The psychoanalysis of stuttering, *International Journal of Psychoanalysis*, 4 (1923), 282–89.

BRUTTEN, E. J. and D. J. SHOEMAKER, *The Modification of Stuttering*. Englewood Cliffs, N.J.: Prentice-Hall, 1966.

BRYNGELSON, B., Method of stuttering, *Journal of Abnormal Psychology*, 30 (1935), 194–98.

———, *Clinical Group Therapy for*

Problem People. Minneapolis: Dennison, 1966.

BULLWINKLE, B. A., Methods and outcome of treatment of stutterers in a child guidance clinic, Smith College Studies in Social Work, 4 (1933), 107–38.

BURR, H. G. and J. M. MULLENDORF, Recent investigations on tranquilizers and stuttering, *Journal of Speech and Hearing Disorders,* 25 (1960), 33–37.

CLARK, R. M., The status of speech correction and pathology (logopedics) in the USSR, *Cameo,* 26 (1959), 40–41.

COOPER, E., Client-clinician relationships and concomitant factors in stuttering therapy, *Journal of Speech and Hearing Research,* 9 (1966), 194–207.

————, A therapy process for the adult stutterer, *Journal of Speech and Hearing Disorders,* 33 (1968), 246–60.

CORIAT, I. H., The nature and analytical treatment of stuttering, *Proceedings of the American Speech Correction Association,* 1 (1931), 151–56.

CORNELIU, F. C., Methodes therapeutiques et correlations pathogeniques dans le begaiement tonique, *Proceedings of the 14th Congress of the International Association of Logopedics and Phoniatrics,* Paris 1968, pp. 62–70.

COZZO, G. and L. GABRIELLI, La therapie du begaiement avec les buytrophonones, *De Therapia Vocis et Loquellae,* 1 (1965), 415–19.

CYPREASON, L., Group therapy for adult stutterers, *Journal of Speech Disorders,* 13 (1948), 313–19.

DAMSTE, P. H., E. J. ZWAAN, and T. J. SCHOENAKER, Learning principles applied to the stuttering problem, *Folia Phoniatrica,* 20 (1968), 327–41.

DANIELSON, H. (Modern Psychotherapy Challenges Traditional Stuttering Therapy), *Nordisk Tisskrift for Tale og Stemme,* 23 (1963), 113–17.

DASKALOV, D. D. (Basic Principles and Methods for the Prevention and Treatment of Stuttering), *Zhurnal Nevropatologii i Psikhiatrii imeni S. S. Korsakova,* 62 (1962), 1047–52.

————, Etude comparative de l'effect curatif de 18 medicaments psycholeptiques lors du traitement complexe du begaiement, *Proceedings of the 14th Congress of the International Association of Logopedics and Phoniatrics,* Paris 1968, pp. 99–104.

DESPERT, J. L., A therapeutic approach to the problem of stuttering, *Nervous Child,* 2 (1942), 134–47.

DEWS, P. B., Psychopharmacology, in A. Bachrach (ed.), *Experimental Foundations of Clinical Psychology.* New York: Basic Books, 1962.

DIAMOND, M., An investigation of some personality differences between predominantly tonic stutterers and predominantly clonic stutterers. Ph.D. Thesis, Syracuse University, 1953.

DiCARLO, L. M., J. KATZ, and S. BATKIN, An exploratory investigation of the effect of meprobramate on stuttering behavior, *Journal of Nervous and Mental Diseases,* 128 (1959), 558–61.

DICKSON, S., Incipient stuttering and spontaneous remission of stuttered speech, *Journal of Communication Disorders,* (1971), 99–110.

DOLLARD, J. and N. E. MILLER, *Personality and Psychotherapy.* New York: McGraw-Hill, 1950.

DOSTALOVA, N. and T. DOSUZKOV, (Aspects of Three Main Categories of Neurotic Stuttering), *De Terapia Vocis et Loquellae,* 1 (1965), 275–76.

DOUGLASS, E. and B. QUARRINGTON, Differentiation of interiorized and exteriorized secondary stuttering, *Journal of Speech and Hearing Disorders,* 17 (1952), 377–85.

DUNLOP, M., Psychologist uses anger to cure stammering, *Toronto Daily Star,* August 25, 1970.

ELLIS, A., Rational psychotherapy, *Journal of General Psychology,* 59 (1958), 35–49.

———— and R. A. HARPER, *A Guide to Rational Living.* Englewood Cliffs, N.J.: Prentice-Hall, 1961.

EYSENCK, H. J., The effects of psychotherapy: An evaluation, *Journal of Consulting Psychology*, 16 (1952), 319–24.

FENICHEL, O. Outline of clinical psychoanalysis, *Psychoanalytic Quarterly*, 2, (1933), 260–308.

————, *The Psychoanalytic Theory of Neurosis*. New York: Norton, 1945.

FERNAU-HORN, H., *Die Sprechneurosen*. Stuttgart: Hippokrates-Verlag, 1969.

FISH, B. H. and E. BOWLING, Stuttering: The effect of treatment with d-amphetamine and a tranquilizing agent, triflueoperazine, *California Medicine*, 103 (1965), 337–39.

FITZ, O., *Schach dem Stottern*. Freiburg: Lambertus-Verlag, 1961.

FLETCHER, J. M., *The Problem of Stuttering*. New York: Longmans, 1928.

FRANKL, V. E., Paradoxical intention, *American Journal of Psychotherapy*, 14 (1960), 520–35.

————, *The Doctor and the Soul: From Psychotherapy to Logotherapy*. New York: Knopf, 1965.

FREUND, H., *Psychopathology and Problems of Stuttering*. Springfield, Ill.: Charles C Thomas, 1966.

FROESCHELS, E., Pathology and therapy of stuttering, *Nervous Child*, 2 (1942), 146–61.

————, Stuttering and psychotherapy, *Folia Phoniatrica*, 3 (1951), 1–9.

FUJITA, K., The diagnostic statistics of 80 cases of stutterers, *Japanese Journal of Otorhinolaryngology*, 67 (1964), 343, Abstract No. 297 in G. Kamiyama, *Handbook for the Study of Stuttering*. Tokyo: Kongo-Shuppan, 1967.

GLASNER, P. J. and M. F. DAHL, Stuttering: A prophylactic program for its control, *American Journal of Public Health*, 42 (1952), 111–15.

GLASSER, W., *Reality Therapy*. New York: Harper & Row, 1965.

GLAUBER, I. P., Dysautomatization: A disorder of preconscious ego functioning, *International Journal of Psychoanalysis*, 49 (1968), 89–99.

————, The psychoanalysis of stuttering, in J. Eisenson (ed.), *Stuttering: A Symposium*. New York: Harper & Row, 1958.

————, Psychoanalytic concepts of the stutterer, *Nervous Child*, 2 (1943), 171–79.

————, The treatment of stuttering, *Social Casework*, 24 (1953), 162–67.

GOLDMAN, R. and P. Guth, The effects of psychotherapeutic drugs on stuttering, *De Therapia Vocis et Loquellae*, 1 (1965), 411–14.

GOODSTEIN, L., Functional speech disorders and personality: A survey of the literature, *Journal of Speech and Hearing Research*, 1 (1958), 358–71.

GRAY, B. and G. ENGLAND, (eds.), *Stuttering and the Conditioning Therapies*. Monterey, Calif.: Monterey Institute for Speech and Hearing, 1969.

GREENE, J. S., Functional speech and voice disorders, *Journal of Nervous and Mental Diseases*, 95 (1942), 299–309.

————, Interview group psychotherapy for speech disorders, in S. R. Slavson (ed.), *The Practice of Group Therapy*. New York: International University Press, 1947.

GUTZMANN, H., Experiments with treatment of speech disorders with glutamic acid, *Folia Phoniatrica*, 6 (1954), 1–8.

HALE, L. L., Consideration of thiamin supplement in prevention of stuttering in preschool children, *Journal of Speech and Hearing Disorders*, 16 (1951), 327–33.

HANICKE, O. and R. LEBEN (Contributions to Modern Views on the Treatment of Stuttering), *Deutsche Gesundheitswegen*, 19 (1964), 545–49.

HATFIELD, M. L., *How to Stop Stammering*. Oakland, Calif.: Fox, 1910.

HEFFRON, M., Stuttering—need for organization, *Asha*, 8 (1966), 167–69.

HEJNA, R. F., *Interviews with a Stutterer*.

Danville, Ill.: Interstate Printers and Publishers, 1963.

HIRSCHBERG, J. (Stuttering), *Orvosi Hetilap,* 106 (1965), 780–84.

HOGEWIND, F., Medical treatment of stuttering, *Journal of Speech Disorders,* 5 (1940), 203–8.

HOLLIDAY, A. R., Effect of meprobramate on stuttering, *Northwest Medicine,* 58 (1959), 837–41.

HOLLINGSWORTH, H. L., Chewing as a technique of relaxation, *Science,* 90 (1939), 385–87.

HOMMERICH, K. W., and M. KORZENDORFER, Untersuchung uber die anwendung von chlordiazepoxyd (Librium) in der stottertherapie, *H.N.O.,* 14 (1966), 211–18.

HONIG, P., The stutterer acts it out, *Journal of Speech Disorders,* 12 (1947), 105–9.

HOOPER, F., Group therapy with stammerers, *Journal of the Australian College of Speech Therapists,* 14 (1964), 8–14.

HORNEY, K., *The Neurotic Personality of Our Time.* New York: Norton, 1970.

————, *New Ways in Psychoanalysis.* New York: Norton, 1939.

HUNT, J., *Stammering and Stuttering, Their Nature and Treatment.* Original Ed. 1861. Reprinted by Hafner, New York, 1967.

IMAZEKI, Y. et al. (The Effectiveness of the Tranquilizer Astyn with Stutterers), *Japanese Medicine,* 14 (1960), 784–88.

INGHAM, R. J. and G. ANDREWS, A description and analysis of a token economy in an adult therapy program, Convention Paper, *Asha,* Chicago, 1971.

JAMESON, A. M., Stammering in children —Some factors in the prognosis, *Speech* (London), 19 (1955), 60–67.

JESSLER, F., Kurse für stotterers, *Neue Bl. Taubat.,* 16 (1962), 202–6.

JOHNSON, W., Perceptual and evaluational factors in stuttering, *Folia Phoniatrica,* 8 (1956), 211–33.

————, *People in Quandaries.* New York: Harper & Row, 1946.

————, Some practical suggestions for adults who stutter, *Speech Pathology and Therapy,* 1 (1961), 68–73.

————, *Stuttering and What You Can Do About It.* Danville, Ill.: Interstate, 1961.

JONES, M. C., Elimination of children's fears, *Journal of Experimental Psychology,* 7 (1924), 383–90.

KAMIYAMA, G., *Handbook for the Study of Stuttering.* Tokyo: Kongo Shuppan, 1967.

KENT, L. R., Retraining program for the adult who stutters, *Journal of Speech and Hearing Disorders,* 26 (1961a), 141–44.

————, Stuttering and endocrine malfunction, *Journal of Speech and Hearing Disorders,* 28 (1963), 197–98.

————, Use of tranquilizers in the treatment of stuttering: Reserpine, chloromazine, meprobamate, atarax, Bibliography, *Journal of Speech and Hearing Disorders,* 28 (1963), 288–94.

————, Carbon dioxide therapy as a medical treatment for stuttering, *Journal of Speech and Hearing Disorders,* 26 (1961b), 268–71.

————, and D. E. WILLIAMS, Use of Meprobramate as an Adjunct to Stuttering Therapy, *Journal of Speech and Hearing Disorders,* 24 (1959), 64–69.

KENYON, E. L., Peripheral physical inhibition of speech: An essential phenomenon and an important causal factor of stammering, *Oralism and Auralism,* 10 (1931), 15–31.

KOCHERGINA, V. S. (Drug Treatment of Stammering in Adults), *Zhurnal Nevropathologii i Psikhatrii imeni S. S. Korsakova,* 65 (1965), 753–56.

KOSH, Z. H., An integrated course for stutterers and voice defectives, *Quarterly Journal of Speech,* 27 (1941), 97–104.

LACZKOWSKA, M., Painting in stuttering

children, *De Therapia Vocis et Loquellae*, 1 (1965), 367–69.

LANYON, R. I., Behavior change in stuttering through systematic desensitization, *Journal of Speech and Hearing Disorders*, 34 (1969), 253–60.

LAZARUS, A. A., Case history of a stutterer treated as an obsessive-compulsive disorder by broad-spectrum behavior therapy, in B. B. Gray and G. England (eds.), *Stuttering and the Conditioning ..Therapies*. Monterey, Calif.: Monterey Institute, 1969.

LEANDERSON, R. and L. Levi, Stuttering, stress and psychotropic drugs—a clinical and experimental study, *Proceedings of the 14th Congress of the International Association of Logopedics and Phoniatrics*, Paris, 1968.

LEITH, W. R. and M. R. Uhlmann, The shaping group: Theory, organization and function, Unpublished paper, *Asha*, Convention, 1970.

LEMERT, E. M., Sociological perspective, in J. G. Sheehan (ed.), *Stuttering: Research and Therapy*. New York: Harper & Row, 1970, pp. 172–87.

———— and C. VAN RIPER, The use of psychodrama in the treatment of speech defects, *Sociometry*, 7 (1944), 190–95.

LENNON, E. J., *Le Begaiement: Therpeutiques Modernes*. Paris: Doin et Cie, 1962.

LEVY, D. M., Release therapy in young children, *American Journal of Orthopsychiatry*, 9 (1939), 387–90.

LOVE, W. R., The effect of pentobarbital sodium (nembutal) and amphetamine sulfate (benzedrine) on the severity of stuttering, in W. Johnson (ed.), *Stuttering in Children and Adults*. Minneapolis: University of Minnesota Press, 1955, pp. 298–312.

LUCHSINGER, R., Die vererbung von sprach und stottern, *Folia Phoniatrica*, 11 (1959), 7–64.

———— and G. E. ARNOLD, *Voice-Speech and Language*. Belmont, Calif.: Wadsworth, 1965.

LUPER, H. and R. MULDER, *Stuttering Therapy for Children*. Englewood Cliffs, N.J.: Prentice-Hall, 1964.

MAHL, G., Disturbances and silences in the patients' speech in psychotherapy, *Journal of Abnormal Social Psychology*, 42 (1957), 3–32.

MARTYN, M. M. and J. SHEEHAN, Onset of stuttering and recovery, *Behavior Research and Therapy*, 6 (1968), 295–307.

MAXWELL, R. D. and J. W. PATTERSON, Meprobamate in the treatment of stuttering, *British Medical Journal*, 179 (1958), 873–74.

McCORD, H., Hypnotherapy and stuttering, *Journal of Clinical and Experimental Hypnosis*, 3 (1955), 210–14.

MEDUNA, L. J. *Carbon Dioxide Therapy*. Springfield, Ill.: Charles C Thomas, 1950.

MEFFRET, M. L., *The Effect of Serpasil (Reserpine) on the Severity of Stuttering*, Master's Thesis, University of Virginia, 1956.

MIELE, J. A., Group psychotherapy with stutterers, in D. Barbara (ed.), *The Psychotherapy of Stuttering*. Springfield, Ill.: Charles C Thomas, 1962.

MILISEN, R. B. and W. JOHNSON, A comparative study of stutterers, former stutterers and normal speakers whose handedness has been changed, *Archives of Speech*, 1 (1936), 61–86.

MILLER, C. H., Psychotherapy in action: A case report, in D. A. Barbara (ed.) *The Psychotherapy of Stuttering*. Springfield, Ill.: Charles C Thomas, 1962.

MITCHELL, B. A., *An Analysis of the Effect of Reserpine on Adult Stutterers*, Master's thesis, Western Michigan University, 1955.

MOGREN, D. and R. LEANDERSON, A layman's self-help experiment, *De Therapia Vocis et Loquellae*, 1 (1965), 447–50.

MORENO, J. L., *Sociometry and the Science of Man*. New York: Beacon House, 1956.

MOWRER, O. H., *Learning Theory and Personality Dynamics.* New York: Ronald Press, 1950.

————, *Learning Theory and Behavior.* New York: Wiley, 1960.

————, Stuttering as simultaneous admission and denial, *Journal of Communication Disorders,* 1 (1967), 46–50.

MURPHY, A. and R. FITZSIMONS, *Stuttering and Personality Dynamics.* New York: Ronald Press, 1960.

NAYLOR, R. V., A comparative study of methods of estimating the severity of stuttering, *Journal of Speech and Hearing Disorders,* 18 (1953), 30–37.

PALASEK, J. R. and W. S. CURTIS, Sugar placebos and stuttering, *Journal of Speech and Hearing Research,* 3 (1960), 223–26.

PENSON, E. M., An exploratory study of the effect of thiamin hydrochloride on adults who stutter, *Speech Monographs,* 19 (1952), 197 (Abstract).

PERLS, F., R. F. HEFFERLINE, and P. GOODMAN, *Gestalt Therapy.* New York: Dell Publishing Co., 1951.

PLATONOV, K., *The Word.* Moscow: Foreign Language Publishing House, 1959.

POLLARD, J. C. and C. BAKKER, What does the clinician want to know? in L. Uhr and J. G. Miller (eds.), *Drugs and Behavior.* New York: Wiley, 1960.

POTTER, S. O. L., *Speech and Its Defects.* Philadelphia: Blakiston, 1882.

QUIDDE, L., Recollections of a stutterer, *Living Age,* 32 (1926), 360–63.

ROBBINS, S. D., The contribution of suggestion and of distraction to the treatment of stammering, *Proceedings of the American Speech and Hearing Association,* 2 (1932), 103–10.

ROGERS, C. R., *Counseling and Psychotherapy.* Boston: Houghton-Mifflin, 1942.

————, *Client Centered Therapy.* Boston: Houghton-Mifflin, 1951.

SACK, L. P., *The Effects of Sodium Dilantin on Stuttering Behavior,* Ph.D. thesis, University of California at Los Angeles, 1968.

SADOFF, R. L. and J. R. SIEGEL, Group psychotherapy for stutterers, *International Journal of Group Psychotherapy,* 15 (1965), 72–80.

SALTER, J. M., *Conditioned Reflex Therapy.* New York: Creative Age Press, 1949.

SCHAUBEL, H. J., and R. F. STREET, Prostigmin and the chronic stutterer, *Journal of Speech and Hearing Disorders,* 14 (1949), 143–46.

SCHILLING, A., Die behandlung des stotterns, *Folia Phoniatrica,* 17 (1965), 365–84.

————, (Adjuvant Drugs in the Therapy of Stuttering), *HNO Wegweiser für die Fachaerstliche Praxis,* 11 (1963a), 300–304.

————, Neuer untersuchungen uber die mitbeleiligung organischer ursachen bei der enstehung des stotterns, *Hals - Nasen - Ohren - Heilkunde,* 14 (1963a), 99–112.

————, Language and speech disturbances, in J. R. Berendes, R. Link, and P. Zöllner (eds.), *Neck, Nose and Ear Therapeutics,* Vol. 2. Stuttgart: Thieme, 1963c.

SCHULTZ, D. A., A study of nondirective counseling as applied to adult stutterers, *Journal of Speech Disorders,* 12 (1947), 421–27.

SCHULTZ, J. H., *Das Autogene Training.* Stuttgart: Thieme, 1964.

———— and W. LUTHE, *Autogenic Therapy.* Vol. 1, *Autogenic Methods.* New York: Gruen & Stratton, 1969.

SCRIPTURE, E. W., *Stuttering, Lisping and Correction of the Speech of the Deaf.* New York: Macmillan, 1931.

SEDLACKOVA, E., A contribution to pharmacotherapy of stuttering and cluttering, *Folia Phoniatrica,* 22 (1970), 354–75.

SEEMAN, J., *The Case of Jim.* Nashville, Tenn.: Educational Test Bureau, 1957.

SEEMAN, M., *Sprachstorungen bei Kindern*. Marhold: Halle-Saale, 1959.

SERRA, M. (Sensory Stimulation for Diagnostic Purposes in 19 Stutterers), *Archivi Italiano Laringologi*, 70 (1960), 355–61.

SHEARER, W. M. and J. D. Williams, Self-recovery from stuttering, *Journal of Speech and Hearing Disorders*, 30 (1965), 288–90.

SHEEHAN, J. G., An integration of psycotherapy and speech therapy through a conflict theory of stuttering, *Journal of Speech and Hearing Disorders*, 19 (1954), 474–82.

————, Conflict theory of stuttering, in J. Eisenson (ed.), *Stuttering: A Symposium*. New York: Harper & Row, 1958.

————, *Stuttering: Research and Therapy*. New York: Harper & Row, 1970, chapter 7.

———— and M. MARTYN, Spontaneous recovery from stuttering, *Journal of Speech and Hearing Research*, 9 (1966), 121–35.

SLAVSON, S. R., *Practice of Group Psychotherapy*. New York: International University Press, 1947.

————, *Introduction to Group Psychotherapy*. New York: International University Press, 1951.

SMITH, A. M., Treatment of stutterers (on basis of psychoneurotic personality) with carbon dioxide, *Diseases of the Nervous System*, 14 (1953), 243–44.

STEIN, L., *The Infancy of Speech and the Speech of Infancy*. London: Metheun, 1949.

————, Emotional background of stammering, *British Journal of Medical Psychology*, 22 (1949), 189–94.

STROMSTA, C., A procedure using group consensus in adult stuttering therapy, *Journal of Speech and Hearing Disorders*, 30 (1965), 277–79.

SULLIVAN, H. S., *The Interpersonal Theory of Psychiatry*. New York: Norton, 1953.

THORNE, F. C., *The Principles of Personality Counseling*. Brandon, Vt.: Journal of Clinical Psychology Press, 1950.

TRAVIS, L. E. (ed.), *Handbook of Speech Pathology*. New York: Appleton-Century-Crofts, 1957.

———— and L. D. SUTHERLAND, Suggestions for psychotherapy in public school speech correction, in L. E. Travis (ed.), *Handbook of Speech Pathology*. New York: Appleton-Century-Crofts, 1957.

TROJAN, F. A., A new method in the treatment of stuttering: The kinetic discharge therapy, *Folia Phoniatrica*, 17 (1965), 195–201.

TUTTLE, E., Hyperventilation in a patient who stammered: Methedrine as an adjunct to psychotherapy, *American Journal of Medicine*, 13 (1952), 777–79.

UHR, L. and J. G. MILLER (eds.), *Drugs and Behavior*. New York: Wiley, 1960.

ULLMANN, L. P. and L. KRASNER, (eds.), *Case Studies in Behavior Modification*. New York: Holt, Rinehart & Winston, 1965.

VAN RIPER, C., *Speech Correction: Principles and Methods*, 5th ed. Englewood Cliffs, N.J.: Prentice-Hall, 1971a.

————, A clinical success and a clinical failure, in M. Fraser (ed.), *Stuttering: Successes and Failures in Therapy*. Memphis, Tenn.: Speech Foundation of America, 1968, pp. 99–129.

————, *The Nature of Stuttering*. Englewood Cliffs, N.J.: Prentice-Hall, 1971b.

————, The role of reassurance in stuttering therapy, *Folia Phoniatrica*, 7 (1955), 217–22.

————, Experiments in stuttering therapy, in J. Eisenson (ed.), *Stuttering: A Symposium*. New York: Harper & Row, 1958.

VLASOVA, N. A., Late follow-up analysis of some cases of recurrent stuttering, *Zhurnal Nevropatologii i Psikiatrii imeni S. S. Korsakova*, 65 (1965), 750–51.

VOELKER, C. H., Incidence of pathologic speech behavior in the general American population, *Archives Otolaryngology,* 38 (1943), 113–21.

WATKINS, J. G., *Hypnotherapy of War Neuroses.* New York: Ronald Press, 1949.

————, Psychotherapeutic methods, in B. B. Wolman (ed.), *Handbook of Clinical Psychology.* New York: McGraw-Hill, 1965.

WEISS, D. A., *Cluttering.* Englewood Cliffs, N.J.: Prentice-Hall, 1964.

WELLS, P. G. and M. T. MALCOLM, Controlled trial of the treatment of 36 stutterers, *British Journal of Psychiatry,* 119 (1971), 603–4.

WINGATE, M. E., A standard definition of stuttering, *Journal of Speech and Hearing Disorders,* 29 (1964), 484–89.

————, Recovery from stuttering, *Journal of Speech and Hearing Disorders,* 29 (1964), 312–21.

WOLPE, J., The systematic desensitization and treatment of neurosis, *Journal of Nervous and Mental Diseases,* 132 (1961), 189–203.

————, The experimental foundation of some new psychotherapeutic methods, in A. J. Bachrach (ed.), *Experimental Foundations of Clinical Psychology.* New York: Basic Books, 1962.

———— and A. A. LAZARUS, *Behavior Therapy Techniques: A Guide to the Treatment of Neuroses.* Oxford: Pergamon Press, 1966.

YANNATOS, G., L'hydroxyzine dans la therapeutiques des begaiements, *Journal Francaise ORL,* 9 (1960), 293–96.

YEARSELY, W. A., *Practical Self-Cure of Stammering and Stuttering.* Yearsely: Accrington, 1909.

ZELEN, S. L., J. G. SHEEHAN, and J. F. T. BUGENTAL, Self-perception in stuttering, *Journal of Clinical Psychology,* 10 (1954), 70–72.

ZERNERI, L., Tentative d'applicazione della voci retardata (DAF) quella terapia della bulbuzie, *Bollettino Della Societa Italiana Di Fonetica, Fonestria e Audiologia,* 14 (1965), 125–30.

Therapeutic Success

and Prognosis

Up to this point we have been describing the incredible variety of therapeutic approaches to stuttering. What kind of a disorder is this that responds favorably, if we can believe those who propose them, to so many differing, even antagonistic, kinds of treatment? How valid are the claims of successful outcome? Shall we be politely gullible or nastily skeptical if the choice must be put in such blunt terms? What do people mean when they claim percentages of cures or percentages of improvement after treatment? We have explored enough histories of persons who were "treated successfully" by the methods we have described to come to some tentative conclusions. First, a very small handful of stutterers do indeed become fairly fluent as the result of almost any kind of therapy. Second, *the large majority of these adult stutterers are not cured*

though they may show little stuttering at the conclusion of treatment. Relapses and remissions are the rule, not the exception for the adult stutterer if long-term follow-up investigations are conducted. Thirdly, claims of improvement are very difficult to substantiate with any exactitude. Undoubtedly many stutterers do improve as the result of any of these different kinds of treatment but our measures of severity and our methods of assessment are so full of flaws as to yield little reliable information. But let us examine the claims and criteria.

How successful is stuttering therapy for the adult?

When the claims of some of our predecessors are considered, we seem to be losing ground. Denhardt (1890) was reported as having cured 93 percent of 2500 stutterers, the highest success rate we have been able to discover in the literature. That our skepticism concerning this claim may have some real justification is supported by the following quotation from Appelt (1929):

Denhardt has treated more than 2,500 stammerers, and claims to have cured 93 percent. The latter figure is more than exaggerated; as a matter of fact, his permanent cures reach an appallingly low percentage. Suffice it to say that the author has twice been treated by Denhardt, and that neither he himself nor any of the many fellow sufferers he met at Denhardt's Institute, and with whom he kept in touch with afterwards, found a permanent cure there. (p. 41)

Some of the other older workers were, by their own accounts, not quite as effective, even though their reports of cures are certainly substantial. According to Potter (1882):

Klencke, in 15 years, treated 148 cases, and claims to have had but one failure. Coen's first 67 cases resulted in 40 cures, 20 improved greatly and 7 failures. Chervin, in 6 months treated 52 cases, of which 46 were cured; 4, failing to apply themselves to the exercises were only partially benefitted, leaving 8 failures. On the other hand, an American teacher, Howard of New York, states that "relapses from partial relief are the rule, permanent cure the distinguished exceptions," and Robert M. Zug, who has a local reputation in Michigan in the treatment of stuttering, reports the result of his own experience of 150 cases, as giving but 15 complete cures. (p. 86)

While most modern therapists seem to be more conservative in their accounts of successes, we find a few of them doing remarkably well. Thus Zaliouk and Zaliouk (1965) claimed to have produced "full recovery" in 37 of 58 stuttering Israeli children in only 20 sessions. Nine others made partial progress and only two failed to profit at all from the treatment. Dostalova and Dosuzkov (1965) in Czechoslovakia report that 60 percent of two groups of 1,811 stuttering children were cured (Balbuties praecox and Balbuties vulgaris) while only 37 percent of a third group (Balbuties tarda) of 189 children were cured. Their failure rates ranged from 19 to 32 percent. Vlasova (1965) insisted that she was able to cure 65 to 70 percent of her Russian cases. Moreover she reports that no recurrence of stuttering occurred later in 60 percent of these children. (Note that most of these were children, not adult stutterers.)

In contrast to these exceptionally high percentages of cures, many modern workers seem to agree with Nadoleczny's (1928) remark that one third of the stutterers are cured, another third are improved and a remaining third should be classified as failures. Luchsinger and Arnold (1965), agreeing with Nadoleczny, say in addition, "It is interesting that all these figures are in exact agreement with the total result of all psychiatric treatment." What is even more significant, perhaps, is that about a third of all neurotics become symptom free without any treatment at all.

The doubters

As might be expected, we also find in the literature some strong challenges to these claims. Among the first to question the permanence of the so-called cures was Bluemel (1913), who attempted to assess the truth of the reported successes produced by the stammering schools of his time. An excerpt from his findings runs as follows:

The writer continued his investigations, and at the cost of considerable labor managed to communicate with a hundred ex-pupils of two other stammering schools —one an American and the other an English institution, and both of them schools that *guaranteed* to cure stammering. Among these one hundred ex-pupils, five pronounced themselves cured. Of these five students, two have, to the writer's knowledge, since relapsed. One of the remaining three the writer met recently in New York, and this cured stutterer was beating time and speaking at the rate of approximately one word a minute. . . . Thus we have apparently two permanent cures in one hundred cases, with one of the cures to be heavily discounted. (p. 265–66)

Elsewhere Bluemel (1957) says "When a stammerer carries his impediment into adult life, it is unlikely that speech therapy will render him facile and fluent." Scripture (1931) says: "Stuttering or stammering is usually regarded as incurable and not more than five percent of treated cases even fully recover, for the pathology of the disease has never been established and no rational methods of treatment have been found (p. 150)." Brill (1923) the famous psychoanalyst who examined 500 stutterers and did long-term treatment with 69 of them, "curing" only five, one of whom had a relapse, expresses his disillusionment thusly: "Like everyone else, I was very enthusiastic in the beginning when I saw the remarkable improvement in some of the patients. My enthusiasm declined with the length of my experience and the number of my cases." "Stuttering," Brill continues, "is the most difficult neurosis that one has to treat. There are very few cures effected among adult chronic stutterers.

Most of these so-called cures are of a temporary nature."

We also find some of the same doubts expressed in the European literature. Hanicke and Leben (1964) say:

Stuttering saps the self-confidence of the stammerer and leaves him with the impression of failure. Because there seems to be no escape, the disorder often assumes the characteristics of a chronic neurosis. It is therefore understandable that Panconcelli-Calzia, one of the greatest of all phoneticians, came to declare almost at the end of his career, "A stammerer will continue to stammer all his life despite the scientist's theories." Certainly stammering can be improved to a greater or lesser extent but the predisposition or the tendency to relapse remains constantly present and it will emerge at the slightest provocation. (p. 545)

In 1938 Bryngelson, who had previously reported that 40 percent of all stuttering children lose their stuttering by the age of eight, expresses his disillusionment about the possibility of curing adult stutterers:

After fifteen years of experience with some 5,000 stutterers, I am forced to say that an absolute cure is very rare. By absolute cure I would mean the elimination of all symptoms, fear, sensitivity, habit patterns, avoidance and postponement devices, psychological and physiologic crutches . . . (p. 122).

Kopp, (1939) is no less pessimistic:

I have questioned every theory of stuttering that has ever been advocated. I have done this because I was convinced that no one method of treating stuttering is sufficient to correct the speech of the majority of stutterers. In ten years of working with stutterers I have never been able to completely cure a single adult stutterer, using one or several approaches. It is true that I have helped to improve the speech of a number of stutterers, both young and old. Dr. West had an apt way of distributing the honors, if any. He would say, "Oh sure, God, nature, the patient, Kopp and myself have helped a few stutterers." (p. 166)

Fitz (1961), in his book *Schach dem Stottern,* also shows some concern about exhorbitant claims:

Certainly it seems both bold and improbable to claim that all stutterers can be freed from their disorder by any reeducation of the voice or speech functions. The limited success shown by the usual ways of treating stuttering in our experience makes such a claim an illusion or an empty assertion. As a rule, of the stutterers who constitute one percent of the general population, only 30 percent can be healed; 30 percent remain the same and 40 percent become worse. When Chemnitz reported 70 percent successes in treating stutterers, the doubts in professional circles were universal. (p. 262)

The late Anton Schilling of Germany, who worked intensively with many stutterers and with success, still expresses caution: "Anyone who boasts of a definite cure for stuttering lays himself open to serious suspicion (1961)."[1] Elsewhere, Schilling (1963) in his account of his own cures is cautious:

On the basis of our experiences, we are very cautious in making the judgment of "healed" with stutterers for good reason. Even when there is freedom from symptom at the end of treatment, we do not consider this as evidence of complete healing. If there still remains an unsureness

[1] This quotation comes from Hirschberg, (1965, p. 783) and is attributed to Schilling's article "Das sprach-und Stimmgestörte Kleinkind und Schulkind" in *Phoniatriekurs fur Kindergartnerinnen,* 1961 which we have been unable to procure.

or shyness in speaking, or microscopic symptomatological differences in accent or tempo or a continuance of other correlated behavior disturbances such as bedwetting, we refrain from judging the patient as healed even if he is fluent. (p. 1190)

Perhaps the basic reason for the skepticism about reported cures is the prevalence of relapse after treatment. There is something very final about the concept of cure. We once worked with one stutterer who said that he had already been cured nine times and wanted to make it ten. It is a bold therapist or one blinded by ego-needs who would use the word "cure" as indicating freedom from stuttering forever. McCord (1955) puts the matter in a saner perspective: "Unfortunately, relief from stuttering can be adjudged 'permanent' only if the individual remains free from the ailment until he dies. Hence, perhaps research in the area should be undertaken only by individuals who anticipate personal longevity (p. 214)."

What is meant by the cure of stuttering

Here once again we meet the difficult problem of definition. In another book, *The Nature of Stuttering* (Van Riper, 1971b), the author has devoted a chapter to this topic. He showed that many different workers in the field of speech pathology defined stuttering differently. This situation in itself would lead to confusion in seeking to equate the results of one person's therapy with that of another's. When one peruses the many reports of clinical successes, we rarely find any mention of the basic criteria by which stuttering may have been defined. In that chapter we also distinguished between a stuttering behavior which we equated with a temporally broken or distorted word and stuttering as a disorder, which is quite another matter. Presumably, most of the reported "cures" are based on the latter, but we find no data which we can use in interpreting the author's standard's of deviance. Neaves (1967) for example says:

The choice of criteria for successful and unsuccessful outcome of treatment was clearly critical and in this case was resolved as follows: (1) All cases to be rated as having responded successfully to treatment either to be completely free from stammering or to show only a very mild stammer. (2) All cases to be rated as not having responded successfully to treatment to have still a moderate or severe stammer. (p. 84)

We would suspect that most of the successes he reports (51 percent) fell in the second half of his first category.[2] We doubt that any person is completely free from demonstrating a few broken words under occasional communicative stress, so evidently this author has a different definition than we have, which is the point we are trying to make. Unless we have some understanding of what authors mean by stammering or its disappearance, we remain in the dark. How perfectly, or how consistently or how permanently do you have to speak fluently to be called cured? We found an old article in the London Magazine of August, 1825, describing Broster's system for the cure of speech impediments, primarily stammering. The author, after examining the treatment and assessing it, makes this pregnant statement, "It is generally effective, but it is not *perfective*." We suspect that most of the so-called cures fall into the former

classification. The stutterers learn to speak more effectively and less abnormally. Some of them become able to "pass" as normal speakers by overcoming the barrier line which signifies deviance.

Long ago, Robert West tried to make some sense out of the various claims of successful treatment of stuttering:

Cure, in the minds of some, is the learning of a technique by which the patient can speak in spite of his tendency to stutter, though his speech is not entirely automatic. . . . Cure, in the minds of others, is a complete return to normal speech with no need for a constant watch lest it slip, in short, to an automaticity of speech. Cure, in the minds of others, is the reduction or elimination of the situations in which stuttering is elicited . . . this by changing the attitude of the stutterer toward these situations. This is the mental hygienist's cure, and assumes that if the old attitudes are brought back again, stuttering will return. (1932, p. 127.)

We do not feel that West's list includes all the various definitions which yield the cure rates reported in the literature. Some successes merely reflect the stutterer's ability to achieve a precarious fluency in oral reading, or speaking in the clinic or laboratory, or to the therapist. Is a stutterer cured if he can speak without broken words but only while tapping his fingers synchronously with each syllable or speaking at a rate of 40 words per minute or only when wearing a wristband? In this connection the Australian, Scott (1969), makes an important point:

If there is such a need to develop "a new psychomotor speech pattern" (Gregory, 1968; Goldiamond, 1965) in the stutterer, this speech must in some way be qualitatively different from normal speech. . . .

2 And we cannot tell from the report how many of these had been "mild" stammerers prior to therapy.

Normal speech becomes confounded (erroneously) with fluent speech. When a stutterer is cured, he should speak normally and not necessarily fluently, if that fluency is only achieved by an abnormal form of utterance. (p. 60)

Some "cures" merely reflect the stutterer's fluency at the time of discharge from treatment. Indeed, some successes are reported merely in terms of the number discharged. Bonafide cures can only be ascertained in terms of follow-up investigations and these pose many problems. As Andrews and Harris (1964) state:

To assess the speech of the subjects at the follow-up clinic only was clearly unsatisfactory, for many learnt to speak fluently to the therapists and yet continued to have difficulty in other settings. The subject's own report of his progress was not reliable, for both denial of symptom and extreme self criticism were common responses. (p. 153)

Few workers have employed the stress interview used by Andrews and Harris to overcome these problems, but even had they done so, there are some stutterers who can rise to the challenge of a reevaluation and present a temporary fluency which, upon investigation, does not characterize their casual speech. Rubin and Cullata (1971) say, "We feel comfortable about declaring nine of the stutterers cured, are optimistic about the outcome of two others, uncertain about two and pessimistic about two." We envy their feeling of comfort but would prefer more information concerning the methods and conditions of their evaluation.

Perhaps another important difficulty in assessing the results of stuttering therapy in terms of cures is that a medical model for the disorder is implied, and may be quite inappropriate. Stuttering is not a disease in the medical sense. Much of its features consist of learned behaviors; perhaps the major bulk of the stutterer's abnormality consist of these. You don't "cure" learned behaviors, you unlearn or you replace them with other learned behaviors. Moreover many of the learned behaviors which characterize stuttering involve conditioned avoidance reactions to multiple and complex stimulus situations. These are notably difficult to extinguish. Others, those characterized by struggle and escape, have also been very powerfully reinforced. While complete extinction of such learned responses is theoretically possible, it is hardly realistic to expect it to occur in a high percentage of the adult stuttering population. The fact that universally more cures are reported for children than for adults is probably due to the fact that this learned fraction of the problem in them is still minute or weakly conditioned. Let us face it—the word "cure" is a very elastic container and various clinicians have crammed a motley array of therapeutic results therein.

Criteria of therapeutic success

It seems to us that if "cures" are claimed, the following questions should be answered since outcome studies will always be regarded with some suspicion if none of this pertinent information is provided. (1) What was the therapist's definition of cure? (2) How was it assessed? (3) When and how often and after what intervals was the stutterer reevaluated? (4) Since such a large proportion of children seem to overcome their stuttering without any therapy whatsoever, how old were the stutterers? (5) How severe was the original stuttering? (6) How many stutterers dropped out of treatment? (7) What proportion of those treated were available for reevaluation? (8) Of those claimed as cured, how many were there who report occasional relapses? (9) Were any attempts made to use no-treatment or placebo-therapy control groups? (10) Was the assessment of cure made by the person who administered the therapy or by the stutterer or by his associates or by some independent assessor? In our review of the literature, only a few studies present the information required to answer even a few of these questions and not one of them answers all of them.

The assessment of improvement

Almost all of the reports of successes in stuttering therapy include the category of improvement. This is often broken down into subclassifications of *very improved* (normal or near normal speech), *improved,* or *somewhat improved.* Although these judgments doubtless reflect the therapist's opinion, which can hardly be viewed as free from some bias, they also are based upon some real changes which may have occurred as the result of therapy. Stutterers do get better, or they stand still, or they get worse. Our concern is not with the concept of improvement but with the criteria used to evaluate it.

Again, as in the case of claimed cures, we usually find no criteria mentioned in the outcome studies reported in the literature. We merely find numbers or percentages, a sorry situation at best for those who seek the truth. All of the unpleasant but necessary questions we posed for the claim of cure are equally important in the assessment of improvement. Or even more important since the claim of cure is presumably capable of validation (e.g., stuttering is not heard, nor seen, nor felt) while the concept of improvement is based upon rela-

tive severity. A person has improved, we might say, when his stuttering is less severe than it was formerly. But this implies that we can measure severity with some reliability and validity and the sad truth is that we cannot. As our review of the severity of stuttering has shown (Van Riper, 1971, chapter 9), neither the frequency nor the duration of individual moments of stuttering are satisfactory measures of severity and they bear little relationship to the stutterer's own view of his difficulty. Moreover, stuttering is very variable in its occurrence in differing situations and under differing stresses and it is greatly affected by interpersonal relationships and intrapersonal emotions. The multiple-factor equation which might truly represent severity has yet to be formulated. We are forced therefore to conclude that these reports of improvement must be viewed simply as the impressions of the evaluators, nothing more. Doubtless they have some face validity but we must always regard reported percentages of improvement with caution.

Attempts to provide valid assessments

Some of these difficulties have been recognized by many workers and perhaps the skepticism with which claims of successful therapy have been met is due to that recognition. One of the earliest attempts to really find the truth about the results of stuttering therapy was carried out by Abrahams and Forchammer (1954) in Denmark where stutterers had been treated in an institute for many years. Rejecting any questionnaire approach as undesirable, they interviewed 144 former patients not only at the institute but at home, saying, "It is our conviction that through home visits one gets a truer and more adequate picture of the patient." They checked the evaluations which had been made at the time of discharge by the institute staff against their own judgments at time of follow-up in terms of the following categories: cured, essentially better, somewhat better, and no change. We do not know what their criteria of cure or improvement were but they concluded that very few stutterers recover totally though the majority make a considerable improvement. Of the 17 persons pronounced "cured," 13 had relapses and 29 percent of all stutterers showed some regression from their "discharge" assessment within six months.

Some other workers have employed the direct interview. To cite but one example, Andrews and Harris (1964) carefully used another member of the staff unknown to the stutterers to provide a stressful situation and recorded the conversation, then made their judgments on the basis of the recording. Far too many workers have relied upon questionnaires, doubtful devices at best, and often with questions phrased so as to encourage favorable answers. For example, Øfstaas (1969) asked 100 stutterers who had previously been treated at the state school for stutterers in Norway how much they had stuttered before undergoing treatment, how much they felt they were helped, and why they thought they were helped (among other items), finding that half of them said they got "good help," one third "very good help," and the remainder "some help." Despite the form of the questioning, over 27 percent reported some relapse from their state at time of discharge.

Attempts have been made to refine the clinical impressions of improvement through the use of rating scales. The ratings have been usually made by the clinician and based upon samples of oral reading or such spontaneous speech as can be evoked by use of the TAT pictures or Johnson's Job Task (see Johnson, Darley, and Spriestersbach, 1963). We find them being used by Frick (1965) and Gregory (1969) among others, but we should remember that both Naylor (1953) and Aron (1967) found little relationship between the ratings of clinicians and the ratings of the stutterers themselves, and we should heed Sherman's warning that "Another consideration in evaluating progress during therapy is the fact that evidence of progress for one type of speaking situation is not necessarily evidence of progress for another type (1955, p. 15)."

One promising approach, which to our knowledge has only appeared once in the literature, was devised by Shames (1952). He recorded pre- and post-therapy samples of the speech of stutterers and then presented them to two experienced clinicians unfamiliar with the cases, asking them whether the speech on the second recording was better, the same, or worse than on the first recording. If we could be sure that the samples were representative of the stutterer's general speech and if the pre- and post-therapy recordings were randomly ordered in the presentation, we might have a useful evaluative tool. Another interesting approach is that by Adams (1971) who used the subject's own original hierarchy of feared speaking situations as his measurement device. Still another is that devised by Prins (1970). Recognizing that stuttering is a multidimensional disorder and that change may occur not only in fluency but in other aspects, he used self-ratings for each of the items in Van Riper's (1971a) stuttering equation, graphing the results in terms of condition at time of therapy termination and at time of follow-up (Figure 7.1). Various other

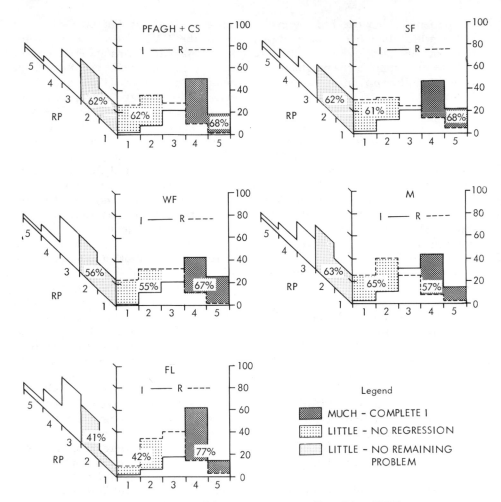

FIGURE 7.1   Multifactor evaluation of therapeutic progress. (From Prins, 1970.)

authors have used physiological or other measures of anxiety. Gray (1968) procured measures of electro-skin-conductance, palmar water evaporation, and the results of the unstandardized Willoughby Test. Gregory (1969) used palmar sweat prints, the Taylor Manifest Anxiety Scale, the Holtzman Inkblot, and other measures. Lanyon (1969) compared pre-therapy post-therapy and follow-up scores on his test of stuttering severity. All of these attempts, like the simple counting of stuttered words per minute, or percentages of nonfluen-cies, or speaking rate, leave much to be desired though they at least are evidence of the recognition that we need more data than the clinician's opinion to support the claim of successful therapy.

We conclude this section with an account of the valiant effort made by Andrews and Ingham (1972) of Australia to measure objectively the success of different kinds of therapy. Using not only frequency counts of stutterings, and syllables uttered per minute, but also the percentages of the stutterings characterized by sound and syllable repetitions as opposed to "blocks, prolongations, interjections, and effortful omissions," they compared pre-treatment performance in conversational speaking with post-therapy performance. They were able to show, for instance, that when syllable-timed speech training was compared with delayed auditory feedback or amplified simultaneous feedback training, "The type of stuttering which remained towards the end of treatment was qualitatively different in each treatment group." Those receiving syllable-timed speech training had "secondary debilitating stutters" whereas those receiving feedback therapy tended to show "simple repetitions." We regard this research as providing a crude model for other outcome investigations we hope will eventually be done. We need more than clinical claims of success.

Recovery from stuttering

Some years ago the author taught a short course on stuttering for speech pathologists attending a national convention of the American Speech and Hearing Association. We lectured and answered questions from the floor for a period of about four hours. Finally one lady could contain herself no longer and challenged us. "What sort of perverse masochism impels you to insist that you are still a stutterer?" she demanded. "I have listened to you for all this time and have not seen or heard a single instance of stuttering and I don't think anyone else has either." We grinned and replied that even if she had not seen or heard any such moments, we had either anticipated or felt hundreds of them but had evidently managed to stutter fluently when they had occurred. Most of them, we said, had been handled automatically as the result of our long self-training but some had been shap-

ed very deliberately so that they would not impede our communication or exhibit unnecessary abnormality. As for our self-definition as being still a member of the clan of the tangled tongue, we said we simply felt more comfortable in the role of a fluent stutterer than in that of a nonfluent normal speaker since the latter might lead to a need to avoid or at the very least to feelings of fraudulence.

We provide this personal anecdote merely to emphasize that the criteria underlying the concepts of cure or recovery are of vital importance. Too often only the outward behavior is scrutinized. We have interviewed persons who claimed to have been cured either by us or by themselves or by others and who certainly appear, at least in the interview situation, to be fluent. However, when we ask them if they ever occasionally stutter or have recurrences under stress, most of them say yes. Some of these no longer think of themselves as stutterers even though they do stutter at times—which is fine. Some view themselves as former stutterers who have a lapse once in a while. Some say that sure they still stutter but that they are no longer handicapped. Others claim to be cured who obviously are still using all the tricks of avoidance and disguise that stutterers have always used to deny their disorder and to pass as normal speakers. We have sought the secret of recovery from stuttering for sixty years and it is our considered conclusion that very few adults recover completely enough to be called cured.

Certain operant conditioners have stressed their procedures as being able to yield "zero stuttering" and have criticized those who would settle for anything less. We would assuredly welcome the demonstration of such successful therapy but, so far as we have been able to ascertain, it has not been so demonstrated in terms of our criteria. We are not impressed by unsubstantiated claims of cure. We are suspicious also of those reports in which improvement is measured in terms of frequency or duration in a few test situations. One very severe and contorted moment of stuttering, even if it is very short or occurs only once in a hundred situations or once in a thousand words can have tremendous impact upon a judging listener or on the stutterer himself. We should also, of course, be extremely skeptical of evaluations based solely on the presence or absence of stuttering if the stutterer exhibits the precarious pseudofluency derived from the use of an extremely slow or measured rate or any other kind of abnormal prosody. A stutterer may be able to speak without stuttering by using such tricks but he will rarely continue to use such an abnormal mode of utterance very long. Moreover, even if he does, he will still speak abnormally. We must also be very alert in scrutinizing the format of the followup investigation. Few of those reported (and we include our own in this context) show any scientific rigor. Let us say it bluntly: very few adult stutterers ever recover completely.

If our conclusions concerning the outcome of therapy sound pessimistic, they at least are realistic. And they point to the need for a different kind of therapy, one that will help the stutterer cope with his stuttering when it does occur. As the second part of this text will demonstrate, we stress the modification of stuttering behaviors so that the stutterer can be fluent even if he does stutter. We seek the elimination of the *handicap* of stuttering. If the stutterer can learn, under our tutelage, to stutter without abnormality and with little interruption to the speech flow, we don't care whether he is cured or not. Nor will he or his listeners.

For twenty years, as we were developing this therapy, we kept careful protocols on what we did with our stutterers and on their outcomes. The results have been reported in our section on Eisenson's *Stuttering: A Symposium* (1958). We are far from viewing this report as a model, for the flaws are obvious, but we would like to quote the set of criteria of successful therapy outcome that we used at that time:

First of all, the stutterer must be speaking better than this author in all situations. This criterion is used for lack of any other effective means of comparison, and I have spoken to groups of my colleagues both formally and informally so frequently and in so many places and for so many years that it seemed to be as good a measure as any I could invent. We might define this as 0.5 on the Iowa Scale of Severity. Secondly, the stutterer must not be avoiding words or speaking situations. Thirdly, his stuttering must not be interfering with his social or vocational adjustment. Fourthly, his situation and word fears must be pretty close to zero. Finally, his stuttering must present no concern to himself or to others. (p. 390)

If we had another twenty years we would revise these criteria and add to them and find independent judges to make the assessments and we hope that others will do a better job. If they do, we hope that they will be just as skeptical of success as we have tried to be.

Prognosis [3]

In the light of our previous discussion of successes and failures in treating stuttering, it might seem that a section on prognosis would have very

[3] Portions of this section were previously published by the author in the *Journal of the South African Logopedic Society*, 15 (1968), 5–17, and are used by permission of the editor, Dr. Myrtle Aron.

little meaningfulness. Yet therapists are optimists or they wouldn't be therapists. Moreover, no matter what kind of therapy they administer, each of them seems to have some successes with some stutterers. Perhaps it is for this reason that we find throughout the literature statements descriptive of favorable and unfavorable prognoses. Clinicians need hope as much as do their cases and sometimes they need prior justification for the possible failures they expect. Whatever the reason, few of us can resist trying to estimate the probabilities of successful outcome. Often we might as well read entrails or palms or tea leaves but still we search for information that may be predictive. Let us survey the literature concerning the embryology of the hunch.

Characteristics of the normal speech of stutterers having prognostic value

Wendahl and Cole (1961) showed that the *normal speech* of severe stutterers is also characterized by temporal irregularities and contains more force and strain than the normal speech of normal speakers. If we can infer that a favorable prognosis is more likely when the normal speech of these stutterers is more integrated than when it is not, some of this information may be of value. The measures of hesitation phenomena such as Mahl's (1957) non-ah ratios might then be predictive. Similarly, Schilling and Goeler (1961), Luchsinger and Dubois (1963), and many others have shown that the pitch range and inflections are more restricted in certain stutterers even when not stuttering and that these features usually indicate a severe problem. Generally, it is felt that the more the pitch and inflectional patterns are restricted, the

poorer the prognosis. Hirschberg (1965) states that a better prognosis is shown when the respiration is not affected. Froeschels (1952) mentioned that the amount of air inhaled prior to speaking is a good measure of prognosis, stating that if it is normal rather than excessive in amount of intake, the prognosis is more favorable. Luper and Mulder (1964) mention good eye contact with the listener as a favorable sign and the presence of excessive tension as an unfavorable one. Robinson (1964) stresses the importance of speech consciousness and concern about communication as important factors in prognosis. These presumably must have their impact on the normal as well as the abnormal speech of stutterers. Other prognostic factors might be the sheer amount of daily talking time, the mean length of normal utterance, the average sound level of the stutterer's normal speech, and even the intelligibility. To our knowledge, no investigator has systematically investigated the incorporation of these leads in devising a prognostic measure, but surely, the normal speech which the stutterer does possess may provide some important information.

Overt features of the stuttering behavior which might yield prognostic clues

There are many statements in the literature to the effect that when the stuttering behavior is confined to simple and regular repetitions of syllables, if few in number, the prognosis is more favorable than when avoidance and struggle behaviors are present. Glasner and Rosenthal (1957) held that the more complex the stuttering behavior, the poorer the prognosis. Using three types of behaviors: excessive hesitation, excessive prolongation and excessive repetition, they found that 51 percent of their stutterers who had only one of these types of behaviors overcame their stuttering whereas only 35 percent of those having two or three of these patterns recovered.

In general it appears that, in children at least, the more frequently the moments of stuttering occur, and the longer they last, the more likely it is that the prognosis will be unfavorable. Often the most grossly severe adult stutterers make the swiftest gains but this seems to depend upon better motivation, less avoidance behavior and more overtness of the symptoms. A very severe overt stutterer has few word or phonemic fears since all sounds and words give him trouble and he has less to lose by confronting and working with his problem than those who have been able to hide the disorder successfully. In these severe stutterers, too, progress is more noticeable.

The openness or visibility of the stuttering behavior, then, may also have prognostic value. Freund (1934) Douglass and Quarrington (1952), and others have stated that internalized or hidden stuttering constitutes a much more severe problem therapeutically than stuttering which is plainly overt, an opinion which has more recently been echoed by Danielson (1963). Quarrington and Douglass (1960) contend that because non-vocal (nonovert) stutterers are typically judged to be less severe than vocal (or overt) stutterers, prognosis is poorer. They appear to be less willing to identify with the therapist due to the strong drives to avoid audibility, the greater personal cost involved, and the feelings that audibility necessarily means a worsening of the condition.

The variability of the stuttering symptoms has also been viewed as predictive, Schonharl (1964) stated that when the stuttering behaviors are highly consistent, the prognosis is more favorable than if they fluctuate in form. We do not agree mainly because of the monosymptomatic picture presented by the neurotic.

The characteristic form of the stuttering behavior has also generated many statements concerning prognosis. Froeschels (1952) mentions the lack of tonic blockings and also pseudotoni (closures without pressure) as indicating less deep-seated problems. He also maintains that if the release from blocking is gradual rather than sudden, the prognosis is better. Diamond's research (1953) showed that predominantly clonic stutterers have a better prognosis than predominantly tonic stutterers. Zerneri (1965) tested the response of 102 stutterers to delayed auditory feedback. Those whose stuttering did not improve under DAF he termed organic and did not test. The remaining 77 became more fluent under DAF and he classified these according to their major behaviors as either tonic or clonic. The tonic group did not respond to therapy, but most of the clonic group made rapid progress. McDowell (1928) believed that one with "a quick hesitant, nervous speech, accompanied by repetitions of single sounds or syllables but unaccompanied by either tonic or clonic spasms" can be expected to "recover quickly" as opposed to one displaying more advanced characteristics. Kenyon (1931) has stressed the point that laryngeal blockings indicate a more severe problem than those where fixations occur in the lips and tongue alone, a conclusion which agrees with our own clinical experience. Multiple fixations also give us more concern than singles. We would also like to add that when vow-

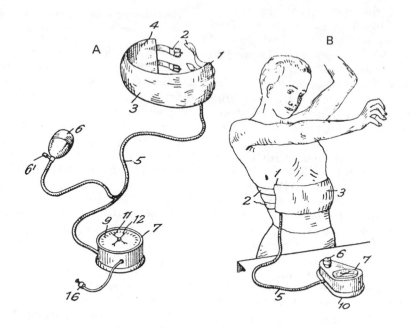

FIGURE 7.2 Azaretti breath monitoring device. (Italian Patent 219761 [1919].)

els are excessively prolonged with a rise in pitch during the moment of stuttering, the clinical problem becomes more difficult. Where stuttering seems to be associated with a strong cluttering component, the prognosis seems to be worse than when either disorder occurs alone (Weiss, 1964), especially when the child is hyperactive or especially "nervous."

Some investigations have sought to investigate the roles of consistency, loci, and adaptation in determining prognosis. Quarrington (1965) and Lanyon (1965) both found that when the stuttering consistently clustered about certain specific sounds and words, less improvement was shown than when more inconsistency in loci was present. This presumably reflects the intensity of word and phonemic fears. Johnson, Darley, and Spriestersbach (1963) also stress the consistency

phenomenon, saying, "in general, it may indicate how strongly his stuttering responses are associated with the stimuli or cues to which they have presumably been conditioned." Lanyon (1965) investigated the relationship between initial frequencies of stutterings and also adaptation rate in repeated readings and improvement after therapy, finding that for severe stutterers, the adaptation rate might have some prognostic value but that the consistency measures or terminal frequencies after adaptation had none. However, Prins (1970) disagrees, writing that, "at this juncture, it appears that adaptation of stuttering is neither predictably nor highly related to speech measures of therapy progress."

Perhaps the most intriguing piece of research on prognosis was performed by Stromsta (1965) who examined the spectograms of stuttering children who had been examined ten years earlier. He found that all those who showed normal changes in formant transitions and no breaks in air flow during moments of stuttering had recovered completely from stuttering whereas those who had shown abnormal formant transitions and airflow breaks were still stuttering. Another interesting study with implications for prognosis is that done by Froeschels and Rieber (1963) who related auditory impercivity to severity. Ringel and Minifie (1966) showed that severity was related to protensity (the ability to judge time). In their study, they used three groups of subjects; normal speakers, mild stutterers, and moderate to severe stutterers. The subjects were asked to estimate the duration of a 10 second period while simultaneously performing the following activities: silence, oral reading, silent reading, listening, or spontaneous speech. Their conclusions were that during communicative activities, the stutterers, regardless of their severity, were less able to accurately judge duration. Performance of the mild group was more similar to that of the normal group than to that of the moderate to severe group. Prognostically, Ringel and Minifie state, "If the protensity over-estimations are related to the stutterer's dissatisfactions with the unpleasant aspects of his communicative activity, the stutterer's protensity-judging ability might improve as he progresses therapeutically."

This review is far from comprehensive but the major positions concerning prognostic clues yielded by the stuttering behavior itself have been stated. The research is obviously inadequate. The clinical observations need to be pooled, organized and rigorously tested. Much needs to be done.

Attitudes or covert behaviors which might have prognostic value

Clinicians have often stressed the importance of motivation, anxiety, guilt, interpersonal relationships, and other similar factors in determining prognosis. To review even a portion of the many statements in the literature bearing upon these would consume far too much space and therefore we confine ourselves primarily to the research findings. Andrews and Harris (1964) in their longitudinal study of British children who stuttered found no significant differences in test results or psychiatric interviews between them and their normal speaking controls. Bullwinkle (1933) treated 23 children who stuttered. Those who failed to progress satisfactorily were found to be more sensitive, shy, withdrawn, with a strong mother attachment and neurotic. Shames (1952) found that social introversion was significantly correlated with a favorable prognosis, while "happy-go-luckiness" was slightly significantly negatively correlated with a favorable prognosis. Buscaglia (1962) suggests that the integration of the self-concept should be considered as a factor in prognosis, a finding also mentioned by Clark and Murray (1965). Lanyon, (1966) using the MMPI found that *ego strength* was positively correlated and *deviant repression* responses were negatively correlated with improvement in therapy. Cooper (1966) showed that the stutterer's positive affective attitude toward his clinicians was related to progress. Sheehan (1954) found that the Rorschach could probably be used to predict psychotherapeutic improvement but not overt speech improvement. He also stated that the Rorschach also had predictive value "in sorting out those stutterers who were likely to drop out of therapy early." In their investigation of recovered stutterers, Zelan, Sheehan, and Bugenthal (1954) using the W-A-Y technique to investigate the self-concepts of 40 stutterers found results indicating that success in therapy was dependent upon starting therapy with fewer negative self-percepts. Naylor and Rosenthal (1968) in a careful study of short-term therapy with army stutterers, failed to find any reliable or valid predictor of progress from either clinician's ratings or personality test data.

Neaves (1967) in a study of 165 stutterers concluded that there was no significant difference in overall personality adjustment between those who responded to treatment and those who did not. In specific traits, the nonresponders emerged as being more dependent, attention seeking, and submissive than the responders who were judged to be more assertive, realistic and self-assured.

If this review of the research appears discouraging, we must point out that it reflects the state of behavioral science generally in the prediction of the outcome of treatment. The clinician, for the time being, must appraise the prognosis of his new patients without the objective tools he will have some day. Nevertheless, we are certain that experienced therapists do use the clues provided by the stutterer's attitudes, emotionality, interpersonal relationships, self concepts, and similar phenomena in making reasonably accurate judgments concerning the probable success of their treatment for a given individual.

Developmental factors important in the assessment of prognosis

Here there seems to be some unanimity. The younger the stutterer, the better the prognosis! We find this statement almost universally recognized. Wulffert (1964) in Bulgaria, Andrews and Harris (1964) in England, Dostalova and Dosuzkov (1965) in Czechoslovakia, Kamiyama (1967) in Japan, and Arnott (1958) in Australia, are but a few of the many writers who agree in general with Glasner and Dahl (1952) in the United States who stated, "The evidence today indicates that if the child's stuttering, as defined by the specialist, is not cleared up by the time the child enters school, his condition will more than likely become progressively worse." There is ample evidence (Milisen and Johnson, 1936; Pollitt, 1951; Andrews and Harris, 1964; Shearer and Williams, 1965; Wingate, 1964 and Sheehan and Martyn, 1966) that a substantial proportion of children who begin to stutter seem to overcome it with or without professional help before adulthood but generally, the opinion seems to be that the longer the stuttering persists, the poorer the prognosis. Daskalov (1962) states that "the best results (of therapy) were obtained in preschool children. The results were more durable with subsequent improvement of speech and an increase in cures with the passage of time." He goes on to state that for adults and school-aged children, therapy was less effective with tendencies for relapse or deterioration. Dostalova and Dosuzkov (1965) in comparing groups by age of onset, found that the group, "balbuties tarda" (onset after age 8) had the greatest resistance to therapy, the greatest severity, and the least amount of spontaneous recovery, in comparison to the "balbuties praecox" group (onset between ages 2 to 4) and the "balbuties vulgaris" group (onset between ages 5 to 7). Saito (1967) in Japan provided similar findings that children whose onset was before four years of age, if brought in for treatment within three months after onset, had the most favorable prognosis. Contrary results have been reported by Jameson (1955) who believes that age of onset has no relationship to outcome of treatment.

Andrews and Harris (1964) found that four out of five stutterers who began to stutter overcame it before the age of ten years but that only one fourth of those who were still stuttering at ten ever overcame it. Freund (1966) reviewed the literature on stuttering which began in adulthood and concludes that it is usually of short duration.

We have already described the effect of complexity and severity of stuttering as factors in prognosis. When these are viewed as developmental features of a disorder which usually begins with simple syllabic repetitions, and then progresses through a series of stages (Froeschels, 1952; Bloodstein, 1960; Van Riper, 1971a), it is apparent that the exacerbation of severity and growth of the disorder should be taken into account in determining the probable outcome. Since the morbid development is usually oscillatory with frequent regressions into an earlier stage and often into periods of complete fluency, the therapist should always view this instability and reversal as favorable signs. Once the disorder becomes stabilized, in an advanced stage, more difficulty in treatment can be expected.

We are certain that the prognosis for an individual stutterer is in large part determined by his basic evaluation of the disorder as a problem and by the positive or negative influences of the significant persons in his present environment and past history. Needless to say, if we determine a prognosis, we need to study intensive-ly this individual stutterer and his history and to do some trial therapy with him. The prognosis (as with the diagnosis) must be constantly reexamined and reevaluated throughout the therapy period. Conditions, attitudes and behaviors never remain constant but are in a never-ending state of fluctuation and change.

In this discussion we have purposely avoided the quagmire of etiology and theory in which the nature of stuttering is presently buried. Does the clutter-stutterer have a better prognosis than the neurotic stutterer? This and other obvious questions of the same ilk cannot be answered at the present time. We can state, however, that a favorable prognosis depends primarily upon the kind of problem presented by the patient. Our successes or failures may help us to assess this particular factor at least, and that is a miserable thought with which to end this chapter.

Bibliography

ABRAHAMS, E. and R. FORCHAMMER (Account of follow-up investigation of stuttering patients and patients with voice disorders), *Nordisk Tidsskrift for Tale og Stemme,* 14 (1954), 78–92.

ADAMS, M. R., The efficacy of reciprocal inhibition procedures in the treatment of stuttering, Unpublished paper, 1971.

ANDREWS, G. and M. HARRIS, *The Syndrome of Stuttering.* London: Heinemann, 1964.

ANDREWS, G. and R. J. INGHAM, Stuttering: Considerations in the evaluation of treatment, *British Journal of Disorders of Communication,* 6 (1971), 129–38.

———, Stuttering: Considerations in the evaluation of treatment, *British Journal of Disorders of Communication,* 6 (1971), 129–38.

————, An approach to the evaluation of stuttering therapy, *Journal of Speech and Hearing Research,* 15 (1972), 296–302.

ARON, M. L., The relationship between measures of stuttering behavior, *Journal of the South African Logopedic Society,* 14 (1967), 15–34.

ARNOTT, D. W. A., Stammering, *Post Graduate Communications in Medicine, University of Sydney,* Australia, 1958, pp. 339–42.

APPELT, A., *Stammering and Its Permanent Cure.* London: Methuen, 1929.

BEASELEY, B., *Stammering: Its Treatment,* 17th ed. Birmingham: Hudson, 1897.

BLOODSTEIN, O., Development of stuttering, *Journal of Speech and Hearing Disorders,* 25 (1960), 219–37.

BLUEMEL, C. S., *Stammering and Cognate Defects of Speech.* New York: Stechert, 1913.

————, *The Riddle of Stuttering.* Danville, Ill.: Interstate, 1957.

BRILL, A. A., Speech disturbances in nervous and mental diseases, *Quarterly Journal of Speech,* 9 (1923), 129–35.

BRUTTEN, E. J. and D. J. SHOEMAKER, *The Modification of Stuttering.* Englewood Cliffs, N.J.: Prentice-Hall, 1967.

BRYNGELSON, B., Prognosis of stuttering, *Journal of Speech Disorders,* 3 (1938), 121–23.

BULLWINKLE, B. A., Methods and outcome of treatment of stutterers in a child guidance clinic, *Smith College Studies in Social Work,* 4 (1933), 107–38.

BUSCAGLIA, L. F., *An Experimental Study of the Sarbin-Hardyck Test as an Index of Role Perception for Adolescent Stutterers,* Ph.D. Thesis, University of Southern California, 1962.

CLARK, R. M. and F. P. MURRAY, Alterations in self-concept: A barometer of progress in individuals undergoing therapy for stuttering, in D. A. Barbara (ed.), *New Directions in Stuttering: Theory and Practice.* Springfield, Ill.: Charles C Thomas, 1965.

COOPER, E. B., Client-clinician relationships and concomitant factors in stuttering therapy, *Journal of Speech and Hearing Research,* 9 (1966), 194–207.

CORNELIU, F. C., Methodes therapeutiques et correlations pathogeniques dans le begaiement tonique, *Proceedings of the XIV Congress of the International Association of Logopedics and Phoniatrics,* Paris, 1968, pp. 62–70.

DANIELSON, H. (Modern psychotherapy challenges traditional stuttering therapy), *Nordisk Tidsskrift for Tale og Stemme,* 23 (1963), 113–17.

DASKALOV, D. D. (Basic principles and methods for the prevention and treatment of stuttering), *Zhurnal Nevropatologii i Psikhiatrii imeni S. S. Korsakova,* 62 (1962), 1047–52.

DENHARDT, R., *Das Stottern: Eine Psychose.* Leipsig: Keil's Nachfolger, 1890.

DESPERT, J. L., A therapeutic approach to the problem of stuttering, *Nervous Child,* 2 (1932), 134–47.

DIAMOND, M., *An Investigation of Some Personality Differences Between Predominantly Tonic Stutterers and Predominantly Clonic Stutterers,* Ph.D. Thesis, Syracuse University, 1953.

DOSTALOVA, N. and T. DOSUZKOV, Aspects of three categories of neurotic stuttering, *De Therapie a Vocis et Loquellae,* 1 (1965), 273–76.

DOSUZKOV, T., On the relationship between stuttering and other neuroses, *Ceskoskivenska Psychiatrie,* 56 (1960), 395–402.

DOUGLASS, E. and B. QUARRINGTON, The differentiation of the interiorized and exteriorized stutterer, *Journal of Speech and Hearing Disorders,* 17 (1952), 377–85.

EISENSON, J. (ed.), *Stuttering: A Symposium.* New York: Harper & Row, 1958.

EYSENCK, H. J., The effects of psychotherapy: An evaluation, *Journal of Consulting Psychology,* 16 (1952), 319–24.

FITZ, O., *Schach dem Stottern*. Freiburg: Lambertus-Verlag, 1961.

FREUND, H. (On internal stuttering), *Zeitschrift Ges. Neurologie und Psychiatrie,* 151 (1934), 591–98.

————, *Psychopathology and the Problem of Stuttering*. Springfield, Ill.: Charles C Thomas, 1966.

FRICK, J. V., *Evaluation of Motor Planning Techniques for the Treatment of Stuttering*, Final Report, Grant 32–48–0720–5003, United States Department of Health, Education and Welfare, Office of Education, 1965.

FROESCHELS, E., *Speech Therapy*. Boston: Expression Co., 1933.

————, The significance of symptomatology for the understanding of the essence of stuttering, *Folia Phoniatrica,* 4 (1952), 217–30.

———— and R. W. RIEBER, The problem of auditory and visual impercivity in stutterers, *Folia Phoniatrica,* 16 (1963), 13–20.

GLASNER, P. J. and M. F. DAHL, Stuttering —prophylactic program for its control, *American Journal of Public Health,* 42 (1952), 1111–15.

GLASNER, P. J. and D. ROSENTHAL, Parental diagnosis of stuttering in young children, *Journal of Speech and Hearing Disorders,* 22 (1957), 288–95.

GOLDIAMOND, I., Stuttering and fluency as manipulatable operant response classes, in L. Krasner and L. P. Ullman (eds.), *Research in Behavior Modification*. New York: Holt, Rinehart & Winston, 1965.

GRAY, B. B., *Some Effects of Anxiety Deconditioning upon Stuttering Behavior*. Monterey, Calif.: Monterey Institute, 1968.

GREGORY, H. H., *Learning Theory and Stuttering Therapy*. Evanston, Ill.: Northwestern University Press, 1968.

————, *An Assessment of the Results of Stuttering Therapy*. Evanston, Ill.: Department of Communication Disorders, Northwestern University, 1969.

HANICKE, O. and R. Leben (Modern views on stuttering and its treatment), *Deutsche Gesundheitsvegen,* 19 (1964), 545–49.

HIRSCHBERG, J. (Stuttering), *Orvosi Hetilap,* 106 (1965), 780–84.

INGHAM, R. J. and G. ANDREWS, The quality of fluency after treatment, *Journal of Communication Disorders,* 4 (1971), 279–88.

————, A description of a token economy in an adult therapy program, *Asha,* 13 (1971), 550.

———— and R. WINKLER, A comparison of four treatment techniques, *Journal of Communication Disorders,* 5 (1972), 91–117.

JAMESON, A., Stammering in children— some factors in the diagnosis, *Speech* (London), 19 (1955), 60–67.

JOHNSON, W., F. L. DARLEY, and D. C. SPRIESTERSBACH, *Diagnostic Methods in Speech Pathology*. New York: Harper & Row, 1963.

JOHNSON, W., *The Onset of Stuttering*. Minneapolis: University of Minnesota Press, 1959.

KAMIYAMA, G. (*A Handbook of Stuttering*). Tokyo. Kongo-Shuppan, 1967.

KENT, L. R., A retraining program for the adult who stutters, *Journal of Speech and Hearing Disorders,* 26 (1961), 141–46.

KENYON, E. L., Peripheral physical inhibition of speech: An essential phenomenon and an important aspect of stammering, *Oralism and Auralism,* 10 (1931), 15–31.

KOPP, G., Treatment of stuttering, *Journal of Speech Disorders,* 4 (1939), 165–69.

LANYON, R., Behavior change in stuttering through systematic desensitization, *Journal of Speech and Hearing Disorders,* 34 (1969), 253–60.

————, The MMPI and prognosis in stuttering therapy, *Journal of Speech and Hearing Disorders,* 31 (1966), 186–91.

————, Relationship of adaptation and consistency to improvement in stuttering therapy, *Journal of Speech and Hearing Research,* 8 (1965), 263–70.

LENNON, E. J., *Le Begaiement: Thera-peutiques Modernes.* Paris: Doin et Cie, 1962.

LUCHSINGER, R. and G. E. ARNOLD, *Voice-Speech-Language.* Belmont, Calif.: Wadsworth, 1965.

LUCHSINGER, R. and C. DUBOIS, Ein vergleich der sprachmelodie und lautstarkekurve bei normalen, ge-hirnkranken und stottern, *Folia Pho-niatrica,* 15 (1963), 28–41.

LUPER, H. and R. MULDER, *Stuttering Therapy for Children.* Englewood Cliffs, N.J.: Prentice-Hall, 1964.

MAHL, G., Disturbances and Silences in the patient's speech in psychotherapy, *Journal of Abnormal and Social Psy-chology,* 42 (1957), 3–32.

MCDOWELL, E., *Educational and Emo-tional Adjustment of Stuttering Chil-dren.* Columbia University Teachers College Contributions to Education, 1928, p. 314.

MCCORD, H., Hypnotherapy and stutter-ing, *Journal of Clinical and Experi-mental Hypnosis,* 3 (1955), 210–14.

MILISEN, R. and W. JOHNSON, A compara-tive study of stutterers, former stut-terers, and normal speakers whose handedness has been changed, *Ar-chives of Speech,* 1 (1936), 61–86.

NADOLECZNY, M. (Stuttering as a manifes-tation of a spastic coordination neurosis), *Archives für Psychiatrie,* 82 (1927), 235–46.

NAYLOR, R. V., A comparative study of methods of estimating the severity of stuttering, *Journal of Speech and Hearing Disorders,* 18 (1953), 30–37.

———— and W. S. ROSENTHAL, *Clinical Investigation of Stuttering: II. Treat-ment and Follow-up of the Adult Stutterer.* Project 3 A–02560–1A826–01–036, U.S. Army Medical Research and Development Command, Be-thesda, Maryland, 1968.

NEAVES, A., Prognosis in stammering. *Brit-ish Journal of Disorders of Communi-cation Supplement:* Speech Pathology: Diagnosis, Theory and Practice. Edin-burg: College of Speech Therapists, 1967.

ØFSTAAS, K (*A Follow-up Study of Former Pupils at the Norwegian Special School of Stutterers*). Oslo: Council of Special Schools, 1969.

POLLITT, J., A review of cases of stammer-ing, *Speech* (London), 15 (1951), 33–41.

POTTER, S. O. L., *Speech and Its Defects.* Philadelphia: Blakiston, 1882.

PRINS, D., Improvement and regression in stutterers following short-term inten-sive therapy, *Journal of Speech and Hearing Disorders,* 35 (1970), 123–35.

QUARRINGTON, B., Stuttering as a function of the information value and sentence position of words, *Journal of Ab-normal Psychology,* 70 (1965), 221–24.

———— and DOUGLASS, Audibility avoid-ance in non-vocalized stutterers, *Jour-nal of Speech and Hearing Disorders,* 25, (1960), 358–65.

RINGEL, R. and F. MINIFIE, Protensity esti-mates of stutterers and non-stutterers, *Journal of Speech and Hearing Re-search,* 9 (1966), 289–96.

ROBINSON, F. B., *Introduction to Stutter-ing.* Englewood Cliffs, N.J.: Prentice-Hall, 1964.

RUBIN, H. and CULATTA, R., A point of view about fluency, *Asha,* 13 (1971), 380–87.

SAITO, H., The analysis of the prognosis of stuttering, Abstract 262 in G. Kamiyama (*A Handbook for the Study of Stuttering*). Tokyo: Kongo-Shuppan, 1967.

SCHILLING, A., Die behandlung des stott-erns, *Folia Phoniatrica,* 17 (1965), 365–458.

SCHILLING, A. (Language and speech dis-turbances), in J. Berendes, R. Link, and P. Zöllner (eds.), *Neck, Nose and Ear Therapeutics,* vol. 2. Stuttgart: Thieme, 1963, pp. 1189–1259.

————, Neuer untersuchungen uber die mitbeleilingung organischer ur-sachen bei der enstehung des stotterns, *Hals-Nasen-Ohren Heilkunde,* 14 (1963), 99–112.

———— and D. VON GOELER (On the question of the analysis of monotony in stutterers), *Folia Phoniatrica,* 13 (1961), 202–18.

SCHONHARL, E. (Change in the type of stuttering with age), *Hals-Nasen-Ohren Heilkunde,* 12 (1964), 152–54.

SCRIPTURE, E. W., Stuttering, Lisping and Correction of the Speech of the Deaf. New York: Macmillan, 1931.

SCOTT, R., The application of modification techniques to the control of stuttering, *Journal of the Australian College of Speech Therapists,* 19 (1969), 58–62.

SERRA, M. (Sensory stimulation for diagnostic purposes in 19 stutterers), *Archiv. Italiano Laringologi,* 70 (1962), 355–61.

SHAMES, G., An investigation of prognosis and evaluation in speech therapy, *Journal of Speech and Hearing Disorders,* 17 (1952), 386–92.

SHEARER, W. M. and J. D. WILLIAMS, Self-recovery from stuttering, *Journal of Speech and Hearing Disorders,* 30 (1965), 288–90.

SHEEHAN, J. G., Rorschach prognosis in psychotherapy and speech therapy, *Journal of Speech and Hearing Disorders,* 19 (1954), 217–19.

———— and M. MARTYN, Spontaneous recovery from stuttering, *Journal of Speech and Hearing Research,* 9 (1966), 121–35.

SHERMAN, D., Reliability and utility of individual ratings of audible characteristics of stuttering, *Journal of Speech and Hearing Disorders,* 20 1955, 58–62.

————, Reliability and utility of individual ratings of audible characteristics of stuttering, *Journal of Speech and Hearing Disorders,* 20 1955, 11–16.

STROMSTA, C., A spectrographic study of

Disfluencies labelled as stuttering by parents, *De Therapia Vocis et Loquellae,* 1 (1965), 317–20.

VAN RIPER, C., Prognostic factors in stuttering, *Journal of the South African Logopedic Society,* 15 (1968), 7–13.

————, *Speech Correction: Principles and Methods,* 5th ed. Englewood Cliffs, N.J.: Prentice-Hall, 1971*a*.

————, *The Nature of Stuttering.* Englewood Cliffs, N.J.: Prentice-Hall, 1971*b*.

VLASOVA, N. A., An evaluation of the treatment of stuttering in children on the basis of the data of catamnesis, in R. West (ed.), *Russian Translations on Speech and Hearing,* A.S.H.A. Reports, No. 3, 1968, pp. 423–32.

———— (The value of the complex method for treatment of stuttering in children), *Folia Phoniatrica,* 16 (1964), 39–43.

———— (Late follow-up analysis of some cases of recurrent stuttering), *Zhurnal Nevropatologii i Psikiatrii imeni S. S. Korsakova,* 65 (1965), 750–51.

VOELKER, C., Post therapy observations on over two thousand cases of speech defects, *Archives of Otolaryngology,* 38 (1943), 261–64.

WEISS, D. A., *Cluttering.* Englewood Cliffs, N.J.: Prentice-Hall, 1964.

WENDAHL, R. and J. COLE, Indentification of stuttering during relatively fluent speech, *Journal of Speech and Hearing Research,* 4 (1961), 281–86.

WEST, R., Similarities and differences in the treatment of stuttering as practiced in America, *Proceedings of the American Speech Correction Association,* 2 (1932), 126–45.

WINGATE, M. E., Recovery from stuttering, *Journal of Speech and Hearing Disorders,* 29 (1964), 312–21.

WULFFERT, N. F. (Recent work in Bulgaria on the treatment of logoneuroses) (*Review of Soviet Medical Science*), 1 (1964), 57–61.

ZELAN, S., J. G. SHEEHAN, and J.

BUGENTHAL, Self-perceptions in stuttering, *Journal of Clinical Psychology*, 10 (1954), 70–72.

ZERNERI, L., Tentative d'applicazione delle voci retardata (DAF) terapia della balbuzie, Bolletino della Societa Italiano di Phonetica, *Fonestria e Audiologia*, 14 (1965), 125–30.

ZALIOUK, D. and A. ZALIOUK, Stuttering: A differential approach in diagnosis and therapy, *De Therapia Vocis et Loquellae*, 1 (1965), 437–41.

OUR

THERAPEUTIC APPROACH

In this section we present an account of our own treatment of stuttering. It will be immediately apparent that we have adopted many of the therapeutic methods described in the preceding pages of this text including some that we have criticized as being ineffective when used as the sole agent of change. We feel that stuttering needs a global therapy, a total push, if it is to yield to clinical intervention and that it must be attacked from every quarter and with every available weapon. Our point of view in therapy as well as in theory is eclectic. We have sought to build upon the contributions of those who came before us, to take from each according to its possible appropriateness for an individual patient, and to revise those which held some promise of therapeutic impact. Thus, although we reject syllable-timed speech as an appropriate method for helping the adult stutterer, we use rhythmic utterances to help the beginning stutterer know again what smooth flowing speech feels like. Although we do not use general body relaxation, we may train the adult stutterer to modify his tremors by loosening his lips. Suggestion, desensitization, punishment and reinforcement, servotherapy, and psychotherapy all find specific applications in our casework. Despite this catholicity, however, the design of our therapy has little randomness in it. We play by note rather than by ear. Ours is a problem-solving approach.

We present it with some reluctance for we are certain that it has grave weaknesses both of design and application. Nevertheless, it has always seemed important to take the risks inherent in exploring new ways of helping the stutterer for only in this way shall we fall forward rather than failing backward. We have sought to blaze a new trail. There may be better ones.

The Design
of Therapy

In this chapter we seek to present the rationale and design of our own therapy for the confirmed stutterer who is in his late adolescent or adult years. (Later chapters will deal with the treatment of the child who has just begun to stutter and the child who has also developed fears and struggle responses but who cannot be treated like an adult.) We have developed this particular therapy over a period of years and though it still leaves much to be desired, we feel it holds much promise. Hoping to find a treatment that would prove successful with more than a handful of stutterers, we have experimented with all the kinds of therapy described in previous chapters of this text, but all of them presented us with far too much long-term failure as compared to short-term fluency. We are not happy with what we have designed. It asks much of the therapist and more of the stut-

terer. It is not a simple, easy form of treatment though in many ways it is primitive, perhaps the forerunner of better things to come. All we can say is that it has given more stutterers more relief and more permanent fluency than any other approach of which we have knowledge. Perhaps someday, when we know more than we know now about the basic nature of the disorder, we may have a therapy that will prevent or eliminate the core disruptions of the motor sequences that perhaps comprise the heart of the problem.

The bases of our therapy

At the present time we do not have this essential information despite all the research that has been performed and so we must exploit to the fullest extent what we do know. Our therapy is founded on learning theory, servo-theory, and the principles of psycho-therapy. With respect to learning, we help the stutterer to unlearn his old maladaptive responses to the *threat* and to the *experience* of fluency disruption and to learn new and more adaptive ones in their stead. In terms of servotheory, since speech seems to be automatically controlled by feedback and there seems to be some real evidence that some failure in the auditory processing system produces the basic disruptions, we train the stutterer to monitor his speech by emphasizing proprioception thus bypassing to some degree that auditory feedback system. The third base of the therapy we advocate is that special kind of learning called psychotherapy. These adolescent and adult stutterers come to us with intense fears, frustrations, and other emotional reactions due to their disrupted speech and feelings of deviance. They show many self-defeating behaviors. Often they are very unhappy, anxious persons. Though most of them show the symptomatic patterns characteristic of what Freund (1966) called an expectancy neurosis rather than those of the classical neuroses, some stutterers show both types.[1] Whatever the presented problem may be in these terms, we cannot ignore the urgent need for relief from the psychopathology that so often surrounds the disorder in adulthood. Accordingly we have designed our treatment so that a psychotherapy appropriate for the secondary, expectancy type of neurosis is interwoven throughout all our interactions with our cases. When we find that a core (primary or *kern*) neurosis also exists, we usually refer the patient to other

selected practitioners as we have discussed in our chapter on psychotherapy. To summarize, the overall design of this therapy and the activities and interactions that comprise it is based upon these three foundations: learning theory, servotheory, and psychotherapy.

There are doubtless many roads to the Rome of fluency, but some are more direct than others. Some meander so far afield that the stutterers who travel them become lost and disheartened. Some end in the swamp of despair. The author of this text wandered long in this therapeutic wasteland and he has known many other stutterers also caught in the labyrinth of the old therapies. These stutterers who have chased the will o' the wisp of easy fluency from clinic to clinic and therapist to therapist are sad souls. They have spent many hours talking with metronomic devices stuck in their ears. They have been hypnotized and psychoanalyzed. They have been exhorted to use more willpower, to watch their language, to chew their breath, to speak like ventriloquists. Their hopes have been raised by a contrived experience of temporary fluency and the promise of quick easy cure only to have those hopes dashed to the rocky ground of reality. Each new generation of therapists seems to have to rediscover the same old tricks, to justify them with new terminology and to apply them to a new crop of stutterers.[2] We have sought to blaze a new trail.

The therapeutic schedule

We have explored many different ways of administering our stuttering therapy and have come to the conclusion that only a fairly intensive program seems to offer a consistently favorable prognosis. In terms of the fre-

---

[1] As we have seen earlier in this text, Fernau-Horn (1969) has described these as *Kern* (primary) and *Rand* (secondary) neuroses with the latter being the one shown by the great majority of stutterers.

[2] It is primarily for this reason that we have written this book.

quency of therapy sessions, for example, we have experimented with many formats: once a week, twice a week, three times, five times, with one hour, two hour, three and four hour sessions. We have used individual therapy, group therapy, and self-therapy, with each of these utilized as the sole mode of treatment and again in different combinations. With some exceptions, the conclusion we have reached is that the *minimum* requirement for most adult stutterers is one hour of individual therapy and one hour of group therapy three days a week and as much daily self-therapy as we can get for a period of three to four months. Were it possible, we would prefer an even more intensive therapy. In addition to this basic program, we have found it wise to include another period lasting about three to four months, during which the stutterer is seen once or twice a week for an hour individually or in a group, this period being devoted to terminal therapy based upon stabilization. While we have been able to treat some stutterers successfully on a much less intensive schedule, our success-failure ratio was highest with this arrangement. Many therapists and many stutterers feel that such a program would be too demanding or time consuming. These are the therapists and stutterers who fail. Stuttering in the adult rarely responds to token therapy. Indeed most severe stutterers know in their hearts that a major effort is required. Too many of them have already experienced superficial therapy and so they welcome, albeit with some reluctance, the invitation to concentrated effort.

The therapeutic sequence

We have also explored several different ways of sequencing the therapeutic activities and their related subgoals. The sequence that seems to have been the most productive of permanent relief is ordered as follows:

1. An *identification* phase in which the stutterer explores, analyzes and classifies the overt behaviors and covert experiences that characterize his particular kind of stuttering.
2. A *desensitization* phase devoted to decreasing his speech anxieties and the other negative emotions connected with his disorder. In this phase we seek to toughen the stutterer to the threat, confrontation and experience of fluency failure.
3. A *modification* phase involving first the varying and then the unlearning of his habitual avoidance and struggle responses, and also the learning, through counterconditioning, of a new fluent, less abnormal way of stuttering.
4. A *stabilization* phase in which we help the stutterer to consolidate his gains, to create generalized sets that will make the new fluent form of stuttering automatic, and to develop proprioceptive monitoring of his normal speech.

This four step sequence has seemed to be most effective of all the variations we have tried in forty years of treating adult stutterers.

We also sequence the various activities carefully in each of these phases of therapy. Generally, we program our therapeutic tasks according to their estimated difficulty for the individual stutterer, beginning with those which can be more easily performed. We will find this hierarchic principle used in identification, desensitization, modification, and stabilization. By using this graded approach in sequencing the activities, the probability of successful performance seems to be greatly increased and motivation remains at a high level.

Provision for individual differences

We wish to make clear that this overall design does not mean that we treat all stutterers in the same way. There is ample room in the program for tailoring the treatment to the clients' special capacities and needs. In the devising of the individual therapeutic tasks for each of the phases of therapy, individual differences are always taken into account. For example, one stutterer may need much desensitization to the public speaking situation while another may speak very well before a group and have little fear of that experience. We would assuredly not seek to give both of these the same desensitizing tasks. For some stutterers, we can pass through the variation part of the modification phase very swiftly. For others, those more rigid and compulsive, this phase may be the most important part of the whole therapy. Certain stutterers need more psychotherapy; some learn more slowly; some show more proprioceptive control of their speech than others. Our program, based as it is upon individually designed therapeutic tasks, is flexible enough to take care of all these differences.

Stuttering therapy as unlearning and new learning

Earlier we have briefly stated that this therapy is based upon learning theory, servotheory, and psychotherapy. We now wish to present in more detail how each of these has contributed to our therapy design. Let us begin with a description of how we apply learning theory in treating the stutterer.

We first pose the essential question: what does the stutterer need to learn or unlearn? The answer of all the old therapies is that he needs to learn to talk normally, that he needs to learn to talk without stuttering. We have seen how our predecessors (and

some of our current colleagues) have sought to facilitate this learning of normal speaking. Having noted that abnormalities in respiration, phonation, and articulation existed during the stuttering act, they drilled the poor devils for hours and months and years in these functions. They taught the stutterer how to breathe, how to produce voice, how to articulate, how to phrase—as though he didn't know how to do any of these things. Therapists asked him to slow down his speech, to sing, to chant, to pace his words and syllables, so that he would be able to speak normally. The basic assumption has always been that by procuring normal speech and then reinforcing it, the stuttering would disappear. We feel that the long history of therapeutic failure with these methods challenges that assumption and we think we know why. It is because these procedures do nothing to weaken or extinguish the motley assortment of avoidance and escape behaviors that comprise the stutterer's chief abnormality.

We believe that the stutterer does not need to be taught to talk without stuttering. This he already knows. He speaks normally much of the time. A large proportion of his words are spoken freely. He usually can talk to himself without any difficulty. He can leave a store where he has had a terrible time getting his message across and then say the same sentences aloud with complete fluency if no listener is present. Does he need to learn how to talk normally or does he need to learn how to stutter? In our view the basic problem involves learning better ways of coping with the stuttering when it is threatened or does occur. This is what the stutterer must learn. Merely giving him a period of fluency will not help him know what to do when he expects or experiences stoppage in the flow of his speech. Indeed such a period of fluency may make him even more helpless when the stuttering does return, as alas it usually does.

The targets of learning and unlearning

Most of the abnormality in stuttering consists of behaviors which are reactions to the threat or experience of interruptions in the flow of ongoing speech. All the intricate habits of avoidance and struggle appear to be learned behaviors that cluster about these fluency breaks. They have been acquired over many years. Beginning stutterers rarely show them. Each stutterer learns his own unique set of these learned coping reactions and if they are learned, then it should be possible to unlearn them. Surely we can teach the stutterer to respond in less abnormal ways to his stoppages than those he habitually uses. Surely we should be able to show him how to respond to the threat or experience of stuttering in ways that will reduce the usual penalty and frustration he commonly feels. Let us find ways of preventing the constant reinforcement of the fear and abnormality that maintain the disorder. If the stutterer can learn to stutter fairly fluently and with little abnormality, both the severity and frequency should decrease. By learning to stutter easily and without struggling he can break up his vicious stuttering circles or spirals of self-reinforcement or at least reverse their course. If he can shave off the excrescences and leave only the core, that core should be a small one, perhaps like that of an onion. Surely we should be able to teach the stutterer better ways of searching for the necessary motoric transitions than the very inappropriate ones he now employs with such devastating conse-

quence. We do not believe that it is necessary to stutter grotesquely, to make faces, or jerk the jaw, or occlude the airway with all one's might. We do believe that it is possible to stutter more easily and less abnormally. A little difficult to learn perhaps, but certainly not as hard (to use the words of one of our clients) as "a one-legged man learning to skate."

What we are saying is that it is folly for therapists to ignore the fact that the confirmed stutterer comes to us with behaviors having a long history of reinforcement. These habitual responses to the expectancy and experience of fluency failure are very, very strong. To hope they will lose that strength when temporary fluency prevents their occurrence seems unrealistic. To hope that, through therapy, we can produce enough increase in the amount of normal speech to prevent any reappearance of the unweakened stuttering behaviors in a confirmed stutterer appears naive. These avoidance and struggle reactions have been linked to too many environmental and internal stimuli; they have been incorporated within the stutterer's language; they have become facets of his sense of self. Any therapist without half trying can get any stutterer to talk without stuttering but should he not instead try to teach him how to cope sensibly with the stuttering when it does appear or is expected? Stuttering can be temporarily suppressed or repressed by a host of procedures ranging from relaxation, shadowing, hypnosis, and operant conditioning to sheer hocus pocus, but unless we *modify* the learned behaviors and weaken them, our efforts will be largely in vain. This the long history of treatment makes very clear.

This position does not mean, however, that we can hold no prospect for relief or that the frequency of stuttering will not be reduced. Indeed we can offer much more than a simple decrease in the severity. By working with the stuttering behaviors and shaping and modifying them into less abnormal forms, we do not prevent the stutterer from achieving the possible "cure" which he might otherwise attain. What we have usually found is that stuttering goes out the same door it came in. As we weaken and eliminate the learned behaviors that were developed as ways of coping with the original speech interruptions, the frequency as well as the severity of stuttering always sharply declines, and in some cases to zero. We have had our share of complete cures and from what we can ascertain, at least as many as those produced by other kinds of therapy. Not very many at that, but certainly enough to keep us from telling the stutterer that he might as well face the fact that he will have to stutter for the rest of his life. Some few of our adult cases stopped stuttering completely though most of our cases continue to stutter, a statement which at least has the virtue of honesty. However, when they do stutter, they stutter easily and their communication is not impaired. They speak fluently despite the stuttering. Stuttering becomes a minor nuisance; they learn to live with it with ease if not with complete grace. If one can stutter easily and without gross abnormality, the disorder does not interfere with most of life's pursuits. In short, we seek to make the adult stutterer fluent whether he continues to stutter or not. We have had stutterers who became successful teachers, airline pilots, salesmen, lawyers, preachers, politicians; we even had one who became a court reporter and another who ended up as an auctioneer. Most of these still stuttered occasionally but when they did they did so fluently

enough to do well in these highly verbal professions.

There are some basic advantages in such an approach as compared with those that immediately set up the goal of "not stuttering" or "zero stuttering." First of all, our therapy presents a significant contrast to all the methods which the stutterer has himself employed in the past to keep from stuttering. All therapists should recognize that the confirmed stutterer comes to us using a host of automatized devices and routines each of which at first seemed to provide some fluency before failing and becoming incorporated into his abnormality. No matter what type of therapy is offered to such a stutterer, that which gives immediate fluency is immediately greeted with some suspicion. Only a very naive and unsophisticated individual could fail to have some doubt concerning the permanency of such stuttering-suppression methods since they remind him of all the other similar things he has himself used in the past. In contrast, when we tell him we want him to stutter and we want him to have fears so that he can change his reactions to them, the prospect is at least novel and different. For years the stutterer has done everything he could to protect a precarious fluency and to keep from stuttering. All his tricks, all his strategies of avoidance and disguise were devised to maintain the constant pretense that he was a normal speaker and they have become an almost intolerable burden. Even when his tricks are momentarily successful, the stutterer feels some shame for having had to use them. And so it is almost with relief that the stutterer greets this new kind of therapy. He is tired of running away, tired of always trying to talk without stuttering, disillusioned with practices which raise his hopes and then dash them. In every life, there comes a time when every man must wrestle with his demon!

But built into this particular kind of therapy there are other advantages as well. The constant dread of relapse, so easily triggered by one small moment of stuttering in the repressive types of therapy is not nearly so potent when a modification form of therapy is employed. If the stutterer has a moment of stuttering, well, all is not lost. Relapse with a capital R has not reared its ugly, well-known head; all that has happened is that he has been presented with another opportunity to do something constructive. In the repressive therapies, the stutterer tends to respond to an occasional stuttering by denial. He tries to forget it, to ignore it. Also, when there is threat of approaching difficulty he tends to use some of his old tactics of avoidance so he can protect the newly found fluency he has worked so hard to get, and, if he does use them, he finds himself in the same old trap again. Such a stutterer tends to feel guilty every time he stutters because he interprets that stuttering as meaning that he has failed to do what he has been taught. No such situation exists in our therapy. Stuttering does not mean relapse. Another moment of fear is no catastrophe. In this therapy we need stuttering behaviors and stuttering fears because they present opportunities for the stutterer to learn new responses to both of them. Each time they occur he has another chance to strengthen those new responses or to weaken old ones.

To cite but one further advantage, this therapy also heals the split in the stutterer's self-concept whereas those therapies that try to get the stutterer to keep from stuttering only enhance it. The role of a person who can speak fluently by stuttering easily and unabnormally does not deny his long-estab-

lished identification as a stutterer. It is easier to define oneself as a *fluent stutterer* than to try to adopt the role of a *fluent or disfluent normal speaker* since he has long tried to assume the latter poses and has always been eventually unmasked. No matter how many people he has hoodwinked in the past into believing that he was a normal speaker, the stutterer has never been able to hoodwink himself. No matter how successful he has been in avoiding overt stuttering in situation after situation, he still considers himself a stutterer. It is not easy to change or erase the adult stuttering-leopard's spots. In other words, when a therapist tries to get the stutterer to talk without stuttering, he is doing what the stutterer has always tried to do, Even when he succeeds, that stutterer will feel like the same old fraud and wonder how soon it will be before that fraudulence is revealed. In contrast, if we can teach the stutterer to be fluent even though he does stutter no false role conflict will occur.[3]

The learning process

In the adult stutterer we find that much of his burden consists of emotional responses that have become conditioned to a large number of sets of external and internal stimuli. We find fears of words, of certain sounds, of certain listeners, of certain conditions of communication such as time pressure, of certain speaking situations. In addition to these fears, we find many other unpleasant emotional reactions as well.[4] Most of these responses have been classically conditioned and therefore in our therapy we apply the well-

---

[3] For a good discussion of role conflicts in the stutterer see Sheehan (1970).

[4] For a more thorough presentation of these responses see the chapter on covert phenomenology in Van Riper (1971).

known classical principles of deconditioning and counterconditioning.
We repeatedly expose the stutterer to
his conditioned stimuli while making
sure that the conditioned response
will not occur, seeking thereby to neutralize the cues that have become
able to trigger the emotional upheaval. By disrupting the linkage between
the conditioned and unconditioned
stimuli, the stutterer loses some of his
chains. He learns for example that
when he knows he must utter a word
beginning with the letter p, that this
perception need not always be followed by distress. He finds that the ring
of the telephone need not signal catastrophe when he answers it. We have
hundreds of ways of doing this essential desensitization by presenting
these stimuli while preventing the
usual unpleasant responses and many
of them will be described in future
pages.

Much of our therapy is based upon
counterconditioning. We constantly
seek to condition more adaptive competing responses to the stimuli that
elicit these fears and frustrations and
the avoidance and struggle responses
which they produce. The stutterer not
only unlearns his old responses; he
also learns new reactions to the same
cues. We follow the counterconditioning principle not only for the classically conditioned emotional responses
but also for the instrumental ones. Instead of avoiding when he fears a word
or situation, we help the stutterer
learn new approach responses. Instead
of recoiling and struggling when he
finds himself unable to integrate a
word, syllable, or sound, we teach him
new searching procedures to achieve
that integration. In essence, we establish and strengthen a new fluent way
of stuttering that can compete with
and replace his old self-defeating behaviors.

Throughout all of these interactions, we apply the basic principles of
contingent positive and negative reinforcement, nonreinforcement, and
certain kinds of punishment to weak-
en the old responses and to strengthen
the new ones. When appropriate, we
use flooding and negative practice
and other forms of desensitization
techniques. Over and over again we
administer reinforcement and punishment so that the stutterer's original
instrumental behaviors can be progressively shaped toward the kind of fluent stuttering we seek. In this therapy
we make strong use of modeling procedures, with the therapist or other
stutterers in the group providing appropriate models so that vicarious
learning can occur.

This emphasis upon conditioning
does not mean however that we ignore the cognitive aspects of learning or that we treat the stutterer as
though he were a nonfluent rat. We
make him an active participant in the
planning of therapy as well as in its
performance. We work constantly for
insightful learning, since we know
that he should be able to devise new
plans and strategies for coping with
his problem when we are not around
to help him. He must "learn to learn"
how to manipulate and control and
reinforce himself. From the beginning,
we get him to set his goals, to devise
his tasks of learning and unlearning,
and to evaluate his performance objectively. In short, we train him to be
his own therapist.

Servotherapy

Since in our chapter on servotherapy we have already presented the basic theory and rationale and some of
our own application of cybernetic
principles in the treatment of the stut-

terer, we shall here provide only a brief review. If motor speech is monitored automatically through feedback rather than by conscious control as it seems to be, any effective therapy must take this into account. Our position is that some of the stutterer's difficulties seem to originate in the auditory processing systems. We feel that if we can get him to concentrate upon proprioceptive feedback rather than auditory feedback we can bypass these difficulties. Accordingly, we use masking noise, DAF, and other methods for facilitating motor control through proprioception. We want the stutterer to stop listening to the gaps and abnormalities in his speech when they occur and when he expects them. We want him to concentrate on the feel of his speech, not on the way it sounds. We believe that many of his abnormalities (apart from those associated with avoidance) are due to a cybernetic searching for integrated motor patterns and so we try to get him to attend to the motor aspects of his utterance. We seek to improve his scanning, to build better models into his comparator mechanism so that error can be recognized and automatic correction achieved. Although we utilize cybernetic principles throughout our treatment, we apply them especially during the stabilization phase. We do this deliberately since we do not wish to prevent stuttering behaviors until we have had a chance to weaken them and to substitute better ways of responding to the threat or experience of word and sound disruption.

Psychotherapy

For many years, as an adjunct to our speech therapy, we experimented with various forms of psychotherapy seeking always to find one most suited to the needs of our stutterers. We began with a somewhat psychoanalytically oriented psychotherapy since we ourselves had undergone analysis, and had found that it provided many useful insights and had helped make us a happier stutterer. Even now we cannot say with Salter that psychoanalysis is an ancient decrepit elephant that should go back into the jungle from which it came and have the decency to lie down and die. In our opinion, most of us, whether we stutter or not, could profit from a long-term, in-depth analysis—if we could afford it. But the question is one of need. Only few of us need to go through such an experience.

Some stutterers are so beset by and tangled in their past conflicts that only an expressive, interpretative, reconstructive psychotherapy can help them. In our long clinical experience, however, these stutterers are few. Perhaps those who desperately need such therapy go, as they should go, to the psychiatrists or psychoanalysts while the others (in our opinion, the great majority) come to us, the speech pathologists. As our earlier review of the research has indicated, most stutterers seem to be pretty normal emotionally and we would agree with Freund (1966) that the neurosis, when it is present, is usually the *result* of traumatic speaking experiences. If it belongs anywhere, it belongs among the expectancy neuroses and it is a secondary, not a primary, neurosis. These stutterers were miserable because they stuttered; they did not stutter necessarily because they once had been very miserable. Were the latter true, most of us would stutter. In history after history in our cases, we found that the neurotic maladjustment appeared years after the onset of the disorder. Even though they stuttered, the stuttering children we studied appeared about as unhappy—or happy—as other normal speaking children until, usually during their school years, they began to feel the penalties and know the stigma applied by others or until they finally reacted to their communicative frustration. Only then did the anxiety, the maladaptive habits, the morbid exaggerations, and neurotic defenses appear. Only then did these stutterers become neurotic. And let us state here that not all of them did so even then.

Some of the most normal, well adjusted persons we have ever met have been stutterers—though usually they were the milder ones. These specimens are not commonly found but they exist. We have also been collecting "stuttering normal speakers" who occasionally show all of the basic characteristics of stuttering. They have excessive syllabic repetitions, prolongations of sounds, blocks in phonation, and are extremely disfluent under communicative stress, yet they do not regard themselves as stutterers nor do they show any of the neurotic features which commonly characterize the disorder. They have no fears, no struggling, no awareness of their interruptions and others do not think of them as stutterers. In exploring the histories of these stuttering nonstutterers we have been struck by the fact that these very nonfluent but well adjusted individuals all had very happy childhoods or possessed, from the first, certain compensatory personality assets which enabled them to escape the usual penalties. They also had parents and friends and teachers who felt no anxiety about their speech interruptions. We have 27 individuals currently in this collection and, in our opinion, any one of them, in a less favorable situation,

could have become a prospective case for a speech therapist.

By these remarks we do not at all desire to leave the impression that most of the adult stutterers with whom we have worked had no need for psychotherapy. Most of them did need some and we had to design a therapy to fill that need. What we are saying is that, though our stutterers commonly had emotional problems unrelated to stuttering, often severe enough to have made them unhappy and inadequate persons, those problems were not of the nature which in our opinion, required deep, long-term, formal psychotherapy but rather one which was supportive. Most of their emotional problems were focused about the stuttering, and, since communication is very vital to adequate living, most of our severe stutterers were still very troubled human beings. Seeking to minimize their hurt and frustration they had erected defenses which imprisoned them. Many had habituated maladaptive patterns of behavior tied to their anxiety that augmented and maintained their miseries.

To provide a brief sampler of the kinds of problems we encountered in addition to the stuttering, we might mention just a few of the cases that come to mind in this connection. There was Evelyn who compulsively talked aloud to herself about how miserable and unworthy she was and not only when she was alone. And Burr, the musician who stuttered on the trumpet when playing any solo, and spent hours each day in his dormitory room conducting, complete with baton, the recorded symphonies of Mozart. And Bob who fainted dead away whenever called upon in class to make a recitation. Or Bill, the very dirty one, who preferred to be rejected because he never washed rather than because he stuttered. Or Joe who always proved his conviction that he would experience very severe stuttering every time the weather changed. Or John who waltzed across the floor when he stuttered and could not help it. Or Anita whose compulsive tongue protruded grossly and impertinently and not always when she stuttered. Or Jim, the hypochondriac, and another Jim whose abulia was so intense he could not even enter a revolving door. And George, the Hermit of the Ozarks, who hated all humans (until he learned to cope with his stuttering). And Jack who was impotent sexually as well as verbally. And Dick, the fat boy, or Wilma who almost died of anorexia nervosa. And Sally who slept only two hours a night. Or Charles whose asthma varied directly with his stuttering. And many others. But the point we wish to make very clear is that all of these assorted neurotic behaviors disappeared once these stutterers learned to cope with their stuttering and became fluent. We have found, as Wolpe and Eyesenck also report, that most of our cases, once they became fluent stutterers, do not develop other symptoms, other neurotic equivalents.[5] Indeed what usu-

ally happens is that as the stuttering declines, so do the other neurotic behaviors.

The great majority of our stutterers did not resemble the ones we have been mentioning. They just stuttered. They truly had no other major concerns. As one of them told us, "No, I don't have any other important problems. I stutter. That's enough. If I could talk all right, I'd be just like anybody else." (And, after some thorough exploration we concluded that he was being objective in his evaluation.) Truly, stuttering is enough, more than enough; the anxiety, the frustration, the fears that dominate the lives of many stutterers are more than sufficient to evoke unhappiness. The disorder pervades all their living space, all their waking time—and some of them even stutter in their dreams. The seeming compulsiveness of the stuttering behaviors shakes the integrity of the self. All interpersonal relationships become colored by stuttering. To exist in a highly verbal world, stutterers almost have to erect defenses to keep from being overwhelmed. The casual onlooker, yes even the inexperienced speech therapist, cannot possibly comprehend how stuttering dominates the lives of these people. What is even more handicapping because they speak so poorly, severe stutterers are denied the verbal expression of their emotions. Travis (1957) writes of the "unspeakable feelings of stutterers." They are unspeakable partly because the stutterer cannot speak easily.

In seeking a type of psychotherapy especially suitable for the majority of our stutterers, at first we were probably naive in hoping that any one form would be appropriate for all of them. But we experimented with various types of psychoanalytically-based

---

5 This is not universally true though it holds for the majority of the cases we have treated. We have had some stutterers who did develop illnesses, marital conflicts, inability to micturate, allergies, and even strabismus as sequellae to their achieved fluency. Most of these cases were older (in their forties) and they had had early histories of other neurotic behavior. A few stutterers showed a reciprocal relationship between their other problems and their stuttering. Thus, one of them broke out into acne whenever he had one of his periods of fluency and the acne disappeared as soon as his stuttering became worse. Another showed the same relationship with her migraine headaches. But these were the rare, unusual cases and not the usual ones.

therapies, Rogerian counseling, most of the forms of directive psychotherapy (see Thorne, 1950), cathartic release therapy (Levy, 1939), group psychotherapies modelled after those advocated by Slavson (1951) and Bach (1954), and even with sensitivity training groups and others. For four years we did only psychotherapy with our stutterers while omitting all speech therapy only to discover that this gave the poorest results of any program of therapy we ever employed (Van Riper, 1958). With some other cases we tried, unsuccessfully for the most part, to concentrate only on a speech therapy based on learning theory, keeping psychotherapeutic intervention at a minimum. We have explored environmental family therapy, taking a total of 13 stutterers into our own home, one or two at a time, for at least a year's residence. For several summers, we sent some of our cases away to a camp (Shady Trails) which offered an intensive program of therapy in an ideal isolated setting.

And what were our conclusions? Simply these: that certain stutterers seemed to benefit from each of these forms of psychotherapy and that others profited minimally if at all. There was no one type of psychotherapy suitable for the majority of stutterers. Each one of them seemed to require a kind of therapy appropriate to his own unique needs, experiences, and problems. Accordingly, we evolved a treatment which would permit a variable approach.

As we have said earlier, our therapeutic program was an intensive one requiring at least three hours daily for four months and then followed by a terminal therapy period of another four months in which the stutterers met twice a week (once as a group and once individually with us). During the first four months, the program was divided into group therapy, individual therapy, and self-therapy, with the group therapy beginning a week or two after the others. We found we needed this preliminary period to learn enough about our individual cases so that we could structure the kind of psychotherapy appropriate to their needs.

Our groups were kept fairly small, ranging from six to ten stutterers. They met daily and, for the first month, only with the therapist. Then our stutterers who were receiving terminal therapy were included. Then, even later, student therapists and, finally, visitors invited by the stutterers or therapist joined our sessions. We found this use of transitional groups to be very effective. First of all, the management permitted the basic identification to be primarily with the therapist, then it came to include some identification with stutterers who had made marked improvement; then, as the normal speaking student therapists and visitors joined the group, one could see marked shifts in the stutterers' distorted perceptions of interpersonal relationships—shifts which were very healthy ones. But always we made sure, even by the seating plans, that the core group consisted of the stutterers and their therapist.

Ours was an activity-oriented combination of speech therapy and psychotherapy. On the first group session of each week the basic goals for that week with suggested methods for achieving them were jointly evolved by the stutterers and the therapist, the rationale of the tasks was discussed, and possible difficulties in their accomplishment described. On this same day, in the *individual* sessions with the therapist, the assigned activities and experiences were structured individually in terms of maximum and minimum goals. For any one stutterer, the goal setting was achieved only after thorough discussion with the therapist and it was a joint decision when finally reached. These planning sessions often provided some highly significant psychotherapeutic interchanges since they necessitated self-confrontation and often produced remarkable expressions of emotion.

Since the *performance* of the self-administered tasks of therapy were also reported to the group or to us personally, we found in this reporting an excellent opportunity for catharsis and analysis. Encouraged to recount not only what they had done in performing their assignments but also how they felt before, during, and after the tasks, the stutterers often came to confront themselves on very deep levels.

In the group sessions the stutterers in turn verbalized a portion of their autobiographies and reported their experiences in *self-therapy*.[6] The others in the group asked them challenging questions or made comments on the stutterer's performance in illustrating the new speech and interpersonal behaviors he was supposedly trying to learn. Our own role in these interchanges was that of clarifier and occasionally, when needed, that of protector. We reflected; we rarely interpreted. At times we amplified what the stutterers contributed by providing similar or contrasting examples from our own fund of personal or professional experiences. Through this sharing, a strong feeling of group unity was usually created and as this occurred, the stutterers became less defensive and more honest. Strong feelings about self and others were ventilated, one person being triggered by another as the discussion grew hot

6 Written reports of the self-therapy were required and these also included the expression of the feelings and emotions experienced.

and significant. Every session demonstrated some abreaction and the beginnings of insightful change—if one dare use these terms sans couch. Admittedly, this psychotherapy was not very deep but it was needed and it was enough. Certainly new important learnings took place.

In the stutterer's daily individual sessions with the therapist, the latter used the kind of psychotherapy he deemed most appropriate to the stutterer's specific needs and problems. Many needed no more than was inherent in the speech therapy. With some stutterers we used the Rogerian approach exclusively. With others, we employed a challenging, verbal analytic approach similar to the rational therapy advocated now by Ellis, or the activity therapies of Glasser and Perls. And we used other psychotherapies. Only a very few stutterers found us primarily interested in uncovering repressed material and submitting it to scrutiny and interpretation. With a few we even employed free association and dream and behavior analysis. Some came to know us only as a gentle, supportive father figure. Others, to put it mildly, saw us quite differently. But whatever therapeutic role we played and whatever methods we used, we were consistent with that particular stutterer.

Diagnosis

Let us now outline our diagnostic procedures. If we are to tailor the therapy to the stutterer's unique needs —and they are always unique—we must be able to appraise the kind of a person and the kind of a problem he presents. This is not to say that it is possible in the initial examination to encompass all the scope of his difficulties, strengths, and weaknesses. We believe that diagnosis is an ongoing process. In every session, from the beginning to the end of therapy, the clinician must repeatedly ask the old questions: "What does this person need now? Why does he do what he does? What does this behavior say about him as a person? Where is he now and where must he go next? How best can I help him?" However skillful the therapist may be, all the answers to these questions will never be found in one session. New answers and new questions constantly present themselves throughout the entire duration of therapy.

Nevertheless over the years we have worked out a fairly standard procedure for the initial examination. After the usual greeting, we outline in a business-like fashion a play-by-play account of what we intend to explore and hope to accomplish during the diagnostic session. We also verbalize some of the stutterer's probable feelings as he enters this confrontation and appraisal. Then we proceed immediately to the speech analysis, in the belief that one should always begin with the complaint, with the presented problem. By so doing, we also show the stutterer immediately that we know a great deal about his disorder; we demonstrate our analytical objectivity, our freedom from qualms about touching or sharing his stuttering; in short, we reveal our competence.

We may (possibly but not always) begin by asking the stutterer to read some passages and to paraphrase what he has read. This usually provides sufficient stuttering for us to make a preliminary estimate of the overall nature of the problem and to provide a crude differential diagnosis of stuttering from cluttering or from normal disfluency or other problems. Then after our client has stuttered obviously

on a word, we interrupt to ask him if, in his opinion, the stuttering he had just shown was typical or unusual, of average duration, or shorter, or longer than that which he ordinarily would experience. In this we seek his subjective estimate of severity as compared with our own. Next we comment on the kinds of stuttering behaviors shown, seeking to analyze them in terms of what the stutterer might say about their probable strategic function, namely as avoidances, postponements, starters, release devices, and the like.[7] As together we scrutinize the stuttering behaviors, we seek to determine those that seem to be most prominent and consistent. We note any hierarchic sequences which may be evident, for example, those in which the stutterer first tries one coping device, then if this gives no release, a second, and another, and another.

We are especially interested in the stutterer's core behaviors as opposed to the avoidance and release responses. We observe the characteristics of his syllabic repetitions, their speed, regularity, and coarticulation, noting their variations as they finally eventuate in the utterance of the word. We are interested in how the stutterer hunts and searches for the proper timing of the simultaneous and successive motor components of that word and how he finally finds it. When fixations occur, we seek to determine how his tremors begin and how they end and what abnormal mouth postures or sudden jerks or surges of tension trigger them. We try to discover in what ways the synergy of utterance is disrupted in terms of the timing of respiration, phonation, and articulation (the *ablauf*). We seek to identify what seems to be awry in the initiation of phona-

[7] For a more detailed account of this analysis, see Van Riper, 1971.

tion, and what the stutterer does when he finally achieves it.

We also explore the loci of the stuttering moments in terms of sounds, words, or position within the sentence. We try to discover whether airflow is being impeded and where the occlusion exists—at the level of the larynx, the tongue, the lips, or in several of these simultaneously. We make estimates of the variability and consistency of the various avoidance and release behaviors. The stutterer's normal speech is also our concern. How fluent is he when he is not stuttering? What are the characteristics of the normal speech in terms of rate, pitch, intensity, and quality? How much does he actually talk during a day? Some of what we discover we share with him so that he can actively participate in the analysis and we make clear that we welcome his commentary.

Next we attempt to explore how well the stutterer can predict his moments of stuttering, having him underline feared words on a passage before he reads or by asking him to signal expectancy during propositional speech. Then through interviewing, we try to get some understanding of the kinds of phonemic cues or situational characteristics which usually are viewed as fearful or difficult. We ask him to tell us of experiences in which his stuttering was most traumatic or severe. In this investigation we try to get some impression of the hierarchies of situation difficulty for this particular stutterer.

We also explore the onset and development of his stuttering, the penalties and rejections, the possible profits and secondary gains, the other kinds of therapy he may have experienced. In all of this communication all sorts of other information are being fed into the clinical computer in our head.

We note his postures and body movements. We make tentative judgments about his emotionality, about his attitudes toward himself, us and others. How does he *really* feel about his stuttering? What other problems may be present? Every bit of information must of course be checked but first it must be stored. Since our diagnostic interview is recorded on tape, we retain much of this information for later review.

When the probing becomes too stressful, or when he needs a break, we take the stutterer to another room and ask him to fill out the Lanyon (1967) and the Erickson (1969) scales of stuttering severity. We also routinely use the Woolf (1967) *Perceptions of Stuttering Inventory* (PSI), an instrument which has real value in assessing the responses of fear, struggle, and avoidance. As he is filling out these tests, we play back our recording of the interview so we can check our previous clinical impressions and plan our further investigation.

When the stutterer returns, we test his response to masking noise and to delayed auditory feedback, seeking in the latter situation to determine those volume settings and delay times which appear especially to facilitate or to disrupt fluency. We check his fluency in singing, and whispering, and in unison speech or shadowing. We note his response to the use of the electrolarynx. If breathing abnormalities are apparent, we may take a polygraphic recording of his breathing in silence, normal speech, and during the expectancy of stuttering, and post-stuttering periods. Next we have him listen to the recordings of some of his stuttering and explore his reactions to this experience.[8] If it will not be

8 A description and outline of this analysis is found in Van Riper (1971), pp. 233–34.

too traumatic, we may ask the stutterer to watch himself in the mirror or on videotape while stuttering and to comment on the confrontation.

By this time we have a fairly adequate first impression of the amount of anxiety, shame or hostility the stutterer apparently feels, and we know pretty well the level of his frustration tolerance. However, we also do some further checking to see how he responds to communicative stress, to hurry, interruptions, listener loss, and the like. We may therefore ask him to make a telephone call in our presence or, if this is necessary and appropriate, to speak before a small group of strange listeners. We see how well he adapts to such situations and also to repeated readings of the same material or to repeated utterances of the same stuttered word.

We also find it important to do some trial therapy, asking the stutterer to attempt to modify certain of his behaviors such as eyeclosing or lip protrusion or clonic repetition. We determine how well he can duplicate some of his moments of stuttering after they have occurred. We ask him to prolong a moment of stuttering until we give the signal for its release. We request that he attempt a feared word without one of his usual approach behaviors, e.g., an inhalatory gasp, the use of "um," or whatever starter device he characteristically employs. We ask him to predict and comment on his performances of these tasks. This trial therapy also helps us make some appraisal of the stutterer's motivation, his ability to relate to us, and the strengths of his stuttering behaviors. Often it reveals some of the difficulties we both will experience once therapy begins.

Throughout this examination, as we have said, we make frequent comments to the stutterer concerning our discoveries, but we also make sure, before the session is concluded, that we present to him a summary of our impressions. We do not tell him all that we have observed but we share enough material so that he sees the main picture of the presented problem as we view it and its implications for treatment. We stress that this view is tentative and always subject to revision. It is important that the stutterer participate from the first in the therapeutic process.

We usually end the diagnostic session by assigning the stutterer the task of preparing a fairly thorough autobiography centered about those important experiences which in his opinion shaped him, and about the significant people who influenced him. We then may make arrangements for the stutterer to complete such tests as the MMPI, the Taylor Manifest Anxiety Scale, or the Willoughby Questionnaire after he leaves us and to have a complete physical examination. Where indicated, we may also arrange for projective tests such as the Rorschach, or perhaps the Bender, the Rotter, the TAT or other special tests. If there is a strong cluttering component or the case presents some moments of stuttering that resemble petit mal lapses, we of course refer him for an electroencephalographic examination.

The organization of all this information presents some difficulty but by keeping in mind that we must know our stutterer if we are to design an appropriate therapy for him, the pattern of the problem soon achieves some definition. An equation which we developed (Van Riper, 1971) provides some assistance:

$$S_s = \frac{PFAGH + Sf.WF + C_s}{M + Fl}$$

in which P designates the amount of and vulnerability to penalties the stutterer receives for his stuttering;

F, the frustration which he feels when stuttering; *A,* the amount of generalized anxiety from any source; *G,* the amount of guilt and shame he feels; *H,* the amount of hostility toward himself and others. *Sf* and *Wf* represent the present strengths of his current situation and word fears; *Cs,* his vulnerability to communicative stress.[9] Some assessment of each of these factors can be made as the result of the diagnostic examination.

The *M* factor in the divisor represents our estimate of the stutterer's morale or ego strength or the overall sum of his assets divided by his liabilities. It can also include the stutterer's motivation to overcome his stuttering. The *Fl* factor represents the fluency he does possess and recognizes. By appraising the apparent strength of each of these factors, a profile of each stutterer's unique problem can be achieved and the *Ss* might be said to represent the overall severity of stuttering in terms of prospective therapy. As we have said, this equation is admittedly crude. It does not take into account the strength of the component habits of avoidance and struggle nor the frequency or duration nor any factor of possible organicity—but it can serve as a nucleus for the general assessment of clinical difficulty and this is what the therapist needs.

We suspect that most therapists use some sort of similar profiling of the clinical needs of their patients in their continuing diagnoses throughout therapy. There is always the need for assessment and reassessment in terms of the kinds of factors we have mentioned. We cannot rely solely on frequency counts of stutterings. The

disorder is too variable, too influenced by too many external and internal stimuli. We cannot treat the stuttering alone. We must treat the stutterer.

Bibliography

BACH, G. R., *Intensive Group Psychotherapy.* New York: Ronald Press, 1954.

ERICKSON, R. L., Assessing communication attitudes among stutterers, *Journal of Speech and Hearing Research,* 12 (1969), 711–24.

FERNAU-HORN, H., *Die Sprechneurosen.* Stuttgart: Hippokrates-Verlag, 1969.

FREUND, H., *Psychopathology and Problems of Stuttering.* Springfield, Ill.: Charles C Thomas, 1966.

LANYON, R. I., The measurement of stuttering severity, *Journal of Speech and Hearing Research,* 10 (1967), 836–43.

LEVY, D. M., Release therapy in young children, *American Journal of Orthopsychiatry,* 9 (1939), 387–90.

SHEEHAN, J. G., *Stuttering: Research and Therapy.* New York: Harper & Row, 1970.

SLAVSON, S. R., *Introduction to Group Psychotherapy.* New York: International Universities Press, 1951.

THORNE, F. C., *The Principles of Personality Counseling.* Brandon, Vt.: Journal of Clinical Psychology Press, 1950.

TRAVIS, L. E., The unspeakable feelings of stutterers, in L. E. Travis (ed.), *Handbook of Speech Pathology.* New York: Appleton-Century-Crofts, 1957.

VAN RIPER, C. Experiments in stuttering therapy, in J. Eisenson (ed.), *Stuttering: A Symposium.* New York: Harper & Row, 1958.

————, *The Nature of Stuttering.* Englewood Cliffs, N.J.: Prentice-Hall, 1971.

WOOLF, G., The assessment of stuttering as struggle avoidance and expectancy, *British Journal of Disorders of Communication,* 2 (1967), 158–71.

9 For a more detailed account of this equation see Van Riper (1971), pp. 374ff. It is often useful to ask the stutterer to draw up his own profile of the relative strengths of the component factors in the equation.

Motivation

Of all the various skills and competencies needed by the therapist who works with stutterers, none is more important in the determination of success or failure than the assessment and management of motivation. We know of no easy road to fluency that can be traversed by the confirmed stutterer. Because there are no quick and painless cures, the tasks of therapy are often onerous, demanding much of both therapist and client. The unlearning of highly automatized avoidance and escape behaviors conditioned to a host of complex sets of external and internal stimuli is not to be accomplished with ease. New responses to the fear and experience of stuttering must be acquired; new discriminations mastered; new ways of perceiving himself and others must be taught the stutterer. The route to fluency has many obstacles and pitfalls

and there will be times when the stutterer, seeing them, will balk or sit down and ask to be carried. Often we have envied the animal psychologist who can deprive his rat subject of food or water to the degree necessary for efficient learning, who knows exactly what barriers, blind alleys, and electric grids are in the goal pathway, and who can administer the reinforcements and punishments appropriately, and precisely control the amount of motivation required. Unfortunately, our stutterers were not raised in the learning laboratory nor can we confine them there. They come from different strains; their stuttering behaviors have intricate reinforcement histories which we may never know. Often our notion of the drives and deprivations and incentives that impel them is unsatisfactorily vague. As Smith (1966) writes, "Motivation is the first essential: men learn what they want to learn. What a person says about his motivation, however, is no safe guide to what it is." Usually we must gather the information we need as therapy proceeds, since the only sure test of a reinforcer or incentive is in its effect on behavior.[1]

The stutterer's motives

Why does the stutterer seek therapy? Some obvious answers to this question have included the following: to free himself from social inadequacy; to get rid of the fears of words and situations which plague him; to increase his self-esteem; to decrease the inconvenience of communicative frustration and the visible and audible abnormality which accompanies his attempts to speak; to enable him to get a good job or better job; to make him more attractive to members of the opposite sex, and so on. The list could be endless but we should remember that the lowest common denominator of all the components in the motivation equation is the stutterer's difficulty in communicating easily and without abnormality. This is the basic source of his distress. He hungers for effective communication; he thirsts for speech uncolored by the frustration of temporally broken words, syllables, and words. He is fluency deprived. From this basic behavioral deficit stem other deprivations: social participation, economic success, sexual satisfactions, self-esteem, and the like. The intermittent inability to speak fluently also leads to the instigation of the learned

[1] One instrument which we have found useful is described in "A Reinforcement Survey Schedule for Use in Therapy, Training, and Research" by J. R. Cautela and R. Kastenbaum, *Psychological Reports*, 20 (1967), 1115–30.

drives of anxiety and frustration. Much of the stutterer's internal misery is due to this communicative frustration and fear and he is motivated to do what he can to reduce both. Much of his external abnormality is due to his struggle or avoidance behaviors and the fears that trigger them. Also, of course, there is the unpleasantness of social rejection for deviance. The stutterer seeks therapy to free himself from stigma, from assessed and penalized abnormality. He wants to speak without fear or struggle. These are such powerful motivating forces that it is surprising to find that the therapist cannot always count upon them to make therapy easy for there are counterforces as well.

"When we deal with the free ranging person we cannot specify exactly what will be reinforcing to him, and to what extent. Different people have different goals, aims, interests, incentives, and reinforcement values. What is strongly positively reinforcing to one subject may actually be aversive to another." This quotation from Buchwald and Young (1969) though referring to experiments in behavior modification, should be remembered by all clinicians who deal with stutterers. Motives cannot be assumed; they must be discovered, nurtured, and sometimes created. Different stutterers present different motivating pictures. While all of them come to us to relieve their distress, and most of that distress focuses about their fluency deprivation, their motivational hierarchies differ markedly one from another. Halfond (1965) provides a vivid illustration:

For example, a young doctor with a mild stuttering problem showed concern about his speech disorder to a clinician who was psychotherapeutically oriented. Counseling was circular and superficial until it became apparent to the clinician that the patient was essentially worried about one aspect of his stuttering problem which was his use of the telephone in professional matters. The clinician eventually realized this . . . and a number of alternatives were considered. The patient's goal was further clarified when it became evident that he did not want to eliminate his stuttering but rather to circumvent it in using the telephone. Therapy was terminated by mutual consent when the patient decided to use a secretary to handle telephone calls. (p. 292)

The costs of therapy

We cite this illustration to make the additional point that motivation varies not only in kind but in amount. We do not agree with Halfond's interpretation that the doctor probably did not want to eliminate his stuttering. We feel instead that the costs of therapy designed to eliminate it altogether were greater than the anticipated payoff. Most of that doctor's discomfort centered about his inadequacy in telephoning. If his drive to free himself from that specific unpleasantness could be reduced by hiring the secretary, that drive was not very powerful, certainly not strong enough to undergo the costly misery involved in the exploration of his dirty little psyche. The strength of motivation can be measured in many ways but always it involves the ratio between costs and payoff. The competent clinician therefore tries not only to assess the strength of the stutterer's drive to be rid of his disorder but also to ascertain his expectations both of relief and of the amount of work and stress he must undergo. Much of the clinician's skill resides in his ability to create more payoff than cost. In the literature we find many statements to the effect that stutterers want and expect to be cured in a very short time and without having to do much work.

Over a hundred years ago, Klencke (1862) had this to say:

Stutterers have certain characteristics which are associated with an inclination towards secrecy, indolence, suspicion, passive opposition to any inconvenience required by the treatment, and a sanguine devotion to anything which seems to point toward an easy and rapid cure. The battle against these characteristics is always most difficult at the beginning of treatment, and if the physician does not succeed in overcoming them in the first six weeks, he might as well send him home.

More recently, Barbara (1954) gives us some explanation for these traits:

Since many stutterers may have gone from clinic to clinic, consulted with various specialists, or, in the case of the more unfortunate ones, been subjected to so-called "miraculous cures," some doubts and feelings of doom and helplessness will have become fixed. As a result, when they are initially interviewed for what they may feel to be "another new and futile attempt, among the many others," they are often skeptical, cautious, and may by this time have little real incentive for receiving help toward solving their problems. It is in relation to this difficult area of resistance that the therapist must give a great deal of himself by way of encouragement. (pp. 272–73)

In our experience, this picture seems to be that presented more often by mild stutterers than severe ones. For those who have a substantial amount of fluent speech, the apparent goal distance seems so short that they find it difficult to expect that they may have to put out much effort to overcome their disability. One of the reasons that severe stutterers often seem to have a better prognosis than the milder ones is that they know they have far to go and so they work harder. Their expectations of the costs of therapy are more realistic and of course, being more miserable, they have greater drive. Their *expected* payoff is greater. We once did a little pilot study on 20 adult stutterers in which we asked them prior to treatment to estimate how long therapy would have to last to be effective if they were given therapy sessions once a week, twice a week, three times a week, and for a varying number of hours daily. The results showed that they were more realistic than we had suspected. All 20 checked the term "forever" for the "one hour a week" scheduling; 15 checked "two years" for therapy offered one hour daily; 14 checked "one year" for "three hours daily." None of them felt that effective therapy could be accomplished in less than four months under any schedule. A comparison of their estimates with their adaptation rates and severity ratings showed that those stutterers who were less severe or who showed the greatest adaptation were the more optimistic ones. The stutterers who were more severe or who had previously attended other clinics showed longer estimated therapy times. However, the results were interesting in indicating that stutterers believe that they need longer and more frequent therapy sessions than are commonly provided in most schools or clinics. Certainly, they make clear the need to assess the stutterer's expectations of the payoff and costs of treatment.

Let us say again that our clients will not work without the promise of payoff. They insist upon getting something for their pain and labor and woe to the therapist who does not keep this fact in mind. Any therapeutic task that entails more loss than gain is simply not going to be carried out. This means that if the therapist is to hope for any success he must be able to assess the probable costs of each suggested activity. Far too often we fail to make this assessment and then, when he refuses or sabotages or makes only a token attempt, we are tempted to conclude that he is weak or lazy. What we should do instead is to increase the expected payoff or to lessen the cost or do both. We can revise the assignment so that it can be done with less loss of time or labor or face, or we can contrive additional rewards for its performance. Sometimes the wisest course is to postpone the task for another day when more profit can be anticipated. Every competent clinician scans his case carefully at the beginning of each session trying to ascertain how much morale currency the latter may have in his pockets on that particular day. Some days those pockets are almost empty; some days they are full and the wise therapist revises his goals and activities and reinforcements accordingly. Whenever our stutterers have demonstrated a "lack of motivation" we feel that we have failed to comprehend his cost-profit ratio and we know that we must observe him and identify with him more closely.

Varying levels of motivation during the course of therapy

This assessing of motivation is not a task we perform only at the beginning of therapy once and for all. It must be done continually for motivation wanes and waxes daily. It varies with different tasks and with new problems that arise during different stages of the treatment. This daily fluctuation in motivation is found in all striving. The athlete must get up for the game. He has his bad days as well as his good ones, and much of the difference between them has to do with the strength of his drives. In therapy we have noted how often our cases fail to work very hard at the tasks of therapy because of other experiences unrelated to speech which have reduced their morale. They had to go to the dentist that day. They were up too late the night before. The girls they were dating had to study. A thousand reasons, many of them good ones, account for the ebbing of their urge to progress in their speech therapy. Clinicians must always make some estimate of the current motivation in every treatment session.

All clinicians also soon become aware of the "honeymoon effect." At the beginning of therapy, once hope has been aroused, a stutterer may work very hard and run very fast toward his goals. Later on, once the novelty of the therapeutic situation has worn off, the same stutterer may show a marked decrease in effort. In part this is due to satiation of the exploratory drive but primarily it is due to the fact that the treatment itself allays some of the distress which drives the stutterer to seek therapy in the first place. Driven to do something about his problem because of listener loss and rejection, he may find in his therapist an almost perfect listener, one who does not penalize his stuttering. Previously bedevilled by constant communicative frustration, he now discovers that at least in one situation, the therapy room, he is much more fluent. Why then work hard? Things are getting better. The hurt is less; the therapist is patient; perhaps time itself will do the healing. The wise clinician will recognize what is happening and will program himself so that this does not occur. For learning and unlearning, love is not enough.

We have come to expect motivational crises to arise at any time but certainly they seem to appear fairly often during the confrontation, desensitization, and stabilization-maintenance stages of therapy. In the therapeutic maze which must be run, the stutterer tends to slow down as he encounters each of these choice points or grids and the clinician must recognize the need at these times to mobilize all the motivating forces that he can control. Fortunately, the first of these crises comes very early in treatment at a time when the urge to get relief is very strong. Confrontation of the stuttering as a problem to be accepted and dealt with directly rather than by avoidance and denial is a high hurdle. Some stutterers try to detour around it by becoming passive clay in the therapist's hands. Often they try to seduce the therapist by attributing to him capacities of magical omnipotence and omniscience which permit them accordingly to refrain from accepting any personal responsibility for the course or outcome of treatment, a situation which if consummated will certainly prevent any learning or unlearning. They may prefer to intellectualize or to discuss their miseries at great length rather than to do anything about them. They may restrict their confrontation to the therapy room while still pretending outside it that they do not stutter. We must understand their needs at this point. For years they have lived in the land of the Emperor's clothes where most of the persons closest to them pretended to ignore the stuttering. They were taught to deny their disorder and that denial gave them some temporary surcease from their suffering. So we should understand that the confrontation stage of therapy may present some motivational difficulties.

A second major locus of decreased motivation appears when the stutterer starts to enter feared situations or deliberately to attempt feared words in learning how to modify his stuttering behaviors. To have to touch the untouchable; to have to speak the unspeakable; to enter the arenas where he was so grievously wounded requires strong motivation.

Finally, the clinician can expect some decreased motivation, especially in the severe stutterer, when enough gains have been made to permit him to communicate with some effectiveness despite the presence of considerable abnormality. For the first time in his life, he can say what he wants to say. Though they now speak laboriously, and with far too much abnormality, such stutterers are so exhilarated with relief they find it hard to put forth the added effort to go any further. When the stuttering that was such a curse becomes merely a nuisance, motivation lags. Again they tend to ignore and deny the small facsimiles of the old abnormality that infest their speech and, when this happens, these miniature stutterings begin to occur more frequently and to become more severe. We meet much this same motivational problem in the terminal stages of therapy when the stutterer has indeed become remarkably fluent. He then is enjoying his newfound ability to speak so much and seems to be so far removed from his old unpleasantness that there is little drive to do things he should do to maintain that fluency until it becomes automatized. None of these problems is insurmountable. All of them should be recognized.

Motivation difficulties in therapy

In light of our preceding discussion we can understand why the beginning speech therapist is often bewildered and shocked to find that even severe stutterers seem to have little motiva-

tion to do the things they have to do to improve their speech. Often the same stutterers who profess a willingness to do anything and everything under the eternal sun and moon to get relief from the impediment, will resist all our efforts to help them. Their ingenious sabotage of clinical assignments is at times almost worthy of our reluctant admiration. They open the therapeutic bottle and sniff lightly of the contents but they will not take the medicine. Often their performance is more token than real. In short, the therapist cannot assume that the stutterer has the necessary motivation for successful therapy. It is necessary to understand the dynamics of his resistance.

Goal-setting difficulties

First of all, we must remember that a person with a long history of stuttering has had a long history of failure. The cumulative effect of hundreds of instances each day in which the person tries and fails to utter a word at the proper time is bound to leave some trace. This is something very difficult for the normal speaker to understand. To try and fail, to try and fail, to ttttry and fffffail again and again to do something which should be accomplished without any effort at all, is to undergo a brainwashing of incredible thoroughness. Why try if you always fail? Most of the research has indicated that stutterers have lower aspiration levels than normal speakers even on tasks which are not speech-related. We are not suprised.

Nor are we astonished to find that some stutterers paradoxically insist upon setting goals for themselves that are unrealistically high, or that they have Demosthenes complexes and unrealistic vocational objectives (becoming politicians, teachers, salesmen, preachers, etc.). This is not an uncommon defense reaction to repeated failure. It creates, however, a real problem for the therapist who must structure treatment in terms of subgoals. He finds that such a stutterer demands instant relief, complete relief and without having to earn it. Accomplishing a small goal, making progress, moving in the direction of the long-term goal appear to have little attractiveness at first.

Related to this matter of goal setting is the stutterer's self-concept. Certain stutterers and perhaps the majority (though we have no research bearing directly on the problem) show a morbid sensitivity to the flaws in their speech perhaps because the latter threaten the illusory perfection of their ideal self-percepts. They are, as several writers have put it, "giants in chains." These stutterers feel that if only they did not have these fluency flaws, they could do all the wondrous deeds characteristic of their many moments of private fantasy. Such stutterers find it difficult to recognize or to prize those little modifications of behavior which are so crucial to final success.

We must also recognize that some stutterers resist the confrontation of their stuttering, not only because of its frustration and stigma, but because it further threatens the basic integration of the self-concept, an integration which is at best precariously unstable. The fluent Dr. Jekyll self does not appreciate being asked to look hard at stuttering Mr. Hyde. The basic need for ego integration, which serves as a mandate for all of us, is thwarted in the stutterer when the therapist insists upon activities which make the split between the fluent and stuttering selves more obvious.

The clinical handling of denial is always difficult. We should be careful not to put the stutterer into the *cul*

de sac position of denying the denial which is what usually happens when he is confronted with the mechanism too soon or too drastically. When therapy becomes argument, the basic therapeutic relationship is threatened. We must realize that this denial behavior has usually had a long history of powerful reinforcement because it in truth did yield some meager relief. Often, only by shutting off awareness of the all too painful reality of his verbal impotence and social deviance, the stutterer was able to maintain a precarious equilibrium in a world full of ego threat. One of the quickest ways of losing motivation is to strip the client bare of needed defenses. Our own policy has usually been based on the fact that denial is seldom consistent. Like love or the weather it fluctuates. There will be times, if the therapist can create the appropriate conditions, when the stutterer will momentarily be able to confront the traumatic behavior that ordinarily he denies. Alert to this possibility, we are always ready to strongly reward each little instance in which that confrontation occurs and we set up hierarchies of self-contact so that more and more acceptance of the stuttering may be tolerated. By so doing, we can bypass this obstacle.

The aversiveness of stuttering

To escape from this level of abstraction, we can also point to the natural reluctance of any human being to be required to touch something which has hurt him in the past. Stuttering behaviors have been painted and repainted with the black pigment of unpleasant emotion thousands of times in the adult stutterer. Therapists must understand the stutterer's reluctance to touch this evil stuff. To put stuttering into his mouth deliberately, to mold and shape it, does not at first seem entirely reasonable. We might say that he does not show enough motivation, that he will not cooperate, or that he resists, but surely we can understand why he shows these behaviors.

In the same vein, we must also recognize that most advanced stutterers come to us with a long history of avoidance reactions that also have been strongly reinforced. They have often spared the stutterer much pain. As numerous psychological researches have demonstrated, conditioned avoidance responses do not extinguish easily. They occur even despite the stutterer's desire to inhibit them. For years he has endeavored to hide his speech difficulty and there have been many instances when he has managed successfully to avoid exhibiting it, enough of them to keep these avoidance behaviors very strong. Though we may persuade him intellectually that avoidance reduces fear only temporarily and in the long run adds to his misery, we must expect him to continue to avoid feared situations, words, and even therapeutic tasks for some time. When he does so, we should not interpret this necessarily as a sign of no motivation. The spirit may be willing but the flesh trembles. The stutterer comes to us as a person who has had to learn ways of minimizing the extreme discomfort of his abnormal and frustrating speech interruptions. To hope that he will suddenly be able to give up his avoidance of feared words and speaking situations, the only strategy which has ever provided him with even partial relief, is unrealistic. Motivation is not to be assumed.

Lack of trust in the therapist

Some of the apparent lack of motivation may also be due to the stutterer's very real fear of placing himself in the hands of a therapist who may drop him. Most adult stutterers have had some unpleasant experiences with other therapists or with parents, teachers, or friends who practiced token or unwise therapy. We cannot expect that such stutterers will trust us immediately. We should know that they must test our competence and commitment before they will willingly accept our guidance. Much of the resistance in the early stages of treatment may be viewed as part of this testing process. The intimate relationship between the stutterer and his therapist is one to be entered with caution and with some reservation on the stutterer's part. However, once we have proved repeatedly that we are both competent and committed, that we have signed the therapeutic contract even if he hasn't, usually the stutterer's attitude suddenly changes. Suddenly we find motivation which we did not know was there.

Reluctance to surrender secondary gains

Many writers have attributed the resistance and lack of motivation shown by the adult stutterer to the latter's reluctance to surrender the secondary gains which the disorder has given him. They feel he clings to his symptoms because of the neurotic profit they bring. There is no doubt that such secondary gains exist. As one of our cases said, "Sure, I get what good I can out of my stuttering; I get out of many responsibilities; I've got a good excuse for not trying, for not succeeding. Because I stutter, I don't have to do a lot of unpleasant or fearful things. But let me tell you something: the little good that I get out of it isn't worth the agony." We would agree with this statement. Sheehan (1970) has a good passage on secondary gains. He writes:

. . . we still hold that with the onset of the problem called stuttering, the primary loss far outweighs anything that may later be rationalized as a secondary gain. An amputee veteran may experience some sympathy (most of it unwelcome) along with a multitude of frustrating social reactions. But does the gain exceed the loss? Would he trade back, given the opportunity? These are the questions that must be asked of the stutterer. (p. 270)

While there are neurotic stutterers as well as neurotic normal speakers, we have not found that these acknowledged secondary gains are sufficient to explain all the motivation difficulties shown by the ordinary stutterer. They may account for some of the resistance in the neurotic stutterer but not for most of it in the majority of the cases with whom we have worked so intensively.

Stuttering as a minor nuisance

We cannot conclude this section without emphasizing another source of lack of motivation. There are some stutterers, usually the milder ones and the younger ones, who have not been hurt enough by their stuttering to feel any strong need to do anything about it. Blessed by having lived in a very favorable environment that was relatively free from penalties, and perhaps being possessed of personality assets sufficient to compensate for their communicative liability, these stutterers find the results of the hard labor of therapy not worth the cost. The cheese of fluency at the end of the maze is far, far away and besides they prefer other available foods. To these stutterers their stuttering is just a minor nuisance, one that they can live with, so why should they be expected to strive so mightily? They are not at all desperate. They get along. Often they come to the therapist only because

others insist. In a vague way, they would prefer to be fluent but only if they could get that fluency without much effort or pain or discipline. So let us face the fact: in some stutterers the motivation to overcome their stuttering is not very strong. They have other more important needs.

Revealing the therapists' competence and commitment

We feel perhaps that we have painted the motivation picture too blackly. Many of our stutterers work eagerly and hard and it has been a delightful experience to guide them. None of the motivational problems we have been describing are insoluble, and in the following sections we describe some of the things that therapists can do to remove the shackles that bind the motivation that we feel lies latent in all our clients. Let us begin at the beginning. While the necessity for demonstrating one's competence and concern for the client must be confronted repeatedly throughout therapy, we have always viewed the initial contacts with the stutterer as the time during which this motivational factor is most crucial. First judgments may often be incorrect but such imprinting is not corrected easily. In our first contact with the stutterer we try very hard to make sure that he senses that we probably know more about stuttering than he does, that we have worked with other stutterers with some success, that we strongly desire to understand his particular problem, and that we intend to do whatever we can to help him. How to accomplish these aims varies, of course, with the individual client—and the individual therapist.

Therapists should be aware of the importance of the opening gambits.

We personally refrain from asking the stutterer very many questions in these first sessions and certainly we do not immediately ask his name and address, those nuclei of a thousand wretched memories. We do not plunge instantly into the depths of his wretched conflicts. Instead we do most of the talking at first, describing the diagnostic goals of this first meeting, explaining why we must do what we do, expressing some of the feelings that this particular stutterer might be having at the moment. Then we might casually mention why we have been doing all the talking, why we haven't badgered him with questions, thus showing that we understand the stutterer's usual greater difficulty in such communication. But as soon as possible we explore the presented complaint, the stuttering. Again we do not do this by asking questions but by describing and imitating the tremendous variety of stuttering behaviors of the stutterers we have known and suggesting that he indicate which of those demonstrated are similar to his own. Usually this is sufficient to provoke some speech and some stuttering and when it does, we then can explore whether the kind of stuttering he has just shown us is more or less typical of his problem in other situations. At this point, he often finds us imitating his stuttering either in pantomime or aloud and we explain that we wish to do it ourselves so we can know just what it feels like, that we must put it into our own mouth to understand it, that to diagnose it we must study it, etc. We also provide a running commentary on what we have observed, thereby sharing with him our analysis of this overt behavior. This both surprises the stutterer and impresses him and probably for the first time in his life he becomes interested in, rather than traumatized by, his stuttering.

Next we turn to the covert features of the disorder. Again we describe the variety of fears and frustration and guilt reactions of other stutterers we have met, showing the stutterer by our verbalization that we are experienced and competent. We invite him to help us know which of the feelings we have expressed are similar to his own. During this phase of the initial examination we do not imitate or share the stuttering but reflect in our own words (often even better than he can) the private emotional aspects of his disorder which he has felt able for perhaps the first time to reveal. There will be other sessions in which similar interactions will occur but none where the revelation of the therapist's competence and commitment have such a profound impact. There are of course many other approaches which can accomplish the same ends and we certainly do not use this gambit with all our cases. If the therapist *is* competent and committed, he will find his own ways of showing these traits.

The inevitable challenge

One of the stutterer's first tests of the therapist's competence presents itself very early. Implicitly or explicitly he will ask the question: "Can you cure me?" How the therapist responds may determine the course and success or failure of the treatment. The answer of course is that stuttering is not a disease in the medical sense, that most of it is learned behavior and that no one can guarantee a cure for such a problem. This is the time to structure one's role as a therapist. He is to be viewed as an experienced guide. He knows what most stutterers need to do to become more fluent and he is willing to share that knowledge. As a guide he can point the way, serve as companion and supporter, but he cannot carry the stutterer. Stuttering is not conquered easily but surely the stutterer can learn to talk more fluently. We tell him that some stutterers achieve complete fluency, at least equal to that characteristic of most normal speakers. We say also that some do not profit at all from treatment, usually because they refuse to assume any responsibility for their own improvement but that those who really try do get better. We say that our goal is fluency and we demonstrate that it is possible to stutter without fear or abnormality and that this at least is within the reach of any confirmed stutterer. The stutterer's job is to unlearn his old ways of reacting and to learn new ones so that he can communicate fluently. We have found that this direct answer to the old question is very reassuring to the stutterer. He knows only too well that his problem has no magical solution. Sooner or later he will surely doubt the competence of any therapist who would have the incredible gall to say point blank that certainly he can cure him.

We do not wish to leave the impression that any therapist can allay all the stutterer's doubts in these first sessions. Throughout the course of therapy there will be many other moments in which the therapist will be challenged, tested and evaluated. Often this is done covertly as well as directly. We soon learned that the appropriate response to this testing was to verbalize his doubts and his need to be certain of our dedication and concern. We showed our acceptance of his hidden feelings that he might not be able to trust us or that we might not really be able to help him and we tell him that most of the stutterers who have come to us had the same misgivings.

Providing hope

The stutterer usually comes to us confused and lost. His previous efforts to find his way out of the morass of stuttering have failed. Often he has little real hope that he will ever be able to overcome his disability. Recognizing that hope is the very essence of motivation, the therapist must either create it or at least blow upon its faint embers until they glow. To do so, the therapist must himself have some confidence in his own abilities to help his client. If molehills or mountains are to be moved, some of the energy necessary to move them will be found in the therapist's faith in himself. This is not to say that one can always be certain of the outcome, but any therapist knows in his bones that he can do much to ease his client's suffering. Like fishermen, good therapists are optimists. Most of them have come to have a profound respect for the latent potential for self-healing that exists in all troubled souls. They resemble Michelangelo who, when asked by a bystander how he could carve such glorious angels from just a slab of stone, replied, "Oh they're already in there. I just have to chip away the stone that surrounds them." Out of the therapist's faith can come the stutterer's hope.

For those defeated stutterers whose hopes hover around the zero mark we have found no better strategy than to have them meet a real live recovered stutterer. Repeatedly we have seen how even a brief contact with such a person can make a profound impact. Unfortunately most of the individuals whom we have treated successfully hie themselves away to other parts as quickly as they can. It is the chronic failures who return to roost, who hang around. There have been times when we envied the Oracle of Delphi whose therapeutic prescription for Battos the Stutterer was to exile himself forever and never return, but fortunately many of our former successful clients come to see us occasionally to brag of their achievements. When they talk to the stutterers with whom we are currently working, we always note a remarkable spurt of progress. Since we routinely record the progress of our clients at regular intervals with audio or video tape, these too can also serve as a useful surrogate. They help the stutterer see and hear both the minor and the dramatic changes throughout the course of therapy.

Recognizing that stuttering is modifiable. One of the impacts of such recordings is that the stutterer vividly perceives that the form of stuttering can be changed, that the behaviors are modifiable. He notes that the stuttering of the person on the tape gradually decreases in its abnormality from segment to segment and that as it does so the person becomes more and more fluent. Then we replay a recording of the new stutterer's speech asking him to observe the variability of his own stuttering and to note that occasionally a very fluent kind of stuttering occurs on a few words. Even in the initial sessions we can demonstrate that he already possesses the model of a variety of stuttering which would impede his communicative progress very little, one which he need not fear, one that most listeners would never penalize. This too is a taste of the distant goal. Also, we often ask the stutterer to experiment with different forms of stuttering, omitting one of the common features, or to change yet another one according to our directions or demonstration. When such an experience takes place while repeating a word previously stuttered, or when echoing himself on a record-

ed sample of speech in which severe stuttering has occurred, the contrast becomes especially vivid. The stutterer begins right then to realize that his behavior is not as involuntary or compulsively strong as he had believed it to be. He discovers that he has some choice, some control of his behavior. We have also used some brief operant conditioning procedures to weaken or eliminate one of the characteristic abnormalities of the stuttering behavior such as eye closing or lip protrusion. Stuttering may still be present but its form has been modified so that it is less abnormal. There are other ways of convincing the stutterer that he need not surrender all responsibility for his behavior when word fear threatens, that he need not automatically struggle in the throes of his contortions, that the behavior may be touched and manipulated. We cannot stress enough how motivating such experiences can be. The stutterer has felt helpless for such a long time. He has felt possessed by his stuttering, unable to control it. Now for the first time perhaps he finds that much of what he does he can change. For many stutterers this is a truly crucial experience. It is certainly a highly motivating one.

Closely related to this anticipatory goal perception of oneself as being responsible for one's own behavior and able to control it, is the glimpse of one's adequacy as a social being. Most of our adult stutterers need much more than fluency. The constant stuttering with its attendant societal reactions has not only restricted their social activities and attitudes but often has also warped them. Since the stutterer's interpersonal relationships have formerly been achieved with difficulty, have often been less than satisfactory, and occasionally have resulted in much misery, the acquisition of fluency may sometimes create more problems than it solves. Anyone who has lived as a chronic avoider for years does not suddenly become outgoing. Fluency can help the stutterer to become an adequate person but it does not guarantee it by any means. Accordingly from the very first sessions onward, we seek to structure our therapy so that the long range goal is not merely relief from stuttering but the acquisition of those behavior patterns which characterize an adequate human being.

How do we give our stuttering clients such a vision? In part we do it through the identification process, by being adequate ourselves. A wound does not heal through contact with a dirty bandage. If we are reasonably healthy and happy, our stutterers tend to become that way too. Call it transference or empathy or learning new responses to old stimuli or modeling or what you will, it is certain that changes occur in the stutterer which reflect not only the therapist's directives but his basic attitudes and values. We are shaped by all those with whom we have had intimate relationships. The therapeutic situation is rarely free from modeling influences.

But we also help our stutterers to glimpse the goal of personal adequacy by differential reinforcement of such behaviors when shown during the course of therapy. We reward by our approving appreciation those behaviors or statements which show honesty, courage, responsibility, and the like. We withhold such reinforcement from other behaviors which are less socially desirable. The work of Shames and his associates at the University of Pittsburgh (1969) shows clearly that the number of positive self statements can be increased and the number of negative ones decreased by operant conditioning procedures. The clinician is trained to positively reinforce the former (example: "I think I might just be able to talk pretty good some day.") by providing approving reflective responses (example: "Yes, you feel you can do it."), and to decrease the frequency of negative self statements such as "Something just gets stuck and I'm helpless," either by not responding at all or by some verbalization of mild disapproval. Thousands of small opportunities present themselves in the interaction that is the essence of treatment to modify much more than the stutterer's speech. Indeed we do this whether we realize it or not and it is better to know what we are doing if we are to do it effectively.

At the same time there are limits to the amount of instrumental shaping we can do and certainly none but the most arrogant therapist would desire to create an exact duplicate of himself even if he could. These human beings who stutter are not made entirely of clay. There are parts that are malleable and other parts that have already hardened into stone. The sensitive therapist soon learns to accept the limits of his capabilities. And yet we have repeatedly come to see that much more potential for modification exists than is at first apparent. For years we always accepted one stutterer for treatment who, in our opinion, had almost a "zero prognosis" at the time of the initial examination. Some of them surprised us by achieving much more than those whose prospects were infinitely more favorable.

Motivational arousal through planning

We have said that a long-range goal appears closer when the person sees the route to that goal. Accordingly we attempt early in therapy to provide for our clients a sketch of the probable sequential course of therapy. We explain that each stutterer's map differs from those of his fellows. Certain paths open to one may not be open to another but there are many roads to relief. Nevertheless, though the therapy must be tailored to individual needs and capacities, there will be some common obstacles that the stutterer will meet and must overcome. He needs a cognitive map of the route he must follow and on this map some of the hazards and difficult places must be evident. In the day of Columbus, old maps often contained such terms as "Terra Incognita" (Unknown land) or "Here be monsters!" While the equivalents of these monsters are always to be found on the cognitive maps of therapy, we feel that the route to fluency rather than the terrors should be more prominent. What are the landmarks on this road to fluency? Specifically, the stutterer must be able to confront his stuttering and himself realistically and honestly, specifying the behaviors, overt and covert, which must be modified and replaced. He must desensitize himself to many forms of communicative stress including those he has interiorized due to past trauma. He must learn to vary his behaviors, then to change them to more appropriate reactions, to those that are conducive to fluency and personal adequacy, and finally he will have to find ways of stabilizing these new ways of fluent talking and effective living. We do not, of course, put the plan of therapy to him in such abstract terms but we do make sure the stutterer realizes that we have a map even if he does not, a map that will show where he is, where he must go, and the major landmarks along the path between. In these first sessions—or even later for that matter—we do not feel it neces-

sary or wise to fill in all the details on the map; we could not do so even if we wished. All we can say is that we have guided others with some success and that we know the terrain.

Subgoals and motivation

The sort of therapy which we advocate is primarily a psychotherapeutically oriented activity therapy. Tasks and experiences are devised jointly by the therapist and the stutterer so that old maladaptive reactions can be extinguished and so that new learning may occur. They involve not only the stuttered speech but other interpersonal interactions as well. Much of the essence of this therapy is to be found in the discussions between therapist and the stutterer as the tasks are devised and reported. We agree with Hollis (1964), a social worker, who writes:

. . . the client will more surely move toward his objectives when he is conscious of what they are. Goals are finally implemented only when they are shared by both client and worker. The objectives of treatment must be thought of as fluid, changing with changes in the client's understanding of his own needs and as the worker's understanding of the clients' needs and capacities develops. (p. 216)

It is also necessary in our opinion, to use this mutual goal-setting approach to counteract the stutterer's all too evident feelings of helplessness. We must not wait until the end of treatment to hand over some of the responsibility for the success of therapy. If we do this we invite regression and relapse. The realization that he is responsible for his own behavior does not come easy to the stutterer and it does little good to try to persuade him intellectually that this is true despite

the valiant attempts of the semantical-
ly oriented clinicians. Better to have
him learn that responsibility by repeatedly having the responsibility for
participating in goal setting and the
devising of therapeutic activities.
Wright (1960) says much the same
thing in writing about the treatment
of the physically disabled:

> The effectiveness of rehabilitation,
> whether it involves physical, vocational or
> emotional adjustment, depends largely
> upon the degree to which the client has
> made the plan his own. Barring special
> circumstances, this effort on the part of
> the client in the long run is enhanced
> when he takes an active part in the de-
> cision making; it is often weakened when
> he feels that his life is being manipulated
> behind the scenes. (p. 345)

Wright wisely mentions "special circumstances." There are times, of
course, when the therapist must dominate the goal setting, clarify the subgoals, relate them to the end goals,
provide a choice of activities, revise
unrealistic aspiration levels, restruc-
ture the activity so that it will not demand too much effort or so that it
can be objectively reported. But always he keeps in mind the require-
ment that the stutterer should participate in the design of his treatment,
and progressively increases his responsibility for goal setting.

The stutterer always seems to have
more motivation when he participates
in the structuring of these subgoals.
For example, in a hypothetical planning session the stutterer and his therapist might be engaged in planning
an activity for each of these subgoals:

1. to enter difficult speaking situations;
2. to devise a self-assignment which will
   reduce his tendency to use subvocal
   self-derogation;
3. to increase his ability to verbalize emotion;

4. to give fluently spoken words some
   stimulus value;
5. to increase his talking time;
6. to weaken the eye closing behavior just
   prior to the release from blockage.

In the discussion during this planning session, opportunity is always
present for ventilation of feelings, for
scrutiny of the self-concept, for examination of aspiration and probable performance levels, and many other similar items. Prediction of probable reactions during the actual performance
of these tasks is discussed along with
their pertinence to the long-range goal
of fluency and personal adequacy.
Provision is made for objective reporting of performance and the feelings experienced. The tasks are so
structured that maximum and minimum achievement criteria are specified. This brief glimpse of the therapeutic process should show not only
that such interaction can be highly
motivating but also that the therapy is
far from superficial. Few stutterers can
undergo such a regime day after day
without making marked progress and
this too is motivating. Moreover, dependence upon therapist reinforcement by way of his approvals is not
so important when the stutterer can
bestow his own rewards.

Again we wish to stress that successful stuttering therapy must be a
joint endeavor of both therapist and
client. It is an interaction, not an injection with the syringe held in the
hands of the clinician. Both must participate actively. No therapist is om-
niscient; he needs the information
that can be provided by the case. We
view therapy as a cooperative process, always. We do not believe in the
clinical philosophy that "You are the
patient. I am the therapist. You are
sick. I am not—and let's not forget
it." If we leave the stutterer out of the

planning, we ask for passivity and non-responsibility. When we include him in goal setting, in the decision process, we mobilize latent motivation which otherwise would remain completely hidden.

Reinforcement

We must not forget that there is more to motivation than goal setting. No one learns or unlearns any behavior unless he profits from that learning. With great drive, the necessity for immediate or complete relief from the impelling tensions can be deferred. To some extent, the very act of working for the ultimate goal becomes invested with goal attractiveness. Positive movement toward a goal is rewarding in itself. Nevertheless, anyone who has had to work with stutterers during prolonged therapy will recognize the need for creating accessory ways of reinforcing them immediately for progress toward that goal. The skill of the therapist lies largely in his ability to handle reinforcement. Since he must weaken and extinguish certain responses and shape and condition others, his ultimate success/failure ratio will be determined by his manipulation of contingencies.

Available reinforcers

Much psychological research (Mandler and Kaplan, 1956) has demonstrated that human beings differ greatly from one another in how responsive they are to different reinforcing stimuli and even to the same stimuli. This is especially true of verbal stimuli. To cite but one instance, Spielberger, Levin, and Shepard (1962) interrogated their subjects at the end of their operant learning experiment, asking them the crucial question:

"Would you say that you wanted me to say 'good'?" Those who replied that they wanted very much to have this sort of reinforcement learned much faster than those who were less desirous. Such experimental verification of what seems only too obvious (though it is often forgotten by operant conditioners and therapists alike) points up our need to scrutinize the kinds of reinforcements we use. They may not be as reinforcing as we think.

As we have said earlier, the major reinforcer used in therapy has always been the therapist's approval. Its reinforcing value, however, depends upon the degree to which the therapist's presence and interaction satisfied the stutterer's current needs, and also upon the stutterer's past experience with similar approvals. We have known stutterers who reacted violently against any hint of verbal approval but who, at the same time, would work hard to gain an approving nod or smile. They had been enslaved by parental approvals or they had experienced verbal approval along with covert rejection. And we have known other stutterers for whom the only effective reinforcement that we could mobilize was escape from punishment. However, most of our cases came to prize our approvals once they found that we could satisfy their need for companionship or serve as a nonpunitive listener or could relieve their anxiety and other tension states. But we could not arrogantly assume that our approbation was valuable in itself. We had to earn its value as a reinforcing token.

The need to please the therapist presents other difficulties. Very useful in the initial stages of treatment, it can become an obstacle in later ones. If the stutterer is ever to maintain his gains, he cannot hope to do so only in the context of therapist support. The therapist cannot be with him always and forever to dispense the candy of approval. Psychoanalysts have long been aware not only of the importance of transference in effecting basic behavioral change but also of the need to work through it and to be able to operate without it. Our job is to set our clients free from us, not to enslave them. We were appalled once to discover that a male colleague, when therapy was being terminated, had given his female case a locket containing his picture as a reminder "to keep working on her speech." Doubtless too much countertransference had taken place and he had forgotten that the therapist's role should be that of a catalyst. Such procedures have only temporary and minimal effectiveness at best, and at worst they doom the client to eternal dependency and failure.

Self-Reinforcement

Since we are always highly aware of the dangers inherent in a "pleasing the therapist" kind of motivation, as soon as we can, we seek to make the transfer from therapist approval to self-approval. Some of this transfer will happen anyway as the client internalizes and generalizes the approving statements of the clinician but we have also been able to aid the shift. One way of doing this is to encourage verbalized self-statements of approval when the stutterer is away from the therapy room. Here is one stutterer's report in this connection:

I had nine times today when I congratulated myself out loud for doing something that I felt was pretty good. I think it's better when I say it out loud than when I just think it. For example, I went up to my instructor after chemistry class today and asked him a question though I was scared silly and had some

hard blocks. But I went to the bathroom right afterwards and told myself aloud that I really had faced my fears for once and had done what I ought to have done. I felt pretty proud and it was good to hear me say so.

Another is to use Premack's Principle which, expressed crudely, is that for any pair of responses, the more probable one will reinforce the less probable one. For example, if a rat dislikes running but likes eating, we can soon teach him to like running by following it with a chance to eat, and after sufficient pairing, the rat will do other things just so he can have a chance to run. In our therapy with stutterers, we train them to defer pleasant activities until after they have done things for which they can verbalize self-approval. Here is one short account:

This morning when I was lying in bed before I got up I told myself I wasn't going to eat any breakfast at all until I had been able to stutter without my head jerk on at least three words. It took me two hours and six people before I ate and I bought ham and eggs and sure had a good meal but it was even better to know that I had finally been able to keep that head from jumping around. Don't think I could have done it though if I hadn't kept getting hungrier all the time.

By learning to reward himself, the stutterer becomes less dependent upon the therapist's approval. What happens finally is that he does what he should do to make therapeutic progress because his own self-approval becomes valuable.

Approval for what

Whether the therapist or the stutterer does the approving, it is essential that it be contingent upon therapeutic *progress* and not just upon any single performance. This very vital principle should govern all therapy and it is often violated. We have seen student therapists reward performances that reflected no progress at all, even those which clearly showed regression. This is folly. "But he at least tried, didn't he?" they protest when we bring this to their attention. "Of course he made a half-hearted attempt," we answer, "and, at the beginning of therapy, such a token attempt might very well have deserved the payoff of your warm smile and nod. But as you know and he knows, he has come a long way from that early beginning. Where is he now? How far has he come on the route that leads to effective communication? What does he have to do now to move further toward his goal? Perhaps he's lost sight of the landmarks that lead to the end goal. Perhaps he needs to have it more clearly defined but, more probably, he is just testing you to see if your approval is worth working for."

Much of the real work of the clinician is spent in definition and discrimination, in the clarification of the meaningfulness of anticipatory-goal activities. We cannot expect the stutterer at first to see that he has made any real progress when he stutters with open eyes rather than clenching them shut. Indeed, according to his scale of values, the view he then gets of the listener's impatience may be painful. Unless we can help him identify this eye opening as progress toward the end goal, he will have no motivation toward revising this stuttering behavior. If the therapist rewards only fluent speech and punishes moments of stuttering, any instance in which the stutterer does manage to open his eyes during his struggling will get no reinforcement at all. If, on the other hand, the stutterer realizes that ther-

apist and self-approval comes, not just because he opened his eyes, but because opening his eyes indicates further progress in reducing his handicap, the contingent approval will enhance that progress.

In many ways, our therapy is a shaping process. The stutterer's perceptions of his own behavior tend to be shaped to coincide with those of his clinician and it is here that the role of the latter's reinforcement is of immense importance. Presumably, the clinician, if he is competent, knows the direction of the route to be traversed or he shouldn't be a clinician. Somewhere in the crannies of his head there must be that map. The stutterer comes without this knowledge and must acquire it. He certainly comes without any ability to evaluate goal progress. To him, there are only two alternatives: to stutter and not to stutter, with the first being evil and the second being good. Conditioned as he is, and being so vulnerable to stress, any other alternatives are not open to him or he wouldn't be a stutterer. If the therapist simply rewards fluency and punishes stuttering, even though temporary suppression of the disorder may occur in the safety of the relationship, nothing is gained thereby, the stutterer still having the same two alternatives and no other choice. In our therapy, we present a third alternative, one that can serve as a true option: the ability to stutter differently and less abnormally. It is the therapist's job to program reinforcement so that the kind of stuttering shown becomes cumulatively less abnormal and less frustrating. In short, what the therapist does is to help the stutterer know when he is modifying his behaviors in a direction that means progress. As a result of the therapist's reinforcement, the stutterer's perceptions of his stuttering behaviors become more and more like the former's and so too do his evaluations. Reinforcement should be given for progress.

Other positive reinforcers

Besides the social reinforcement provided by the therapist or other stutterers in the therapy group, we have experimented with a variety of other reinforcers and incentives including the use of tokens. Tokens have been widely used as motivating devices in many learning experiments and they have some remarkable advantages. They can be given immediately; they can be saved; they are easily administered; they resemble the currency rewards of our monetary-centered culture; they can be exchanged for a wide variety of rewards and permit the subject to choose those which are most attractive to him. Once, for a month, we created a token economy in our clinic for stutterers. Each day we gave the stutterers cards resembling meal tickets which could be punched variously for different achievments. All successfully performed therapeutic tasks earned points; some achievements more than others; and each stutterer had his own individually tailored set of tasks with their values. One stutterer, for example, got three points for making a phone call to a store; five points for making one to a strange residence and asking for himself; ten points for a job interview, and so on. He could earn fifteen points for speaking before a college class if he managed to do so without any avoidance. Each successful cancellation was worth one point; each good pull-out two points. Other stutterers had other activities and other values for the points accumulated. For two hundred points, the stutterer could choose among (1) the phone number

of a girl who would accept a blind date with a stutterer; (2) a free ticket to a movie; (3) all the beer he could drink. Five hundred points when earned in a single day entitled the stutterer to a weekend trip with the therapist to his forest cabin. While the stutterers responded enthusiastically to the program and made rapid advances under these incentives, its management became increasingly laborious and it possessed a fundamental disadvantage which made us finally discard it. Token reinforcers have some use in establishing new responses but they are not very good at maintaining them. Their value is artificially inflated; they have no value in the real world. The learning they motivate rarely persists very long. Social reinforcers work better. The therapist's approval for example can transfer into self-approval and this is the kind of positive reinforcement that is most useful. Nevertheless we have occasionally continued to use token reinforcement in special circumstances.

We have employed many other kinds of positive reinforcers, even those related to the primary drives. For example,

In the morning, Don was always starved. He would fix himself a good breakfast and then bring it into my study. I would then set up a bit of behavior to be rewarded by one small bite of egg or toast or one sip of coffee or orange juice. Often the food got cold before it was eaten and sometimes the conference period ended with much of it untouched. As he gradually became more successful, however, we set up small quotas which had to be achieved before he took food. By this approximation to operant therapy (or a therapeutic infantile feeding situation, etc.), we attacked his eye closing, jaw jerks, abnormal mouth postures, tongue protrusions, the "um-but" starters, and many other of the instrumental responses which formed so large a part of his abnormality. Significantly, we did not apply it to the tremors themselves. Occasionally, I would eat my breakfast with Don, and he could deprive me of a bit or sip by being able to say a word, phrase, or sentence without demonstrating certain of these reactions even though stuttering occurred. He enjoyed those sessions. (Van Riper, 1968, p. 106)

We hope we have not left the impression that such extrinsic reinforcers are our preferred answer to the motivation problem. When the therapist serves as a feedback mechanism and provides evidence of progress toward the goal, that awareness of progress in itself is reinforcing. Also, the opportunity to speak, to communicate without fear of punishment is probably one of the most attractive incentives any stutterer can have. The permissive therapist's open ear is better than any M and M candy. By occasionally making it available but contingent upon successful performance of a task, our stutterers worked very hard at their learning tasks. Stutterers want, above all else, to be able to talk.

Always it is necessary to determine the kinds of reinforcers each stutterer seemed to find desirable. We have always had to try a variety of them before we knew. For example, with some very hostile stutterers, the opportunity to penalize the therapist seemed to be more highly motivating than any other reinforcer we employed. The important thing was to get them moving and to keep them progressing but in retrospect we wonder if our dedication had a bit of masochism in it. Nevertheless they improved. Here are two accounts which illustrate the variety of reinforcement strategies we have used:

We had a gangling freshman, weak and immature, with an incredible variety of avoidance tricks, who seemed unable to make a real attempt on any feared word but had to postpone and filibuster until the pain of his long wait exceeded his fear of being unable to utter the word if he did try. Tremors traumatized him. He was also aware of his expectancy of rejection. At the time we had a student therapist, a senior girl who had no objection to kissing boys in the interest of scientific research. We enlisted her aid. The stutterer and this student therapist were placed before a mirror and he was required to read some isolated words which he feared. For every three words on which he stuttered but did not avoid or postpone, she kissed him gaily and enthusiastically. After three or four of these very vivid experiences, he was unable to stutter. We then used consecutive material, which procured a few more kisses before the stuttering disappeared. Then the stutterer made some phone calls. The boy went back to his dormitory exhausted but with his first free speech for years. He was back the next day seeking for more and avoiding as usual, but the experiment was over. He reported, however, that stuttering was never so feared again, and he was later able to do considerably more therapy than previously. . . . (Van Riper, 1958, pp. 338–39)

One of our stutterers was a very negative 13-year-old, big for his age and full of hostility. He hated his stuttering, his listener, himself, his parents, and especially this therapist who was trying to help him. He had very few avoidance tricks and few word or phonetic fears, though he was fearful of certain situations. He characteristically blundered into tremors of the lips and jaw, increased his tension tremendously, then attempted to jaw-jerk his way out of them. He was full of frustration. Unable to establish any real rapport with him, we took him into the laboratory, gave him a strong electric shock, then told him he could fasten us onto the coil and give us a stronger shock for every five stutterings he could collect in oral reading. He collected his five in a hurry, pushed up the coil, and shoved on the juice, whereupon we jumped and screamed though we actually had broken the circuit with an unethical foot. He loved it. We saw him smile for the first time, the little stinker. And he returned enthusiastically to his reading. We had to jump twice more before his stuttering disappeared, but it did so quite thoroughly. We continued this for several days with marked transfer into his ordinary communication. When he stuttered he would tend to smile slightly in memoriam. Then he discovered the cut-off switch. (Van Riper, 1958, p. 339)

Our discussion of positive reinforcement should not fail to include some mention of the principle of embedding, a technique well known to parents and to therapists of all persuasions. By incorporating the therapeutic task as part of a highly desired activity, it is more likely to be performed than if it is not. Thus with a stutterer in his early teens we found that by having him verbalize continually and putting short easy prolongations into his speech while he was learning to drive our automobile, and refusing to let him take the wheel unless he did, he was motivated to do so.

Negative reinforcement

One of the stutterer's strongest drives is to escape from communicative unpleasantness. The *escape* from punishment has dominated the adult stutterer's life for many years. He has constantly scrutinized approaching communicative situations and words and the sounds of those words for signs of danger. He has devised strategies of incredible complexity to cope with them so he will not suffer penalty. When caught in the throes of his oscillations and fixations, he has similarly sought escape. Indeed the great bulk of the stutterer's abnormality consists of avoidance and escape behavior. It is only natural, therefore,

that negative reinforcement, which by definition consists of the escape from punishment, should prove to be a powerful therapeutic tool if used wisely.

While the increasing relief from fear, frustration, and penalty gained by the stutterer as he proceeds through therapy is probably the main way by which negative reinforcement has its impact, it is also possible for the therapist to devise special activities and experiences which also exploit its power. For example, if we are attempting to extinguish a tongue protrusion, we might tell the stutterer that he must read aloud to some listener for an unpleasantly long time—say 60 minutes —but for every time he stutters *without protruding his tongue* he can deduct five minutes from that long hour. Or, if we are attempting to weaken his use of an anticipatory "ah-ah-ah" postponement behavior, we could even have him stand on one leg until he has collected a certain quota of stutterings in which no such postponement behavior occurred. We have used noxious sounds, electric shocks, boring perseverative motor activities, and a host of other contrived punishments so that escape from them was contingent upon successful performance of a specified therapeutic task. Again, let us emphasize that the purpose of these assignments was always discussed and that they were jointly devised by both the therapist and the stutterer. At times, we too have shared the punishing activity, taking the shock jointly with the stutterer, standing on one leg, or doing the interminable oral reading together. Occasionally we have begged for the relief that both of us could get only when the stutterer does what is required. Such an experience can clearly illuminate the basic therapeutic relationship. However we do it, the use of negative reinforcement is one of the most powerful tools in what Robert West liked to call the therapist's armamentarium.

Punishment

In our therapy, we use punishment very rarely and then only with great discretion—never when we feel the flicker of personal irritation at the stutterer's refractoriness or resistance. Our feeling is that the stutterer has been punished enough. All his life he has been punished—not only by others but by himself. The penalties with their resultant anger, shame, and embarrassment reactions have flowed into an internal pool of guilt that sloshes continually within his skin. We do not want to add to that pool. No, not even when he hands us the whip and invites us to the flagellation! Indeed much of our effort has been devoted to reducing the invisible self-beating which characterizes many confirmed stutterers. We have never forgotten what C. S. Bleumel told us once when we asked him how, late in life, he had been able to "cure" himself of his stuttering. "I changed in two ways," he said. "First, I learned to be kind to myself and second, I learned that I was responsible for what my mouth did." If stutterers have a punitive therapist, they find it very hard to be kind to themselves.

There is much that we do not know about punishment though the psychologists have been investigating it for many years. It is not the direct antithesis of reward as many think it to be. It often (but not always) does seem to be able to suppress a response especially if that response is weak. Punishment can temporarily decrease response rate and amplitude but that it usually has very little lasting effect has been shown by many studies except when counterconditioning of an antagonistic response also concurrently takes place. Punishment does not weaken strong habitual behaviors; it merely buries them for the moment.

Nevertheless there have been times when we have found it advantageous to program some punishment into our therapy. For example, it has served us as an alerting device. When we reach the point in therapy in which we attempt to teach our stutterers to substitute a more normal preparatory set instead of the usual covert rehearsal of blind anticipatory struggle, we find some stutterers so compulsive that they cannot scan ahead for such an opportunity. They blunder headlong from one blocking to another, doing nothing to accept the opportunities presented for modifying their stuttering behaviors. We have found punishment useful with these individuals primarily because the expectancy which results therefrom can be changed. It is not the punishment but the *threat* of punishment for one behavior, when another more adapting behavior is available, that enables these stutterers to exert some choice. Since the compulsivity resulting from old stereotyped, overlearned sets can often be terrifically strong, the threat of punishment has some utility in such an instance. Moreover, we have considerable evidence that calling attention to stuttering (in the adult at least) seems to decrease its frequency as Wingate (1959) and others have demonstrated. The threat of punishment can serve very well as such an alerter. Since awareness of the behavior to be modified is often dependent upon this expectancy, contingent punishment accordingly can give the stutterer a chance to do that modifying. We can provide that chance when he has available not just one old response but two competing responses (an old and a new one) to the same set of stimuli and one can be punished as the other is rewarded. Usually we have tried to confine our use of punishment to such counterconditioning procedures.

Even in this context we are careful to make sure that the stutterer realizes that it is not he who is being punished but a specific bit of behavior. This convincing can take some doing! We always take the utmost pains to help him understand the rationale behind its use. Sometimes, despite all our efforts, we do not succeed and then we lose more than we gain. It does not seem appropriate to jeopardize the basic relationship between therapist and case merely to get the bit of extra motivation that punishment can provide. There usually are other tools which can be used. Nevertheless, as we have said, there are times when punishment can help us and these opportunities usually involve counterconditioning.

Perhaps the most effective punishments to use in suppressing certain behaviors are those which have always been especially noxious to the stutterer: silence, listener loss, the necessity to repeat what has already been spoken, time-outs to block further communication. To illustrate: Recently we were having great difficulty trying to get a stutterer to assume a lip closure posture in starting words beginning with bilabials. Always he would open his mouth very widely agape then suddenly snap it shut repeatedly. All other attempts to weaken this compulsive behavior had failed. Finally we told the stutterer that whenever he showed this wide mouth opening on a word beginning with p, b, or m, we would shut our eyes and cover our ears for 30 seconds whereas *no matter how long he stuttered on these words but kept his lips closed* we would give

him our full and undivided attention. We enlisted his wife and 16-year-old daughter in the same program and within three days this particular behavior which always had been the most grotesque and abnormal of all his stuttering features had disappeared.

Ordinarily we prefer to use penalties that are less drastic, more token than real, those which have little hurt in them. They then serve as alerting devices and are primarily intended to help the stutterer become highly aware of his approaching stuttering moments as opportunities for modification. More forfeit then punishment! We try to invent penalties that have a bit of bizarre humor in them. For example, to eliminate a compulsive rhythmic lip popping, we required one stutterer to observe a goldfish in a bowl for 15 minutes whenever he stuttered five times using these abnormal movements. Anyone who has watched the mouths of goldfish will understand. At this point we feel some temptation to provide other examples but feel it wiser to leave them to the reader's imagination lest they be applied inappropriately and without discrimination. If we use punishment with a stutterer, let us use due care. He has had enough.

We do not wish to end this chapter with the discussion of reinforcers and punishers lest we give the impression that motivation should be viewed simply in terms of conditioning. Many of the most vital problems to be met in therapy seem to us to require structuring in terms of cognitive learning theory. To cite just one example, successful therapy often requires the creation of plans, strategies, and hypotheses related to problem solving. As these are formulated, tested, and accomplished, the stutterer's motivation increases quite apart from any external contingent reinforcement. Self-actualization, the fulfillment of one's potential, is itself immensely rewarding as the existential psychologists and philosophers have proposed. When the stutterer, so long inhibited and constrained, finds himself expanding his activities into ever widening areas of functioning, he discovers the age old truth that growth is very, very good.

With respect to motivating stutterers in therapy we have known some excellent therapists and some poor ones. Somehow the difference seemed to lie in the former's ability to get the stutterer involved in the design of therapy as well as in its performance. As George Shames (1970) writes, "The idea that stuttering can be manipulated in part by the consequences provided by the therapist may help the clinician to organize his therapy, and may even suggest specific clinical techniques. But, with these sound principles tucked away close by and available for application, sound clinical judgment is still the rule for clinicians (p. 34)." But there is always something more than reinforcement and judgment. Perhaps it is found in the wise words of Zaddick (Kopp, 1969), words which the author of this text keeps before him on his desk:

Certainly, as therapists we may advise, teach, interpret, support, offer models, selectively reinforce, and undo with counter-strategies. But if all of this occurs outside the context of genuine personal engagement, in the absence of loving, then all we do is teach new games, perhaps more effective games, but games nevertheless.

We have tried to present some of the principles of motivation in this chapter but we know deep down that some of their essence has escaped us. Somehow we blow the trumpet that sends the stutterer forward into the battle

for his freedom and somehow we get him to blow it himself. Faith is said to move mountains but it is the therapist's dedicated care and concern, if not love, that moves stutterers.

Bibliography

Barbara, D. A., *Stuttering: A Psychodynamic Approach to Its Understanding.* New York: Julian Press, 1954.

Buchwald, A. M. and R. D. Young, Some comments on the foundations of behavior therapy, in C. M. Franks (ed.), *Behavior Therapy: Appraisal and Status.* New York: McGraw-Hill, 1969, pp. 607–24.

Cautela, J. R. and R. A. Kastenbaum, A reinforcement survey schedule for use in therapy, training and research, *Psychological Reports,* 20 (1967), 1115–30.

Halfond, M. M., Patient-oriented goals in speech therapy, *De Therapia Vocis et Loquellae,* 1 (1965), 291–93.

Hollis, F., *Casework: A Psychosocial Therapy.* New York: Random House, 1964.

Ingham, R. J. and G. Andrews, A description of a token economy in an adult therapy program. Convention Paper, A.S.H.A., Chicago, 1971.

Klencke, H., *Die Heilung des Stotterns.* Leipsig: Ernest Keil, 1862.

Kopp, S., Zaddik, *Psychology Today,* 2 (1969), 26–37.

Mandler, G. and W. K. Kaplan, Subjective evaluation and reinforcing effects of a verbal stimulus, *Science,* 124 (1956), 582–83.

Shames, G. H., D. B. Egolf, and R. C. Rhodes, Experimental programs in stuttering therapy, *Journal of Speech and Hearing Disorders,* 34 (1969), 34–37.

Shames, G. W., Operant conditioning and therapy for stuttering, in C. W. Starkweather (ed.), *Conditioning in Stuttering Therapy.* Memphis: Speech Foundation of America, 1970.

SHEEHAN, J. G., *Stuttering: Research and Therapy*. New York: Harper & Row, 1970.

SMITH, H. C., *Sensitivity to People*. New York: McGraw-Hill, 1966.

SPIELBERGER, C. D., S. M. LEVIN, and M. C. SHEPARD, The effects of awareness and attitude toward the reinforcement of the operant conditioning of verbal behavior, *Journal of Personality*, 30 (1962), 106–21.

VAN RIPER, C., Dave: A clinical success, in H. Luper (ed.), *Stuttering: Suc-cesses and Failures in Therapy*. Memphis: Speech Foundation of America, 1968.

VAN RIPER, C., Experiments in stuttering therapy, in J. Eisenson (ed.), *Stuttering: A Symposium*. New York: Harper & Row, 1958.

WINGATE, M. E., Calling attention to stuttering, *Journal of Speech and Hearing Research*, 2 (1959), 336–35.

WRIGHT, B. A., *Physical Disability: A Psychological Approach*. New York: Harper & Row, 1960.

Identification

Since it is our view that the great bulk of stuttering consists of learned responses to the experience or anticipation of broken fluency, it follows that our therapy is designed to unlearn these responses or to modify and shape them in such a way as to facilitate ongoing speech. Moreover, we regard the inadequate personality characteristics of the stutterer as also having been learned. Since we consider them to be consequences of the communicative interruptions as evaluated by the significant persons with whom the stutterer has interacted, our task is again to extinguish and replace these through new learning experiences. The therapeutic situation creates the opportunity for this learning. Stuttering therapy involves unlearning, relearning, and new learning.

Identification

We begin our therapy by training the stutterer to identify the overt and covert behaviors that constitute his disorder. We have experimented with many different initial approaches to treatment and beginning in this way has resulted in our greatest successes. There seem to be many reasons for starting with identification activities. They present an opportunity for establishing the basic therapist-client co-worker relationship. They specify the therapeutic problem in terms of what must be unlearned. They immediately place upon the stutterer the responsibility for doing something about his stuttering, namely, to explore it analytically so as to define its components. By collecting examples of these component behaviors, not only in the clinic but outside it, we prevent the insularity that impedes generalization. By starting with identification, we avoid placing too much demand upon our cases for immediate modification. To ask a stutterer to begin immediately to change the way he stutters is to ask for failure, if only because he rarely knows how he stutters. Instead, when we ask him to scrutinize what he does when he says he's stuttering and to seek out opportunities to stutter so he can find out, we strengthen the approach gradient immediately. What is probably of greatest value is that, in this collecting and analyzing process, the stutterer soon discerns that the therapist does not reject or punish his stuttering but instead welcomes it as necessary for its analytical confrontation. Identification aids desensitization. There are many other reasons which we shall spell out later. Here let us say merely that by beginning in this way, we solve many of the problems that usually arise in the first few days of therapy.

One of the curious features in the stutterer's perception of his stuttering is his tendency to lump together a host of disparate behaviors ranging all the way from nose wrinkling to saying "ah-ah-ah" and to call that lump stuttering. When you ask him what he did, he will merely tell you that he stuttered. Moreover, he rarely recognizes what he does, perhaps because that recognition would be too painful or perhaps because the accompanying emotional upheaval prevents the discrimination. Without training, the stutterer cannot duplicate, even immediately afterward, the abnormality that he has demonstrated. Sadly, clinicians and researchers alike regard stuttering in the same way. They speak of moments of stuttering or stuttered words. They count these words

or moments. They use them in operant conditioning although one set of stuttering behaviors may be as different from another set as apples and onions. The component behaviors shown on different words may serve completely different purposes. Even on the same stuttered word, the stutterer may use a bit of vocalization such as a prolonged "ah" as a strategy for postponing the actual moment of utterance or as a timing device for initiating vocalization or for other reasons. How does he stutter? This is the basic question that must be answered if we are to change that "stuttering" or extinguish the individual responses that comprise it. Surely we should begin by seeking its answer.[1]

Although it is possible to change certain behaviors through contingent reinforcement without the subject's awareness that this is being done, learning proceeds much more swiftly when the learner knows and cooperates in the learning process. Certainly, the experimenter or therapist must specify for himself the responses to be altered or extinguished if he is to schedule reinforcements or punishments appropriately. Since we view therapy with the adult stutterer as usually necessitating a co-therapist approach, with the therapist and the

---

[1] Brutten and Shoemaker (1967) have strongly advocated this point of view, claiming that using the term "moment of stuttering" covers up basic differences in the constituent behaviors of that moment, specifically the differences between operant and respondent behaviors. Lohr (1969), Webster (1968a), and Zenner (1971), using motion pictures, all showed the wide variety of behaviors that tend to be masked by the labels "moment of stuttering" or "stuttered words." Not only do some of these different behaviors seem to serve different functions; they also show different effects when punished (Webster, 1968b).

client both participating in its programming, the earliest and most continuing of therapeutic activities consists of confronting and specifying the behaviors to be changed. The stutterer must become aware of what he does when he is stuttering.

But is not this awareness already too morbid in the stutterer? Are there no dangers of increasing an already undue concern about his disfluency? In the beginning stutterer we seek to prevent his attention from focusing on broken sounds and words. Why then in the confirmed stutterer do we ask him to scrutinize his actual stuttering behaviors?

We have several answers to these questions. First of all, in the advanced stutterer who has long been keenly aware of his speech difficulty, who has learned to anticipate and react to it, our clinical attention to its details will add very little increment to its total unpleasantness. Secondly, we must combat the defense mechanism of denial. If one has a problem (and stuttering is a problem, not a mysterious curse) it is better to face it. Thirdly, the sort of awareness which the stutterer does possess is often chaotic and undifferentiated. All he senses is that he has "got blocked" or that a storm of emotion has swept over him. He does not recognize and cannot analyze the specific component behavior which characterized that particular episode of stuttering. If we hope to get him to modify his stuttering behaviors he must be able to discriminate them. Moreover, the identification process provides an excellent opportunity for desensitization. Since our aim is also to reduce the attendant emotionality, the analytical examination of the displayed behavior *in the context of the therapist's genuine interest and freedom from punitiveness* reduces anxiety. For once, the experience that he has always avoided is sought and desired. The untouchable can be touched.

But there is something more. By beginning in this way, we immediately structure therapy as a conjoint process. The stutterer is immediately given the responsbility for participating actively in his treatment. It is he who must collect the various kinds of stuttering behaviors that comprise his disorder and bring them to us so that we can help him recognize their features and the purposes they serve. Often the sample of stuttering that we find in the therapy room is far different from that which characterizes his performance under the stress of outside communication. Only the stutterer can provide this information and to do so he must accept some responsibility for the identification and analysis when we are absent. This immediate delegation of responsibility counteracts the passivity that stutterers often show at the beginning of treatment. "Help me, O wise one!" they silently beg. "Do thy will unto me! I am clay in thy hands. Savior, heal me!" While we can understand why they feel that way, we will not be seduced into assuming any magical role. "There is work to do," we tell him. "You, the stutterer, must do much of it. Let us begin. Here is where we begin. Your job is to stutter and to find out exactly what you do when you stutter and why you do it. Not only here in the clinic where I can observe but everywhere! Bring me your stutterings and the feelings that accompany them so that we can clearly know what we must change."

Identification procedures

"First catch your fish," advised Isaac Walton. If we are to analyze the stuttering behaviors so that we can start programming our learning and un-learning schedules, it is first necessary to capture and to hold them long enough to study them. This then is one of our earliest subgoals: to collect specimens of stuttering behaviors. But we do not only collect. We also catalogue the fauna and flora of stuttering always seeking to find commonalities in the variety, discovering, for example, that the anticipatory interjection of "ah" or the compulsive clearing of the throat or the licking of the lips all belong to a species we might call postponement behaviors included in the genus of avoidance. This designation of categories of stuttering behaviors is not schematic. These categories reflect the dynamics of the stutter's ways of coping with his problem. Some workers prefer to stick to the observable behaviors and to ignore the purposes served by the stutterer's coping reactions. We do not. We consider verbalizations as observable behavior. Too many stutterers have told us why they do what they do, that they pause before a feared word to postpone the abnormality and frustration they expect to experience if they say it, that they jerk their jaw, or gasp, to try to release themselves from a tremorous closure of the lips, that they time the moment of speech attempt with an arm movement so that they can finally get started, that they use a synonym so that they will avoid stuttering on the word it replaces. Most of the stutterer's component behaviors originated in purposeful activities. They helped him; they minimized his difficulties. To ignore the payoff they still may produce seems to us to be unwise. The stutterer needs to know not only what he does but why he does it.

Furthermore, the process of identifying and analyzing the stuttering behaviors inevitably leads to the revelation of the feelings that the stutterer has about his disorder and himself. Storms of emotion occasionally arise. These too can be identified and accepted and the part they play in the problem can be ascertained. Moreover, in the permissive atmosphere of the therapy session, they lose some of the strength they have acquired.

We have discovered that this collecting and classifying process is anxiety-reducing in itself. It decreases avoidance because to collect stuttering samples one must seek them. Through their confrontation and analysis the mystery begins to diminish. When the stutterer demonstrates these behaviors to the therapist or they both listen to them on tapes or watch them on the video-screen, these stutterings are re-experienced with little or no unpleasantness, a process which is fundamental to desensitization and extinction. We have tried many different ways of beginning therapy but this approach seems to have been most effective. It makes no exorbitant demands upon the stutterer. He needs only to stutter. It creates the kind of interaction between stutterer and therapist which permits testing of the latter's competence and commitment. It displays and defines the problem.

The hierarchy of identification therapy

In exploring methods for helping the stutterer to begin his collecting and cataloguing of stuttering behaviors, we found it necessary to provide some guidance. Left to his own initiative, he tended to concentrate his attention on those that were most abnormal and when this occurred, he soon found the experience too traumatic. Accordingly, after some trial and error we finally devised a sequence that has usually been quite satisfactory. By getting the stutterer first to identify his fluently spoken words, we present the easiest and most palatable of all the tasks he will encounter. Usually he is surprised to find how much fluency he possesses and his morbid misconception that he cannot speak fluently is exposed as erroneous. Next we ask him to identify those short, easy stutterings which serve as our temporary primary target and which already exist unrecognized in his speech. When he can do so consistently and without negative emotion, we proceed to the next step on our hierarchy, the collection, confrontation, and analysis of avoidance behaviors. When these can be identified with some objectivity and calmness, we do the same for the postponement, timing, verbal cues precipitating expectancy of stuttering, and all of the other items in the hierarchic sequence. Again let us emphasize that in this beginning stage of therapy we do not ask the stutterer to eliminate or to modify these behaviors. His role is that of a collector and cataloguer, not corrector or extinguisher. We want to know and we want him to know what he does when he says he stutters. We are defining the learning problem.

Identifying the target behaviors—the fluent stutterings

Every stutterer, no matter how severe, will occasionally emit a word in which the amount of temporal alteration is minimal. Perhaps the first sound or the vowel is slightly prolonged, or the transition is elongated, or an easy unforced single syllabic repetition is exhibited, but no avoidance, recoil, or struggle behaviors are present. These tiny stutterings do not interrupt the forward flow of speech and

certainly they are not sufficiently noticeable to evoke either frustration or listener penalty. Stutterings come in all sizes and shapes. Some are long, some are short. Some are grotesquely abnormal, some are not. It is difficult for some of our cases to recognize this variation at first or to accept our definition of these little distortions of sound sequencing as belonging to the stuttering category. We do not argue. We merely fill our own speech so full of them that their presence is unmistakable and we point out those we hear and see in the stutterer's speech as the kind of stuttering he can learn to use someday instead of the unpleasant kind he now exhibits all too frequently. He doubts us of course and we accept his doubt but we still hold that there are many ways of stuttering, that there are some that are better than others, and that it is possible to stutter without impairing fluency or incurring listener penalty. If the stutterer can learn this, he will not have to fear communicating.

Usually at first the stutterers are unaware of these little abnormal stutterings until they listen to them on recordings or see them on video tape or have the therapist insert his imitation of them into his own speech. Sometimes they first must recognize them in the speech of other stutterers. As soon as our cases become able to identify these consistently in the clinic we send them out hunting for them in other speaking situations, writing down the words on which these fluent stutterings occur and then practicing them retrospectively so that they can demonstrate them to us at the next therapy session. This assignment usually has great impact. It also puts the goal model right in their mouths; they taste the eventual reward at the very beginning of the therapeutic maze. We reward them with our approval and ask them to visualize how they will feel when all of their stutterings are of this sort. "If I could stutter like that all the time, which I can't, at least now, I wouldn't be afraid to stutter. I could say anything." This is a typical comment. It has been interesting to observe how such a project immediately begins to alter the old malattitudes. Instead of attending to the worst of their speech abnormalities as they usually do, instead of reliving over and over again their abnormality, frustration, and shame, the stutterers begin to adopt an exploratory objective set. The morbidity starts to subside.

We have seen a few rare stutterers who immediately discarded all their old abnormal behaviors after such a project and learned this new easy variety of stuttering in only a few weeks, then became completely fluent and remained so. We suspect that these individuals are those who respond favorably to any treatment involving suggestion. They are probably the ones that any quack can cure. Most of our cases have profited greatly from this task but we know well that therapy has just begun. We hope only that the stutterers will start to examine and confront their stuttering behavior, that they will come to realize that it is possible to stutter in many ways and that some of the latter may interfere very little with communication. Even for those who seem to be able to collect only a very few of these short fluent stutterings, such a project is useful for it clarifies the goal. It strengthens the approach and decreases the avoidance gradients. It provides opportunity for much discussion between the therapist and stutterer. For example, with one of our very severe stutterers who claimed that he never could collect a single instance of easy stuttering anywhere

(and proceeded to demonstrate that we couldn't find any either in his conversation with us) we used some recorded adaptation readings, in which he had to repeat any word on which he stuttered ten times. As we had expected, great variability occurred on these repeated attempts, and some of them were very short and easy. As we listened to the recording and he heard the latter ones, he finally blurted out: "OK, Yeah, I've had some like those. Why do I hate to admit it? Why do I always have to pump up my horribleness. Maybe, I'm afraid to hope." This led to a discussion which laid bare for the first time some of his basic feelings about self. It proved to be one of those crucial experiences which every therapist treasures.

Identifying avoidance behaviors

As soon as we have made sure that the stutterer has come to recognize these models of fluent stuttering in his speech, we next proceed to help him confront his habitual reactions of avoidance. Again we jointly set this up as a subgoal. We do not ask him at this time to stop avoiding feared words or situations. We ask him merely to start collecting the types of avoidance that he uses. Our aim in this is to help him become aware of his whole repertoire of dodges. These serve as the basic topics of our discussions. He writes down those that occur in other situations; he demonstrates to us how he fled the scene of approaching stuttering, how he substituted an easy word for another one that was feared, how he revised his sentences, etc. We listen to tape recordings; we model the identifying processes ourselves. The stutterer tells us, often at first with some expressed pride in his ingenuity, how he managed to keep a listener from knowing that he was a stutterer, and by so doing, he defines for us and for himself the specific avoidance behaviors which later we will seek to extinguish. We come to recognize those which occur most frequently and those which are strongest. We begin to recognize the cues which evoke them. This is vital information for any therapist.

But also during this period of collection and identification the stutterer suddenly becomes vividly aware of the tremendous burden that this avoidance has imposed upon him. He comes to discern how deviously he lives, how much the threat of stuttering tyrannizes him. The constant necessity to hide, to disguise, to flee—the incredible chore of always having to scan for danger, to be ever alert lest he be exposed for what he is, the sham of the pretense of not being a stutterer, all these suddenly seem to overwhelm him. In our conferences we hear sentences such as these: "Why must I live like this?" "Why must I keep pretending?" "I'm nothing but a damned coward; I've been running away all my life." Though all we have asked him to do is to collect and classify his avoidance behaviors and have rewarded him for so doing, what happens is that the stutterer begins to confront himself on a much deeper level. When he does so, the therapist is understanding and supportive; he encourages the expression of long suppressed feelings; and he helps the stutterer to see that if he can learn to stutter fluently there will be no need to avoid or pretend. We have found repeatedly that, once the stutterer begins to confront these avoidance behaviors and has to report or demonstrate them, they begin to decline in frequency.

There are some stutterers, however, usually the very severe ones, who show little avoidance of feared words, though they still avoid speak-

ing situations. These are the individuals who have found no profit in substituting synonyms because they simply had just as much or more difficulty in uttering the substitute word. Less severe stutterers, those who possess substantial amounts of fluency, are the ones who show the most intricate strategies for reacting to the threat of stuttering by altering words or rephrasing sentences. Some of these persons have become incredibly adept at avoiding and disguising. Not only are they able to fool the usual listener but also the therapist and themselves. Sometimes one can detect the avoidance only by the fact that the utterance seems spoken somewhat strangely. A word or two, a pause, a change in tempo seem slightly askew. Only after the collecting and searching process has been under way for a time do these stutterers begin to recognize these behaviors for what they are. Oral reading before an audience often unmasks these avoidances since the words of the text cannot be altered. When these subtle avoidances shown in conservation are pointed out by the therapist, the stutterer will tend to deny them, arguing convincingly that he had merely shifted his thought. We make a practice never to challenge such argument; we gently accept the explanation but we also show that we watch for them and the stutterer knows it. When he realizes that we are not punishing his avoidances but only seeking to recognize them, he too finds it possible to scrutinize them without defensiveness.

Along with his identification of substitution of synonyms and the aleration of word order, the stutterer usually reports many of the other devices he also uses to bypass and avoid the expected stuttering. He describes how he managed to keep from stuttering by speaking in a different voice or with exaggerated inflections. He may now be able to recognize his use of laughter or anger displays to counteract his fears in the hope of avoiding disfluencies. He tells us how he distracted his audience or himself so that his stutterinrg would not be noticed. There are literally hundreds of these avoidance and disguise strategies, and each stutterer has learned a few of them.

These early experiences in confronting avoidance often evoke emotional outbursts which seem surprisingly disproportionate to the stress of the activity since all the stutterer is doing is collecting samples. However, when we understand the underlying processes involved, his emotionality seems quite reasonable. We must remember that, due to the punishment the stutterer has received in the past for exhibiting his speech difficulties, avoidance has been his basic coping reaction. Must he give it up? He does not really want to avoid but he knows he will and he prefers not to know how much avoiding he does. Most stutterers interpret avoidance as cowardice, thus this confrontation of avoidance behaviors involves the self-concept. Although often, through avoidance, the stutterer can occasionally pass as a normal speaker, even when successful, his use of the tricks reminds him again of his other conflicting self-role—the stutterer. Since he will be meeting this same problem again and again throughout therapy—the reconciliation of the two selves—the therapist will be understanding and accepting when this conflict first shows itself during the identification of avoidance behaviors.

Collecting postponement behaviors

Postponement behaviors should be viewed as a subspecies of avoidances.

Though the stutterer eventually utters the word or enters the situations he fears, he seeks through postponement to avoid the experience of communicative frustration or abnormality by putting it off as long as possible. Moreover, he has discovered that often the delay does seem to prevent the anticipated stuttering. As Selye (1950) says, "No living organism can be maintained continuously in a stage of alarm (p. 31)." The stutterer finds that his fear waxes and wanes and that if he can make the speech attempt during the waning phase he may be able to say the feared word fluently. Postponement is an avoidance in time.

Again we make clear that all we wish the stutterer to do at this stage in treatment is to explore his communicative behavior, to hunt for all the varieties of postponement behaviors he can find. A new therapist is often astonished to discover how many they are. So is the stutterer, once he begins his search. Some of these postponement strategies are very common: the use of an "ah" or other interjections, the repetition of a previous word or phrase, the elaborately casual clearing of the throat or licking of the lips. Others can be involved and intricately complex. To cite one example, one of our clients showed a most peculiar and stereotyped sequence of behaviors which called more unfavorable attention to him than did his actual stuttering. First he would cock his head to the right, look up at the sky, then suddenly jerk his head down to the left, then rapidly say "Well-well-well," then speak the word he had feared. At times he would repeat this entire sequence several times, usually when the fear was strong. The response chain had become so powerful as to appear involuntary and it comprised the major part of his abnormality. Yet, when we studied and analyzed it, we found it to be all filibuster. It was used in an effort to wait for the precise moment in time when he felt he might not stutter. The behavior had been shaped by the occasional reinforcement of not stuttering. We remember him as resembling one of Skinner's pigeons.

As with the other avoidance reactions mentioned earlier, the collection and study of postponement responses is extremely valuable for the therapist. It enables him to specify the behaviors to be weakened or replaced. It helps him assess their strengths and the cues which trigger them. The factor of time pressure can be evaluated. In no other type of stuttering behavior can the approach-avoidance conflicts be seen so clearly. For the stutterer too there are equal advantages. The mystery of stuttering begins to fade. He begins to understand why he does what he does. He comes to realize that much of his abnormality has nothing to do with the actual utterance of the word, and that he cannot possibly say the word he wishes to say while he is filling his mouth with other irrelevant vocalization. He learns that his "stuttering" is not random spasm, that most of it consists of accumulated habitual responses so overlearned as to have become automatized. And what is equally important, he uncovers his pretense. In this benign therapeutic situation, he can touch and examine all the transparent disguise reactions he has used but hidden from himself for years. A sort of cleansing takes place which results in great relief. At last he has found one person, the therapist, with whom he can confront himself.

Identifying timing behaviors

As the stutterer begins to observe and analyze his stuttering, he discovers another set of behaviors antecedent to the real speech attempt which differ from those used to avoid or postpone it. These behaviors are not stallers but starters. They represent the stutterer's effort under time pressure to terminate the delay and to begin speaking. In this sense they are similar to what one does when he has to jump a ditch which seems too wide and yet one which he must cross. Commanding himself to commit himself to the leap, he counts to three, then makes the effort. Or he uses some other verbal or bodily gesture to signal the moment when he must take off. Similar timing behaviors reflect the stutterer's need to solve the approach-avoidance conflict. He must speak and yet he fears to speak. He dare not wait longer. The die must be cast. To aid him at this precarious moment, he uses some accessory behavior, some device to say "Now!" We do not find these postponement behaviors in the very young stutterer. They develop with awareness and, as with the other secondary reactions, they become strengthened every time they succeed, however intermittently this occurs. Even at worst, when they do result in stuttering, they at least terminate a long ambivalent postponement which itself has become punishing; at best, they occasionally result in fluency. This combination of negative and positive reinforcement is sufficient to maintain them at high operant levels.

Some of the most grotesque features of the stuttering picture are due to these habituated timing devices. The sudden head or jaw jerks, the flailing of an arm, the gasp of air, all these can be used as timers. We once compiled a collection of over 70 different types of starter behaviors from a group of only nine stutterers. One of those we found most frequently was the forced exhalation of all the breath, the speech attempt being timed to the sensing that even the complemental air was about exhausted. It was, as one of the stutterers said, "Speak then or have to do the whole damned thing over again."

The reader will have noted that we have listed the identifying of fluent stutterings, avoidance, postponement, and now timing behaviors sequentially. Again we say that this ordering is not academic. Through experimenting, we have found that a hierarchy of confrontation difficulty exists. By deliberately programming the identification tasks in this order we proceed from the least difficult to the more difficult and so we avoid difficulties which otherwise would occur. When we come therefore to the collection of timing behaviors, the stutterer must confront some of the features of his speech abnormality that have produced the most listener penalty and personal distress. We find that he prefers to tell us about them rather than to duplicate them. He finds it difficult to watch them in the mirror or on videotape. He hates to see other stutterers using them. They are the stigmata of his disorder, the sign of the beast.

A competent therapist will of course recognize that this phase of identification creates a real opportunity for progress once the emotionality has been evoked and managed. Yes, at times even a breakthrough occurs at this point. Self-hate and self-disgust are ventilated there in the safety of the therapy room. The untouchable is touched. If the therapist can share the confrontation, can put the same behaviors into his own mouth, can contort his own face and jerk his body yet remain untraumatized as he makes a demonstration phone call, the stutterer's shame and misery begins to melt away. He begins to recognize that

stuttering is behavior. He comes to understand why he does what he does. As the therapist calmly scrutinizes these important components of the stuttering act objectively and provides a running commentary on what he has observed, much of the stutterer's attendant emotionally decreases. Stuttering actually begins to become interesting.

Identifying the verbal cues

All of the behaviors we have been describing are those that occur prior to the actual speech attempt. They have been responses linked to antecedent sets of stimuli, to features of the communicative situation, or to characteristics of the words to be uttered. They are expectancy reactions and the expectancy is colored with unpleasant autonomic upheaval. Since we must find ways of weakening them, we must be able to identify the cues to which they are linked.

Although confirmed stutterers are usually able to describe some of the cues that trigger the fears and the consequent behaviors of avoidance, postponement, and starters, we find that the description often lacks specificity. "I just knew I would stutter; I don't know why," is a common comment. "When she called me, I knew I'd have a hard time." "H-words are always hard for me." "It's having to break the silence and begin the talking that starts the butterflies in my stomach." We have found it wise to introduce the exploration of these perceptions and their accompanying feelings at this later point in the therapy sequence. By this time the stutterers learned to hunt, to collect, to report, to demonstrate. They have become interested in exploring their behavior, in understanding themselves. Perhaps now they may be able to trust the therapist enough to share some of their private burdens of anxiety and shame.

We have found it advisable first to have them hunt for the phonemic and positional cues that signal approaching stuttering and, outside the therapy room, to write down the words on which they have anticipated difficulty. At the same time, however, we jointly devise projects to test the reality of those fears. For example, one of our stutterers, who claimed always to have trouble on words beginning with *m* and who feared such words intensely, discovered by listening to tapes on his speech that he had really stuttered only eighteen percent of the words that began with that sound. Another one who greatly feared words beginning with *p* and *b* sounds but had little anxiety about words beginning with *m* or *n* came to us excited by finding that he had expected stuttering on the word "pneumonia" because it began with a *p*, then suddenly realized that it really started with his easy sound, the *n*. His comment was: "I've got scarecrows in my head!" We do not minimize these fears; they are all too real. Sometimes the stutterer may try to seduce us into pooh-poohing them. He wants us to tell him that they are irrational, nonsensical. We answer that they are not, that they have been conditioned and are being maintained by partial reinforcement. We ask him to collect specimens of the cues that trigger stuttering expectancy, and to find out for himself how valid they are. As he continues to explore, the stutterer identifies other verbal cues that set off fear such as the length of the word, its position within the sentence, its meaningfulness, its history of past unpleasantness, and all the rest. It is especially important to structure the exploration so that as he collects, he checks. How often does this particular cue really evoke fear of stut-

tering? How great is the correlation between the expectancy and the actuality of stuttering? How well can he really predict that he will stutter? Let's find out! How far ahead does he see the feared word coming? Let's see! What little rehearsals of stuttering behavior occur in the period prior to the speech attempt? Does the fear fluctuate in intensity? What specifically is he afraid will happen? These are the questions that arise during the discussions between therapist and stutterer, and their answers are found through the exploration of actual communication.

Some difficulties are occasionally found in this project. The stutterer at first may be so aroused with emotion that he seems to be unable to discriminate at all. This can be solved by using adaptation procedures or by using long delays on the auditory feedback apparatus or by recording and then using playback. With an interested, permissive therapist, this initial difficulty in discrimination soon fades, especially if the therapist will call the stutterer's attention to some possible cues and then have him select the most probable ones. There are also the few severe stutterers who have little or no word or phonemic fears. (With these we skip this phase and proceed directly to the analysis of the situation fears.) A more common problem lies in the stutterer's fear of fear itself. For years he has tried to distract himself so he will not be afraid, trying always to keep from anticipating his abnormalities of speech. Though usually he is unsuccessful, there have been enough instances in which his distraction tricks have been successful to make the process of attending to fear-colored stimuli very distasteful. We are now asking him to seek what he has fled from. Nevertheless, if the therapeutic relationship is rewarding, the stutterer will soon overcome this temporary obstacle. This is why self-therapy is so difficult; this is why stutterers need therapists. Over and over again the support of the therapist is essential if the stutterer is to be desensitized to the stimuli that evert their evil control over his behavior.

Identifying the situational cues

We deliberately postpone this item in the hierarchy of identification processes until this time because it involves the direct confrontation of self. Though the stutterer has merely to identify those features of communicative situations which arouse his speech anxiety, he soon finds himself examining instead his relationships with others. Many of these, of course, have been far from satisfactory. He discovers, for example, that he fears speaking in a given situation because of the potential threat to his self-esteem. Old traumatic memories flood over him. Though he has long felt the sting of stigma—as represented by the evaluation of others—now he is having to verbalize it. He has long repressed these feelings. He has tried to forget his ancient wounds. Now they are reopened. Why did he fear phoning that attractive girl? "She probably thinks I'm a freak, a living zombie. After she hangs up, she'll laugh to her roommate and I can hear the remarks she'll make." Why does he keep collecting older women as sources of his situation fear? He may not know or want to know. This is dangerous territory to be exploring so early in therapy. At this time it is wise to keep to the main roads and not to plunge too deeply into the swamps. There will be opportunity later on, if such investigation is appropriate. Now we are merely guides. We accompany our cli-

ents; we do not push them into the mire even if we think they need to get dirty. The neurotic stutterer finds it hard to resist the opportunity presented by this phase of the investigation but the ordinary garden variety of stutterer will not want to explore too deeply too soon. Nevertheless, the clinician must recognize that when the stutterer begins to explore the phenomena related to situation fears he can be expected to show some emotionality and resistance. He is exploring himself.

The reports brought to these therapy sessions by the stutterer usually refer to the conditions of communications (telephoning, speaking to a group of people, asking a favor, etc.) and to the expected listener reactions. The stutterer, when asked why he expected to stutter in these particular situations, at first can only say that they have always been difficult. If pressed, he will remember specific instances in similar situations wherein he had experienced such communicative frustrations or listener penalties. "Every time I have to make a telephone call, I fear that I'll get blocked and then they'll hang up on me." "I'm afraid they'll get impatient and turn away, or laugh, or make some smart crack." "I'm afraid they'll think I'm stupid or insane." "I'm afraid they'll pity me." These are just a few of the common verbalizations.

Once again, we explore to test the reality of these expectations. In ten phone calls, how many times did the listener actually hang up the receiver? How many listeners on a given morning did laugh when he stuttered? How many showed signs of impatience or rejections and how did they show them? Usually the stutterer will be surprised to find that the validity of these expected unpleasant listener reactions is very low, that most casual listeners have very little interest in any but their own concerns, that at most they seem surprised rather than shocked, more curious than rejecting. There will be a few in the collection who do demonstrate the expected aversive behaviors, usually (as the therapist may suggest) those who are themselves insecure or harried, but this reality testing almost always demonstrates that the expectancy was exaggerated. It is wise here to provide some feared speaking situations with the therapist being present and in which the stutterer analyzes his expectations beforehand and then later identifies the actual consequences. It is often useful too if the therapist will do some severe pseudostuttering in these situations and be able to comment calmly and objectively on the listener reactions.

Identifying the core behaviors

Most of the behaviors, overt and covert, that we have previously been having the stutterer identify are those that occur prior to the attempt to utter the word. Now we explore the manner of the abnormal utterance itself. We wish to discover what abnormalities exist in its motor sequences. Again we face the confronting of old traumatized behavior, the frustrating oscillations and fixations, the loss of integration, the felt inability to proceed, the verbal impotence. About these frustrating core experiences the disorder has been built. As one of our cases said, "The stuff is too hot to tackle. It's burned me for years." Nevertheless it must be touched if it is later to be manipulated or shaped. We have been spending time and energy exploring the peripheral reactions of stuttering. It is time to go to the core.

The stutterer often finds the discrimination of these core behaviors difficult unless he compares the way he speaks the stuttered word with the way he says it normally or stutters on it fluently. As we did at the beginning of our identification, we again seek as models those moments of easy, forward-moving stuttering which can always be found in his speech. Again we collect these samples, but now, for comparison purposes, we also need to examine the motoric features of the normally spoken word as well. Therefore, we seek triads—the abnormal utterance, the fluent stuttering, and the normal utterance—comparing each with the other to identify the features that characterize them. (Note that we are not interested in how they sound but how they are produced!) Even this early in therapy we are seeking to alter the stutterer's usual bias toward monitoring his speech acoustically rather than proprioceptively. We want him to stop listening to the gaps and abnormal sounds in his speech and to start finding out what he is actually *doing*. Eventually we want him to learn to do what normal speakers seem to do—to monitor speech primarily by proprioception. And so we focus our attention and his attention on the abnormal motoric aspects of his stuttered utterances as compared with the fluent ones. If we are to hope for corrective feedback, we must make provision for such comparison.

We must remember that this sort of analytical comparison is foreign to the stutterer. He has seldom examined what he does when he stutters in contrast to that which he does when he speaks normally. Instead he characteristically examines how he sounds or looks. All he knows is that sometimes he speaks freely and at other times he gets miserably stuck. As he now comes to observe the contrasts in behavior between stuttering utterance and normal utterance on the same word, he will be surprised, even shocked to note how different they are. "It's crazy, man, the things I do —like trying to say the f-word with my mouth wide open. Never knew I did that." He is also impressed by the close resemblance that his fluent stutterings have to the normal utterance. They at least begin with normal rather than abnormal articulatory postures. Their sequences are similar though the fluent stutterings seem slightly dragged out with slower transitions between sounds. As he collects these triads, and observes their motoric features, other important differences become apparent. At this point in therapy, the stutterer may make some attempts at self-correction despite our urging that he not do so. This is probably a good prognostic sign and the therapist is not unduly concerned. An occasional success may even help motivate the stutterer and his inevitable failures will help him to continue to accept our guidance.

In devising the tasks and subgoals for this phase of identification, we concentrate first on those articulatory postures which are most visible. Accordingly for the first time we use the mirror, snapshots, or videotape. For stutterers who show grotesque mouth formations and contortions we often begin the visual confrontation by using a facial shield with eye openings and a large space through which only the mouth area can be seen, explaining that we wish to concentrate the attention on mouth movements alone. A therapist must be alert to the trauma that visual self-confrontation can bring to a severe stutterer. He has never really known how he appears to others. Though he must finally come to confront this picture, we

must not overwhelm him. For most stutterers, even the milder ones, it is usually wise for the therapist to prepare them for the experience by verbalizing some of the reactions other stutterers have had and by redefining the purpose of the task. Once the stutterer realizes that he must examine three things—not only the abnormal stuttering utterance but also the normal utterance and the fluent stuttering on the same word—he becomes more curious than appalled. By isolating the word, repeating it several times, and detecting the changes in motoric behaviors that take place during its adaptation, the stutterer is helped to face the reality of his behavior with much of the same analytic attitude shown by the therapist. What does he do first in attempting the actual speech attempt? Does he shape his lips in the same way for the *m* sound which initiates a normally spoken word that he does when stuttering upon it? "What differences are there? Didn't the jaw seem to be contracted to one side when he stuttered on that word 'good?' Let's try it again and see. No stuttering this time? All right, was there any difference in how you form the word when you said it normally as compared with how you did it before? Let's hunt for some more differences." So the therapist's part of the colloquy might go.

In this exploratory stage, we look for gross differences, not the minute ones. We discover abnormal and inappropriate preformations, those that make it almost impossible for anyone other than a ventriloquist to produce the initial sound of a word, those in which the lips or tongue block the airway so completely that no one could emit the vowel being attempted. "It looks like I'm trying to pour my speech likker out of a corked bottle, doesn't it?" one stutterer said. Or the lips are observed to protrude, snout-like, in the attempted utterance of an *f* or *v*. The stutterer compares this with the normal utterance and is astonished at the discrepancy. "What am I doing? What am I doing? Why don't I do it on those easy stutterings? I'm not a human. I'm a pig grunting . . . in the dirt." We do not then ask him to explore the dirt though doubtless there may be much of it . . . unless he so wishes. "Let's not evaluate now. Let's see what you're doing. Let's explore."

It is fascinating to be present at some of these discoveries. One stutterer who had great trouble beginning words that started with the *t* sound, found that when he stuttered, the upper surface and tip of the tongue was curled concavely so that its tight contact was made far back in the mouth whereas when he did not, the surface was convex and the tip make a brief brushing contact against the upper gum. "I've been looking in my mouth and putting my fingers and things in it and that's what I find," he insisted. "When I stutter, I'm doing things upside down." We gave him no lecture on kinesiological phonemics; it was enough to have him making some motoric discriminations. It was good to find him interested rather than covered with fear and shame. Therapy was progressing. Desensitization was taking place.

In this exploration, trigger postures —those to which tremors have become conditioned—become defined. The stutterer notes that he almost seems to cock his mouth for stuttering, that there are certain preformed mouth or jaw or lip postures that, when assumed, almost guarantee that he will have trouble. Something very similar is also discovered about the contacts made by tongue or lips, i.e., that there are certain spots—often different ones than those used normally in sound production—which, when contacted strongly, almost always result in fixation or the recoils of repetitive syllables. "I've got a mouth full of booby-traps," one of our stutterers commented. Several others have phrased the same discovery in terms of the doorbell or buzzer analogy: "I've got stutter-buttons in my mouth and on my lips. If I press them, boy, then my stutter-buzzer sure starts ringing. If I don't, I don't." We wish we could remember more of the colorful phrases in which our stutterers have expressed similar discoveries. It has been interesting to us that, though they may verbalize it differently, most of them find the same basic things—that when they stutter on a word, they use different motoric behaviors than when they say it normally or have some fluent stuttering.

They also become very curious about their tremors. "You know, it's when my jaw, my tongue, or my lips start shivering that I feel really stuck. It's a kind of feeling of helplessness then. My mouth gets wound up so tight it starts vibrating. Why do I do this only when I stutter? I never do this when I say the word all right." We have heard so many similar statements from our clients that we have almost become convinced that the stuttering tremor comprises the heart of the disorder in the advanced stutterer. Even more than the social penalties, it is this experience of finding a tremor running on perseveratively that they dread. For a moment they feel seized, unable to move forward, unable to do anything but continue to vibrate. As we shall see in our next section, most of the abnormal escape responses of the stutterer seem tied to the noxious experience of the tremor. And so we explore this stuttering tremor, studying its beginning, its variations, how it is terminated.

Because the experience of tremor has so many implications of impotence, of inability to control the self, we structure other forms of tremor in ourselves, setting our knees to vibrating or duplicating the finger tremors which produce a violin vibrato and so on. We observe how these are voluntarily initiated, how they are sustained, how they are ended. Then we seek to set similar tremors to vibrating in our own lips, jaws, and tongue, the therapist sharing and demonstrating that he too can tremor. Next the stutterer begins to examine his own tremors, first studying how they end, then how they vary, and finally how they begin. Note again in this sequencing the presence of a desensitization subhierarchy here—as in all the programming of identification tasks that we have described earlier. We work on each step of identification and description until the accompanying negative emotion subsides, and only then do we move to discriminations that are more highly charged with unpleasant emotion.

The stutterers are usually very curious about how their "blockages" are terminated. Some of the mystery of stuttering seems to be focussed here. As one of them said, "What bugs me is I don't know what happens. There I am stuttering hard and all of a sudden my stuttering is over and I can say the word. And it comes out *easy!* Oh sometimes I seem to have to force it out but often it just seems to run its course and then quit. I don't understand." What the stutterer finds, when he systematically collects and analyzes some samples of tremors visually and kinesthetically, is that there are three characteristic terminal features:

1. the tremor decreases in amplitude and slows down;
2. a sudden jerk or timed surge of tension seems to interrupt the rhythmicity of the tremor; and
3. the localized state of hypertension subsides.

He also notices that in the latter, the sudden jerks or bursts of hypertension may sometimes effect momentary syllabic release but that he bounces back into the tremor again. When he compares these phenomena with the models of normal utterance, he finds none of them present; when he compares them with those of the little fluent stutterings, he notes that the latter's short tremors, when present, always follow the first course and slow down and decrease in amplitude; and that very little hypertension is present.

As the stutterers investigate the tremors themselves in this phase of identification, they discern first that they vary more in duration than they do in frequency. The durations seem to be proportional to the antecedent fear and to the amount of localized tension present. One stutterer remarked. "I've been resting my chin in my hand with my elbow on the table and watching my tremors in the mirror. I find that they aren't even. They seem to get bigger and then smaller. Sometimes they spread to my lips and tongue, usually when I start forcing. They wobble." Far more important than the stutterers' observations is their experience in making benign contact with the tremor. The burnt child finds that the stove may not be as hot as he remembered. The rat, held in contact with the electrified grid, finds that it can tolerate the shock, that it need not freeze or shake when the tone comes on. We are beginning to extinguish some of the fear and frustration.

Identifying loci of tension

One of the later subgoals in the hierarchic set that deals with this stage of identification focuses on the discrimination of tension. Each stutterer seems to show a fairly unique set of tension foci. These patterns of tension foci and overflow are almost as individualistic as his fingerprints. The loci of hypertension also vary phonemically—with the mode of sound production. We seek to get the stutterer to become vividly aware of these focal areas and structures that are so highly tensed. As he compares the stuttered production with the normal utterance he comes to understand how hard he works to cause trouble for himself. One of them watching himself on videotape exclaimed, "Look at me. Look there how I'm squeezing my spout. . . . And now, I'm saying it, the same word, without any. . . . That's nuts. I'm going to quit doing that crazy stuff. If I can!"

Stutterers find more difficulty locating their tensions during the tremor state though the latter seems to be dependent upon tension as well as upon the simultaneous contraction of antagonistic musculatures. As we have said earlier, tremor behaviors seems to be especially difficult to confront objectively. When tremors are occurring the stutterer tends to detach himself from his own actions. As one of them said, "That's when I blot everything out. That's where I leave my skin behind and go off somewhere until my stuttering has left me." Other stutterers speak of blackouts. Froes-chels and Rieber (1963) called it auditory impercivity when they found that their stutterers seemed to be unable to respond to an auditory signal while in blockage. Again, however, we have found much variability in this trait. Those stutterers who are biased toward being more visile than audile or kinile seem to be able to recognize foci of tension during tremoring better than the others can, perhaps only because in therapy we usually employ much visual scrutiny in identifying them. However we also have the stutterer feel and palpate the facial and neck areas in this identification of tension and have found some curious benefits resulting therefrom. It certainly seems to eliminate the detachment. It also heightens awareness that stuttering is not just happening to him but he is doing it. In a few stutterers this self-contact through self-touching has been a turning point in therapy, one of those crucial experiences we seek. We are reminded here of the old technique of Wendell Johnson's that we mentioned earlier and that he termed semantic relaxation. Johnson had his stutterers gently feel and rub their hands together as they talked. Perhaps when they do this the stutterers are merely learning to be kind to themselves; perhaps the soft strokings bring back old memories of being fondled in infancy. Whatever may be the explanation, we know that this technique tends to induce relaxation and thereby to facilitate better identification of the tension foci so characteristic of advanced stuttering. We can see and feel the tensions disappear.

Identifying repetitive recoil behavior

Few stutterers show only complete stoppages or fixations; most of them have another variety of core behavior which is oscillatory in nature and for some stutterers it is the major kind of core behavior they possess. Stutterers often call those compulsive syllabic repetitions "runaway blocks." Much faster than the repetitive behaviors of early stuttering, these moments of stuttering almost seem to represent the kind of oscillations that characterize other servosystems under overload. The systems detect error and recoil, then automatically return. Over and over again this happens until the necessary alteration in the system takes place. Stutterers sense this repetitive recoil behavior very vividly. They report that they seem to have lost control of the speech musculatures. They tell us that once the recoiling "gets started circling it won't stop right away." "My jaw gets to bouncing like a ball." "I begin to say a word and the first syllable keeps chugging like a steam engine." "It's scary when you find you can't stop doing what you don't want to do." The experience seems to be very difficult to express in ordinary objective terms; almost always the stutterers use animistic analogies in their attempt to communicate what they think is happening to them. The experience however is very real. It is also traumatic. "I've been stuttering like that all my life and each time I have one of those runaways, it shakes me up. I can't get used to them. I can't accept them. They shake me to the bone."

Our tentative explanation for the behavior is that the servosystem is thrown into oscillation because the timing of simultaneous and sequential movements has been disrupted but we don't tell our stutterers that. We merely ask them to examine the behavior and report what they discover. We ask them as best they can to observe and analyze it. How fast do

they recoil? From what do they recoil? (Some report that they do so when they sense a tremor, hard contact, or abnormal articulatory posture.) If the repetitive behavior is syllabic, as it usually is, what vowel appeared in the abortive attempts? (They usually report an inappropriate schwa vowel.) What variations occur in the recoil behavior? (They tell us that often they sense none, that they "automatically" repeat the same inappropriate movement or syllable in exactly the same way each time except that some changes occur just before the release.) So it goes, this exploration, with few of the questions answered completely or satisfactorily. As therapists we are not too concerned. This is early in the game. It is enough for now that the stutterer is in contact with his behavior without being flooded with anxiety. It is sufficient that he is making discriminations, that he is specifying his behaviors. Most importantly he is recognizing how differently he behaves when he stutters than when he is fluent. Some light pierces the dark mystery.

Identification of the post-stuttering reactions

We also explore the *feelings* which result from the *experience* (not the anticipation) of stuttering last in the sequence of the identification hierarchy because these feelings seem to be most unbearable and hardest to identify. Our stutterers have always found it most difficult to express these feelings in words. Essentially, as reported by the great majority of our cases, the basic feelings that a stuttering act evokes are frustration, shame, and hostility. Occasionally anxiety is also felt but this arises some time later as the stutterer moves on to find other feared words or situations. It is probably because of these emotional consequences that the stutterer hurries onward so compulsively and swiftly after moment of stuttering. He desires, if he can, to escape their impact. He hates to remember them. He finds it hard to put them into words.

Identifying feelings of frustration

Most of the intense frustration is reported as occurring during the moment of stuttering, but immediately after it, the stutterers tell us, it is the lag in communication that bedevils them. Speech is felt to be labored, each moment of stuttering adding to its sluggishness. The sentences plod. One of our stutterers told us after a short phone conversation, "I thought I'd never get done. All I said was two sentences. Somehow I slugged my way through them but oh, it took so long. I think I felt more impatient than the person on the other end of the phone. Block after block after block. And then they say, 'Huh? What? What did you say?' and I've got to go through all that hard work again. It's like walking with such heavy weights on your shoes that you can hardly move. I get tired stuttering." We have seen little boys cry with frustration and stop talking altogether. One of them said, "It's too hard to talk. It's too hard!" These feelings dominate the private world of the stutterer. They need to be ventilated and shared. This phase of identification provides the opportunity.

Identifying feelings of shame

Feelings of shame are much more easily verbalized than those of frustration, an observation which shouldn't have surprised us, knowing the culture we live in, but it did. Words have been made available for

such feelings by all the culture carriers who have bestowed them throughout the gauntlet of childhood. There are few words for verbal impotence, though there are many for shame. At any rate, our stutterers seem to be able to express with some precision the intensity of the feelings that are distributed along the continuum of embarrassment, shame, and guilt. Always there is the implication that these feelings are due to past or present listener penalties, overt or covert, real or imagined. In this early stage of therapy, no deep verbalization of shame or guilt occurs though we sometimes hear the stutterers "breaking trail" for real revelations to follow later. During this identification training, stutterers usually seem content merely to skim the surface of their shameful feelings. Often we find them watching us closely, wondering if we are accepting or pitying or rejecting when they disclose how shameful they feel when they stutter. One of them almost shouted at us: "Why don't you say there's nothing to be ashamed of? That's what the others have always said. And they're all liars." We replied that we were interested in knowing how he felt and why he felt the way he did. "I'm not ready yet," he blurted, and so we went on to other cabbages and things. There are, however, a few stutterers who from the first seem to love this particular phase of identification. They revel in their breast beating, in their exaggerated self-pity, in their self-disgust. Again we show our interest but without providing the kind of reinforcement which they doubtless have experienced from too many other people. If they insist upon wallowing interminably in the mire of self-reproach, we let them do so of course and then we wait patiently on the bank until they finally come out and start moving again, which they always do. We must remember that this identification process proceeds throughout all the therapy and that we are just beginning to train the stutterer to discriminate. There will be other opportunities. Nevertheless, we feel it very important to program some initial confrontation of such feelings early in therapy so that our cases will understand that we are concerned with more than the feathers of the broken wings of broken words.

Identifying feelings of hostility

In identifying their feelings of hostility stutterers reveal reactions of wide variability. The milder cases show very little hostility, their affect seemingly being colored mainly with anxiety. Once the moment of stuttering has passed, their basic experience is one of relief, one that soon transforms itself into another anxious scanning for the next threat to fluency. It is those whose stuttering is characterized by complete stoppages and tremors who are more likely to be the ones reporting anger. In part this is due to the frustration of being unable to communicate, to complete the message. Word after word arises as an obstacle to give these stutterers trouble. Each struggle generates some frustration. Summation of emotion takes place leading finally to blow-ups which surprise the stutterer almost as much as they do his listeners. The mother of one of our ten-year-old advanced stutterers asked for a conference. "Bobby seems to be changing in personality," she complained. "He's always been a sweet child, happy, eager to please, easy to handle. But lately he's getting onery—even mean. The other day, for instance, after trying to tell us what had happened in school, he just went beserk. He put

on a terrible temper tantrum. He knocked over chairs, broke a vase, and even tried to hit me. He was crying all the time but he was just furious. I don't understand it." We understood it. From many stutterers older than Bobby we have had reports of inner feelings of fury that are surprising in their intensity. "All she did was to say kindly that she was sorry but she didn't understand me. A nice little old lady but I could have killed her. I mean *killed!* I was so mad!"

Not all the hostility comes from frustration however. Perhaps even more comes from resentment due to listener penalty. Convinced that they are completely innocent of any crime against society for which they should be held responsible, some stutterers acquire deep hatreds for those who reject them. Some of them, like Tam O'Shanter's wife in the poem by Burns, nurse their wrath to keep it warm. We have heard some astounding reports of rage during this phase of identification—and from the most unlikely testifiers. One little mouse of an adolescent girl, demure and polite, told us of fantasies in which she subjected a store clerk (and others) to the most exquisite and diabolical tortures. As she spoke, her face was as livid as her language. We have rarely examined such an essence of highly distilled hate. As hostility begins to pour forth, the therapist must expect to become the target of some of this long repressed aggression especially in those stutterers who have turned their hatred inward upon themselves because they couldn't project it outwardly for fear of being clobbered some more. We are not appalled when this happens. The therapist's receptacle should be large enough to receive such evil. Better to have it come out than to keep it within. Better to have it expressed in words rather than in stuttering behavior. Good therapists are self-flushing anyway.

Bibliography

BRUTTEN, E. J. and D. J. SHOEMAKER, *The Modification of Stuttering*. Englewood Cliffs, N.J.: Prentice-Hall, 1967.

FROESCHELS, E. and R. W. RIEBER, The problem of auditory and visual impercivity in stuttering, *Folia Phoniatrica,* 15 (1963), 13–20.

LOHR, F., Visible manifestations of stuttered speech, Convention paper, A.S.H.A., 1969.

SELYE, H., *The Physiology and Pathology of Exposure to Stress*. Montreal: Acta, 1950.

SHAMES, G. W., Operant conditioning and therapy for stuttering, C. W. Starkweather (ed.), *Conditioning in Stuttering Therapy*. Memphis: Speech Foundation of America, 1970.

VAN RIPER, C., *The Nature of Stuttering*. Englewood Cliffs, N.J.: Prentice-Hall, 1971.

WEBSTER, L. M., *A Cinematic Analysis of the Effects of Contingent Stimulation on Stuttering and Associated Behaviors*, Ph.D. Thesis, Southern Illinois University, 1968a.

————, A methodological investigation of the contingent stimulation of stuttering moments, Convention paper, A.S.H.A., 1968b.

ZENNER, A. A., *A Molecular Analysis of Stuttering and Associated Behaviors During Massed Oral Readings of the Same Material: The Adaptation and Consistency of Behaviors*, Ph.D. Thesis, Syracuse University, 1971.

Desensitization:
The Reduction
of Negative Emotion

In this chapter we describe some of the ways by which we seek to reduce the stutterer's speech anxieties and other disturbing emotional states. We say reduce rather than completely eliminate because we doubt that in most confirmed adult stutterers they can ever be brought to a permanent level of zero. Secondly, we seek reduction rather than complete elimination at this time because we would not really want to eliminate them completely even if we could, for we need some fear and we need some stutterings if we are to teach the stutterer more adaptive ways of responding to both of these experiences. Again we wish to emphasize that in stuttering we find two classes of stimuli, those that govern avoidance and those that govern escape. There are stimuli that

signify threat of approaching unpleasantness (such as the perception of a certain feature of a certain word in a certain speaking situation) that lead to avoidance, disguise, or various anti-expectancy behaviors. There are others inherent in the stuttering itself (such as the realization that a fixation, tremor, or perseverative recycling of a syllable is being experienced) that trigger various searching, coping, or interrupting responses as well as emotional upheaval. Both of these classes of complex stimulus sets are able to release strong emotional responses in the confirmed stutterer. Our goal in this desensitization phase of therapy is to disassociate the responses from their stimuli.

Although we shall attempt to avoid the terminology of learning theory as we describe what we do in desensitization, it will be apparent that our endeavors are based upon the following concepts:

1. nonreinforcement and response prevention;
2. counterconditioning of new and incompatible resposes to the same sets of stimuli;
3. flooding and adaptation;
4. reconfiguration of stimulus sets;
5. conditioned inhibition.

There is an old Japanese poem which, crudely translated, runs as follows: "The first time I looked on evil, I said, 'It is horrible. Take it away!' The second time I looked on evil, I said, 'It is curious but it belongs to others. I will avert my eyes.' The third time I looked on evil, I cried out, 'It is my own!'" This same sequence seems to occur in successful stuttering therapy and we would hope that a fourth look will lead the stutterer to exchange his evil for something better. Nevertheless, anyone who works with the problems of confirmed, fully developed stuttering soon comes to realize that much of his real success will depend upon his ability to desensitize [1] the stutterer to his stuttering and to its controlling stimuli. This is not an easy task.

Some students of the disorder have claimed that the stutterers' fears reflect its essential nature as a logophobia but phobias are by definition *irrational* fears in which the expectations bear no reasonable relationship

[1] In this chapter, we use the term *desensitization* in a broader sense than that of the *systematic desensitization* technique popularized by Wolpe and Eyesenck. In our discussion we will describe all the ways by which we attempt to allay the stutterer's sensitivities concerning his disorder.

to the possible consequences. In stuttering, on the other hand, the fears are not at all unreasonable or unrealistic. They have been based upon very real experiences of communicative frustration and listener rejection. They are as justified as the highly appropriate fear of an approaching grizzly, though, we would admit, perhaps neither so rare nor so intense. (We have known a few stutterers who might argue the latter point.) Similarly, the feelings of embarrassment, hostility or shame, and guilt triggered by stuttering have also been determined in large part by actual experiences. Stutterers feel shame because others have placed a stigma on the disorder, because the impacts of scorn and other penalties have been keenly felt. Although the psychopathology of stuttering depends not only on the presence of these reactions in the stutterer but on his morbid exaggeration of them, some, even much of his concern, may be rooted in actuality. With his history of hurt and the attitudes of society toward communicative deviancy the stutterer *should* be afraid or ashamed. Our purpose in desensitization therapy is to reduce the strength of the attendant emotional upheaval enough to enable the stutterer to learn new ways of coping with the expectancy and experience of broken words.

In the kind of therapy that we advocate this desensitization takes place. The host of cues to which unpleasant emotions have been linked, one after another, are reexperienced, actually or through recall, in a situation which is benign. With a warm and accepting and interested therapist, the amount of anxiety elicited by these old stimuli progressively decreases. Over and over again, the fear-laden cues are experienced without being followed by penalty or other unpleasantness. In the therapist the stutterer not only has a non-punitive listener but one who minimizes the urgency of communication so far as time is concerned. The therapist does not interrupt or hurry him. The therapist will wait. Time pressure is reduced in this situation and so the amount of felt frustration is markedly reduced. Since the fears of the stutterer involve the expectancy of frustration and listener penalty, and both of these are minimal or absent in the therapy situation, deconditioning begins. The conditioned stimuli are experienced but the punishment is not.

It may be objected that this is all well and good but the stutterer cannot live in such an ideal world with such an ideal listener and that as soon as he leaves the therapy room he is again naked in a world of knives. This is quite true but we must begin somewhere. Somehow we must create a nucleus situation in which unlearning can start, in which new learning may be attempted. The stutterer will not be the worse for discovering at least one spot in time and place wherein he can talk without distress even though he stutters. An ancient book speaks of the valley of Ephraim where one goeth to restore one's soul. Each of us, stutterer or normal speaker, requires an Ephraim too from whence we can sally forth and to which we can return. Those who have been hurt most grievously need one most.

By speaking in this vein, we do not mean to imply that the therapy situation must always be so structured as to involve no stress, no fear, no stuttering. Desensitization implies stress. It requires, though, that the amount of stress can be controlled by the therapist. A person with hayfever can probably imprison himself in a completely filtered, air-conditioned room and never have a sneeze, but to live a normal life it is better that he be administered the pollen in progressive amounts to enable him to build up his defenses and reduce his hypersensitivity.

The therapist's role

What then should be the therapist's role in desensitization? First of all, as we have said, he must be able to create in the therapy room the zone of safety and security, where basically the stuttering is felt with little frustration and where the listener is not punitive. Secondly, however, the therapist must be able to control the conditions of communication so that stress can be programmed into contrived speaking situations in the appropriate degree. By this we mean mainly that the therapist and stutterer must explore the limits of the latter's stress tolerance so that, through the joint devising of a graded hierarchy of speaking tasks, the stutterer becomes progressively able to modify his stuttering behavior without becoming so emotional that he cannot do so.

Note that we are not desirous that with us he can always speak without any stuttering. Were our goal merely to give him some temporary fluency devoid of any stuttering behavior, we could do so without having to do any desensitization therapy. For the unlearning and learning that must be done, if more permanent gains are sought, we need, as we have said, some stuttering behaviors; we need some fear and frustration, but we need them at levels of frequency and severity which will permit modification. Were the stutterer to remain in the therapy situation overwhelmed by noxious emotion, were he to stutter compulsively on almost every word, we could do very little to help him. He wouldn't even be able to understand what we were saying. He could not discriminate. He could not participate in the structuring of therapy. He could not learn or unlearn anything.

In essence, then, we seek a therapeutic relationship that will enable the therapist to exert some control over the stutterer's covert behavior. As therapists we should be able to create an atmosphere of tolerance and calmness for the stutterer there in the therapy room with some consistency. We must also, however, be able to inject into this therapy situation increments of stress that will evoke tolerable amounts of stuttering and emotionality. By tolerable we imply only that the stutterer can continue to work meaningfully on his problem. When the communicative stress is too great or the task too difficult, the threshold of his tolerance will have been exceeded and he will show this by marked increases in anxiety, shame or hostility and by the kind of stuttering behavior that occurs. And by failing!

How can the therapist identify these thresholds in such terms? In the present state of the art, the detection of the client's anxiety, shame, or hostility levels can hardly be said to have much objectivity. In the laboratory we can wire our clients for galvanic skin responses, or electromyographic records, or dip their fingers in a solution to compute Palmar Sweat Indices, but even these imperfect instruments are hardly suitable for clinical therapy. Perhaps someday clinicians will be able to implant electrodes in the hypothalamus and reticular formation of their clients and do their desensitization by reading dials, returning to basal levels whenever the pointer indicates nearness to threshold; but in this still benighted age, a therapist must use his eyes and ears and em-

pathy. And the process is not really as difficult as it might seem to be.

How to desensitize: Recognizing negative emotionality

First of all we can use the stutterer's subjective reports as our anxiety indicator. He can tell us when his anxiety begins to flare and when it subsides and, if the therapist is a close observer, he can soon begin to correlate other behavioral signs with this testimony.[2] Often the breathing may show it first with higher I/E ratios (longer inspiration as compared with the duration of exhalation), or the stutterer may inhale sharply, then hold the breath before he exhales. Or he may hold the breath at the end of exhalation. These are observable physiological responses to fear. (We can stand a sudden blow better if we are inhaling or have just inhaled much better than when our ribcages are collapsing.) At any rate, as therapists, we watch the breathing of our clients while we increase the stress, and we stop increasing it when these signs appear.

There are also other visible signs of tension that can be used. The gross bodily musculatures lose their fluidity and mobility. Movements become jerky or may overshoot. Postures stiffen. The face begins to become masklike. Occasional twitches appear. As the therapist comes to know his client, these and many other little cues, some almost subliminal, signal emotional overload. It is difficult to generalize since almost every stutterer has his own characteristic ways of signalling

[2] Lanyon and Mansevitz (1966) subjected the validity of self-reported fear to experimental test using physiological measures of emotional arousal and concluded that generally the self-reports of fear were corroborated.

his emotional states, but if the therapist becomes tuned in, has done the preliminary checking of the validity of his perceptions and interpretations, he can sense the feelings of his client pretty well. As practicing therapists we work at this. We deliberately work hard to "read" our client's hidden feelings for we know that much of our success will depend upon how well we do so.

The speech itself is probably as good a barometer of the client's feelings as any other indicator. By this we refer not alone to the stuttering but rather to what Mahl and Schultze (1964) and others have referred to as the "non-ah" ratio, and to the pitch, intensity, and quality variations shown by the stutterer in his moments of fluency. Again, we cannot generalize, but a given stutterer will reveal much about his inner emotionality by the way he speaks even when he is speaking normally. Thus we learn to listen not merely to his thoughts but to his inflections, to the tempo of his speech and its pauses, recalling the features which formerly characterized his obvious emotional states. Close observation, enough contact, and this checking can provide much useful information for the clinician. Clinical sensitivity is almost impossible to describe in words but there is no doubt that it exists and can be learned at least by some persons (Truax and Carkhuff, 1967). Moreover, when the clinician does misinterpret the signs, he soon finds out, and this perception of error itself leads to better understanding.

Constructing hierarchies

Assuming that the therapist has learned to gauge the level of his client's emotionality with enough accuracy to keep from exceeding the threshold of excessive emotional arousal, how then does he proceed to desensitize his client? First, in conjunction with the stutterer, he must construct hierarchies of stimulus sets, or clinical tasks, that are progressively graded in terms of the anticipated intensity of emotional arousal. The lowest rung of the hierarchy of tasks, for example, will have the least probability of evoking emotional disruption of performance. The next rung of the desensitization ladder will increase that probability and with each higher item of the hierarchy, more stress can be expected to be felt. Our basic purpose is to devise the hierarchy so that, as each item is experienced over and over again, the attendant emotionality is not reinforced but instead is extinguished. We repeatedly work on one task or confront one set of unpleasant stimuli until the anxiety it elicits, for instance, decreases nearly to zero. Then we move to the next higher item step on the hierarchy and again work on that one until its emotionality subsides. And so on, until we find a task which exceeds the threshold, one which the stutterer cannot handle without having negative emotion disrupt it.

If possible we always try to stop before this threshold of emotional discharge is reached, but if we do ask more of the stutterer than he can handle, we then return to an earlier item on the hierarchy and start climbing again. What happens is that eventually the stutterer becomes able to do easily the same tasks or to confront calmly the same stimuli that formerly evoked too much emotion to permit learning or unlearning to occur. Desensitization inserts filters or buffers into the stutterer's system so that excessive amounts of emotional noise or static can be blocked out. Desensitization is the process of response prevention, of gradually building barriers against autonomic disturbance. It is in essence a toughening process. The stutterer learns that he can experience greater and greater amounts of anxiety or frustration or shame or hostility laden stimuli without having these trigger emotional upheaval. By carefully programming the incremental dosages of stress so that he is never overwhelmed, the stutterer's ability to tolerate stress is increased. He discovers finally that he can function well in the presence of stimuli which once would have rendered him helpless.

We should point out that some of the fear decrement effects may be due to the positive reinforcement provided by the therapist for progressively attaining success on each consecutive step of the hierarchy. Lang, Lazovik, and Reynolds (1965) recognize this:

Desensitization subjects received regular feedback concerning progress through the hierarchy. Clearcut success experiences (as well as failures) were part of the therapeutic interaction. In this context, a good therapeutic relationship may be one in which a therapist has gained the properties of a reinforcer, and this capacity is in the service of a specific program of behavior change. Desensitization would then progress more rapidly if approval is given for the completion of items. The better the relationship, the more effective such reinforcement is likely to be. On the other hand, it should be pointed out that the completion of an item is in itself reinforcing and many subjects compliment themselves on their own progress. (p. 398)

Let us give some specific examples of the process in desensitizing a stutterer to the confrontation of the disorder.

A very attractive girl stutterer showed some very unattractive behavior when stuttering. Her eyes shut tightly, her face contorted and her tongue protruded spasmodically. Often she would avert her face or cover her mouth with her handkerchief. She had seen all too often the shocked surprise of listeners when they witnessed these reactions. She had felt their rejection. She was becoming a recluse. It was impossible even to begin the identification of her behaviors because of her storm of revulsion. Though intellectually she understood the necessity for confronting and analyzing the stuttering if she were ever to modify it, her emotionality made this quite impossible. Accordingly we began by devising the following hierarchy of confrontation: (1) Observing the therapist stuttering in a fluent way; (2) Observing the therapist as he imitated the stuttering behaviors of other stutterers which were presented in a rank order of progressive abnormality; (3) Observing the therapist as he imitated her eye closing; (4) Observing the therapist as he imitated the eye-closing facial contortions and tongue protrusion. In this step of the hierarchy substeps were used in that the duration or extent of contortion or protrusion were progressively increased. (5) Observing the therapist as he showed the behavior while he made a phone call. All the preceding items of the hierarchy were performed in the privacy of the therapy room. (6) Observing the therapist as he imitated the behavior while speaking to a store clerk.

In this segment of the hierarchy we used a modeling approach. The therapist is not a passive observer but an active participant. Modeling is a more powerful procedure than is often realized. When the therapist, with whom the stutterer has come to identify closely, performs the fearful acts and the stutterer observes that he shows no reluctance and does not seem to be bothered by the listener reactions, the stutterer vicariously learns to be less afraid. As Bandura (1969) says:

Repeated modeling of approach responses decreases the arousal potential of aversive stimuli below the threshold for activating avoidance responses, thus enabling persons to engage, albeit somewhat anxiously, in approach behavior. Direct contact with threats that are no longer objectively justified provides a variety of new experiences that, if favorable, further extinguish residual anxiety and avoidance tendencies. Without the benefit of prior vicarious extinction, the modification of severely inhibited behavior generally requires a tedious and protracted program. (p. 192)

In this account of therapy we also emphasize the way that this kind of desensitization differs from the systematic desensitization of Wolpe's. This is *in vivo* desensitization. The patient is not asked to imagine himself in stress situations. He actually enters them. He is not trained in relaxation. We have experimented with Wolpe's techniques with stutterers and find great difficulty in getting any adequate transfer.

The above set of six experiences comprised only the first segment of the desensitization process, as we will make clear later. The girl did nothing but observe. Nevertheless, as soon as we came to Step 3, the girl said and showed that she was becoming emotional, though not markedly. We had her watch us. Over and over again we closed our eyes as we imitated very short blockages until she signalled that they weren't bothering her any more. Then we went back to Steps 1, 2, and 3, and then moved upward to Step 4 wherein we imitated her own behavior fairly closely but at first very briefly. Again she showed some emotionality, even though our tongue was barely protruded and the facial contortion and eye blink very short in duration. We continued until her tension subsided, then we increased the imitated abnormality progressively, always making sure to keep within her limits of tolerance. Finally she was watching us almost with amusement so we then began to make phone calls. Again the flareup of emotion occurred and was extinguished.

On Step 6, when we went out together to a store for the first time, we did not judge her threshold correctly and she fled from the situation when we imitated *her* characteristic stuttering behaviors. We bought her a cup of coffee and talked it over. She suggested that we climb the hierarchy from Step 3 in consecutive store situations and that perhaps she might then be able to tolerate our exhibition. This we did and again she found it quite possible to observe us showing her symptoms even though one of the clerks gave some very unfavorable responses. "How can you be so calm?" she asked in astonishment. "Didn't you see how she looked at you?" We talked it over. "How did *you* feel?" we asked. Again she looked surprised. "Say, that's right. I wasn't upset. I was wondering why that clerk reacted like she did and I was wondering also if you really were feeling as calm as you looked. But *I* wasn't upset. That's right." Our clinical notes mention that the first hierarchy's desensitization with this unusually hypersensitive stutterer had taken four therapy sessions to complete.

We next devised a new hierarchy which followed much the same sequence as the former one for the first five steps except that both of us read prepared sentences silently, then spoke them in unison while watching ourselves in the mirror. It was necessary on some of the steps to introduce the extra substep of having her keep her eyes only on the therapist's mouth at first, then later to watch her own before her emotion subsided to manageable levels. This entire second hierarchy was completed in two more sessions. By this time, she was duplicating her own characteristic stuttering behavior with remarkable calmness, but again only when speaking in unison with the therapist. We then ran another hierarchy in which we faded out our own model by speaking more softly, then whispering, then using pantomime while she continued to speak and stutter at normal vocal intensities. It was at this point that she said, "Oh, let's not do any more of this being so careful. Let me talk and watch the real stuff." We suggested that she hold a manila folder before her face whenever she thought she might stutter and to lower it to view herself only if she felt she could stand the sight, that if she felt she were becoming emotional to put up the shield. She agreed but used the shield only once to blot out the picture of contortion and tongue protrusion. This turned out to be another crucial experience. From this time onward, we had little difficulty. She eagerly went through the identification phase of therapy. The tongue protrusion bothered her a bit but interestingly this behavior disappeared before we ever really got to modify it. Though the desensitization had taken part of seven consecutive therapy sessions (we did other things too) it was well worth the time and effort. We feel pretty sure that had we not used it in the way we did, therapy could not possibly have been successful with this case.

We fear that this long illustration may possibly give an erroneous impression that desensitization training is unduly laborious and time consuming. Sometimes it is, but usually, if the subgoal experiences are structured appropriately, it proceeds much more swiftly. Most hierarchies need not be graduated in such small steps. The stutterer is a pretty tough animal. He has had to live with anxiety and other forms of stress for years. Indeed those who treat him too carefully and gently often make a serious mistake for he will interpret the cautious gingerliness as reflecting the therapist's covert dislike of contacting stuttering. He respects a therapist who expects him to be able to touch and work directly with the stuttering behavior. He does not want to put himself in the hands of one who flinches from the contact. Nevertheless, a competent therapist will always try not to make unreasonable demands for performance. He must be able to assess the probabilities of success and devise his therapeutic assignments so that it can occur. If he is sensitive to the stutterer's burden of emotionality, he will al-

ways take this into account. Desensitization provides a means for coping with the emotional disruption which retards progress in learning a better way of stuttering.

The targets of desensitization therapy

Now that we have described the process of desensitization generally, let us point to the features of the stuttering problem which usually require its application. The first of these is of course *the confrontation of the disorder*. Though very few stutterers demonstrate the exceptional hypersensitivity of the girl with the tongue protrusion, most advanced stutterers find some early (though temporary) difficulty in facing up to the reality of their abnormal speech behavior. They have always fled from self-scrutiny when they could. Whenever it was possible to do so, they have disguised and hidden the fact that they stuttered. Some denial always seems to be present. No therapist can expect any stutterer to contemplate his disorder with equanimity. Confrontation always generates some emotional arousal though its intensity varies widely from one client to another. This confrontation then is our first target, and we have dealt with it through identification activities.

The second major object of desensitization therapy is what we have termed the *core behavior* (Van Riper, 1971). The experiences of feeling blocked in a fixation or of compulsively oscillating in repetitive behavior are extremely traumatic to the stutterer. They trigger emotional arousal. They provide the original sources of much of the stutterer's fears and frustration. We have therefore found it necessary to do all we can to desensitize our clients to this basic experience. If we can raise their thresholds of tolerance for fixations and oscillations, an immediate reduction in avoidance and escape behaviors often occurs. The frequency and severity of the moments of stuttering will decrease. The fears subside. The stutterer will know that he is making progress.

Let us state here again, however, that we do not hope that desensitization will eliminate all of the emotion surrounding the core behavior. What we desire instead is to be able to reduce the intensity of the attendant emotion enough so that the behavior becomes manageable. Usually this presents no great problem; the stutterer has had too long and traumatic a history of communicative frustration to permit our desensitization therapy to reduce the highly charged recoil and struggle behavior completely. We have had some stutterers who did respond in this way but only temporarily and only in the therapy situation. Their flight into fluency presented some real problems while it lasted but usually it didn't last long. One of the few exceptions that we can report was a man who, following desensitization to his characteristic complete stoppages, became completely fluent in all situations and remained that way for seven months. All stuttering and all fear disappeared completely. Then suddenly it reappeared (at 7:30 P.M. of July 4, 1947) in exactly its old form and as strong as ever. It was obvious that we had not modified or weakened the basic stuttering responses at all. Other experiences of this sort have taught us to use desensitization with some discretion. We do not wish to leave the impression, however, that this is a common result of desensitization when aimed at the core behavior. More frequently, the converse is found. Stut-

terers adapt very slowly to the confrontation of their fixations and oscillations because they are too loaded with emotionality. Let us now illustrate the procedure.

Jim C., aged 24, was a very severe stutterer with long silent fixations accompanied by lip, tongue, and jaw tremors. The longest one we timed lasted for 70 seconds on the word "paymasters." Often he would have to stop and inhale before returning to the same hypertensed closures. There were very few avoidance reactions of any kind. He reported instances of fainting while stuttering though we never observed this. In a severe moment of stuttering, however, his eyeballs would gradually roll upward under the eyelid, showing white. He had few fears of sounds or words but he spoke as little as possible and then in short telegrammic foreshortened sentences. Each one of these long fixations, as he said, "crucified" him.

Consulting together, we worked out this desensitization hierarchy, focusing first on interruption and silence: (1) Jim administered at will an auditory, visual, or tactual signal that stopped the therapist in the course of his utterance and the therapist could not continue speaking until a second signal was given. (2) The procedure was reversed, the therapist giving Jim the signal to stop but it was administered only during fluent utterance. The silence period after the signal was progressively lengthened but the second signal to continue was given only when Jim appeared fairly calm. (3) Up to this point, the cessation of utterance was complete, but in this third step, as Jim talked he was *to hold the posture or sound he was making* at the moment he heard, saw, or felt the signal. The therapist lengthened the period of the stuttering fixation progressively. We found some strong emotion coming in at this step and continued to work on the step until it extinguished. Jim finally became able to stop the forward progress instantly upon signal and to hold the sound or posture until our preset criterion of five seconds had been reached and to do so without showing or reporting frustration.[3] (4) We next administered the signal during Jim's stuttering fixations. This item of the hierarchy had to be broken down into several substeps: (a) having the therapist assume some prolongations with Jim doing the signaling; (b) having the therapist give a visible signal as Jim watched himself in a mirror, first stopping completely, then maintaining the posture (first with and then without tremor), and for increasing durations; (c) having the therapist use a tactual signal (touching the lips or jaw) in the same kind of activity. All in all, we worked on this item of the desensitization hierarchy for five sessions until Jim was consistently able to maintain his abnormal articulatory postures occurring at the moment of stuttering without much emotion for at least ten seconds before continuing. (5) In this, the final step, Jim gave himself the signal. We used several substeps in this item: (a) Jim signalling complete cessation during normal speech; (b) Jim signalling complete cessation during a stuttering fixation but with the therapist signalling its end; (c) Jim signalling both the beginning and ending with the latter signal to be given finally only if no tremor activity or emotion was being felt. (6) Doing the last item in the presence of various listeners.

The outline of this stutterer's desensitization process does not include many of the interactions between therapist and client which actually occurred. Various observations were discussed in the therapy session. At different times, we had to return to an earlier step on the hierarchy before we could move forward. Frustration and other emotions often flared up unexpectedly and had to be worked down. We reinforced progress and withheld reinforcement for failures. At times we were highly supportive, verbalizing his feelings and getting him to do so too. But what is important in all this interplay of forces is that this stutterer was touching the core behavior of stuttering. His glands were learning not to squirt when he was stopped by a broken sound, syllable, or word. The emotion which had been overwhelming him at these moments was no longer so intense. He now could tolerate that which formerly he could not bear. To some degree he had become desensitized to the core of his stuttering.

Desensitization to listener reaction

Another major focus of desensitization therapy is the stutterer's vulnerability to the stress created by the listener. This stress includes more than the social rejection or the other forms of punishment that are bestowed upon the stutterer by the people with whom he talks, though these of course tend to arouse strong emotional responses. In addition, however, we find desensitization useful in building resistance to the disruption caused by such communicative pressures as hurry, sudden challenge, interruptions,

---

3 Note that in this situation, the stutterer is prevented from responding with maladaptive struggle to the stimuli produced by the *experience* of stuttering. He is prevented from avoiding or escaping this experience while at the same time he is being fed the therapist's approval which presumably he desires. Baum (1970) describes the use of such techniques as follows:

Response prevention or flooding is administered after the avoidance response has been learned, and it can be effective in eliminating the learned behavior. Response prevention consists of forcing the animal to remain in the presence of the stimulus or situation which it fears while avoidance responses are prevented or blocked. It can be likened to forced reality testing. . . . A frequent finding is that the avoidance response extinguishes very rapidly following a period of response prevention. (p. 227)

noise, questioning, being misunderstood, being asked to repeat, and other similar factors. Each stutterer has his own particular vulnerabilities and it is necessary for the therapist and stutterer to define what they are and to identify the ones for which desensitization would be most likely to produce therapeutic dividends. Usually we prefer to begin with a type of communicative stress which promises rather quick desensitization. Interruption, or the threat thereof, has often seemed to be one of these. Once desensitization to interruption has been accomplished, then we select some negative listener reaction which tends to evoke strong emotion. We rarely have to desensitize the stutterer to very many of these stresses, often only two or three, because we have found that the increased resistance to one stress seems to carry over or generalize to others of the same class. After a few experiences in desensitization it seems that the stutterer *learns* that he need not yield to listener pressure. This generalization effect is fortunate. We would hate to have to desensitize the stutterer to every specific disturbing listener reaction to which he is vulnerable.

Again we devise some appropriate hierarchies; again we make it possible for the stutterer, through repeated experiences at each consecutive level, to reduce his anxiety or orther negative emotionality until finally he is able to tolerate communicative stresses which formerly would have thrown him for a loop. We may once again illustrate with some case material.

One of our recent clients, an older woman, was especially vulnerable to direct *questioning*. She attributed her feelings of panic, which were highly consistent and vivid and quite independent of the nature of the questioner, to a series of early traumatic experiences at home and in school. "The moment someone asks me a question I go into a tailspin. Usually I can't talk at all or stutter hard but even when I don't I'm upset and all churned up. It's almost like terror. I know it's foolish to feel like that but that's how I feel." To hope to do effective speech therapy with such a client without using desensitization is unrealistic.

We therefore devised the following hierarchy: (1) Reading sentences (statements) dealing with early school and home experiences first silently, then whispering, then in unison with the therapist. Stuttering was ignored but this item was not accomplished until she reported little emotional arousal. (2) Completing unfinished sentences on the same material begun by the therapist. (3) Reading sentences, as in Step 1, but some of these were questions, and the proportion of questions increased. (4) Writing down and then reading questions to be answered by the therapist. (5) Reading questions devised by the therapist. (6) Answering the written questions. (7) Answering spoken questions by the therapist by writing her response, and later by reading it. (8) Answering the therapist's questions orally but only after a silent delay interval. She was not to answer until she felt relatively calm. (9) Answering questions put to her when she appeared before a group of other stutterers. (10) Answering questions from a university class of normal speakers. We were able to complete the program in six sessions (We should again mention here that other therapeutic activities were also taking place during these periods) and she was responding very well to the stress. Indeed, although we concentrated our effort solely on her feelings of panic, her stuttering also showed a marked decrease in frequency and severity. What is more significant, she finally became able to speak more fluently when being questioned than when making statements.

At the risk of belaboring our point, let us give one more illustration, this one dealing with desensitization to listener penalty.

Jack E. was a short, cocky, belligerent man who met one of our former cases after a fight in a bar on Guam during World War II. After leaving the service he came directly to our clinic and demanded to be fixed up pronto. Born in Alaska, cradled in half a whiskey keg, he was one of the toughest men we have ever met. When he stuttered, he exploded with frustration. Jack showed no word or situation fears. He talked and stuttered anywhere and to anyone. His negative emotionality was rage, not anxiety. He looked you in the eye and kept his fist cocked. He was always in trouble. Within the first two weeks, we had to bail him out of jail three times for hitting people. If only to keep from going broke, we had to use some desensitization. The one listener reaction Jack could not bear was any hint of mockery or amusement. When Jack stuttered, you smiled at your peril. He'd poke you in the nose, swiftly and most competently. We confess that we began the desensitization with some trepidation, mitigated to some degree by his evident affection for us. "You're a good little bastard, Doc!" he would reassure us repeatedly though we towered nine inches above him, and insisted that we were not little. "Ok, a big bastard but a good bastard, see?" We remember Jack with affection, and not only because he was one of our successes in therapy.

We structured the desensitization part of therapy carefully and made sure that he helped us do so and that he understood that much of his stuttering behavior was due to the explosive anger that flooded him when he got stuck. It would be a hard job to stop being so quick triggered but this is what had to be done. We began with desensitization to the feeling of being blocked rather than to listener reaction and after some difficulty this was accomplished successfully. Since we have illustrated this before, we shall not describe it now but turn instead to the subsequent program that dealt with listener amusement.

Fortunately, it was very easy to tell when Jack was becoming angry. First, a red flush would begin to creep up his neck. Then he would stiffen, his hands would clench, and his eyes would narrow. When his thumbs would begin to move against the fists, he had become consumed with fury and look out! An easy person to read.

The hierarchy we designed was as follows: (1) He was to smile and then laugh as the therapist stuttered in a fashion quite unlike that of his own abnormality. (This proved to be too difficult. Stuttering was no laughing matter to Jack. We had to back up and do our own smiling as we faked our stuttering before he could tolerate this first item.) (2) We took some snapshots of Jack smiling and had him look at the photographs when he was fluent. (3) He was to look at himself smiling in the picture whenever he stuttered in the therapy situation. Even this provoked some strong anger at first but by having him first look at the picture after the stuttering had passed and then moving forward to view it during a stuttering episode, he finally came profanely to accept the experience. (4) We provided a smiling picture of ourself to contemplate as in item three and made sure that we kept a sober clinical countenance while he was forcing himself to examine it. (5) We brought one of our better looking girl clinicians into the therapy session (Jack didn't hit women; he just cursed them) and had her smile at him, first during fluent and then during stuttered speech. This turned out to be of little desensitizing value because Jack and the girl turned it into a kidding counterconditioning session. (6) We made a tape loop of raucous laughter and the girl turned it on when Jack pointed to her. He first gave the signal during fluency and later during stuttering. We controlled the volume and duration of the laughter and made sure that both were reduced if the telltale signs of anger appeared. (7) Jack was to smile, first after he stuttered, and then during stuttering. (8) The therapist and Jack both smiled during stuttering. (9) The therapist laughed aloud and Jack smiled while stuttering. (10) Jack took part in a heckle session in which he instructed other stutterers and student clinicians to try to get his goat by laughing at him whenever he stuttered. (This proved more than he could take at first and we went back three items before trying it the second time.) Despite the barrage they gave him, this time he kept his cool and didn't turn a hair. He felt very good as he grinned after the experience. "Those #!!_____ bastards can't get to me any more! I've got 'em licked."

As we recall, this was a turning point in therapy. It is certain that the severity of his stuttering decreased remarkably as a result. How much carryover was there? Well, he had only one more fight during the rest of his stay with us and that was when he was drunk and it concerned things other than his stuttering. Though he returned to Alaska and his reports were sparse, in his file we have a letter three years later that thanked us not only for helping him "learn to talk" but also for teaching him to control his temper.

As we have said, we aim our formal desensitization procedures primarily at the three targets of confronting the abnormality, tolerating the fixations and oscillations, and resisting communicative stress and listener penalty. As we shall recount, we have also attempted to desensitize the stutterer to his word and situation fears but even when we have apparently succeeded, we have trouble with generalization. Far too often the desensitization effect seems limited to the specific word or situation—which helps only a little. It is possible, for example, to work up an elaborate hierarchy to desensitize the stutterer successfully to the telephone but we must remember that it is not the instrument which is the primary source of his emotional arousal so much as the anticipated listener reaction. Fortunately we have other tools, adaptation being only one of them. Moreover, fears of certain words or sounds diminish rapidly when the stutterer becomes able to tolerate the stoppages or repetitions and learns how to handle them when they do occur.

Counterconditioning

Desensitization is based upon extinction. When the stutterer is repeatedly exposed to stimuli that produce *weak* anxiety or other negative emotionally tinged responses, the latter will decrease and finally extinguish under appropriate conditions. The word *weak* is italicized since extinction occurs very slowly, if at all, when the anxiety, for example, is strong. This is why we set up hierarchies—to present first the stimuli which are near the edge of the generalization gradient, those which will evoke only a weak response. However it is clear that most desensitization procedures in stuttering therapy involve much more than simple repetitive exposure to unpleasant stimuli; some counterconditioning is also required. By this we mean that we try to link some other anxiety-inhibiting response to the same stimuli that usually evoke the anxiety. This is the principle of reciprocal inhibition. We seek to condition a competing response to threatening stimuli, a response which is antagonistic to negative emotionality. This is nothing particularly new. Mothers have probably caressed or fed or comforted their frightened children since the dawn of mankind. Reciprocal inhibition is certainly one of the common ways for reducing anxiety. It is found in the physician's bedside manner, in religion, in group membership, and a host of other human interactions. Relief and fear cannot sleep in the same bed.

In stuttering therapy we never escape the constant challenge of anxiety, guilt, and hostility as they are reflected in the stutterer's behavior. How successful we are as therapists depends directly on how well we deal with these features of the problem. Accordingly it is necessary that we remain constantly aware of the potential healing effects which counterconditioning possesses.

The therapist as a counterconditioner

There seems to be no doubt that the therapist's presence, his attitudes, and behaviors play a large part in this counterconditioning. He must structure the therapy situation so that when the stutterer experiences stimuli colored with anxiety or threat, the ensuing unpleasantness is less intense than he expected it to be, primarily because at the same time he is also responding to the warmth of the therapist's interest, approval, and companionship—among other things. The confrontation of his stuttering is not nearly so unacceptable when the therapist accepts it. When the stutterer's need to communicate is blocked by his closures and repetitive syllables, the resulting frustration occurs in the context of the therapist's vast fund of patience and lack of time pressure and he relaxes in spite of himself. Indeed he finds the therapist not only nonpunitive but actually inviting him to have these core behaviors. As Wolpe (1958) and others have shown, neurotic cats can unlearn their anxiety reactions if they are fed at the same time that stimuli formerly associated with the anxiety were presented simultaneously.

The stutterer has many hungers even stronger than that for food. He hungers for acceptance, for companionship, for a good listener, for hope, for guidance, and when any of these is

offered he feeds voraciously upon them. The therapist provides this "soul food" (as one of our cases called it) and does so at the very moment when the old anxiety evoking stimuli are being experienced. Herein lies much of the therapist's so-called art. We cannot doubt the undoubted effectiveness of some therapists' "magnetic" personalities or charisma. But there is no mystery here, no magic! The skilled therapist simply uses every possible means at his disposal to produce the reciprocal inhibition of his client's anxieties. He carefully feeds his stuttering cats when their anxiety is weak and then does it again at each successive higher step of a desensitization hierarchy. We wish to make it very clear that unless the stutterer does feed (does find in his interactions with the therapist the reliefs he hungers for) no counterconditioning will occur. Somehow, at the moment when the dread or frustration is upon him, the stutterer must also be experiencing other responses that are antagonistic to his fears or frustrations if the latter are to be weakened.

Assertive responses

One of the most appropriate therapeutic measures for overcoming the stutterer's approach-avoidance conflicts with their attendant anxiety is to mobilize more energy into the approach gradient. Anxiety is the father of ambivalence but the son of ambivalence again has the features of the parent anxiety. Most advanced stutterers get caught in the avoidance whirlpool, and every time they swirl around, the avoidance with its associated fear is strengthened. Strongly assertive behavior, as Salter (1949) has shown, can actively inhibit anxiety. Much of our own therapy is based upon this counterconditioning principle. We try to get our stutterers to stop avoiding, to stop postponing or being ambivalent, and to tackle the words and situations they fear. As models, we confront the problem assertively. We examine the behavior directly, hear it, look at it, feel it. We (both the therapist and the stutterer) seek out stuttering so that we can modify it. We go out of our way to look for the stimuli that trigger it. The listener who laughs, the one who rejects, are those we need. We help the stutterer learn to beat the disrupting stress of delayed feedback machine. We teach him to stutter on purpose. In a hundred ways, we employ assertive responses in our therapy—and we find that by so doing, the stutterer's speech anxiety decreases.

One of the best approaches we have found for teaching the stutterer to use assertive behavior as a countercorditioner to his fears is that found in Kelly's (1955) fixed-role therapy. In this approach, the therapist writes a personality sketch of an assertive, aggressive individual. This is then reviewed and revised in the joint interaction between the therapist and his client. Then the therapist models the role both in the therapy room and in a graduated series of real life situations. Next, the stutterer enacts the assertive role in a similar way. We do not exhort the stutterer to be assertive. We ask him instead to experiment, to try the new role on for size, first in the safety of the therapy session, then in carefully contrived situations, and finally to play the role continuously for several days in most situations. We have also used Moreno's psychodrama procedures to create on the clinical stage the kinds of situations that often pose the greatest threat to the stutterer (Lemert and Van Riper, 1944). Serving both as director of the roles to be assumed by the other partici-

pants and also as the assertive actor, the stutterer often finds that his communicative fears markedly decrease. The kind of interaction we also use in training the stutterer to be more assertive is clearly portrayed by Wolpe and Lazarus (1967):

While being trained in assertive behavior, patients are told to keep careful notes of all their significant interpersonal encounters and to discuss them in detail with the therapist. It is necessary to know the circumstances of the encounter, the patient's feelings at the time, the manner in which he reacted, how he felt immediately after, and his own subsequent appraisal of the situation. The therapist, upon identifying disabling inhibitions, firmly stresses assertive, as opposed to aggressive reactions, whenever applicable. Play-acting, of prescribed behavior, known as *behavioral rehearsal,* is often helpful. Where the patient's reaction is considered deficient or inappropriate, he is required to re-enact the incident while the therapist plays the role of the other person(s). The therapist may then switch roles and act the part of the patient, sometimes presenting a deliberately overdramatized picture of assertion, thus affording the patient an opportunity for learning adaptive responses by imitation. (p. 46)

Disinhibition

Certain stutterers, perhaps most of them, show much inhibitory behavior. They live constantly on guard, scanning for approaching trauma, holding back until the way seems clear ahead, and only then taking tentative steps forward—as though tip-toeing through rotten eggs. Stutterers need freedom from this constant burden of inhibition; assertive behavior is disinhibiting. That sad sack of an interiorized stutterer described by Freund (1966) and Douglass and Quarrington (1952) is caught in the moose-trap of constant inhibition. He needs to let go, to let fly, to act and speak spontaneously. We help him bang the gong, and when he does, his anxiety lessens. Others have criticized us as advocating an unduly heroic form of therapy, one far too demanding of courage which may not be there. But one can bang a small gong lightly at first, then move to a louder one—and there is some hero in every man. By using a desensitization hierarchy, assertive behavior can be developed. Indeed, one of the advantages of using assertive behavior to countercondition is that it is probably operant by nature. It has instrumental effects. By carefully scheduling the reinforcements, assertive behavior can be developed, shaped, and brought through self-talk under self-control.

Perhaps an actual report of some of this use of assertive behavior to countercondition anxiety would be illustrative here. The writer of this account, a very severe stutterer, 47 years old, and a very successful businessman despite his speech handicap, responded very well to this kind of therapy. Some excerpts from his account are as follows:

It was suggested that a new type of *strong assertive speech* should be initiated and used consistently, one that entailed feeling the tip and jaw movements, making a conscious effort to use increased volume (not to the extent of loudness), and slow and firm speech. These items represented the physical aspects of the new therapy. The change to strong assertive character or role entailed the following: *assertive action during any moments where anger, hostility, or resentment situations arose;* in other words, to express my feelings, no matter what they were, rather than retain the feelings; this was to be done regardless of results. As an example, while having lunch at the Pacific Club with my district manager and a fellow auditor, the waitress approached us as we were leaving and remarked to me that one of the local accountants (he had left earlier) wanted to know if all state employees took longer than an hour's lunch at nite spots where drinks were served. I told her to tell him "to go to hell" the next time he came in and to be sure to tell him that I had said so. My first feelings were those of anger and rather than hold in these feelings and say something nice or apologetic or make some form of explanation, I expressed my feelings loud and clear. In fact my district manager was somewhat surprised at my outward expression since I was normally easy going; he even tried to apologize for the accountant, but I told him it was none of the guy's damn business where I ate. The feeling afterwards was very good and I could feel my chest being thrown out and my head lifting.

For several weeks I had been auditing one of the large wholesale businesses in town. As auditor-in-charge I had two fellow workers assigned to assist me in the audit. These fellows were cooperative and followed instructions but many times they asked so many questions about auditing procedures and tax laws that I found myself constantly taking too much time explaining things. I resented their questions deeply. When I came in to work one morning, I gave the usual instructions and turned away; one of the fellows began questioning the procedure. I told him quickly just to do what I told him to do, that I did not have time to explain every detail to him, and besides I did not care if he understood or not. Needless to say, they both crawled into their shells and I had no more trouble. The branch manager at this business was one of those types that consistently made digs about the state and anything connected with it. Earlier during these times I had always acted as a self-appointed public relations man and tried to appease him and hold up for the state, so he had me on the defensive most of the time. During this present week at a coffee break, he began his usual griping, whereupon, I told him that he was wasting his time griping to me; rather he should gripe to his legislators or go back to Illinois where he came from. I was riled and he knew it;

he then became very apologetic, but I did not accept this. That same day I also had to jump at one of the women employees who made some digs about having to look up records, etc. I told her I thought she was being paid to work at the business by doing anything that she was told. I had no further trouble out of her. Heretofore, I had been firm and forceful at the outset of an audit, though when the taxpayers began questioning my decisions I always took excessive time in explaining the law to them and showing an apologetic feeling towards them in having to tell them that they were wrong in their tax applications. Using this new therapy I was beginning to feel that I did not have to take anything off of anyone, that I did not have to feel apologetic, and constantly feel on the defensive; I decided to put them on the defensive. I held an earlier than usual conference with the general manager so I could try out my new concept. At the outset of the conference I defined my role as an auditor for the state, auditing their records for taxes as requested by the state. Any pertinent tax laws would be explained. However, if they wanted to argue the case they would have to take it up with the state. With this approach I was able to put them on notice from the start that I would not take any guff and I was also able to put into practice the use of the strong speech, using slow and firm speech. With this new therapy I was also able to maintain good eye contact which heightened my effectiveness. Needless to say, I had no further difficulties at this business.

In the operation of my apartment-rental business it is necessary to make many telephone calls; to local servicers in regards such things as garbage, pest control, furnace repairs, etc., and to answer calls involving vacancies. This entails a great deal of talking and over the years I have depended upon my wife to handle the telephone calls, mainly because I have much more trouble talking over the telephone. As I progressed using strong speech I decided to handle my own telephone work. When someone called about an apartment I gave them the information myself and made all appointments to show the apartments. Recently, I started a pest control service for all of the buildings; this was all done over the telephone, giving the addresses and names of all tenants. The garbage service had been rather slow, so I called and gave the company hell, threatening to change service if they did not do a better job. Several calls were made to furnace repairers also. Over the years, as mentioned above, I would have relied on my wife to make the calls; calls that were sometimes made at her own pleasure. There was a great feeling of relief being able to handle the telephoning myself. One aspect proved very interesting; the more calls I made the less fear I had so that when I knew I had a call to make I just picked up the phone and made it, of course having a number of blocks but being able to use strong speech to pull out of them. And for the first time I did not care how the person at the other end felt; as far as I was concerned they just had to wait until I got the words out and while in a block my mind did not wander to their feelings, that is, how they were reacting to my stuttering; I just didn't care. This forceful and assertive attitude was very rewarding in that *I felt very calm* and much more secure. This feeling is in contrast to the usual apologetic way that I felt. And I stuttered very little.

Systematic desensitization using relaxation

We have intensively explored the use of relaxation as a counterconditioner to the stutterer's speech anxiety. We have employed both therapist-induced visualization of feared words and situations arranged hierarchically while the stutterer is deeply relaxed, and also graded presentations of actual speaking situations experienced *in vivo*. We have used relaxant drugs and hypnotic suggestion. Regretfully we came to the conclusion that none of these was useful in our stuttering therapy.

We say regretfully because the

technique at first seemed very promising. Moreover, a reduction in the frequency and severity of the situation and word fears could be produced immediately and with it an accompanying decrease in stuttering. The effect was so striking that we could not ignore it. Unfortunately, the effect was also temporary and transfer was most unsatisfactory. Try as hard as we could and using all the ingenuity at our disposal, we always failed to be able to train our stutterers to the point where they themselves could induce the necessary deep relaxation when situation or word fears raised their ugly heads outside the therapy room. No desensitization hierarchy that we could devise seemed to help them remain relaxed when they began to block. When they feared a word or situations (and all of them eventually did), or *if* they got stuck, they became tense. The speech anxiety reciprocally inhibited the relaxation. There were many times when we had hopes that certain stutterers, usually the more suggestible ones, would be able to maintain their lack of muscular tension under threat, but in the long run they always broke down. We found it incredibly easy to produce fluency through relaxation, complete freedom from any stuttering and occasionally (with our support) in situations that formerly had provoked much abnormality in speech. In a few cases, periods of fluency and without fears would last for weeks but always, sooner or later, the stuttering would return. When it did, it appeared in full force and as severe as it was before we began the systematic desensitization.

In the literature that we have reviewed in our chapter on relaxation therapies, the reported success rate of systematic desensitization using relaxation with stutterers was not impressive but some workers have evidently done a little better than we have. We cannot understand why we failed so abjectly. One possible explanation is that stuttering is not a monosymptomatic disorder and does not seem to be triggered by single sets of stimuli. Many responses are chained to many sets of stimuli and the sequences involved are often staggering in their complexity. Luper (1968) says in this regard:

A person in the act of stuttering encounters a large number of behavioral choice points. He may come up to a word and debate over whether to avoid it or to plunge ahead and attempt to use it (an approach-avoidance conflict). Once he has made one response, other stimuli and responses are set off, each having the potential of being reinforced. In a short time, he comes to another behavioral choice point—another place where he sees an option to his behavior—and again he sets off a chain of response-correlated stimuli. As I have been trying to point out, stuttering is an extremely difficult kind of behavior to describe in learning theory terms. It is very intermittent, it varies a great deal from one individual to another, and it appears to be a type of sequential behavior, consisting of many stimuli and responses, rather than an isolated event. (p. 88)

Or perhaps our use of systematic desensitization failed because there were just too many scenes to visualize and too many fearful speaking situations to order hierarchically. As we have seen earlier, Rosenthal (1968) had to design a hierarchy of 215 items for his stutterer and complains about the difficulty in constructing one. He also notes that just to achieve two successive "tension-free responses," as many as 17 presentations of the visualization were required. Moreover, in spite of all his work, Rosenthal never did eliminate all of his patient's anxiety or stuttering. We have experienced similar difficulties. Perhaps confirmed stutterers dare not live relaxedly in a world so full of stimuli that signal danger. To try to train them to be thoroughly relaxed as they run this gauntlet is perhaps a demand that they be psychotic. As Martin Palmer once said, "Who can be a rag doll in a steel world?"

We must also report in this connection that, though we no longer attempt to train our stutterers to be relaxed when they fear speaking or attempt to speak, we find that they actually become relaxed once our therapy had taken hold. As they learn to stutter fluently and without their old struggle and avoidance, their former tension states have clearly lessened. Perhaps this is the key: that relaxation should be a byproduct, not the tool, that it should come as the *result* of successful coping, not as an instrument for coping. Self-induced relaxation can only be produced by self-suggestion and, as the hypnotists have discovered, such suggestion has never been particularly effective in producing permanent relief from stuttering.

Pseudostuttering in desensitization

Speech therapists have employed the deliberate use of stuttering-like behaviors in their therapy for many years and for many different purposes. Here we discuss pseudostuttering, sometimes called "faking" by the stutterers, as a technique for producing anxiety reduction and for lessening the word and situation fears. The use of negative practice as a psychotherapeutic technique has had a long history. One of its first formulations was by Dunlap (1942) in his *beta* and *gamma* hypotheses, developed as the result of his observations that practicing errors in spelling or typing caused them to decrease. Various researches

by Fishman (1937), Case (1960), Meissner (1946), Fahmy (1951) and Sheehan and Voas (1954) on the use of negative practice with stutterers showed no consistently beneficial therapeutic effects when this technique was the sole vehicle of therapy. Some stutterers improved; others did not; some got worse. Much of the discrepancy in the findings was probably due to the kind of pseudostuttering used, or to how it was taught, or to the kind of stuttering behaviors exhibited, the "tonic stutterers" profiting less than those whose stuttering consisted primarily of syllabic repetitions. In accounting for the success in unlearning habitual errors, Guthrie (1935) felt that the real value of negative practice lay in its vivifying of the cues which lead to the error. To eliminate the seemingly uncontrollable responses, the person must become aware of the stimuli that trigger them. The relationships between the members of the response chain can be brought under control once they are perceived and one way of recognizing them is to practice them. Sheehan (1970) attributes the efficacy of voluntary stuttering to its substituting of an approach response instead of the usual avoidance one. Our own use of pseudostuttering, as will be made clear, is somewhat different. We employ it first in desensitization and later as a means of teaching the stutterer a fluent form of stuttering and both uses are only a part of a comprehensive therapy program. In the present context, what we want the stutterer to learn is that he can demonstrate and experience his communicative abnormality without becoming excessively emotional. We want him to feel stuttering in his mouth without having it trigger anxiety or revulsion.

Most advanced stutterers have made avoidance almost a career, developing very elaborate rituals to escape the revealing of their stuttering. Though the avoidance is only intermittently successful, its occasional success occurs often enough to maintain it. Unfortunately avoidance does nothing to weaken the fears. If anything, it strengthens them. If the telephone rings, and the stutterer refuses to answer it, fearing that he will experience listener rejection or personal frustration if he does so, that telephone will acquire an added increment of threat because he did avoid its signal. Avoidance permits no reality testing; as we have previously pointed out, the correlation between the amount of fear and the amount of stuttering is far from perfect. There always exists the probability that a particular listener might not be punitive or impatient, but the stutterer who avoids will never find out. Instead he generally tends to exaggerate when predicting noxious listener responses. He remembers the few listeners who were most cruel and uses these as representing all listeners. Accordingly, whenever he avoids successfully he feels he has managed to escape an experience that would have been highly traumatic. Avoidance is the pump of fear. We want to keep the stutterer from constantly pumping. Through pseudostuttering we can teach him that he does not always have to flee.

When we suggest that the stutterer employ pseudostuttering in desensitization so that he will not succumb to his usual compulsion to avoid feared words and speech situations, or so that he can bear its unpleasantness without struggling, we must make certain that the kind of stuttering he first assumes is not unduly traumatic. Usually simple repetitions or unforced short prolongations are the first kinds taught. Also, we make sure that he does his "faking" on nonfeared rather

than feared words and that he first practices inserting these fakes in nonfeared situations such as the therapy room, then gradually into other more fearful speaking situations. It is therefore evident that our use of pseudostuttering differs from the negative practices commonly recommended wherein the person is asked to duplicate as closely as possible the behavior he seeks to eradicate.

We feel it is unwise to ask the stutterer to display his abnormality voluntarily before he has become somewhat desensitized to it. Accordingly, we set up a hierarchy of experiences so that the kind of stuttering to be practiced voluntarily on the nonfeared words begins with behaviors quite unlike his own and only gradually are they programmed to resemble it. For example, we might use the following sequence: (1) Using the stutterer's characteristic behaviors, the therapist stutters to a certain listener as the stutterer observes to see how soon the listener responds by looking down or gives some other type of negative response. (2) The therapist stutters with easy repetitions of one, two, four, and six syllables, then with short to longer prolongations, then with various forms of avoidance or release reactions until finally he uses the kind of stuttering typical of the stutterer. As he demonstrates, the therapist remains calm and unaffected no matter what listener response is shown.[4] (3) Next, the

4 Bandura (1969) has summarized the literature concerning the vicarious extinction procedures used in these first two steps. He writes, "Vicarious extinction of fears and behavioral inhibitions is achieved by having persons observe models performing fear provoking behavior without experiencing adverse consequences (p. 175)." He reports numerous experiments with animals as well as humans that have shown the effectiveness of modeling in extinguishing fears.

stutterer attempts the same three sequential steps while the therapist observes. Always the pretended stuttering should be voluntary and on those words that the stutterer has previously declared to be free from word fear. If real stuttering occurs on other words, these are ignored for the time being. The task is to remain calm only on the fakes. As soon as emotionality does occur on these, the stutterer returns to an earlier step on the hierarchy, or the therapist demonstrates again that it is possible to manifest the behavior without emotional disturbance. This assumes, of course, that the therapist is capable of doing the pseudostuttering without also becoming emotional, but this can be achieved through training.[5]

Most of our stutterers have been able eventually to learn to remain calm while stuttering voluntarily on nonfeared words first in the therapy room and then later in the real world when we have desensitized them hierarchically in the context of our warm support. When this has been accomplished we follow the same procedures on the words they fear, strongly rewarding them for maintaining voluntary control of the abnormality they exhibit at each step of the sequence. Often at first the pseudostuttering on these feared words tends to turn into real stuttering but with practice they learn to control the uncontrollable, to be able to turn the stuttering on and off at will. These experiences have tremendous impact and are very meaningful to the stutterer. One of his worst experiences has been the loss of control over his behavior, the feeling that he has suddenly been seized by

mysterious forces that manipulate him and render him helpless. By deliberately assuming stuttering behaviors and resisting their automaticity, he directly attacks this vital feature of his problem. He becomes the master of his mouth and, if not the captain, at least the sergeant of his soul. As the success-failure increases, one can see the fears subside. He has deliberately held his mouth on the electrified grid and has found that he can bear it, that he need not panic. There is also an important spin-off since through these experiences he also learns that most listeners are not nearly so punitive or rejecting as he had thought. They evidently can bear stuttering and so can he. One of the most surprising discoveries this author ever made in his own self-therapy was that most of his listeners were indifferent when he stuttered. A few were bothered but the great majority simply waited for him to struggle through his blockages and then went their way. With some few exceptions, most were indifferent, kind or at worst mildly impatient. They could tolerate stuttering to a degree which astonished him and as a result of this reality testing through pseudostuttering the author found that he could tolerate not only his faked but also his real stuttering enough to start modifying it.

Assigned experiences in pseudostuttering are especially effective desensitizers when a pair or a small group of stutterers work alternately as performers and observers and have the opportunity to discuss what happened immediately. Often we have sent them out into the city to "collect" quotas of different kinds of listeners. One of our groups (four members) set their maximum goal as the collection of four hostile listeners, three laughers or smilers, and two permissive strangers as they stuttered voluntarily on a

---

[5] In this connection Sheehan (1970) says, "The Achilles heel of most normal speaking therapists who try to work with stutterers is simply that they are not willing to do what they ask their stutterers to do (p. 283)."

nonfeared word of the standard sentence: "Can you tell me where the railroad station is, please?" All in all they asked the questions of 30 strangers, finding only 1 hostile, 3 who smiled (but pleasantly, not mockingly), while all others had to be classed as patient and permissive even though the type of stuttering used was an unforced prolongation of the initial sound which lasted for approximately five seconds—a relatively long time.

Pseudostuttering as self-disclosure

One of the continuing traumatic experiences that afflict the stutterer and produce much anxiety is the threat of exposure. When he is not talking, he looks, feels, sounds, and smells like anyone else. It is only when he talks that he discloses himself as being different. A large share of his intricate strategies of avoidance is due to his desire to keep from revealing this deviancy. Jourard (1964), in his book *The Transparent Self,* has shown very clearly how much anxiety and emotional sickness can stem from the need to hide and cover up the features of the self that are unacceptable, and he insists that the way to health is through disclosure. This is far from being a radical idea. Most psychotherapies are based upon self-revelation in a relatively safe situation. What we wish to point out here is that when the stutterer deliberately exhibits that side of self, the stuttering side, by assuming on purpose the behaviors he has tried so hard and unsuccessfully to hide, a great relief is experienced. No longer need he spend his energies in pretending to be that which he is not—a full-time normal speaker. As Sheehan (1970) points out, he is a part-time normal speaker and a part-time stutterer. Through pseudostuttering the stutterer demonstrates his acceptance of his problem as a problem since he does it on purpose. The evils of denial, of self-alienation, are mitigated. By learning to stutter voluntarily, by disclosing this side of his being, his split self comes together. As Selye (1950) has shown, all sorts of human ills can stem from stress, and one of the most intensive stresses to which the stutterer is subjected is this need to hide his disorder. Jourard (1964) has a fine passage:

Every maladjusted person is a person who has not made himself known to another human being, and in consequence does not know himself. Nor can he be himself. More than that, he struggles actively to avoid becoming known by another human being. He works at it ceaselessly, twenty-four hours daily, and it is work. In the effort to avoid being known, a person provides for himself a cancerous kind of stress which is subtle and unrecognized, but none the less effective in producing not only the assorted patterns of unhealthy personality which psychiatry talks about, but also a wide array of physical ills that have come to be recognized as the province of psychosomatic medicine. (pp. 32–33)

Misuses of pseudostuttering

We find no utility in the indiscriminate use of pseudostuttering. It should be employed for a specific purpose, one well understood by the stutterer. We have found some stutterers using it to punish themselves masochistically or their listeners sadistically. Certain stutterers have revealed much of their basic personality dynamics by turning the assignment into listener torture, an assertive behavior that did decrease their anxiety temporarily. One of them only collected little old ladies and, refusing to go up the hierarchy, insisted on smearing them with prolonged, highly abnormal stuttering much worse than he ever had shown before. Though it was hard on his victims, his gleeful report turned finally into some real understanding of the sources of his hostility when the experience was subsequently discussed with his therapist. We do not advocate this practice, though we have experimented with it as another means of counterconditioning, simply because what these few stutterers gain in anxiety decrement they lose in increasing guilt. Similar insights result when the stutter uses his faking to punish himself. At times we have had the impression that the deliberate use of pseudostuttering brings to the surface many of the deepest needs for resolving interpersonal conflicts. Free stuttering seems to be as revelatory as free association.

Another variation in the way that certain stutterers misuse pseudostuttering is found occasionally in the deliberate assumption of the most exaggerated and ludicrous stuttering behaviors. These stutterers cannot even help laughing while they perform in this way and they often defeat the serious purpose of the assignment by so doing. Listeners react in three ways to the evident clowning: either they are offended at the put-on; or they laugh at, rather than with, the performer; or they are frightened, thinking that the speaker is crazy. Though humor and fear are antagonistic to each other, we have seldom found much lasting value in encouraging such behaviors. We have known some very sad laughing-stutterers, always quick to tell a stuttering joke, always smiling, apparently always gay. While these persons often gain thereby the reputation of being a jolly good fellow or pleasant companion, and manage to gain some fringe acceptance within groups by virtue of their humor, we have found in most of them a profound self-hate and revulsion for the comic role they have doomed themselves eternally to play. One of them told us how he greatly had despised himself when he had to call a physician to report a very serious injury to a friend and found himself compulsively laughing and joking as he gave the message. Another said, "I'm so tired of my smiling mask but it's the only one that has a hole I can talk through." One of them confessed that he could not bear his masquerade: "Oh it's a good trick all right. If I can get them laughing at me or with me or just laughing because I hee-haw, well then they won't hit me. Sometimes I almost enjoy seducing them with my fake happy disposition because then I'm on top and in control. But most of the time I despise them for getting sucked in and even worse, I despise myself for always playing the fool."

The conquest of self is no laughing matter. This does not mean, however, that we cannot use humor in stuttering therapy. Any competent therapist will use it often to allay anxiety, to reduce stress, to permit time for recovery when the stutterer's defenses collapse too soon or too completely, but we do not reinforce the stutterer positively when he uses pseudohumor in his pseudostuttering.

Although few stutterers greet the task of learning to stutter voluntarily with any alacrity, they become much more willing to insert pseudostuttering into their speaking when they discover that the payoff is very real. Often they find that the number and severity of their real stuttering behaviors decrease dramatically. As they become able to bear the faked stuttering without emotional upheaval, they find themselves less distressed when the "real" stuttering is experienced. They find themselves no longer avoiding as much and their struggles are less severe. They have become more desensitized.

Adaptation

Remembering that, because of his long history and practice of avoidance, the stutterer's fears have become unduly magnified and exaggerated, we have built into our program of therapy what some of our cases have called "the bath of stuttering." This flooding kind of experience seems to be most useful for those who are chronic avoiders, who spend their lives always dodging feared words and situations, for those whose existence is ruled by flight. It has no utility for the severe exteriorized stutterers who struggle from one word to another, plunging from one minor verbal catastrophe into the next. These poor devils live in the stuttering bathtub. But for those who are constantly using synonyms, postponement, and disguise whenever the remote possibility of stuttering exists, a period of constant stuttering can produce a surprising amount of anxiety reduction. Generally this experience is structured so that the stutterer must collect a certain quota of stutterings in a certain period of time and perhaps in certain specified types of communication. Again we use the hierarchic principle, designing the particular sequence of steps according to the stutterer's vulnerability, courage and so forth. A typical hierarchy for one week's bath of stuttering project ran like this:

First day, A.M.: You will collect 40 real or faked stutterings in reading aloud to a friend for five minutes (the friend does the counting). P.M.: You will collect 20 real stutterings (no fakes) before you can have your evening meal. (Use hand counter to record these.)

Second day: The basic assignment is to read aloud to your friend for a full hour, doing real or pseudostuttering on *each* word. This reading will be done in the afternoon, but one minute of that quota can be subtracted for every time you stutter (no fakes) during the morning period.

Third day: Collect 7 moments of stuttering and 13 pseudostutterings before you eat any breakfast; 26 real and 14 faked stutterings before you eat any lunch; and a total of 200 recorded stutterings of either variety before you eat the evening meal.

Fourth day: Do not leave your room until you have collected 50 moments of real stuttering while phoning. You may escape a repetition of this assignment this afternoon if you also can collect an additional 50 faked stutterings.

Fifth day: Collect a total of 500 moments of real stuttering before you go to bed tonight, writing down the word on which you stuttered, the time, and the situation in this notebook. Telephone me when you are finished even if it is late at night.

The whole week's project described above was designed by both the therapist and the stutterer jointly and undertaken with some understandable trepidation by the latter. He was afraid he could not do it, afraid that he would cheat, afraid that it would make him worse. He asked for additional motivation. "Tell me that you won't see me again for therapy until I do." We wondered if this was his way of terminating our relationship, but we acceded, primarily because he had said "until I do it" rather than "if I don't do it." We also asked for a daily conference late each afternoon where he could report his problems, achievements, and feelings. Much to his surprise and ours, he went through all the assignments, not without difficulty but successfully, though that last day he phoned us at midnight to tell us profanely and very fluently that he had finished his quotas. The cumulative effect of these experiences was very apparent from that time on. His fears of situations and words markedly diminished. Most of his avoidance tricks extinguished and a great spurt of progress ensued.

What actually occurs in this sort of saturation therapy to produce such a marked reduction in anxiety and stuttering? On the face of it, one would expect just the opposite result. It seems to be true that the more you stutter the more you fear, and the more you fear the more you stutter. But there are several important differences between this saturation program and the stutterer's usual situation. First of all, we are strengthening the approach and decreasing the avoidance gradients. Stuttering to some degree loses a bit of its old unpleasantness when each newly collected moment of stuttering brings the stutterer closer to fulfilling his quota which in turn leads to food, sleep, or therapist approval. It's hard to fear something you very much desire. As one of our clients told us over the phone early one morning, "Well, I've finished my quota and I'm going to bed, damn you. For two hours I've been going around to filling stations and bars trying to get those last few stutterings and you know something, it's been hard to get them. I've been wanting so much to stutter I can't. These last two hours my only fear is that when I talk to that cop on the corner, I won't stutter, not that I will. Strange . . . but listen to me now. I'm not even stuttering to you." For one of the first times in his life the stutterer is truly willing to stutter.

Many of the desirable effects of these therapeutic procedures may be explained as being due to conditioned inhibition. The strength of any habitual response seems to be momentarily decreased once it occurs and by massing these responses these reaction inhibitions can accumulate, thus eventually preventing the response. Moreover, it is possible to attach this inhibitory state to certain controlling stimuli, thus producing conditioned inhibition. In the language of the layman, you can finally become weary of being anxious or ashamed; you can stop avoiding out of sheer fatigue. An you can learn thereby to do both.

Also important is the stutterer's relief from the constant scanning for danger, from having to be constantly vigilant, from always having to avoid and flee. Many stutterers become very tired of always having to run away. Why constantly avoid, dodge, hide, disguise, and contrive endlessly? Our stutterers have almost universally reported that this rejection of avoidance is one of the dominant features of their therapeutic experience with us; they also report that the actual stuttering or listener reactions were not nearly as unpleasant as they had expected. Fear diminishes when it is not corroborated. When stutterers begin to realize how exaggerated and morbid their expectations have been, they come to recognize that they themselves are tougher than they thought, that no one dies of stuttering in a paroxysm of dysphemic pain. As the stutterer counts his blocks: "365, 366, 367" and "133 yet to go before I sleep," one more moment of stuttering hardly seems very traumatic. All this time, the old cues are being presented in a context of minimal anxiety and many of them without being followed by any stuttering as the stutterers testify with astonishment: "Over and over again I thought I would stutter but I couldn't." Deconfirmation is the best fear extinguisher man has yet discovered.

We have also used other forms of this saturation therapy to extinguish some of the fears of certain sounds. The stutterer reads orally a long passage of perhaps 45 pages, *doing pseudostuttering on every word,* a task which becomes very boring and irritating after a time. If, for example he especially feared words beginning with the *k* or *g* sounds, we would make a bargain with him that whenever he had real stuttering on any word beginning with these sounds, he could stop doing the pseudostuttering for the rest of the paragraph. Were stuttering merely an instrumental or operant response, one would expect that stuttering on such words would markedly increase, but this is not what seems to happen in most of our cases. They seek these words, hope that they will stutter on them, and are a bit disappointed when they do not do so, for then they must keep on pseudostuttering for what seems like an eternity. Since few stutterers ever consistently stutter on every word, and the adaptation effect usually causes a progressive decrease anyway, the stutterer discovers to his surprise that these feared sounds are not nearly as much to be feared as he had thought.[6]

Another approach requires the stutterer to collect and write down all words on which he had expected to stutter and did stutter upon during an entire morning or some other period. These, mixed with an equal amount of neutral words, then are typed and are underlined on the reading list. The stutterer reads them one by one through a public address system with strong amplification, pausing before each word to signal when anticipation of stuttering is experienced. The therapist turns down the volume for five seconds whenever an underlined word is stuttered upon but not if the stutterer stutters on one of the neutral words. Since he hates the very loud amplification, and is rewarded for stuttering on the words that he had feared and stuttered upon that morning by having the volume turned down, every time he sees one of those underlined words, he comes to hope that he might be able to stutter upon it. Often he finds that he doesn't, more often than not, and again the word fears are not corroborated and are less unpleasant. He is really being rewarded for stuttering on these bugaboo words and being mildly punished for saying them fluently, but most of our stutterers find that these particular words lose much of their fearfulness as a result of the experience.

An alternative and somewhat similar procedure is to turn the volume down or to insert masking noise on all words on which the stutterer signals that he expects to stutter. Since any stuttering which does occur is thereby muted and loses stimulus value, the usual correlation between anticipated severity and perceived severity is lowered. When one expects and anticipates unpleasantness and then does not experience the amount expected, the anxiety decreases. Much of the effect of masking in facilitating fluency in the stutterer is due to this presentation of danger signals (as rep-

---

6 Brutten and Shoemaker (1966) provide this pertinent commentary:

If an instrumental response is called forth infrequently and for short periods of time, then little or no conditioned inhibition will develop, and the minimal reactive inhibition will dissipate. On the other hand, if the occurrence of an instrumental response is massed over long periods of time, the patient will find it increasingly difficult or virtually impossible to continue to respond in this way. (p. 129)

resented by all the cues which signal approaching stuttering unpleasantness) and the prevention of the subsequent auditory perception of communicative abnormality. The Russian word for masking noise can best be translated as "muffling," a term that probably represents more clearly the diminished stimulus value of stuttering when heard under noise. We use masking noise in many ways in stuttering therapy but it can be used also in reducing the stutterer's word fears.

Nonreinforcement

Still another method for extinguishing specific word fears requires the stutterer to repeat certain words on which he stutters over and over again until he says each of them fluently and then to continue to say that word louder and louder until some criterion —perhaps three or five trials of consecutively fluent utterance—has been met. Not all stutterers show the adaptation effect in this repetition task and for them, this technique would be inappropriate but, for those who do (the majority in our experience), some very evident decrease in fear occurs on those words which have been worked over in this way. Often we structure the task hierarchically with the following representing one such sequence:

(1) Repeat the stuttered word instantly but repeat it only one time. Continue this until you can repeat it fluently. (This takes advantage of any reaction inhibition which might occur.) (2) Repeat it once instantly, then again after a short pause and fluently this time if possible. (3) Repeat the stuttered word fluently in *pantomime* one, two, three times, then say it aloud. (4) Repeat it in pantomime once then say it aloud fluently a specified number of times but slowly and deliberately. (5) After the moment of stuttering, do not repeat it until the therapist has given his suggestion that you will stutter severely every time you reattempt it, but then repeat it five times and try to show him that he is wrong. (6) After each moment of stuttering, tell yourself aloud that you will probably stutter severely if you try the word again, and then repeat it several times fluently in spite of your self suggestion.

As in the other use of hierarchies, if the stutterer fails on any step of the sequence, he returns to an earlier step and then works up the ladder. When the stutterer successfully accomplishes the final two items of the hierarchy, we find a marked decrease in the fear of that particular word and some generalization to other similar words.

Negative suggestion and flooding

This use of negative suggestion by the therapist and the stutterer himself can often produce some startling reductions in anxiety. We do not employ it however until we are fairly certain that the stutterer can resist it. What we really do is to present the kinds of negative self-suggestions characteristic of the stutterer's fears and we employ words and phrases which he has previously used to describe them along with our own improvisations. For example: "Though you've been able to make your phone calls pretty well of late, on the one I'm going to give you now, I bet you'll have a very hard time. You are to call my wife and tell her I won't be home for lunch. On the word 'lunch' you'll have your worst stuttering. You'll shut your eyes and lips like you used to do, force and then try unsuccessfully to jerk out like this. It will probably last even longer than the one I just showed you. See, already you're getting afraid. Your heart is pumping a bit faster. You're stiffening. You'll have a terrible block on that word. She'll probably have to say it for you. You'll be anxious and upset, etc." Note that the therapist's suggestions are deliberately exaggerated beyond his real expectations of the stutterer's performance. He really expects the stutterer to have very little trouble on that final word and he knows that *his* wife will not interrupt. Nevertheless some anxiety is generated in the stutterer by the suggestion and if, as expected, no stuttering occurs or much less than had been so eloquently predicted, the stutterer will find that anxiety deconfirmed. He will also do his utmost to prove the therapist wrong and usually does. Later on, he can give himself the same exaggerated negative suggestions, verbalizing them to the therapist, or to himself, and then subjecting them to test.

This technique bears some resemblance to the implosive therapy of Stampfl and Levis (1967) in which the therapist deliberately floods the patient with verbal cues evocative of anxiety in a situation where no unpleasant consequences are forthcoming. Hogan and Kirchner (1967) for example demonstrated that rat-phobic patients could be brought to pick up the animals after an intensive program of imagining scenes in which the subjects touched the rat, "having a rat nibble at their finger, or feeling one run across their hand. Then the rat might bite them on the arm. The S's might next experience the rats running rapidly over their body. The rodent could pierce them viciously in the neck, swish its tail in their face, or claw about in their hair. It might even devour their eyes. The S's might be told to open their mouths. Suddenly the rodent jumped in, and

they swallowed it. . . ." And so on. Flooding the subjects with the repeated evocation of anxiety-laden cues without unpleasant consequences diminishes that anxiety. What is more important in this flooding kind of negative suggestion is that the stutterer learns to doubt not only our own but his own self-suggestion of approaching misery. The reality is never as dire as it can be pictured, and rarely as unpleasant as he usually imagines it.

Response prevention

Much of the abnormality of stuttering consists of escape responses that have been conditioned to the experience of fixation or syllabic reverberation. The gross facial contortions, the head and body jerks, the sudden surges of tension, the gasping inhalations, and hundreds of other reactions were first used to escape, to interrupt, to terminate this distressing experience. The perception of his tense closures or blockade is very traumatic to the stutterer. So too are the tremors or runaway repetitions of syllables. Many therapists fail to recognize that these too are stimuli to which many instrumental responses are conditioned. If we can eliminate these coping responses we will have done much to reduce the stutterer's handicap. Our task then is to get the stutterer to experience these stimuli (those we have termed the core behaviors) and to prevent him from reacting in the old abnormal ways.

But how can we prevent the stutterer from responding by maladaptive struggle? It would seem that we have no barriers to place in his cage, no escape doors to close. Again we use the modeling approach and pseudo-stuttering. The therapist voluntarily throws his lips or jaws into tremor occasionally as he talks and asks the stutterer to signal when he can cease and continue. Then the stutterer tremors on nonfeared sounds of nonfeared words, holding these tremors until the signal for release is given. The stutterer is next asked to throw himself into a real block on purpose and to maintain whatever he is doing until the therapist gives the signal for termination. He is not to try to interrupt it, to jerk out of it, to do any of the things he usually does when he feels blocked, at least not until the therapist's signal has been given. The same procedure is used on the clonic "runaway stutterings." By gradually lengthening the duration of the core behavior by postponing the signal for release, the stutterer learns that he can tolerate it much longer than he had realized. He finds that the grid was not as hot as he had thought it would be; that it is possible to stutter without jerking or contortion. It is forced reality testing. Rachman (1966) states, "It has not been satisfactorily demonstrated that the immediate or rapid introduction of very disturbing stimuli is always or necessarily harmful. There are indeed cases in which the gradual chipping away of intricate and extended hierarchies present such a tiresome prospect that recourse to a quicker 'confrontation' has considerable appeal (p. 1)."

Adaptation with negative suggestion

We now describe another method that we have used successfully to diminish the stutterer's emotional reactions to the experience of stuttering. Again we begin by asking the stutterer to prolong a moment of *pseudostuttering* until we give the signal for him to terminate, usually while read-

ing a passage in which previously designated words are underlined. During the prolongation we verbalize as vividly as we can, and in his typical language, the sorts of feeling which he has reported his real fixations. For example, "Oh, God, I'm stuck again. I can't get it out. I can't get it out. I'm helpless. Will it never quit? Wonder what my listener is thinking? He's thinking, 'Poor devil. He sure stutters hard. Why does he have to make those faces? Wish he'd hurry and get it out. Oh, come on! I can't wait all day!'" And so on. We begin with comments which are fairly mild, then use ones which are specially vivid, even exaggerated. Even if we fail to verbalize exactly what the stutterer tends to feel, we come close enough to arouse some genuine feeling in a situation which is without actual penalties. As we have said in our discussion of pseudostuttering, the resemblance of these methods to those of implosive therapy is obvious though they were used in speech therapy many years before Stampfl and Levis (1967) described them. The basic principle is stated by Hogan and Kirchner (1967):

As the subjects become accustomed to experiencing intense anxiety in the absence of primary reinforcement (real occurrence of the feared stimuli), as they comprehend that nothing actually is happening to them, their anxiety to the imagery diminishes. This reduction of anxiety transfers to the actual feared stimuli, and fear conditioned to them extinguishes. (p. 106)

After we have done this for a time, we ask him to go through the same procedure but to prolong his *real* stutterings until we give the signal to terminate. We have found it wise to have a preliminary period in which we do not use any commentary; but merely train the stutterer to prolong beyond the probable duration of the actual abnormality. Sometimes we have him give a gestural signal when he thinks he might be able to say the word and then we delay our own signal for increasing lengths of time. This by itself seems to reduce much of the emotionality attached to the behavior. The stuttering behavior continues (until we give the signal) but the frustration is gone, because he now expects that he can say the word. If we can get the stutterer to experience his stuttering behavior without the attendant emotionality, we help him greatly. Many students of the disorder have failed to realize that stuttering is itself a stimulus. They see it only as a response to antecedent cues. But much of the emotionality in stuttering is linked directly to the behavior itself. We try very hard to get the stutterer to break this linkage.

After he has learned to prolong his stuttering behaviors beyond their normal course, we introduce our negative suggestion commentary as we did in pseudostuttering. We seek to generate some speech anxiety, frustration, and shame reactions concurrent with stuttering behaviors that he knows he can terminate at any moment. We withhold the signal to end the deliberately prolonged stuttering and to say the word until we discern that the emotionality has faded. The stutterer usually comes to resist and reject our negative commentary. By so doing, he also builds up barriers to his own negative self-suggestions of helplessness and deviancy. At any rate we have been impressed by the effectiveness of this flooding procedure.[7] One of our

cases said to us, "You know, at first you used to be able to get my goat when you kept talking about how terrible I was feeling when I was holding those blocks but then I got so it didn't bother me at all. And you know something funny? Lots of times when I'm in a real block, really stuck, I don't get worked up like I used to—almost feel calm and courteous." Later on we also use these procedures during the period prior to speech attempt with good success.

Adaptation to stress

Man, like other organisms, learns to adapt to stress. He can live in the Arctic, in the Sahara, and even in Kalamazoo, Michigan. We learn, by enduring and coping, to function reasonably well under a variety of unpleasant conditions. With repeated exposure, we come to tolerate smog and pollution until finally we hardly recognize it. We build buffers against a host of different noxious stimuli. If the combat veteran can learn to live with fear, cannot we hope somehow to use the adaptation principle in stuttering therapy? Is it not possible to build some tolerance to situation and word fears in these cases of ours? The blind learn to accept their lack of sight, the deaf their inability to hear, the crippled their limited locomotion or coordination. Why then does the stutterer remain so vulnerable?

One answer, of course, is that stuttering occurs intermittently and so he

---

[7] The contrast between these procedures and those of systematic desensitization is expressed clearly by Baum (1970): "Unlike 'desensitization therapy' where exposure to the fear stimulus or object is gradual and through progressive steps, response prevention 'floods' the animal with the full-strength fear stimulus for a protracted period of time (p. 197)." The efficacy of flooding therapy is usually explained in terms of Pavlovian extinction of classically conditioned fear responses or on the basis of the forced learning of new responses.

can't get used to it. The fears of stuttering come and go. We would suspect that were a stutterer to have no fluency whatsoever, his fears would diminish. He would adapt. Indeed we often see this adaptation in the surprising lack of word fears of very severe stutterers. If, then, it is the constancy of the unpleasantness which is crucial in building the adaptation barriers, we might be able to reduce the stutterer's fears by creating an environment in which communicative stress is the rule, not the exception. Our studies of stutterers who "spontaneously" recovered from their disorder without therapy indicate that, among other factors, one of the most important was that they found themselves in situations where they had to do a lot of talking, often under extreme stress. For example, one of them, deciding that fear was the cause of his stuttering, got a job (how he did so, we do not know) as a radio dispatcher for taxicabs. He said that at first he had great difficulty under the time pressure but within a few weeks was able to handle the communications effectively, and after about six months had cured himself. Another got a job as a house-to-house salesman and after great initial difficulty, found himself fluent. We have collected many similar accounts. Some stutterers do seem to have overcome their fears by repeatedly and consistently exposing themselves to communicative situations which produced strong fear in them.

Accordingly we have explored the use of similar methods in therapy with selected stutterers. Interestingly, we found that those stutterers who showed more than the ordinary amount of embarrassment, shame, and guilt seemed to profit more from jointly devised tasks which required them to enter a series of very difficult situations day after day for a two or three week period than did those for whom the stigma was not the dominant feature of the problem. Perhaps they were expiating their guilt, paying the penance for their stuttering or other sins. At any rate, we found that after entering these hard situations, all ordinary ones seemed to have lost their former capacity to elicit much fear. For example, one stutterer who underwent 52 consecutive job interviews, and stuttered severely in each of them, found for the first time no fear in class recitations and very little stuttering. "It's as though my fear yardstick is now about nine feet high," he reported. "I used to stutter badly whenever my fear was two feet high. Now it has to be seven feet high before I stutter. In most ordinary situations now it never gets up in that range. I'm just not afraid of them after all those tough interviews. They hardened me." Another stutterer gave himself the assignment of making phone calls, one after another and to strangers, for five hours a day for a week. We tried to convince him that this would be unwise but he insisted he wanted to find out if he couldn't "lick the fear of phoning" in this way. Using a hand counter he recorded all instances of stuttering and then plotted the curves. Each day showed an initial rise then decline but by the end of the week, a marked decrease in stutterings was demonstrated and he reported that most of his usual speaking situations generated little fear. "I've worn it down!" he commented. Some few specific situation fears remain pretty well extinguished but usually once the intensive adaptation period is over, they tend gradually to return. However, we have learned to take advantage of the time when the fears are of low strength to make real progress in modifying the old overt stuttering behaviors.

We have said that this adaptation training seems to be most suitable for those stutterers who view their disorder as especially shameful. At least they seem not to resist the stress adaptation experience as much as stutterers in whom anxiety is the most dominant characteristic, the stutterers who show much avoidance, and those who might be termed interiorized or masked stutterers. In general these latter cases do not seem to profit much from heavy doses of feared speaking situations, if indeed it is possible to get them to experience them. They already hurt too much to be hurt more. All that occurs when they enter very feared situations is the corroboration of their already exaggerated fears. With such a stutterer, we find we can achieve much of the same adaptation effect by setting up only a few stress situations, or even a single challenging situation, that the stutterer has always viewed as beyond his courage to undertake, one which he has always avoided. With the proper motivation, he may be able just for once to summon up all his courage and to enter it. Even though he may stutter severely, we have found repeatedly that merely entering such an experience can be a turning point in therapy. A great surge of pride suffuses the stutterer. For once, he finds he can stop running away and face up to his fear, that he can bear the stuttering and still survive, that he is tougher than he thought. The scale of situation difficulty can be altered drastically by even one such experience. To this sort of stutterer, the chronic avoider, situations that formerly seemed very difficult now appear easy by comparison.

For the self-punitive stutterer the use of such assigned adaptation experiences is contraindicated. The stutterer who regards himself with complete loathing because he stutters, or who is full of hatred for his listeners but dares not show it, may enter a program of consecutive hard situations solely to punish himself further. When anxiety and guilt have transformed themselves into self-hate, we find little advantage in asking such a person to whip himself harder. We have had stutterers who attacked such adaptation situations (and themselves) ferociously, almost reminding us of a bulldog we once had who chewed right through a porcupine. The more the dog hurt the harder it chewed. We find little healing in such activity.

Of course, such cautions are difficult to feed into the computer of clinical judgment. Most advanced stutterers show some hostility, guilt, and anxiety and we have no objective way of doing an assay on a specific stutterer to determine whether it is certain that he would benefit from this deliberate exposure to stress. Nevertheless we have made such judgments and have the illusion at least that we have been right more often than wrong. Some human steel must be forged in fire and no therapist should fear the heat if good can come from the processing. Some of the most significant gains made by our cases have come from what one of them called "this trial by fire." We would prefer to think of it in less dramatic terms, i.e., he who works hard with his hands first knows blisters and then calluses. Stutterers are a tougher breed than they appear. They have had to be tough to survive the trauma of living with a tangled tongue in an all too verbal world. They respect a tough therapist who has faith in their ability to endure threat but who will bind up their wounds, share their pain, and send them back to the fray again, yet never ask more of them than they can give. It is not easy to be a competent therapist with stutterers but if one becomes truly involved, the mistake in clinical judgment can be kept to a minimum. When they do occur, selah! So be it! To paraphrase Anatole France, if our hearts are pure, it doesn't hurt too much if our clinical hands occasionally become horribly red. Most of our cases forgive our occasional mistakes.

Eliminating other sources of anxiety

The clinician should not forget that the stutterer's fears of stuttering may be drastically reduced by solving some of the other personal problems that are generating negative emotionality in him. Into his funnel of stuttering, all of his other anxieties or guilts or hostilities seem to be poured and they emerge through the spout as fears of situations or words or sounds. If we can help him solve these other problems, help the stutterer get a job, help him find a girl, help him lose his isolation, or eliminate any other sources of what, in another book, we have called Pfagh, his stuttering fears will diminish. Often we can accomplish much more by working indirectly than directly on these fears. The more healthy the stutterer's emotional life, the less intense those fears will be. We are not saying that successful psychotherapy can wipe out all of the stutterer's verbal fears. They have been conditioned too specifically to let us hope for such an outcome. But we can at least try to reduce the overload of emotion, which, when it exceeds certain limits, overflows into disrupted speech. We who stutter must learn to live better lives than normal speakers if only so that we can keep from amplifying our stuttering fears. Even after we have learned to speak and stutter fluently, we cannot afford to let other sources of guilt, hostility, or anxiety convert themselves into precipitants of stuttering. Sad as the prospect may seem, we must deny ourselves the human privilege of wallowing in the muck of sin and folly. If we do, then we pay the price in fear and in stuttering. If there is any injustice involved in having to be a stutterer and to be fluent in spite of stuttering, it is in this denial of the right to live foolishly. This author has always resented this constraint.

Reassurance

We must not forget our childhood experiences with anxiety and the reassurance given us by our parents that we need not be afraid of the dark or of thunderstorms or the things that go thump in the night. Just the presence of a loving, powerful protector allayed our fears. Anxiety decreases when one knows he is not alone. If that parent were not afraid, and if we could cling closely, all was well. Thorne (1950) long ago pointed out that direct verbal reassurance by strong, significant persons with whom the client can identify should not be discounted as having no value in diminishing fear. But all reassurance need not be verbal; it can be communicated in many other ways. Doubtless some of this reassurance occurs in all successful therapy. The placebo effect of doing anything about one's problem, anything at all, owes much to its inherent reassurance. When the therapist, as a model, shows that stuttering can be tolerated or demonstrates that the stutterer's fears have a substantial fraction of exaggeration in them, the latter's anxiety goes down. Long ago we wrote this:

As in the psychiatric relationship, the patient is assured that the therapist is sharing his experience and can bear it. The therapist may also stutter and share the case's feelings of ambivalence, of anxiety, of struggle, but with the basic difference of objectivity and the attitude of problem solving. He will be with the case in his struggle for mastery of a tangled tongue and an unruly self. He will be able to touch the snake and thereby demonstrate that it is touchable. With the therapist by his side, the case can come to scrutinize the moment of stuttering without upheaval. (Van Riper, 1955)

We never give our stutterers any false reassurance. We promise them no quick and easy cure. We do not poohpooh their fears or tell them that they are unsupported. We do not brainwash them through suggestion. What we do give them is our dedicated concern for their welfare. They know that they are no longer alone and this special kind of reassurance is one of the most potent attenuators of negative emotion ever invented.

The anxiety reduction effect of modifying stuttering

Finally, we wish to stress that the best way to reduce the stutterer's fears and other negative emotion is to help him learn a new way of stuttering that will not evoke those penalties and frustration that are the main sources of his distress. All we have written heretofore in this chapter has been designed to facilitate *this* learning. If our cases can stutter easily and without pain, ache, or frustration; if they can stutter and still be fluent and unabnormal, they will have little rea-

son to be afraid or ashamed. As a rat finally perceives that the grid that formerly was electrified no longer shocks him, that the cues that signified sudden misery no longer do so, it no longer jumps spasmodically or freezes in a tense immobile posture in the floor of the cage. True, this learning to stutter fluently is a difficult learning task. So much more then do we need first to desensitize the stutterer as much as we can. He comes to us full of anxiety and shame, unable to confront his problem, disguising it, avoiding contact with it. Through a preliminary period of desensitization we calm him and gentle him enough so that he can do this new learning. And as he realizes he is coming to grips with his problem and making progress, his morale goes up and his fears go down. And so does his stuttering.

Bibliography

BANDURA, A., *Principles of Behavior Modification*. New York: Holt, Rinehart & Winston, 1969.

BAUM, M., Extinction of avoidance conditioning through response prevention, flooding, *Psychological Bulletin*, 74 (1970), 276–84.

BRUTTEN, E. J. and D. J. SHOEMAKER, *The Modification of Stuttering*. Englewood Cliffs, N.J.: Prentice-Hall, 1966.

CASE, H. W., Therapeutic methods in stuttering and speech blocking, in H. J. Eysenck (ed.), *Behaviour Therapy and the Neuroses*. London: Pergamon Press, 1960.

DOUGLASS, E. and B. QUARRINGTON, The differentiation of interiorized and exteriorized secondary stuttering, *Journal of Speech Disorders*, 17 (1952), 372–88.

DUNLAP, K., The technique of negative practice, *American Journal of Psychology*, 55 (1942), 270–73.

FAHMY, M., Stuttering, *Egyptian Journal of Psychology,* 3 (1951), 399–404.

FISHMAN, H. C., A study of the efficiency of negative practice as a corrective of stuttering, *Journal of Speech Disorders,* 2 (1937), 67–72.

FREUND, H., *Psychopathology and Problems of Stuttering.* Springfield, Ill.: Charles C Thomas, 1966.

GUTHRIE, E. R., *The Psychology of Learning.* New York: Harper & Row, 1935.

HOGAN, R. A. and J. H. KIRCHNER, Preliminary report of the extinction of learned fears via short-term implosive therapy, *Journal of Abnormal Psychology,* 72 (1967), 106–9.

JOURARD, S. R., *The Transparent Self.* New York: American Book Co., 1964.

KELLY, G. A., *The Psychology of Personal Constructs.* New York: Norton, 1955.

LANG, P. J., A. D. LAZOVIK, and D. J. REYNOLDS, Desensitization, suggestibility and psychotherapy, *Journal of Abnormal Psychology,* 70 (1965), 395–402.

LANYON, R. I. and MANSEVITZ, M. Validity of self-reported fear, *Behavior Research and Therapy,* 4 (1966), 259–62.

LEMERT, E. M. and C. VAN RIPER, The use of psychodrama in the treatment of speech defects, *Sociometry,* 7 (1944), 190–95.

LUPER, H. L., An appraisal of learning theory concepts in understanding and treating stuttering in children, in H. H. Gregory (ed.), *Learning Theory and Stuttering Therapy.* Evanston, Ill.: Northwestern University Press, 1968.

MAHL, G. F. and G. SCHULTZE, Psychological research in the extra linguistic area, in T. A. Sebeok (ed.), *Approaches to Semiotics.* The Hague: Morton, 1964.

MEISSNER, J. H. The relationship between voluntary non-fluency and stuttering, *Journal of Speech Disorders,* 11 (1946), 13–23.

RACHMAN, S., Studies in desensitization: Flooding, *Behaviour Research and Therapy,* 4 (1966), 1–6.

ROSENTHAL, T. L., Severe stuttering treated by desensitization and social influence, *Behaviour Research and Therapy,* 6 (1968), 125–30.

SHEEHAN, J. G. and R. B. Voas, Tension patterns during stuttering in relation to conflict, anxiety-binding and reinforcement, *Speech Monographs,* 21 (1954), 272–79.

SHEEHAN, J. G. *Stuttering: Research and Therapy.* New York: Harper & Row, 1970.

SALTER, J. M., *Conditioned Reflex Therapy.* New York: Creative Age Press, 1949.

SALTER, A., *The Case Against Psychoanalysis.* New York: Holt, Rinehart & Winston, 1953.

SELYE, H., *The Physiology and Pathology of Exposure to Stress.* Montreal: Acta, 1950.

STAMPFL, T. G. and D. S. LEVIS, Essentials of implosive therapy, *Journal of Abnormal Psychology,* 72 (1967), 496–503.

THORNE, F. C. *The Principles of Personality Counseling.* Brandon, Vt.: Journal of Clinical Psychology Press, 1950.

TRUAX, C. B. and R. B. CARKHUFF, *Toward Effective Counseling and Psychotherapy.* Chicago: Aldine-Atherton, 1967.

VAN RIPER, C., The role of reassurance in stuttering therapy, *Folia Phoniatrica,* 7 (1955), 217–22.

————, *The Nature of Stuttering.* Englewood Cliffs, N.J.: Prentice-Hall, 1971.

WOLPE, J., *Psychotherapy by Reciprocal Inhibition.* Stanford, Calif.: Stanford University Press, 1958.

———— and A. A. LAZARUS, *Behavior Therapy Techniques.* New York: Pergamon Press, 1967.

Modification

We are now ready to work directly on the shaping and modification of the stutterer's abnormal responses to the fear or perception of disrupted fluency. We seek to teach the stutterer that it is possible to stutter and yet to be very fluent. We want him to learn that he need not yield helplessly or avoid or struggle aimlessly when he anticipates trouble or finds himself fixated or oscillating. We want him to realize that he can change his old maladaptive reactions into adaptive ones, that he is responsible and accountable for the kind of stuttering he exhibits, and that there are better ways of stuttering than those that have tyrannized him in the past. We hold out to him the vision that it is possible to stutter fluently and that if he can learn to do so, there will be no need to fear or avoid speaking. We insist that he can learn to stutter without forcing or struggling and that then he will know little frustration or listener rejection. We remind him that he has already collected and identified many of these easy, unforced stutterings. It is now time to learn how to use them deliberately.

Since to many therapists and stutterers this view that stutterers must be taught to stutter seems strange, perhaps we may be permitted the inclusion of a personal anecdote that changed this author's whole life. Once, while hitch-hiking on a back road near Rhinelander, Wisconsin, he was picked up by a very old man in an old car. Though the old fellow was very fluent and garrulous, he spoke in an unusual way with many little jerky prolongations of the first sounds of his words, as he talked about the weather and such. Finally he ceased his monologue and asked the author a whole barrage of questions. We remember stuttering terribly as we tried to answer them, even flailing around in the car with body contortions. The old man began to laugh outrageously and so interminably we almost hit him. Finally recognizing our furious anger, he suddenly stopped and said, "Now take it easy, son. Take it easy. I know how it is to stutter like you do. That's why I was laughing. It's crazy to stutter like that but when I was your age I used to spit and sputter and jerk and stutter just the way you're doing. But no more! I'm too old and too tired to stutter hard any more so I don't. I just stutter and let them leak out." For the rest of that ride and for hours afterward, the author was in a daze of revelation. All of his life he had been trying to talk without stuttering and the more he tried the more he had failed. The old man had by chance found out how to stutter without struggling. It was incredible but it was possible to stutter and yet to be very fluent. Even now, after almost fifty years, we remember the vividness of that insight, that flash of bright light in the darkness of despair. And we recall our immediate vow not to wait until we too were too old and too tired. We would start right away to try to learn the old man's way of easy stuttering—and even to improve it. This we have done. We know personally and professionally that it is possible to learn to stutter with a minimum of interruption and abnormality, and that when the stutterer learns to do so, most of his troubles disappear.

This is not to say that the task is an easy one. Avoidance and escape behaviors acquired by the stutterer over the course of many years do not extinguish easily. No token therapy will change them. We have found that only a concerted all out attack is required, a total push. We must not only decondition old learned responses: we must also change the ways the stutterer perceives himself and others; we must help him revise his strategies for coping with the threat and experience of interrupted communication; we must even alter his attitudes and thinking. The stutterer must be changed as well as the stuttering. This set of "musts" looks so incredibly demanding that successful therapy with the adult stutterer would appear almost impossible. Yet we, like other therapists, have been successful with many of these individuals perhaps only because these stutterers came to us desperately seeking relief from the tyranny of their fears and frustrations. Given half a chance, the body, mind, and soul will heal themselves. In each of us, no matter how troubled we are, the potential for favorable change always exists. Changing oneself is hard but it is easier than trying to change all of the world. Given a therapist who hungers to help and knows what to do, even the most formidable obstacles to change can be overcome by a determined stutterer and a dedicated therapist.

Variation

In this phase of the sequence of stuttering therapy the hallmark is *change*. Somehow we must help our stutterers to free themselves from their *stereotyped* patterns of behavior. Fear, frustration, shame, and hostility, the four shadows that follow stutterers wherever they go, all tend to create constraints and these produce constant limitations on freedom of choice. Anyone who has worked intensively with many adult stutterers will recognize this picture. To protect themselves, stutterers walk with extreme care through the mine fields of a communicative world. As the years pass by, the constant inhibition and excessive vigilance result in a progressive narrowing of their repertoire of responses to a wide variety of stimuli. Few adult stutterers know how many options they really possess. For years they have lived restricted lives, imprisoned by the defenses they have erected to fend off threat and hurt. These constraints affect not only the speech of stutterers but also their thoughts, attitudes, and interpersonal relationships. Somehow we must help them to get out of their ruts, to know how many choices they really have.

Unfortunately for both the therapist and his client there seems to be a built-in reluctance to change. Neale Miller (1964) says, "One of the most striking features of the human personality is its ability to maintain what might be described as psychological homeostasis in the face of many vicissitudes (p. 161)." We cling to the familiar even if it is unpleasant. Somehow its evils seem less threatening than those of the unknown. Our stutterers are miserable but they know their misery and have been able to endure it. When we formulate therapy as the exploration of new ways of behaving and feeling, we find not only the lag of inertia but often active opposition. Eric Hoffer writes, "It is my impression that no one really likes the new. We are afraid of it. It is not only as Dostoyevsky put it that 'taking a new step, uttering a new word is what people fear most.' Even in slight things the experience of the new is rarely without some stirring of foreboding." [1]

Another source of the resistance to change may lie in Huygen's Principle —that a system reacts to a disturbance in such a way so as to minimize that disturbance. This ancient homeostatic view finds modern representation in

1 Hoffer, E., *The Ordeal of Change*. New York: Harper & Row, 1968, p. 1.

congruity theory (Osgood and Tannenbaum, 1955) and Festinger's (1957) *cognitive dissonance* formulation. Basically, these positions hold that a person's beliefs about himself and his world are organized into a consistent system. His behavior should be congruent with his beliefs, and consistency is the glue that holds the system together. Each stutterer has his own system of beliefs about himself. For example, one might be that he must constantly protect himself against verbal dangers; another that he cannot answer the phone; another that he is helpless or cowardly. Unpleasant as these self definitions may be, they form a consistent system. As Shakespeare wrote, "A poor thing but mine own!" In the confirmed stutterer, the disorder permeates all of his being. He builds himself, his system of beliefs and social attitudes about it. Any challenge to that system, any invitation to change it creates dissonance and incongruence and is therefore rejected.

Accordingly, we begin, not by immediately trying to modify the stuttering behavior itself, but by first trying to introduce some modest changes into the stutterer's usual mode of living. The basic goal of this phase of therapy is variability. In our individual conferences with the stutterer we discuss the rationale for exploring and experimenting with new ways (not necessarily better ones) of behaving, thinking, and feeling and then we invite him to formulate specific assignments which might implement these changes.

The exploration of self

The goal of these first assignments is designed to help the stutterers to recognize the way they characteristically behave, to identify the idiosyncratic patterns of thinking, feeling, and acting which comprise their identities and styles of living. Among some of the experiences they have designed, undergone, and reported are these. They have silently watched themselves in a mirror for an hour at a time alone—often a devastatingly revealing experience—and then reexperienced it again for another hour but this time with verbalized self-commentary. They have watched films and videotapes in which they were shown sitting, walking, talking, eating food, or reading a book. After they had recorded their autobiographies they have listened to them not once but several times, usually adding supplementary or evaluative comments into the microphone of another recorder. They have explored their study habits, their diurnal rhythms, scrutinized how they ate, and slept, and combed their hair, even how they looked and acted when intoxicated. They made collections of their reverberatory negative thoughts and recurring unpleasant memories. They studied their habitual postures, their responses to startle and interruption or demand. They explored their role-taking behaviors. In this account we have given only a glimpse of the variety of the exploratory tasks designed by different stutterers and it should be obvious that their planning and reporting provided a useful vehicle for psychotherapy. Nevertheless, our major aim at this time has been primarily to produce an analytical self-awareness of the things the stutterer might be able to alter. If we wish to effect some changes, we must know what can be varied.

Varying behaviors

Our next set of therapeutic experiences are those in which the stutterers deliberately *vary* the habitual patterns which they have previously identified. They call these self-assigned tasks "rut breakers." One group of such assignments deals with changing some facet of the body image. Thus some of the stutterers have grown beards, changed their coiffeurs, purchased and worn hats or ties that ordinarily they would never have considered owning. Some have even changed the way they walked; habitual body postures have been altered. Assuming different facial expressions for a morning or two, they explored their own responses and those of others to the difference. Other tasks found them using different gestures, new tones of voice, new inflections. (One stutterer discovered 16 different ways of getting out of bed in the morning!) They tried new foods; they made new acquaintances. Seeking unusual patterns of living, they explored new activities; they visited places where they had never been before; they took new routes even to and from the clinic. They whistled as they walked, occasionally breaking into song and, as one of them said, "to hell with the person who wonders why." They surprised their friends—and themselves.

Role playing

In effecting change, one of the therapist's important tools is role playing. Janis and King (1954), Harvey and Beverly (1961), and Janis and Gilmore (1965) have shown that role playing can significantly alter the *attitudes* of the person assuming the role, and since attitudes tend to influence behavior, role playing should be a useful aid for the clinician. Other research (Wolpe, 1958; Sturm, 1965; Lazarus, 1966) has shown that role playing, termed *behavior-rehearsal* by Lazarus, (1963), can indeed change characteristic behavior patterns. Speech therapists have been using these methods for a very long time. In another article, Lazarus (1965) describes how he trains his patients to do this behavioral rehearsal, a procedure remarkably similar to our own:

In this method patient and therapist role-played various scenes which posed assertive problems for the patient . . . expressing disagreement with a friend's social arrangements, asking a favor, upbraiding a subordinate at work, contradicting a fellow employee, refusing to accede to an unreasonable request, requesting an increment in salary, criticizing his father's attire, questioning his father's values, and so forth. Commencing with the less demanding situations, each scene was systematically rehearsed until the troublesome encounters had been enacted to the satisfaction of the patient and therapist. The therapist usually role-played the significant persons in the patient's life according to description provided by the latter. The patient's role was shaped by means of constructive criticism as well as modelling procedures in which the therapist assumed the patient's role and demonstrated the desirable responses. (p. 82)

In the group meetings during this phase, role playing was encouraged and we often put on psychodramas in which the stutterers in turn served to set the scene and direct the action. Most of these concerned old traumatic experiences or difficult situations that they were anticipating. One of the latter, which we very vividly recall, dealt with the stutterer announcing to his prospective father-in-law that his daughter had agreed to marry him. Another rehearsed the asking of his employer for a raise. In this stage of therapy, we have even had professional actors coach our stutterers in assuming new roles. One group invited an instructor to teach them modern dance, so the stutterers could learn new movements. The stutterers would also observe strangers in a variety of situations and then imitate their behaviors before the group. In their "Guess who?" group objects they even caricatured their therapist, each other, and themselves. Trojan's (1965) kinetic discharge therapy, in which the stutterer acts out and verbalizes his basic feelings toward the significant persons in his past and present, proved highly useful at this stage. In this experimental role playing some of the stutterers resorted to caricature and burlesque to escape any real identification and they insisted on playing only those roles which enabled them to do so. Others initially rejected the whole project. Some played the parts only superficially. These reactions, of course, are the reflection of the resistance to change that all of us show. Like most new shoes, most new roles are not very comfortable at first. Truax and Carkhuff (1967) describe their encounter with these problems in their attempts to train professional psychotherapists through role playing and say that the difficulties are usually temporary. Most of our clients manage eventually to overcome their resistance to this sort of change, though often we have to help them by setting up a hierarchy of roles which can increase their tolerance. There are always certain costs to be paid in taking on a new role. Thibaut and Kelley (1959) in this connection state, "It is fairly apparent that no person should perform a role that overloads his perceptual or motor capacities. This is ultimately a matter of minimizing costs, since these costs probably rise sharply as the limits of a person's abilities are approached (p. 278)."

Most therapists who have had to work with confirmed adult stutterers have been struck by their behavioral rigidity. They tend to play one role exclusively—the stutterer's role. They need some taste of freedom and spontaneity; they need to explore other ways of living, other roles. Cameron (1950), a sociologist, speaks to this point:

. . . the member of any organized society must develop more than a single role, or role behavior, if he is to reciprocate and cooperate effectively with his fellows. To the behavior pathologist, this implies further that the person whose repertory includes a *variety* of well-practiced, realistic social roles is better equipped to meet new and critical situations than the person whose repertory is meager, relatively unpracticed and socially unrealistic (p. 465).

Training in role enactment does seem to free stutterers to a remarkable degree. Moreover, it has its own built in reinforcement, since stutterers often speak much more fluently when playing some other part. And they become more spontaneous, less constrained. As Sarbin and Allen (1968) say, "Spontaneity occurs more often, and is approved more often, in the course of valid role enactment than one might at first assume (p. 503)."

Attitudinal change

The stutterers did not confine their variation activities to their overt behaviors. In our individual conferences they reported instances in which they had deliberately shifted from one mood to another, from depression to exhilaration, or the reverse. They experimented with attitudinal changes. One stutterer who could not bear a certain girl made a point of cultivating her despite the fact that she bored him silly. He wined and dined her and reported, much to his surprise, that even stupidity had its fascination.

Another, a black student, made a valiant effort to change his violent hatred of whites by seeking them out as companions.

Having previously recognized the reverberatory thoughts and recurring memories and negative autosuggestion to which they were prone, the stutterers now attempted to alter this thinking, first expressing the thoughts aloud to someone else and then formulating competitive thoughts and memories. Here we helped them by elucidating and applying Albert Ellis' (1962) rational psychotherapy procedures so the stutterers would not fall into the superficial traps of Norman Vincent Peale or Coué. They accordingly experimented by trying to think only negative thoughts for a day, or to spend another day deliberately brooding over their wrongs. One of our groups devised "Paranoia Day" during which they would be suspicious of everything and everybody until the evening meeting when they hilariously pooled and shared their experiences. These few illustrations are far from encompassing all the ingenious and significant ways in which the stutterers attempted to modify their usual patterns but perhaps they help make the process clear. The most important thing the stutterers learned was that it was possible to change.

Varying the stuttering behaviors

In seeking to change the characteristic forms of the stuttering itself the first targets of our attack are the anticipatory behaviors, especially the habituated postponement and avoidance reactions to the immediate threat of stuttering. We have found that these are more easily varied because they are already highly variable. Moreover, they appear apparently to be more under the stutterer's control than the core behaviors or escape reactions. In their habitual form the postponements and avoidances represent old strategies for preventing the appearance of stuttering, strategies that once were highly conscious and voluntary. Though they have often become highly automatized in the adult stutterer, they seem to be more vulnerable to deliberate alteration than the other behaviors.

Since the stutterer by this time has already done considerable work in identifying his stuttering behaviors and knows how he postpones the speech attempt or avoids feared words or situations, we can proceed directly toward the goal of varying these reactions. Again in our conferences we also plan the assignments jointly, structuring each in terms of maximum and minimal performances. Often the therapist needs to offer suggestions concerning the kinds of experiences to be undertaken but we have always made sure we gave more than one suggestion so that the stutterer had to exert some responsibility for choosing the one he preferred. (And we would usually challenge him to devise a better activity than those we had described as possibilities.) Here again we resort to the modeling approach. We demonstrate once again that we can and will do anything we ask of the stutterer. When he finally has made his choice and has set up the maximum and minimum criteria we then discuss his reasons and reluctance.

To show the dynamics of this interaction we might provide an example:

One of our stutterers had shown very little initiative in his self-therapy up to this point. He had alternated between being completely passive or sullenly resistant. Always he insisted on setting his minimum goals close to zero performance. He did as little as possible and we suspected that in his reports he often lied about what he had done outside the clinic. His most characteristic stuttering abnormality consisted primarily of long series of "ah-ah-ah-ah-ahs," used to postpone the speech attempt on his many feared words. Often this continuous ah-ing, however long it lasted, failed to prevent the actual stuttering tremors. Sometimes he did manage to wait them out but usually they appeared as soon as he finally did begin to make the direct speech attempt. The tremors and fixations rarely lasted more than a second and the great bulk of his speaking disability consisted of the habituated postponement device. It was obvious that if this ah-ing could be modified or discarded, only a very minor abnormality would remain.

Accordingly, in our planning conference, we had the stutterer listen to some recorded samples of his speech and then asked him what he might do to vary the constant "ah-ah-ah-ing." Somewhat surly, he refused. So we gave him three suggested ways that other stutterers had used to alter their similar postponement behavior: to deliberately vary the duration of the component ah's in the sequence; to begin with ah but change to oh or oo; or to vary the loudness of the ah's. Again we asked him if he could not invent a better way. No! Then what choice would he make of those we had suggested? "I'll choose the last one and vary the loudness and my maximum goal is ten for the day and my minimum goal is just one." We nodded acceptingly. "OK, now why did you pick that assignment and why did you set your minimum goal so low?" we asked. "Do you think you can achieve the ten per day you set as a maximum?" We are certain that we were permissive and accepting and that no note of sarcasm appeared in our voice. We can be patient. We can wait. We knew that eventually this stutterer would begin to move. We were therefore a bit surprised by the torrent of emotion that poured forth. It went about like this:

"Oh damn you, damn you, damn you! Why don't you give me hell? Why don't you tell me I'm a lazy bastard, that I've been sitting on my butt doing nothing for over a month while the other guys are really making headway? Why do you always have to be so damned patient with me? You know I always do as little as possible—if that! You knew I picked that assignment about changing of the loudness of my braying so I would make it softer not louder, and I try to do that anyway. And I picked one as a minimum hoping that it would bug you. And it didn't. What do I have to do—spit in your face before you'll tell me what a louse I am? Wasting your time and mine. I'm never going to get anywhere and you know it. So why don't you be honest enough to tell me so?"

We forget how we responded but we must have done so adequately because he raged some more, then fought back some tears as he told us all about his relationships with his father. He recounted many incidents, only two of which we recall. Once when he was eight years old and needed an extra quarter to buy a kite, his father had made this contract with him. The boy was to weed a row of carrots in the garden and would get the quarter for doing so, but for each weed that remained, he would be docked a penny. And it had to be done that morning. The boy had done his best but at noon the father counted the weeds remaining and said that the boy owed him one dollar and forty-three cents which he would take out of his dime allowance at the rate of a nickel each week. That was one tale. Another concerned the time when the boy was on a high fence and the father held out his arms to catch him as he jumped down. As he leaped, the father pulled his arms away and said, "That'll teach you to trust nobody!" Anyway, we do remember how we responded to his recounting of this last incident. We said simply, "And your world has ever since been full of fathers—except for me." For some reason, this session proved to be the turning point in that stutterer's therapy. The session ended by his revising his planned activities so that they included not only quotas of 50 each of the three suggestions we had given him but also an extra one in which he said he would wobble the inflections of every ah that he used as a postponement when talking to

a minimum of ten strangers. We were tempted to persuade him to set less exorbitant goals but thought better of it and were glad we did because he exceeded his maximum goals on all four assignments. Moreover his speech the following day was vastly improved, most of the ah's having disappeared. Some regression of course occurred later but from that time on he made consistent progress and we have seldom had so cooperative a client.

We have constantly been surprised by the ingenuity shown by the stutterers in devising pertinent assignments. Once they understand that by varying their stereotyped behaviors they might be able to weaken them, they demonstrate remarkable inventiveness. Thus one stutterer who characteristically postponed the speech attempt on feared words by backing up several words and beginning again, a very common delaying reaction, assigned himself the task of repeating first the immediately antecedent word, then the one before it, and so on until he ended by repeating all the prior words—and then he reversed the sequence. This took tremendous concentration but he managed finally to collect over 100 instances in which he had used this variation. The result was that most of the retrials disappeared from his speech. He still stuttered but not in the same old way. Another stutterer with the same problem gave himself the assignment to do pseudostuttering on each word of the retrial if he found himself repeating preceding words and not to say the feared word until he had done so. Still another one inserted a long pause between each word of the phrase repeated. Another used humming instead of his typical "ah" postponement. We could never have had enough imagination to devise the wide variety of tasks that the stutterers have formulated.

Many of our cases use certain stereo-typed words or phrases either as post-ponements or as starters. They inter-ject such words as "well," "why," or such stereotyped phrases as "You know . . ." or "Let me see now . . ." At times these words or phrases (used to gain time or to get a running start for the feared word) have become so automatized they almost resemble non-sense. Thus one of our stutterers char-acteristically used the utterance "um-see-umsee-umsee" over and over again before tackling the word on which he expected to stutter. We suspect this curious interjection was the automa-tized distortion of "Let me see." In another context (Van Riper, 1971) we have described how a stutterer's compulsive utterance of "andohdoh-dohanddohdoh" had derived from "And don't you know?" At any rate, whenever such words or phrases are typically used in approaching feared words, we help the stutterer learn to vary them. Thus one of our stutter-ers, who used "umuh-umuh-umuh" (occasionally as many as 18 times se-quentially) before making a real ef-fort to say an especially feared word, varied this automatic behavior by put-ting in some "umpas" in with the "umuhs," and in another assignment used different vowels instead of the "uh" so that he would say "umuh-ummo-ummee-ummoo" and so on.

We wish to emphasize here that these variations were used in live com-munication, not only with us or other members of the group of stutterers, but also with the person's friends and with strangers. At first, it was often difficult for some of the stutterers to use these deliberate modifications when they were under strong com-municative stress but they always man-aged finally to surmount their failures and to have enough success to show marked change. Originally we had some initial skepticism that this train-ing in varying the stereotyped behav-iors would indeed weaken them but over and over again we have seen their habit strength diminish. Once the stutterers became aware of what they were doing in approaching their feared words and situations and found that the behaviors they had thought were completely out of their control could be modified, much of the stut-tering behavior almost seemed to melt away before our eyes. We were also pleasantly surprised to find that no reciprocal increase in the duration of the core behaviors or other reactions occurred. They continued to occur but they did not grow.

Varying the escape behaviors

Certain features of the stuttering however proved more difficult to vary than did the postponement or avoid-ance reactions. In the main these were the sudden eye-closings, the abnormal mouth positions, the jawjerks, the breathing abnormalities. They were the responses most closely related to the feelings of blockage or to the run-away repetitions of syllables. They were the mechanisms used to time the moment of speech attempt or to effect a release from tremors, fixations, or oscillations. Often, despite the stut-terers' intention to change, these old reactions prevailed and they knew once again the powerful compulsivity that characterizes this disorder. Some stut-terers after a few such experiences gave up temporarily; others licked their wounded egos and returned to the battle.

Our individual conferences at this time were full of emotional storm but again many new insights were achiev-ed. Certain stutterers needed strong support and we gave it to them in many ways. We showed them how we could assume their own abnormal mouth postures and revise them before finishing a word and in situations that they feared. We stuttered along with them in unison as they made a phone call, adopting the first part of their abnormality but then introducing some variations and asking them to follow our lead. Using a binaural auditory trainer, we fed our variation into one ear as they heard themselves stuttering in the other. We had them shadow us as we duplicated their kinds of stuttering and as we changed them. We had them watch themselves on videotape and stutter differently and in unison with their old reactions. We rewarded any change however small, and stayed with the stutterers until some success had been achieved. We verbalized their feelings better than they could. At this time too the group therapy was highly important. Some of the group members always made faster gains in varying their behaviors and the models thereby presented proved highly motivating to the others. Often the stutterers would work together, demonstrating, discussing, and making suggestions about how to change their stuttering. Few of our cases have been able to resist the forces thus brought to bear.

Those stutterers who had habitually squeezed their eyes tightly shut while in the throes of stuttering became able to open one eye, then the other while it occurred. The inhalatory gasps were slowed or interrupted with exhalations. Jaw jerks were done sidewise, or changed to those resembling chewing, or done in slow motion. Lip protrusions were shifted from one contour to another. The stutterers who attacked words beginning with vowels by forcibly tightening lips learned to open them in different ways or to close them even more firmly. They learned to shift the loci of tension from one area to another, e.g., from the larynx

to the lips, even from the mouth to the left leg. Instead of using their usual abnormal preformations of the articulatory posture of the feared word's first sound, they revised it into another totally different phonemic posture. They learned to make their faces mobile rather than rigid; they even learned to smile as they stuttered.

As we have described in a previous chapter, many of the stutterer's "symptoms" are linked together in definite sequences, certain behaviors being found earlier in the sequence than others. The components of any complex moment of stuttering are not randomly ordered. Instead a definite stereotype is usually very evident. To weaken the linkage of these chained reactions, the stutterers altered these sequences, reversing their order, omitting one of them, or inserting a foreign behavior. Thus one stutterer who consistently showed a three component sequential pattern of (1) closing his eyes tightly, (2) squeezing his lips, (3) jerking his head backwards as he attacked the feared word, would begin the speech attempt with the head jerk, then lip squeeze, and then close his eyes. Or he might omit the eye closure or insert a slow exhalation of air between the first and second of these components. By so doing, their stereotyped sequences were disrupted and weakened.

The net effect of all this manipulative alteration was impressive. It seemed to be impossible for any stutterer to undergo such experiences without losing his sense of helplessness and gaining some feeling of being able to control the uncontrollable. At this time, the stutterers eagerly sought out opportunities to speak in stressful situations so that they could get the stuttering they needed to do their altering. What is more significant, the more they hunted for feared words and situations, the less fear and stuttering they experienced. The feeling of compulsivity during stuttering subsided and so did the shame and embarrassment. No longer did the stutterers feel themselves controlled by their disorder. As they wrestled with their stuttering and manipulated its form and substance, they began to believe that they would eventually master it. They were twisting the tiger's tail. Both in the individual and group meetings, some rather profound psychotherapeutic experiences took place. The stutterers began to increase the repertoire of responses available to their regulating mechanisms. They began to scan their output; they became able to compare it with models other than the abnormal fixed patterns they long had known. In the cybernetic sense, we had taught them how to start "hunting."

Modification: teaching a fluent form of stuttering

Much of the preceding therapy has been preparatory to this most important stage of treatment. The stutterer has now learned to identify his various stuttering behaviors; he has become desensitized, at least to some degree, to the threat and experience of fluency failure and he has found that he can alter and vary his stuttering reactions and himself. By this time he is usually highly motivated. The relationship with his therapist has become a close and meaningful one. The stutterer has come to desire the therapist's approval and to know the value of the guidance the therapist can provide. In short, he is ready to move.

The basic goal in this stage is to modify and shape the form of his stuttering so that it may occur without impairing the stutterer's communication or contributing to the mainte-

nance of the disorder. This target of his learning must be a kind of stuttering that will be neither frustrating nor evocative to listener penalty. The *sequential ordering* of the sounds he produces when stuttering should come as close as possible to that which characterizes normal utterance. Contortions, accessory timing movements, interjected sounds, forcings, and the like are to be progressively eliminated. The stutterer must direct his energies to the utterance of the sequence of sounds that comprise the motor pattern of the word he is attempting. Accordingly he must begin with the first sound of the word and do his searching until he can integrate it into the syllable and the syllable into the word.

This searching must be narrow, not wide or random. It should cluster about the template of the model, the fluent easy kind of stuttering which he has already discovered occasionally in his speech. If he opens his mouth wide in the utterance of a labial plosive, he must shift the posture into that appropriate for the sound. If, in the attempt of a word beginning with a vowel, his mouth is askew to the left, he must change it to a more symmetrical position. If the tongue is retroflexed in a concave contour and its tip pressed tightly against the palate in trying to say a "th" sound, the stutterer should search for a more normal way of producing it, and keep on searching until he finds it. If he is holding his breath, he should recognize that fact and explore ways of starting air flow. If he is emitting air but no sound as he attempts a vowel or sonant consonant, he should hunt for ways of phonating and restrict his efforts to that task rather than perhaps using the maladaptive reaction of jerking his head. If the stutterer finds himself in the co-contraction of antagonistic muscle groups so that tremors arise at the site of the closure, or rapid clonic oscillations occur, he should attempt to slow these down and to smooth them out instead of increasing the tension or trying to jerk out of them. Often the stutterer discovers that his long prolongation of an initial consonant is due to the fact that he is attempting a syllable containing the schwa vowel rather than the vowel he needs. He must then strive for that proper coarticulation and for smooth, slow shifts in the motoric sequences rather than sudden, ballistic ones. If his tongue or lip contacts are very hard and tight, he should attempt to loosen them. Whatever the stutterer is doing that is inappropriate to the normal production of the sound, syllable, word, or utterance should become a vivid error signal so that it can be altered in the direction of the normal production. This is the work of this stage of therapy. If the stutterer must stutter, then let him make sure that he is confining his struggles and searching behavior to attempts which make some sense in terms of the programming of the motoric sequencing of speech.

Clarifying the motor model

To be able to change his stuttering behavior, the stutterer must have clearly in mind the *motoric* model of standard utterance. We stress the word motoric because, although he knows very well how the normally uttered word should sound, he has only a vague awareness of how it should be produced. While it is true that even the speech scientist cannot describe every fine detail of the motor sequencing of speech, the gross features of utterance are easily recognized. Air flow, phonation, and the necessary articulatory postures and movements comprise such features. Though we may not be able to describe in words the

requirements of each of these in order to produce a sound, syllable, or word, we can easily demonstrate that we know what they are. We can pantomine the sound or sequence, whisper it, or say it aloud, time after time, with only minor variations.

The stutterer can do this too but when the fear is on him or when he finds himself stopped or oscillating, most of his attention is focused on the listener's reaction or on the abnormal sounds and silences he is producing. Very little awareness of what he is actually doing motorically is evident. His error scanning is visual and auditory, not proprioceptive. Indeed he doesn't really want to attend to the abnormality of his mouth movements. He is behind his contorted face, not in front of it, and hence he can ignore what takes place in that face motorically though he cannot escape *hearing* what comes out of it or *seeing* its reflection in his listener's eyes. The error signals received by his servosystem tend to be visual and auditory, not proprioceptive, because apparently he insulates himself from further hurt by putting buffers or filters in the proprioceptive circuits. Kinesthetic and tactual feedback are of course present but they too are ignored. This is why it is so very difficult for the stutterer to vary his behavior appropriately. Somehow we must train him to recognize what he is doing motorically and to compare that motor output against the standard pattern of normal utterance. Only then will he be able to search and hunt and vary his output so that the errors will be reduced. His attention must come to be focused, not on what he is seeing or hearing, but on what he is doing. He needs to be trained in matching, in comparing, in hunting and searching, in recognizing when he is not doing what he should be doing and when he is coming closer to the desired target.

We should understand that the stutterer will need help in this new emphasis on scanning his proprioceptive feedback. For years the alarm signals of feared words and situations have set off intense "looking and listening" responses. These signals have triggered the well-practiced strategies and routines of avoidance and struggle that have become so highly automatized as to appear involuntary. Yet we should realize that much of the strength of these stuttering reactions is due in part to their freedom from the automatic controls of proprioceptive monitoring. We can't do much about the sounds or sights which have already been accomplished. Once an abnormal sound is uttered, it is gone; once a listener has made an unfavorable value judgment, it is done. But there is opportunity to modify motoric utterance as it is happening if one is attending to it. It should not surprise us therefore to find that the stutterer speaks with less stuttering when he finds in the therapist a permissive listener whose reactions need not always be scrutinized for signs of rejection. Nor should we be surprised, when we block out his self-hearing, that the stutterer also becomes more fluent under this condition. In large measure, the servosystem will do its job of automatically correcting much of the error if the stutterer will only give it half a chance. Somehow we must help him to reverse his abnormal hierarchy of feedbacks so that, as in the normal speaker, proprioception has dominance over self-hearing in the monitoring of motoric speech.

Proprioceptive monitoring: masking

Accordingly, we usually initiate this phase of therapy by some intensive training in proprioceptive monitoring. One way to do this is to use auditory masking to prevent the stutterer from hearing himself in the hope that he will thereby pay more attention to the proprioceptive kinesthetic and tactual information provided by his speaking. The rationale for this lies in the view expressed by Stromsta (1959), Webster and Lubker (1968), the present author, Van Riper (1971), and others that some of the basic difficulties of the stutterer lie in his auditory processing system. Whenever we can minimize the role of self-hearing and maximize the role of proprioceptive feedback in the automatic monitoring of speech, the stutterer seems to speak better. We have therefore devised and employed various types of masking noise devices having low and high pass filters with the former seeming to be more effective. Tape loops of such noise can be made and fed through earphones at any desired intensity. But we have also used recorded "cocktail" noise, loud laughter from many speakers, and an incoherent melange of shouted statements about the curse of stuttering. We have constructed devices so that the stutterer, wearing the earpiece of a hearing aid, may feed himself the masking noise in outside situations at the moment he expects to stutter or actually does so. We have used a voice actuated masking noise triggered by a throat microphone but find that it fails to be useful when silent fixations and tremors appear. We even built a contraption which would trigger the masking whenever the jaw went into tremor but it was too cumbersome for clinical use. Perhaps the simplest and most useful source of masking noise is the standard electrolarynx. When placed firmly against the ear, the stutterer cannot hear himself and so is effectively deafened for the moment.

Though the masking decreases the frequency and severity of stuttering in most stutterers and as such is highly motivating, we are not so much interested in the gain in fluency as we are in enhancing proprioceptive feedback control, and we make this very clear to the stutterer. To exchange stuttering for deafness is no great bargain and we have found little permanent improvement as the result of masking itself.[2] Let us repeat again that the stutterer does not need to learn to speak fluently. He already does this much of the time. What he really needs to know is how to cope with his stuttering. Any slight increment in fluency that he might get from masking will do little by itself to solve his problem. But if we can use the masking noise to teach him to stop his morbid self-listening and to monitor his speech primarily by proprioception we may be attacking the disorder much more fundamentally.[3]

What we do therefore is to give the stutterer repeated experiences in which the masking noise is first applied, then faded out as he continues talking. We ask him to concentrate on feeling his movements and contacts during the moments of his normal speech and his stuttering. As he speaks a list of words on which he has previously stuttered, we turn on the masking and intermittently remove it. We ask him to try to throw himself into some "real" stuttering or a reasonable facsimile thereof and then to say the same word again noting the discrepancies in how they were produced. Imitating his stuttering as closely as we can, we ask him to shadow us in pantomime so that he can recognize proprioceptively the dominant features of his difficulty while the masking noise is in his ears. We repeat this tracking behavior for normally spoken words as well, often those on which he has had considerable difficulty in the past, such as his name or his address. We have him imitate his own image on the videotape replay while stuttering and while being fluent, turning off the sound track so he can become highly aware of the motoric aspects of both his fluent and disfluent speech. We have him watch himself in a mirror as he makes a phone call and then try to duplicate any stuttering that occurred immediately afterward in pantomime or while under masking noise. We want him to discriminate the motoric features of stuttered words as compared with those same words when spoken normally so that he can tell the differences, not in how they sound, but how they feel.

Enhancing proprioceptive awareness by delayed auditory feedback

The stutterer can also become aware of what he *does* when he stutters through experiences using delayed auditory feedback.[4] In order to resist

2 In this connection it is helpful for the stutterer to read or be informed of the content of the following two articles: Trotter, W. D. and M. M. Lesch, "Personal Experience with a Stutter-aid," *Journal of Speech Disorders*, 32 (1967), 270–72; and Perkins, W. H. and R. F. Curlee, "Clinical Impressions of Portable Masking Unit Effects in Stuttering," *Journal of Speech and Hearing Disorders*, 34 (1969), 360–64. These articles may help convince the stutterer that he should not become dependent upon the masker to produce temporary fluency but rather to use it to learn how to monitor his speech proprioceptively.

3 The reader is referred to chapter 5 of the present text and to chapter 14 in *The Nature of Stuttering* (Van Riper, 1971) for the rational of this training. Other useful references are: Yates (1963), Butler and Stanley (1966), Webster and Lubker (1968) and Martin (1970).

4 Numerous studies (Nessel, 1958; Adamczyck, 1959; Lotzmann, 1961; Bohr, 1963; Webster and Lubker, 1968; Soderberg, 1968, 1969) have shown that when stutterers speak under delayed auditory feedback, many of them become remarkably fluent.

the disturbance caused by the delayed sidetone, one which is felt by most persons who experience it, he soon learns, under our coaching, to ignore the auditory sensations and to concentrate instead upon the proprioceptive ones. The therapist tries to prevent the stutterer from increasing his vocal intensity since he may use this to overcome the delay by getting better bone conduction. We also try to prevent the stutterer from altering his rate and pitch. In this our practice differs sharply from the use of DAF by Goldiamond (1965), Perkins and Curlee (1969), and others who employ DAF to get the stutterer to speak at a very slow and controlled rate. We have very little faith in rate control; its history, as we have seen in an earlier chapter, is both ancient and discouraging. Using DAF as a gadget to slow the stutterer down may merely add the magic of the machine to the procedure. Soderberg (1969) provides this significant bit of support for our remarks: "In a personal communication with the writer, Goldiamond indicated that DAF was not necessary in establishing the prolonged fluent speech patterns. When stutterers were instructed to voluntarily prolong their speech (DAF omitted), the results were found equivalent with those obtained under DAF (p. 263)." For the same reasons we discourage the stutterer using the DAF echo as a device to time his utterance of words. One might more efficiently use Columbat's metronome if this is what is desired. We therefore disagree with Soderberg (1968) who states that "the stutterer should be encouraged to speak along with the cadence of the delay time." We use the DAF in the same way that we use masking—to deemphasize auditory monitoring and to increase proprioceptive controls. We do not want the stutterer to use any artificial way of talking but we do

want him to become aware of the motoric aspects of his speech.

We therefore have found it wise to have the stutterer watch himself in a mirror at first as he speaks under the delay and then intermittently to close his eyes so that he can attend to the feeling of the movements. We also gradually alter the delay time from that delay which seems to be able to produce the most fluency to the other delay time which seems most able to produce maximum disruption. This desensitization process requires more and more proprioceptive control and the therapist must program his reinforcements so that progressive mastery is attained. There is no value merely in flooding the stutterer with confusion. We seek rather to teach him to beat the machine, the DAF apparatus, and to do so by enhancing the scrutiny of proprioceptive cues.

As we have described in our chapter on servotherapy, we also use a similar desensitization procedure by gradually bringing up the *volume* of the delayed feedback in gradual steps, working always to keep below the threshold of breakdown, but using repeated dosages of DAF which increase in stress (intensity) until the stutterer is able to tolerate more and more. Once the stutterer has had some success in resisting the stress induced by the delay and is monitoring his speech primarily by proprioception (which can be perceived by the appearance of slightly exaggerated and more precise mouth movements), we then interrupt the delay, the stutterer now hearing himself as he usually does. We ask him to continue talking in the same fashion whether the delay is present or not, and, if we intermittently shut off the delayed feedback, we soon will find the stutterer continuing to monitor his speech much more proprioceptively than before.

In order to consolidate this new

learning however, we have him speak in hierarchies of communicative situations carefully graded in terms of his past history of fear. Also to insure better carry-over, we have the stutterer record his speech while under DAF, then listen to it, and try to revise his DAF manner of speaking until he can sense no difference between the DAF condition and the direct feedback. As we have indicated, we do not want the stutterer to learn an abnormal way of speaking, and at first his efforts to overcome the delay often result in a louder, exaggerated, or a slower drawling form of speech.[5] Therefore, he must continue to work on the DAF apparatus until he sounds no different under the delay, when this is played back, than he does when talking without it. Only then can we hope for effective carry-over of the proprioceptive monitoring. The prime object of this training is to apply the controls he learns during his DAF experiences to his ordinary speaking. Let us say again that we want him to stop eternally listening for abnormal speech. We want him to *feel* what he is doing. The use of this intensive DAF training, in our opinion, has been most effective in accomplishing this end. We have also tried to build a portable DAF which can be used outside the clinic and we are certain that sooner or later an adequate one will be invented though our own efforts have failed. One which we saw at the University of Utrecht in Holland was made in Prague but it failed to have either sufficient volume or the variable delay times so necessary for adequate clinical use. Perhaps by the time this book is published, it will be available.

5 MacKay (1969) has shown that it is possible for normal speakers to resist the disrupting influence of DAF by speaking very nasally. So can stutterers but our aim is to reduce abnormality, not to add to it.

Proprioceptive monitoring using the electrolarynx

Still another way of emphasizing the motor aspects of speech can be found through the use of the electrolarynx. The stutterer works with it until he becomes highly intelligible. This requires very precise articulation and concentrated attention to the formation of sounds and syllables. We have found only one stutterer who ever showed any stuttering while employing the instrument even when speaking in situations which were usually feared. When used properly, the electrolarynx can train the stutterer to be highly conscious of proprioceptive feedback. We work also, through varying the pressure on the device's trigger, to get more normal phrasal, accentual, and intonation patterns, an experience which many severe stutterers have seldom recognized in terms of motor sequencing.

In using the electrolarynx we constantly stress the purpose involved, not the artificial fluency which it creates. In this regard, we have found that asking our cases to read the article by McKenzie (1955) "A Stutterer's Experience in Using an Electrolarynx" helps to show them the limitations of the device. We don't want them to feel that it is any magical panacea. As we have said, what we are after is to increase the stutterer's awareness of what he is doing motorically both when he speaks normally or when he stutters. Thus we often ask the stutterer to say the feared words that he has been collecting during that day and to use them in sentences with and without the electrolarynx, trying hard to note the differences in postures and movements which occur in stuttered as compared with normal production. At times we have the stutterer repeat over and over again the words on which he stutters in our conversation, alternating the use of the electrolarynx with pantomimed utterance, and then with vocalization, again trying to heighten the differing tactile and kinesthetic features. Or, while using the electrolarynx, we may have him say his hard words first in the usual way, then next with concurrent voicing, then while whispering, and finally when holding his breath. The discriminations thus formed seem to be highly effective in initiating automatic correction of error signals and some carry-over into ordinary communication usually ensues.

Proprioceptive monitoring through pantomiming

But the use of masking, DAF, and the electrolarynx are merely teaching aids in this heightening of proprioceptive feedback and it is wise to have the stutterer also learn to scrutinize his motor speech production without relying upon them. Therefore, in this phase of therapy, we use a lot of pantomimic and whispered speech in the stutterer's rehearsal of attempts on his feared words, and again after the stuttering has occurred. The therapist first, and then the stutterer, notes and comments on the differences between normal and stuttered utterance. As we did under masking or DAF, we take his feared words (isolated or in phrases or sentences) and use them repeatedly until adaptation produces enough normal speech to enable him to compare the initial stuttered rendition with the final normal one. We have the stutterer practice stuttering in pantomime, sometimes working on a single word as many as 20 or 30 times, until he can go through its motoric patterning with a high degree of accuracy. And then we do the same procedure as the stutterer pantomimes

the normal utterance of the word. Then we might pick up the telephone and have him use both in live communication.

Again in this pantomiming, videotape recordings provide a most useful means of helping the stutterer to know what he is doing differently when he stutters. We first record him on videotape when stuttering severely, then play it back, asking him to suspend value judgments for the moment, and to pantomime each moment of stuttering as he observes it. When he can do this with some fidelity, we then ask him first to pantomime the normal utterance of the word *as he sees himself speaking it stutteringly,* then to whisper it, and finally to utter it aloud in one replay after another. We also feed our imitation of one of his stuttered words into earphones worn by the stutterer and have asked him to demonstrate through pantomime the kind of stuttering behaviors which would parallel the auditory experience. We have had the stutterer alternately pantomime stuttering and normal utterance of words collected during the day on which stuttering had occurred and to do this alternately many times. These are but a few of many possible ways for enhancing the stutterer's ability to attend to the motoric aspects of his speech.

It is obvious from this description that we have been approaching the problem from a cybernetic point of view.[6] First of all, we have been training the stutterer to open his scanners for proprioceptive information and doing this by minimizing the intrapersonal auditory feedback and the interpersonal visual feedback. We have been trying to establish vivid standard patterns in terms of the move-

[6] For another presentation of the stutterer's problem from the cybernetic point of view, see the references by Mysak (1960, 1966).

ment and tactile features of normal utterance so that when the motoric errors are sensed by the comparator, variations in output can be created by the regulating mechanism so that the errors can be reduced. What is significant is that this error reduction then often occurs automatically in many instances and marked increases in fluency occur. However, it is also clear that the stutterer usually finds some real difficulty in operating his servosystem in this unfamiliar way when he is afraid of stuttering. Old abnormal standard patterns of stuttering dominate his awareness. He auditorily rehearses them; he listens for them. For years the stutterer has looked for rejection and listened for gaps and uncouth sounds in his speech. For years he has filtered out the proprioceptive information he needs so badly if he is to speak with less abnormality. It is not easy to change old ways of perceiving and behaving. But it can be done by this voluntary and deliberate training program.

What may not be so apparent in our description of the methods used to emphasize proprioceptive feedback is that a very intensive learning process is also involved. We structure this phase of therapy as a learning experience, jointly setting up a careful series of subgoals, discriminating the stimuli, specifying the desired and undesired responses, and providing the necessary differential reinforcements. Quite catholic about the kind of learning which takes place, we program our approval and other token kinds of reinforcements so that they are contingent upon specified performances. We attempt through operant procedures to shape, for instance, the kind of strong, overly articulated speech produced by DAF into a form more like that of normal utterance yet still maintaining the motoric awareness.

Pantomimed stuttering when introduced under the benign conditions of therapist approval and the subject's exploratory curiosity illustrates the application of classical deconditioning and so do many of the other techniques we have mentioned. Finally, we seek, through these learning experiences, to facilitate those flashes of insight that are so important in behavioral change. As one of our cases said, "You know, I've been behind a kind of puppet's mask all my life. Felt someone or something else was pulling the strings when I stutter. But it's my mouth. What *I'm* doing, I'm doing! I can pull those strings differently but only if I keep them in my hands and move those hands the way I should."

As the above quotation also illustrates, these experiences in self-confrontation can also be highly psychotherapeutic. Hope increases; fear diminishes. The split between the stuttering and the normal speaking self begins to narrow and to fuse. The stutterer begins to exert some choice, to assume some direct responsibility for his own behavior, at least to get some self-control. Needing many moments of stuttering to carry out his exploration, he seeks out that which he has always avoided or repressed. Any neurotic profit or secondary gains which have accrued to the stuttering no longer have their old value. The relationship with the therapist in this stage of therapy becomes less supportive and more challenging yet always the stutterer feels the impact of the therapist's conviction that change is possible. Each stutterer has his own particular set of dynamics, his own unique responses to those inevitable failures (or successes) which always accompany the revision of one's behavior, and the ventilation and verbalization of these in the individual conferences or group interactions can be very healing.

Cancellation

We are now ready to help the stutterer shape his stuttering behavior so that even though it occurs he can be more fluent and so that what he does will not contribute to the maintenance of the disorder. We are ready to teach him a new fluent way of stuttering, a new way of coping with the fear and experience of fluency disruption. We call this process *cancellation*. Superficially considered, cancelling is very simple: once the person emits a stuttered word, he simply pauses deliberately and then says it again before going on. With all the vehemence we can muster, let us emphasize that there is much more to the cancellation process than the mere repetition of a stuttered word. Many therapists have not understood that cancellation is designed primarily as a vehicle for learning new responses to the stimuli that trigger the abnormal stuttering responses. It is a miniature learning laboratory and it's portable. We see very little value in merely saying a stuttered word again fluently. Most stutterers can do this anyway—say it again on the afterbeat or say it again after someone else has said it for them.

Cancellation as a preventive of stuttering self-reinforcement

Stuttering probably becomes self-reinforcing for several reasons but primarily because, following all the avoidance and struggle behavior, the word the stutterer so desperately wants to speak is finally spoken. It therefore appears to the stutterer that his struggles and avoidance have helped him to transmit his message. We must understand that the basic drive which impels the stutterer is to get the listener to comprehend what he is trying to say. This need to complete his communication is primary; it is basic; it is the prime essence of his need. Also we must remember that the listener comes closer to perceiving the meaning of a message with each consecutive word the stutterer speaks, as Shannon's (1951) guessing technique shows clearly. Thus when a person stutters and finally emits the stuttered word, some progress in communicative closure is achieved. This is what the stutterer hungers for—communicative closure. Accordingly, any behavior that immediately precedes this fractional goal achievement is reinforced by that progress. If the stutterer has trouble on the first word, at least the listener knows that he is trying to speak and with each successive word (uttered normally or stutteringly) the message being transmitted becomes clearer. Of all the built-in reinforcements which maintain stuttering, this one of communicative progress is probably the most important because, for one thing, it is always contingent and always immediately delivered.

If then we are to prevent this built-in reinforcement, we must find ways of eliminating the communicative payoff that stuttering produces. It is well known that any reinforcement loses much of its contingent effectiveness if it is delayed too long. Stutterers usually flee as swiftly as they can from the scene of their abnormal performance. They hurry to say as much more of the message as they can before being blocked again in the forward flow of their speech, and the more words they can utter after a moment of stuttering, the more that prior stuttering behavior is reinforced. Sooner or later of course, they meet stimuli that threaten disruption or they experience unexpected breaks in their fluency and once again they avoid and struggle until the word is uttered. Then again the same automatic reinforcement in terms of communicative progress is self-administered. There are many vicious circles to be found in the disorder of stuttering but this is certainly one of the most important.

The Pause

Therefore, to remove the immediate communicative profit from a moment of stuttering, we teach the stutterer to insert a deliberate delay after the word has finally been spoken. Despite his own urgency or fear of listener loss, he must train himself to stop and wait for a moment after each instance of stuttering. He is not to plunge onward. He is to stop, to pause. This is our first subgoal.

This cessation of any further speaking as a time-out consequence of a moment of stuttering prevents the usual reinforcement of communicative progress which the abnormal behavior ordinarily produces. If anything it is now the pause which gets more reinforcement than the avoidance or struggle behaviors since these are further away in time. The stutterer is no longer *immediately* rewarded for jerking his head or screwing up his face or uttering some inappropriate sound. It is the pause that gets the most communicative reinforcement.

One might wonder if this would be wise. Would not the number of gaps in the flow of speech be expected then to increase? There is indeed a slight tendency for this to occur but, as we shall soon describe, we use these pauses in cancellation to change the stuttering behaviors. We need these pauses after the stutterings to show

the stutterer he can react less abnormally and more fluently. Therefore, if they show some increase, we are usually delighted.

However, the contingent pause also seems to serve as both a punishment and as an alerting device. Wingate (1959) found that when stutterers spoke over a communication system and the connection was temporarily broken (and signalled by a warning light) every time a stuttered word was finally spoken, the frequency of stuttering decreased. Haroldsen, Martin, and Starr (1968) also found the same decrease when a mandatory time-out (TO) from further communication was made contingent upon stuttering. That silence may be aversive to the stutterer is shown by the research of Gould and Sheehan (1967). Having to pause after a stuttered word thus serves to suppress stuttering and acts like a punisher. The effect, however, is temporary. The use of the contingent pause alone does little to solve the problem of stuttering. It is what the stutterer does during that pause, before he continues transmitting his message, that is of vital significance. If we can use the time-out interval to develop new, more appropriate behavior and more adaptive competing responses, we can hope for more than temporary suppression. But first we must get the stutterer to pause after he stutters, to stop for a moment before he continues.

Resistance to contingent pausing. This simple prescription however is very difficult to fulfill. Stutterers fear silence almost as much as they do the exposure of their abnormality. The gaps in their communication have always been anticipated with dread. The communicative delay inherent in the stuttering itself makes further delay almost seem intolerable for they feel they must get their message across before the listener interrupts or leaves. As Sheehan and others have pointed out, silence for the stutterer can even have overtones of impotence and death. Overt or covert resistance always makes its appearance when we set up this goal of contingent pausing. Strong emotional reactions occur. Perfunctory and token performances are commonly found and here a healthy relationship between therapist and client is of great importance.

This picture of the stutterer's reactions to being asked to pause is one which most psychotherapists will recognize as indicating also a real opportunity to make progress. Resistance is often a sign that a disorder is under strong attack and is vulnerable. All we are asking is that the stutterer stop for a moment after he stutters! Why does he find this task so very difficult? Why all the emotional storm?

The therapist who understands these dynamics persists in his faith that the stutterer can finally bring himself to come to a dead halt after each moment of stuttering and he designs a program to help the stutterer do so. Often the therapist inserts enough instances of pseudostuttering into his own communication and pauses after each one to show that he at least can tolerate them even if the stutterer cannot. Also other stutterers who have successfully undergone the experience verbalize their difficulties and feelings before the group—and their final triumphs. The rationale for the use of the contingent pause is carefully presented. Except for the group meetings and individual sessions with the therapist, all other therapy is omitted at this time. The stutterer finally faces up to the challenge and disciplines himself to pause consistently after each moment of stuttering.

Necessity for completing the stuttered word before cancelling. There are some therapists who train their stutterers to stop instantly upon the first perception of stuttering. For example, Damste, Zwaan, and Schoenaker (1968) state, "The first and most important reaction the stutterer has to master is a preventative reaction. As soon as a block sets in, he has to stop. Then he must reflect on what means are available to him to produce a more adequate responses to the situation." This stoppage is contingent not on the completion of the stuttered word but on the first awareness that stuttering is occurring. Long ago (Van Riper, 1958), we used a similar procedure in devising the "stop-go" response to the perception of stuttering but discarded it for two reasons: it encouraged half-hearted speech attempts and retrials, and it produced too many split words. We therefore insist that once the stutterer begins to stutter, he continues until the entire word has been uttered before he cancels it. We view the essence of stuttering as consisting of the temporally broken word (Van Riper, 1971). We want the stutterer to learn how to unify that word, not to break it up by stopping the moment he feels stuck. The new form of stuttering he learns should at least follow the motor sequencing of the word as normally spoken. It should begin with the same movements and follow the same motor patterns. Though some time distortion may occur, certain sounds or transitions being prolonged, at least the sequential features of the normally spoken word are run through. This is why we *do not want* our stutterers to use a syllabic form of repetition (as in the bounce) when cancelling, and why we do prefer a slow-motion, prolonged sequencing as our target behavior when the stutterer makes the new attempt after the pause. If we are to hope for transfer, let us at least approximate the temporal patterns of the normal word.

We seek to have the stutterer use the contingent pause consistently, not only in the clinical sessions but also in his usual communication. This consistency of course does not imply any 100 percent criterion of perfection. Human frailty and the stutterer's long history of compulsively hurrying away from each moment of stuttering would make this unreasonable. Accordingly we set higher criteria for performance in the group and individual sessions than we do for other outside situations, but we insist that the contingent pause be used to some degree in all of his speaking and occasionally even when he is in great fear or under great stress. Again we try to get the stutterer to set up reasonable subgoal quotas of contingent pauses, and, as he makes progress, to increase the consistency of their use. We prefer to set no general quotas or criteria for the whole group but to tailor the tasks to the individual stutterer's own ability and vulnerability. And, as always, we use their reports in our individual sessions for the ventilation of feelings and the facilitation of insight.

Using the Pause for Calming. As soon as the stutterer is able to be fairly consistent in pausing after his moment of stuttering, we ask him next to use the pause as an opportunity to try to calm himself and to begin the next word slowly rather than swiftly. This too is often very difficult at first but eventually, as a result of our carefully programmed approvals or other reinforcements, he manages to accomplish the goal at least occasionally and sometimes with surprising frequency. We have experimented with the use of various forms of general relaxation training in this post-stuttering pause but have not found them as successful as merely asking the stutterer to try to be as calm as possible. Some covertly verbalized self-suggestion and a slow exhalation seem to be what they commonly use. At any rate this training in pausal calming does seem to be effective in lengthening the duration of the contingent pause if it does nothing else. Let us stress the point that it is important that the pause after the moment of stuttering be sufficiently long—a minimum of three seconds—to have the desired impact.

Most stutterers at first tend to make the contingent pause far too short; almost a token hesitation. It may well be that the stutterer cuts short his contingent pause before saying the word again because he dimly senses the presence of reaction inhibition. Once a response has been completed, there seems to be a subsequent short interval of time during which that response cannot be evoked again. We see this clearly in the knee jerk reflex but it also holds for other responses. If the stutterer says the stuttered word again immediately after its completion, often he can say it fluently. If he waits a bit longer, the reaction inhibition dissipates, and he will stutter on it again. An alternative explanation for this phenomenon is that the stutterer's specific fear of stuttering on that particular word has been satisfied by the stuttering exhibited, and so it takes some time before it builds up again. The need to hurry on may also be due to the stutterer's strong communicative drive; in part to his reluctance to stay in close proximity to his verbal unpleasantness, but also some of his difficulty appears to be due to subjective time distortion. Empty time always seems longer than filled time as many experiments have demonstrated. We are asking the stutterers just to *pause and wait a few seconds* but stutterers almost always overestimate the duration of the pause as they overestimate the duration of their moments of stuttering. A two-second blocking seems to them to last for minutes; five seconds of stuttering seems to go on forever. Accordingly, we have found it very valuable to have them check with a stop watch or the second hand of an ordinary watch to determine just how long their stutterings do last—and also how long they actually pause afterward. (One of our stutterers measured his contingent pauses in "hippopotami." A three second pause was one in which he said the word hippopotamus to himself three times. Once he reported that on the telephone he had had a seven hippopotami block and only a one hippopotamus pause afterward.) Anyway, we have found in this stage of therapy an appropriate opportunity for helping the stutterer become more objective about his dimension of time.[7]

We find that though it is very difficult for stutterers to relax or calm themselves *prior to* or *during* their moment of stuttering, it is much easier to the period just after it occurs. As we indicated earlier, this may be due to reaction inhibition in that the surge of tension once emitted does not tend to occur again for a short interval or it may be due to the anxiety reduction which several investigators (Wischner, 1952; Sheehan, 1958) have claimed takes place once the threat of stuttering has been corroborated and that particular moment of abnormality has ended. Whatever the reason, stutterers seem to be better able to

calm themselves during this post-stuttering period than they can during its anticipation or occurrence.

What also seems important is that through this training the stutterer comes to realize that he need not surrender blindly to his impulsive tendency to deny, disregard, ignore, suppress, and flee from a bit of stuttering behavior. He can confront it, accept it as a *fait accompli,* and perhaps learn something from it. To the surprise of many stutterers, most listeners react more favorably to the contingent pause (especially if the stutterer's attitude is one of calm acceptance) than they do to his usual way of reacting to his fluency breaks. As Bryngelson, Chapman, and Hansen pointed out long ago (1944), listeners scrutinize the stutterer's attitudes toward his stuttering and tend to evaluate his disorder in the same way that he does. If his reactions to stuttering indicate that he feels it is distressing and shameful, they too will tend to accept this evaluation. On the other hand, if his reactions to a moment of stuttering show little distress, the listeners soon come to share that judgment too. Within limits, a stutterer can shape the attitude of his listeners and thereby spare himself some rejection. As stutterers begin to put these pauses into their speech following their moments of stuttering while, appearing relatively unruffled and unhurried, they find much more acceptance from those with whom they are communicating than they had expected. This by itself is reinforcing since it diminishes the threat and decreases the amount of stuttering. Also, since these more favorable audience attitudes and increased fluency occur when they are using the contingent pause, the stutterers find its use not only much more tolerable than before but also somewhat rewarding.

[7] The research of Ringel and Minifie (1966) showed also that the more severe stutterers had the greatest protensity (time distortion) errors.

Filling the pause. Our next step in training the stutterer in cancellation requires the stutterer to do something more positive during the pause than merely trying to calm himself. We now ask him to fill it with two specific behaviors. First, he is to reduplicate in pantomime a foreshortened version of the stuttering behavior he has just experienced and, secondly, he is to rehearse, again in pantomime, *a modified* version of that behavior. Only when he has done both of these two pantomimings is he free to continue talking.

Why do we proceed in this manner? Why stutter again in pantomime? Surely once is enough! These challenges always appear at this time and again we find stutterers resisting our guidance. We explain carefully that behavior as highly automatized as stuttering needs to be brought up to vivid awareness if it is to be weakened and changed. It is difficult to control or modify that which is ignored or disregarded. By duplicating the abnormal behavior again in pantomime, the stutterer becomes highly conscious of the inappropriate things he has done motorically. By the foreshortening, the most prominent features of the behavior are highlighted so that they can serve as discriminative stimuli and can function as cybernetic error signals. In short, by performing the behavior again, the stutterer has to confront both his maladaptive behavior and his disorder objectively. The listener will know very well that the stutterer is doing this confronting because the pantomime makes it obvious—and interestingly enough, most listeners regard this with respect. They seem to feel that the stutterer who stops and goes through some tasting of the word on which he has just had trouble must be trying to do some-

thing about his impediment, that he is not just a hapless victim, helplessly seized by his stuttering. All of us respect a person who tries to cope with his disability even if he has trouble doing so. We pity or turn away from those who merely suffer.

But there are other reasons too. The stutterer soon comes to realize under this regime that his blind, random struggling or elaborate avoidance, timing, and disguise rituals do not help him to make any progress in communication. Indeed, the more stutterers struggle, or the more complicated their avoidance mechanisms, the longer it will be before they are freed to continue talking since in cancelling they must duplicate these behaviors before proceeding. Thus the punishment comes to fit the crime. Moreover, this program of pantomimic reduplication and rehearsal is at first felt as highly aversive. We need no electric shocks or blasts of 100 decibel tones contingent upon stuttering to produce a decrement in frequency of stuttering. Those aversive stimuli are highly artificial. Is it not better, if we are to employ operant conditioning procedures, to use something more appropriate, the reduplication of the stuttering itself?

But most significant of all is the fact that, when cancelling in this way, the communicative continuance is contingent on the *revision* of the old stuttering behavior. The stutterer cannot go on until he first repeats, then revises and modifies his stuttering. The specific behaviors which are immediately antecedent to this freedom to continue talking are the ones that get the most strengthening, and this is now the rehearsal of a different and better way of stuttering, one which progressively can be programmed to come closer and closer to fluent utterance. Thus now the revision rather than the pause gets the most reinforcement. What we strongly desire is to get the stutterer to react to the threat or experience of communicative blockage in a more appropriate way. By having the freedom to continue talking contingent only upon change, upon shifting from an old to a new form of behavior, we strongly reinforce that change as well as the revised attempt. Moreover, from a different point of view, we have the stutterer touch again the behavior he so dreaded, but under conditions of reduced anxiety.

In some stutterers, indeed, we may have them reduplicate the stuttering behavior again and again as many as 20 times or until all the emotion has faded from the motoric act. The principle of negative practice is thus invoked, though it occurs after the stuttering rather than instead of it. The technique thus requires that the subject be exposed to unpleasant stimuli but that he not be allowed to escape and so he must adapt. But the main effect is due to reexperiencing the original traumatic behavior in a pantomimic form which only partially resembles the original unpleasantness. The stutterer thus comes to view this form of cancelling finally as another type of desensitization. Moreover, we must not forget that the successful use of the reduplication and rehearsal is followed also by the anxiety-reducing effects of therapist approval and other positive reinforcements.

Finally, if we consider the process from the view of cognitive learning, what we have here is the learning of a new set of strategies for coping with the experience of stuttering. Following the pantomimic review of the old behavior, the stutterer deliberately attempts to discover a new way of utter-

ing his feared words. Opportunity is thus provided for testing this new approach. He has some time to plan his revision. Indeed it is mandatory that he do so if he is to effect some change.

And what does the stutterer actually do after the first pantomimimg of the prior stuttering behavior when he rehearses the better way of stuttering? Not the word as it would be spoken swiftly and normally! Instead he uses a highly conscious, deliberate, slow-motion, pantomimed rehearsal of the motoric sequence which comprises that word. He must make sure that he begins it with the right articulatory postures appropriate to the syllable, and then shifts gradually from one movement to the next. He must try vividly to *feel* the successive movements and contacts which comprise that word. The contacts must not be abnormally tight; the movements should be slow but strong. As the stutterer performs this second pantomiming before continuing, it will be obvious to the observer that he has not only recognized the abnormality which he has exhibited but also that he is now rehearsing a better way of uttering that word. Nevertheless, at this particular stage in the therapy, the stutterer never utters the word aloud. This will come later. At this time we seek only to build the model for the overt canceling which he soon will be using.

Once the stutterer has been able to respond consistently to his moments of stuttering by this double pantomiming, we then get him to do the reduplication and the rehearsal in a soft, almost inaudible whisper so that airflow can accompany both. This is especially important in those stutterers of the type that Quarrington and Douglass (1960) called the nonvocalized stutterers, but it seems to be of value to all of our cases in that it provides a necessary small transitional step prior to canceling aloud.

Cybernetic aspects of cancelling

From a cybernetic point of view it is apparent that in this canceling we are concentrating on scanning, on comparing, and attempting to build the necessary foundation for changes in the output of the regulating mechanism. The pause gives the stutterer the time to scrutinize the dominant features of his stuttering behavior in terms of their appropriateness to normal utterance. He is also given time to search, to vary, to "hunt" for a better way of speaking. In a very real sense we are seeking to establish a kind of a self-correcting process that we hope will eventually become automatic. Also, through the use of pantomime and whispering, we are emphasizing the proprioceptive rather than the auditory or visual feedbacks.

The overt cancellation

When the stutterer has shown that he can respond to his moments of stuttering in these new ways and with some consistency, we move onward to the final step in cancellation. The goal now is to do something more than what the stutterer has done before, yet the task again is built upon that which has been previously accomplished. Up to this time, you will recall, we have not asked the stutterer to say the stuttered word again aloud before he continues. First he has followed it with a pause in which he tried to calm himself; secondly, he learned to pantomime or whisper softly the original stuttering and its subsequent revision but these were done relatively silently. Now we gradually fade out the pantomiming during the

pause and ask him merely to pause and then to say the stuttered word again but this time he says it aloud. Let us repeat that he is not to say it normally. We prefer instead that he use the strong, deliberate slow-motion kind of utterance in which the sequencing of the motoric components is somewhat slowed and obviously highly controlled. A listener would know immediately in hearing such a cancellation that the stutterer had recognized his error and was obviously correcting it with some care. This is easy to demonstrate but a bit difficult to describe in words. Stutterers soon recognize that it resembles the fluent stutterings which they have observed occurring occasionally in their speech. The cancelled word does not sound the same as it would were it spoken normally. It is slower, stronger, spoken more carefully and consciously.

Though this model should be viewed as the target, it is not necessarily the only criterion of success as the stutterer learns how to cancel. At first it is quite acceptable that on the retrial some features of the old stuttering will be present—some, *but not all of them.* The revisions need not be perfect; it is sufficient that revision is apparent. Indeed at first we prefer to have some semblance of stuttering on the cancellation but always with a significant difference. The retrial must always have less abnormality in it. What we do not want is merely an automatic, fluently uttered word on the cancellation. Stutterers often can, and prefer, merely to say the word again without stuttering. But what we are seeking are models for more fluent forms of stuttering, for better ways of coping with its threat and occurrence. We want the stutterer to learn new and better ways of responding when he fears or feels a fluency failure. Through cancellation, he puts these new models into his mouth.

Shaping

We have therefore found it wise to design a series of progressive approximations which the stutterer can work through sequentially in these overt cancellations. Each stutterer has his own unique set. At first, when he says the word again aloud, for example, he might merely revise the initial abnormal mouth posture on the retrial and he works on mastering this kind of cancellation until he has met the desired criteria of consistency in various situations. Then next, in saying the word again, he might add the opening of his eyes and the smoothing out of the tremor to the change of mouth posture. Then next, he might include a slower opening of the jaw in shifting from the initial consonant to the vowel in his cancelled utterance of the stuttered word. Then finally on other attempts he merely says the word again very carefully in the new way we have described. Often it is necessary to program some of the earlier forms of cancellation—the silent pause alone, or the two pantomimes, or the whispered rehearsals—into this stage of therapy. For some stutterers we may prescribe the use of all these variations in sequence before he says the word again aloud. Or we may even add an extra transitional step, the use of soft vocalization following the whisper. This makes for a long pause but a few experiences of this sort put the emphasis where it belongs— on the act of revision. They clarify what the stutterer has done and must do. As the stutterer succeeds in accomplishing each of these successive types of cancellation, strong reinforcement is provided in much the same fashion that an operant conditioning psychologist would shape the behavior of a pigeon, but with the exception that the stutterer knows from the first what the purpose of the process is and is given a map of the route the successive approximations must undergo before the final target behavior of fluent stuttering is reached. By breaking down the modification of the stuttering into small steps, and employing the period just after the stuttering has occurred when the emotionality is weak, we find that the stutterer soon learns new and better responses to the old stimuli which formerly evoked his abnormal behavior.

The payoff from this training in cancellation is difficult to overestimate. We have seen many stutterers who needed very little additional therapy. Once they learned, through cancelling, other and better ways of stuttering they immediately applied this new knowledge whenever they expected or experienced disruption. The cumulative effect of the powerful reinforcement which the ability to continue talking brings into play often provides dramatic decreases in the frequency and severity of stuttering. The stutterer needs to slay his dragon not once but many times. Every time he stutters he has a new opportunity to do so again. He has a new sense of self-mastery and esteem. He has learned that he need not yield helplessly when feared words or situations come his way, that he need not struggle randomly. He has something specific to do and this in itself tends to counteract ambivalence and panic. Each cancellation is a frank admission of his stuttering; there is no denial, no disguise to leave the residue of guilt. The self-concept, formerly so split, now becomes whole. He is a stutterer but he is obviously confronting his disorder and coping with it and, as a consequence, the responses of his listeners are no longer so punitive. In many ways, the vicious spiral of stuttering is becoming unwound. It no longer automatically regenerates itself.

In a very real sense, cancellation serves as a vehicle for a kind of psychotherapy that we have found to be very effective. Perhaps Bloodstein (1969) expresses it best:

> Cancellation, for example, may be regarded as a basic form of therapeutic self-confrontation and, as the stutterer makes use of his blocks as opportunities to battle for control of his fears, malattitudes, and abnormal initiation and release of sounds, he may be compared with the neurotic person who gradually succeeds in the course of the psychotherapeutic process in taking responsibility for his maladaptive behavior. (p. 252)

Modification of Stuttering During Its Occurrence

Pull-outs

One of the intriguing observations that we have made concerning our treatment of stuttering is that the modifications of behavior learned through cancellation tend to move forward in time to manifest themselves *during* the period of the stuttering itself. What happens is that the stutterer now does not wait until after the stuttering has occurred and the word has finally been spoken before he attempts to correct his inappropriate behavior. Instead, we find the stutterer applying what he has learned *as soon as he recognizes that he is in the midst of a fluency failure.*

As with the word "cancellation," we hold no brief for the term "pull-

out."[8] It was invented by the stutterers themselves as a way of labeling what they did when they felt themselves stuttering and then decided to find a better way of responding to that experience than by using their former avoidance and struggle reactions. As one of them said, "I'm tired of waiting helplessly until my block runs its course and the word comes out. I know now that *I'm* doing what I'm doing and that there are both sensible and foolish things I can do when I get stuck. I'm trying to use the sensible ones and I've already learned a lot about them through cancelling. Now I'm working out of my blocks without struggling. Easing them out."

Nevertheless, we do not rely only upon this automatic self-correction. We need to find ways of facilitating this "easing out of the blocks," ways of teaching a new unabnormal release so that the stutterer will know very clearly what he should do. Though cancellation continues to be used whenever the stutterer stutters and does nothing to modify the course of his abnormal speech attempts, the therapeutic emphasis now shifts to a new goal—the modification of stuttering *during* its occurrence. Moreover, as a motivational aid, we suggest to the stutterer that, whenever he makes a real attempt to pull out of his stutterings, he need not cancel that particular word.

8 Sheehan (1970) has used the term "slide" to label behavior that resembles pull-outs. He specifically states however that the slide should not be used on feared words or on those in which stuttering appears since it is employed primarily to demonstrate the acceptance of the stutterer's role. Gregory (1968) offers this definition: "Pull-outs consist of the person not allowing the speech block to run its course, but modifying the behavior as the word is spoken. Again, the reinforcement of the maladaptive stuttering response is diminished and the adaptive pull-out is reinforced."

In the beginning phases of this pull-out stage of therapy, we reward *any* attempt to change the usual stereotyped stuttering behavior if the change occurs before the word is finally spoken. Then, through a shaping process, we program our reinforcements so that the stutterer is led through a series of progressive approximations which culminate finally in the kind of utterance the stutterer has already learned in the final phase of his cancelling, namely that characterized by the kind of behavior that we call "slow motion or fluent stuttering," a kind which permits an easy transfer into normal speech. As we have said, we try to break the modifying process into small steps to insure that the stutterer fulfills some reasonable criterion of consistency at each level before he moves from one modification to another. If this is operant conditioning, so be it.

Pulling out of fixations. In our conferences we jointly set up a series of subgoals to help the stutterer out of his fixations or syllabic repetitions. First of all, we structure the task as a searching process. The stutterer deliberately prolongs what he is doing when he stutters and uses this as the central focus or take-off base from which he explores new ways of timing and integrating the necessary transitional movements. Thus one who finds his mouth screwed to the left in the prolongation of the "w" sound of the word "woman" would first voluntarily prolong this abnormal posture, then slowly shift it into a more normal position and not attempt to say the word until the latter has been accomplished and maintained. *He does not stop and try again.* He continues the initial behavior and then changes it. For example, if, in trying to say the word "can," he finds he is thrusting his tongue forward and curling it up

against the upper teeth, he first would hold onto this inappropriate contact until he is highly aware of what he is doing and then he slowly and voluntarily changes that abnormal lingual posture to one which makes the utterance of that first phoneme possible. Or, if in the utterance of "Thank you," the airway is completely blocked by the tongue on the "th," he hunts and searches until the tight contact and complete closure are loosened and airflow is evident; only then does he make the slow, smooth speech attempt. If his lips are tightly closed, as on the word "money," he varies their tension and contact until he has searched for and found a more normal way of initiating that word. Or, when the stutterer finds himself lengthily prolonging a continuant such as the sibilant in the word "Saturday" he keeps varying the motoric characteristics of the "s" until he finds those characteristics of the sound which "fit" and are preparatory for the "ae" vowel which follows it in the syllable, rather than remain fixed on those which would be transitional for the schwa vowel. Thus, he hunts and searches; he tries one variation after another, always trying to make a fix, as the radar operators call it, on the proprioceptive target.

On a word beginning with a blend such as the "fl," to give another specific example, such a stutterer might wonder why he cannot say the word "flower." He discovers himself in a long prolongation of the "f" but it is an isolated "f," or one which would only fit the syllable "fuh." Through searching, he will finally find that he must also raise the tongue into the position for the "l" sound, the second component of the blend, and only when he has achieved this simultaneous and joint use of both the labiodental and the lingual-alveolar formation will he discover that he has any chance of producing that first syllable of the word. On words beginning with an "h" such as "he" the stutterer will at first realize that his mouth is shaped for the schwa vowel. If then he hunts around, he will discover that if instead he shapes the mouth for the "i" (ee), he no longer needs to keep prolonging the exhalation of the uncoarticulated "h." We hasten to state that few stutterers analyze what they do in such terms. They need not be phoneticians but they do need to search intelligently rather than randomly for the necessary coarticulation and timing if they are not to remain caught in the throes of their fixations.

In this regard, the research of Maier and his students (1952) has some pertinence. They showed that when rats and other animals are subjected to a very frustrating situation, they developed a rigid stereotyped kind of behavior characterized by abnormal fixations and that these fixations persist unadaptively, despite the application or removal of punishment. Maier found however that he could cure his rats of their abnormal fixations by "preventing the animal from practicing the fixated response, and at the same time, guiding the animal by the hand so as to force it to jump to the correct window." Although we can get the majority of our stutterers to release themselves slowly from their fixations by providing models and directions, there are a few whose fixations are so compulsive and strong that direct manipulation of the lips or jaw may be necessary at first. In this we follow the general principles of motokinesthetic training (Young, 1965).

Pulling out of tremors. Some of the felt compulsivity of the fixations is due to presence of accompanying tremors usually located in the focal articulatory structures involved in the production of the prolonged phoneme. Thus, for the labial sounds, the lips show the tremors; for the lingua-dentals, the tongue or jaw may be in vibration. Vowel sounds usually show a gross jaw tremor. The naive stutterer tries to break out of these tremors by stopping and starting again, or by using a sudden surge of tension, or by employing a jaw or head jerk, inhalatory gasp or some other kind of interrupter mechanism. Occasionally, these interrupter devices do seem to effect a release from the tremor and since therefore they permit the word to be uttered, the intermittent reinforcement is very powerful. Examination of the electromyographic recordings of these interrupters has convinced us that when successful they impose a large out of phase movement upon the structures being tremored, thus breaking up the tremor rhythm which averages about seven to eight per second (Welsh, 1970; Fibiger, 1971; Basili, 1971). However, we also find two other ways in which tremors terminate. They decline in amplitude and they slow down just before the word is finally uttered.

Since we feel very strongly that we should not recommend the use of the out-of-phase jaw jerks or retrials, we usually find ways of getting the stutterer to attempt to pull out of his tremors by smoothing them out and slowing them down and to do so voluntarily once he senses that a tremor has begun. Often we suggest that he voluntarily initiate them in other parts of his body, to set his leg to tremoring or his fingers when pressed against some solid object, and then to slow these tremors down and decrease their amplitude before terminating them. Next, we suggest that he *voluntarily* throw his jaw, and his lips, and his tongue into similar tremors and terminate them in the same way. Then we ask him to create tremors in the articulatory postures of the first sounds of nonfeared, then finally on those of his feared words. We also help him to analyze how his stutterings begin, how they usually start with an abnormal postural fixation, how they often begin suddenly and ballistically, and how important the sudden surge of tension seems to be in their onset. We ask the stutterer to explore ways of varying each of these initiatory factors. Usually he learns to begin slowly, to ease into the feared sound or word, and to do so without the critical surge of tension. Through this experimentation, the stutterer learns that tremors are also modifiable and can even be prevented.

Perhaps an actual therapy report (Van Riper, 1968) may illustrate some of this therapy:

Today was a very interesting day. I attempted to fake tremors so I could learn how to control them and ended up having less control than before. What I felt was interesting was that many of the old mannerisms, escape attempts, lip closures, and sudden jaw movements were apparent. Instead of helping overcome these tendencies, I had a double dose of them. I am rather glad this thing happened today because it gave me a lot of insight into what happens to set off the tremors. I think I was finally learning how to overcome the tremor by relaxation and integration.

The two things which really set off the tremors were the "tremor-smooth-tremor-smooth" turn-on and turn-off sequence and the easy stuttering. Many times these would go off into the real thing. It is interesting to note that I did not complete my quota for integrated words. I know I need to have a real strong dose of the integration. What I want to do tomorrow is to follow every tremor-smoothing sequence with a highly voluntary and integrated production of the same word. I will also try this on the sentence right after I have had a moment of easy stuttering. (pp. 114–15)

We cannot overemphasize the importance of tremor modification in the confirmed stutterer. These tremors seem to lie at the very heart of the feeling of being blocked. They seem involuntary, uncontrollable. They perseverate. Fibiger (1971), a Swedish worker, has shown that when they have large amplitudes they seem to inhibit phonation, and that a period of at least one tenth of a second free from tremor must occur before phonation can be initiated. The following translation from the French text by Lennon (1962) also stresses their importance:

When trying to say a difficult word, the stutterer will sometimes have tremors of the lips, jaw or other articulatory structures. Although these tremors resemble those of certain cerebral disorders, they are actually caused by excessive tension of the articulatory muscles when the stutterer tries to say a word. To him these brief moments of tremor seem much longer than they are in reality. He feels that he is being controlled by some external force over which he has no power. (p. 21)

Once the stutterer learns to escape from these tremors without simply stopping and trying again, or using an out-of-phase jaw jerk, or a sudden surge of tension, but instead by decreasing their amplitude and slowing them down, he is well on the road toward mastering his difficulty. He can also learn to prevent their onset by making slow-moving speech attempts rather than sudden ones, by using loose rather than tight contacts or hypertensed postures, and by rejecting his old preformations. When he is given enough experience in smoothing out his tremors, slowing them down, voluntarily initiating and terminating them, he loses his sense of verbal impotence and helplessness.

Release from laryngeal closures. One of the more distressing kinds of difficulty experienced by some stutterers is in trying to utter a word beginning with a vowel. Often, in this kind of stuttering, the airway is occluded at the level of the larynx with both the true and ventricular folds closed tightly. We have watched these stutterers as they searched for ways of releasing themselves from laryngeal fixation. Some of them vary the tension in the neck area, making it stronger, then weaker. Or they vary their head and neck postures or they may attempt motoric changes that create differences in pitch or intensity; they inhale or exhale silently to free themselves from the felt blockade. In our opinion, these spontaneous searching behaviors have doubtless contributed much to the gross abnormality of stuttering once they have been reinforced by communicative payoff and some of them, such as an interruptive jaw jerk or a gasping inhalation, are dangerously susceptible to abnormal growth for this reason and so we do not encourage the stutterer in their use.

Use of the vocal fry. Many of our stutterers have discovered that the vocal fry provides an appropriate transition from the complete laryngeal blocking into air flow and phonation. It seems almost as though the stutterer has the dim awareness that, by using vocal fry he can loosen and open his constricted glottis. This is why we hear it appearing so frequently just before the word is spoken. Indeed, one can observe this vocal fry occurring toward the very end of any laryngeal blocking in most stutterers as they hunt for phonation but it is usually intermittent, irregular, and involuntary. When we do find this be-

havior, we call it to the stutterer's attention and then begin to shape it into a voluntary method for initiating phonation. We suggest that he explore what happens when he tries deliberately to produce vocal fry, to see if he can discover ways of making it continuous and regular rather than intermittent and irregular. We ask him to experiment with ways of combining it with true phonation.

Some of our stutterers have devised a five-step sequence which they practice by themselves as a model for this searching behavior when they do have laryngeal blocking. The five steps are these: (1) deliberately assume a silent, forced laryngeal fixation complete with tremor, trying if possible to turn it into a "real block;" (2) shift from this into *intermittent* vocal fry; (3) shift from this intermittent vocal fry into a *smooth, regular, and continuous* vocal fry; (4) shift from this into the combined vocal fry and true phonation; (5) shift then to true phonation without the fry, and attempt the word from this last behavior. Once this progression has been run through repeatedly during the pseudostuttering with some precision, the stutterer then applies the same hunting sequence to his real laryngeal blockings. It is a learning process. This searching for the integrations he has momentarily lost can be facilitated if the therapist will provide both models and the appropriate contingent reinforcements for mastery of each step in the sequence.

What usually happens is that the sequence soon becomes foreshortened as it becomes learned. The stutterer finds that he need not go through all five sequential steps, that he can omit first the second step (the intermittent bursts of vocal fry) and then both the second and the third as well. By exploring the terrain he seems to have found a new and better pathway to phonation and so finally he takes this most direct route. It is fascinating to watch these individuals searching for the necessary integration and finally finding it. We prefer, if possible, to have the stutterers discover these things themselves and without any coaching but there are some for whom maps and models must be provided. One way or another, the stutterers must learn how to pull out of their fixations and sometimes they need our help. We rarely say, "Do it this way!" Instead we ask them pregnant questions, offer some insightful comments on their behavior, give them some hints as to the directions their variations may take, hoping always for the time when they come to us with the gleam of discovery in their eyes, holding up the trophies they have collected from their hunting ground.

In this connection, we wish to stress, too, that there are many routes from every here to there, from the initial fixations into the appropriately integrated speech attempt. There is no special virtue in this vocal fry technique. Some stutterers find that they can release their laryngeal constrictions by initiating airflow first or by slowly and deliberately moving the jaw from a prior resting position into the posture required for the vowel as they make the speech attempt. Some of them find that relaxing some focal point of tension in the articulatory structure far removed from the larynx, one that seems to serve as a trigger for the closure, or for the accompanying tremor, helps to open up the airway and to facilitate phonation. And there are other ways. What is vital is that the stutterer do this hunting and searching and do it deliberately and voluntarily.

Release from clonic behaviors

We have thus far been discussing pullouts from fixations and closures. What can the stutterer do when he finds himself in a clonic, "runaway," repetitive moment of stuttering? How can he keep from reverberating automatically, from recycling over and over again the same inappropriate syllables that he has already spoken? We have scrutinized many electromyographic recordings of such clonic stutterings to seek some answer to these questions. We have carefully tried to observe what occurs as these syllabic repetitions terminate in the hope that we might find therein some clues. Although the basic research is still to be done, it seems tenable that these compulsively clonic forms of stuttering may represent some kind of servosystem failure due to overload and overshoot. Self-correcting systems can be set into oscillation in many ways by many forces and once they have begun to reverberate, the oscillations become almost self-maintaining. Our problem is to discover what to do to get them back under control again.

As we tried to see how the stutterers themselves finally stopped their recycling we found that they used several different reactions. We found first that they introduced changes in the rate at which their syllabic repetitions were being produced; these usually became irregular and slower just before the stuttering ended. More rarely a sudden, very fast burst of syllabic emission characterized this critical period just before release. The significant finding was the implication that some change in the rhythm of syllabic utterance during clonic stuttering might be useful and we have accordingly incorporated this into our therapy. But there were other kinds of phenomena that also occurred just prior to the release from these runaway stutterings. Often the stutterers' electromyographic recordings showed marked variations in the timing of antagonistic muscle groups. Formant changes also appeared in the sonographic records of the stuttered syllables at the critical moment just before release. Moreover, as the clonic repetitions continued, these changes seemed to come closer and closer to the patterns of normal utterance. During the course of the long repetitive stutterings the stutterer seemed at times to have almost found the timing or coarticulation he needed—almost but not quite. When this occurred, the repetitions would continue until finally the right timing patterns were approximated and then the stuttering terminated. Observing this variation in the volleys of impulses to the antagonistic muscle groups (which apparently seemed to be occurring automatically) we wondered whether it could be facilitated by trying to perform the variation voluntarily and consciously. Finally, we noted that some of these clonic stutterings were terminated only after the repetition had turned into a prolongation. Could this too be used in therapy? We asked our stutterers to explore the possibilities.

In general, we found again that different stutterers seemed to find different ways of effecting a voluntary release from their clonic blockings. Some of them found release when they deliberately slowed down the rate of syllabic production and especially when they attempted to change the recycled syllable from its usual schwa vowel into the one required for normal utterance of the word. This seemed to be the most useful technique for most of them. The stutterers brought the reiterated syllables under conscious control and they varied the

formant characteristics of those syllables as they did so. For example, they would begin the word "Saturday" with their usual fast irregularly automatic "suh-suh-suh-suh," then slow the syllabic rate so it became "suh . . . suh . . . . . suh . . . . suh," then change the vowel until finally the word was spoken "suh . . . . sih . . . . . . seh . . . . . sae . . . . . sae . . . . Saturday." This process of controlling the seemingly uncontrollable was not easy at first for these clonic stutterers. Often for a moment they would become masters of their mouths then lose that mastery a moment later. But, with repeated attempts, and the goal of integrating the broken word clearly in mind, and with the therapist's encouragement and reinforcement, the stutterers found that they no longer had to let their clonic stutterings run their course. They learned that they could modify the repetitions and shape them appropriately. With each success, they became more and more efficient and soon they were taking charge as soon as the first syllabic repetitions were sensed.

Some stutterers learned to terminate their compulsive recycling by slowing down the utterance of the individual syllables themselves. They began to drag them out, to drawl them. Often the first few syllables of the series would be uttered swiftly and each one terminated with sudden vocal arrest; then, as they sought to slow down the coarticulation of each syllable, it was apparent that airflow was not arrested. When this was achieved and the schwa vowel changed into the appropriate one, they were able to integrate the word. Why some stutterers found one way of release while others found a different one, we cannot explain. Rarely did we suggest a specific method. We simply clarified the goal of finding a better way of releasing themselves from their recyclings and occasionally described several strategies that they could explore.

As we have said, other stutterers seemed to find that by changing their repetitions into prolongations they could interrupt the recycling and enable them to pull out more efficiently. We have often wondered whether this prolongation method for facilitating release from automatic repetition might explain how stuttering behavior so often changes from the clonic to the tonic form during the course of its development. At any rate, we discovered it is very important, when the stutterer does shift from repetition to prolongation, that he makes sure that the prolongation does not become invested with tension or tremor. When it is, the transitional coarticulatory movements are thereby prevented and the stutterer is no better off than he was before. Nevertheless some stutterers find this change from rapid irregular repetitions of inappropriate syllables into a smooth unforced prolongation of a sound or posture gives them an ability to modify their stuttering that they can achieve in no other way. In essence, what they do in this kind of pull-out from clonic stuttering is to use the sort of things we described earlier as ways of getting out of the tonic blockages.

Getting control of the uncontrollable

Other stutterers seem to discover how to release themselves from their fixations or compulsive repetition of syllables by a different process. The moment they find themselves doing either of these, they stop instantly, then slowly and deliberately and highly consciously they utter a series of syllables or sequential sounds that progressively come closer to the motor pattern of the standard word they are trying to say. It is a searching process and a highly voluntary one. We have seen one of them stop prolonging an *s* sound, then drive himself to say *sih*, *seh*, and *sae*, then *sat*, then *sater* before he finally ended with the word he was trying to say—Saturday. We have seen him lose control and go into tremor, then regain that control again as he hunted hard for the integrations required. These were not the automatic repetitions of the "bounce" technique. Each one was a deliberate attempt to improve on its predecessor and to approximate the sequential patterning of the word on which he was having difficulty. Other stutterers who also have adopted this way of searching for proper coarticulation and sequencing have told us that it gives them a profound sense of self-mastery, that by insisting upon voluntary and progressive approximations with each new attempt they learn how to control the uncontrollable. By using this "voluntary searching" they certainly demonstrated to their listeners that they were working hard to overcome their speaking disability and were often rewarded by the reactions of those listeners. In many ways, this approach resembles the "voluntary stuttering techque" proposed by Bryng Bryngelson long ago.

Pull-outs as the consequence of cancellation

As we have mentioned, some stutterers almost immediately seem to be able to apply the modifications they learned through cancellation and need none of this training or teaching. They learn the knack of pulling out of their blocks in much the same way as they learn to skate or acquire some other motor skill. A few falls; a little wobbling, and suddenly they can do it.

With younger children and with mentally retarded stutterers, often all they require are models the therapist can provide by throwing himself into the kind of stuttering shown by the case and then demonstrating how the pull-out can be accomplished. "When you get stuck, do it this way!" By stuttering in unison with the client, the therapist begins by duplicating the beginning of the stutterer's abnormality, and then shifts out of it in a more appropriate fashion. If the identification is adequate, the stutterer tends to follow the therapist's model and so finds himself using the new way almost without realizing it. In this case it is necessary, however, through recording or mirror observation or the therapist's reduplication, to have the stutterer become very aware of what he has done. Also the therapist may throw himself into a good facsimile of the client's stuttering, then ask the stutterers to *show* the therapist how to pull out of it and to do this by demonstrating through simultaneous pantomiming the necessary varying and shifts. By teaching the therapist, the stutterer thus teaches himself.

Other models of very good pull-outs can be collected from the stutterer's own speech. Among all the kinds of stutterings shown by an adult stutterer, there are always a few that are excellent examples of successful pull-outs. If these can be recorded on video-tape, or viewed in the mirror as they are happening, the therapist can help the stutterer to recognize and fix them as the models he can emulate more often. Some of our cases have mastered better techniques of responding to their felt blockages by deliberately flooding their speech with samples of good pull-outs, using them at first mainly on nonfeared words, and then with words on which they expect to stutter. When this approach is used,

it is wise to make sure that the shifts will emerge from behavior which is very close to that typical of the person's usual stuttering. Also, we often suggest that the stutterer in this faking, should demonstrate, not perfect pull-outs but a series of progressively better ones. What we are after, of course, is to use these assumed pull-outs as a way of teaching him that there are alternative responses available to him when he finds himself unable to proceed. We want him to learn how to search for the better ways.

In our desire to be explicit about what happens during this stage of therapy we fear we have made the process of modifying the stuttering seem much more laborious and intricate than it really is. Most of our stutterers do not find it difficult at all, probably because we have done so much preparatory work in identification, desensitization, variation, and cancellation. Or perhaps because by this time the concurrent psychotherapy has begun to make itself felt. While there are some stutterers who again use this new challenge as another opportunity to resist accepting any responsibility for their behavior, most of them greet the need to explore new and better ways of releasing themselves from the tyranny of their impediment with some alacrity.

We have also been impressed by the way that acquiring skill in pulling out of their blocks seems to produce marked decrements in anxiety and fear. By giving the stutterer something specific to do when he encounters a fixation or oscillation, much of the anticipatory stress is relieved. Ambivalence augments fear. This is why the military forces drill their men so hard in stereotyped ways of coping with possible (though not predictable) enemy action such as hand to hand combat. Having available a plan, any plan, for coping with a prospective emergency is fear-reducing. Drinkwater, Cleland, and Flint (1968) make this point vividly in their description of pilot training. They point out that the opportunity to learn certain control behaviors "reduces the anticipatory stress generated to a level where it enhances performance rather than impairs it." We find this same thing happening when the stutterer learns ways of modifying his stuttering response.

The use of motor planning and preparatory sets

In his *Theories of Perception and the Concept of Structure,* Allport (1955) chided his fellow psychologists for their neglect of motor and perceptual sets as determinants of behavior. Since that time modern neurophysiology has contributed major information concerning the bases of arousal, selective attention, and motor planning.[9] The *reticular formation* in the brain seems to be especially important in these functions since it seems to act in part as a screening filter of incoming information from all of these sense modalities, and, as such, probably has much to do in determining the responses based upon this information. Hilgard and Atkinson (1967) describe preparatory sets as follows:

Some of the selectivity in perception is present before the stimulus appears. We prepare ourselves to perceive and to act upon stimuli that we expect to appear. Such a preparation goes by the name of *set,* and it has the same meaning here as in the situation of the runner who gets *set* to run at the sound of a gun. His set

9 One of the best expositions of the role of the reticular formation in arousal and motor planning is found in the reference by French (1960).

includes both the readiness to hear the gun and the readiness to leap forward into the race. When a person is set, the actual stimulus that initiates his action, like the sound of the shot for the runner, is merely an occasion for action that was largely prepared for in advance. Momentary set is an anticipatory adjustment holding certain kinds of responses in readiness. (p. 239)

Frick (1961) says, ". . . one reason why the stutterer's motor plan breaks down is that he puts his articulators into an unnatural position as part of 'getting ready' for the point in the (verbal) sequence which is perceived to be difficult. As a result of this unnatural position, he literally does not know how to get out of it (p. 5)." It is our contention that these abnormal anticipatory postures are due to conditioned motor sets.

It is also our conviction that much of the impression of compulsivity and involuntariness that characterizes so many stuttering behaviors is due to the functioning of abnormal preparatory sets. It is even possible to observe the stutterer covertly rehearsing his struggling before he even attempts a feared word. These tiny motor rehearsals of anticipated unpleasantness are doubtless the source of the stutterer's perception of impending doom. They have been so thoroughly conditioned to various situational and verbal cues that somehow we must design a therapy that will alter and prevent them. In this section we describe how we try to do so.

As stutterers become more adept in the use of pull-outs we find again the same tendency to move forward in time that previously we have seen with the cancellations. The new slow-motion form of fluent stuttering that had been learned through the cancellation and the pull-out modification techniques now appear in the stutterer's speech, not as a response to the actual experience of stuttering, but instead as a response to its anticipation. This means that a new way of attempting feared words is being learned. We seek to condition this new slow-motion approach to the same cues that in the past have triggered avoidance or struggle. As the stutterer scans approaching words for features that indicate the probability of stuttering, he now *prepares* to use the same behaviors he learned in cancelling and pull-outs. Rejecting his old abnormal preformations and tendencies to use hard contacts and sudden surges of tension, he plans to begin the feared word in a more normal fashion, integrating the timing of airflow and phonation and working slowly through the motoric sequence. He plans to use the right syllable rather than one containing his usual stuttering schwa vowel. We help him understand that the new model of fluent stuttering which he will be using as a replacement for the old one is pretty largely a slowed version of the standard utterance. Some writers have misunderstood this and have asked the stutterer merely to prolong the first sound or the vowel of the feared word being attempted. We reject this as being very unwise. We do not want the stutterer to distort the motoric sequence by such prolongations; we want the whole sequence to be slowed down, all sounds and transitions proportionally. We want him simply to work through all the parts of the word slowly. Occasionally, to make this point, we have him perform other activities in slow-motion, scratching his head, lifting a foot, opening his mouth, clapping his hands. We don't care how fast he talks but we do want him to stutter very slowly.

But is it stuttering? Again we meet the difficulty of definition. Our stutter-

ers have called it "fluent stuttering." We care not. It is new behavior, more adaptive behavior, a replacement that becomes conditioned to the same antecedent cues that formerly led to highly abnormal avoidance or struggle. It is also one that transfers very easily into normal speech. The stutterer who stutters in this way can be very fluent.

Why does the stutterer now tend to prepare in advance to try to use this new way rather attempting his feared words in the old ways? First of all he does so because the new "fluent stuttering" receives powerful reinforcement. Repeatedly, during the cancellation and pull-out phases of training, this new, slow-motion utterance has been followed by communicative progress. Unlike the old avoidance and struggle kinds of stuttering behaviors that provoked so much listener rejection and penalties, this new replacement instead seems quite acceptable. If noticed, it gains respect. The listener feels the stutterer is trying to master his difficulty. His former abnormal reactions left the stutterer feeling helpless and impotent; the new ones give him a sense of mastery. The older forms of stuttering generated anxiety, guilt and frustration; the new kind does not but instead builds up the stutterer's self-esteem. To the stutterer, the old behaviors feel involuntary; the new ones are sensed as being under his direct control. It is easier and less effortful to stutter in the new way than in the old. And, of course, the new fluent form of stuttering receives strong reinforcement from the one who has now become a very significant person in the stutterer's life—the therapist.

We have watched the spontaneous development of these fluent stutterings as replacements for the old stuttering patterns with great interest since we hoped thereby to find new ways of helping those stutterers who did not acquire them without training. What seemed to take place was this. Those stutterers who skipped the pull-out stage immediately began to use the same procedures learned in cancelling moments of past stuttering whenever they expected to stutter on an approaching word. They rehearsed both the old and the new forms of stuttering, then chose the latter. Sometimes they pantomimed both forms in sequence in the period just prior to the attempt on the feared word. We did no teach this nor encourage it but these stutterers simply substituted the preparatory set to use the new slow-motion kind of stuttering whenever they expected difficulty. What they did was to change their motor planning for the feared utterance.[10] They chose a newer, easier way of responding to expectancy of stuttering because it seemed better than the old.

Other stutterers began to use this new kind of stuttering (in speaking their feared words) as a result of their experiences in learning how to extricate themselves from their old stuttering behavior with pull-outs. Though at first they deliberately prolonged the old stuttering behavior before they modified it, these prolongations eventually became shorter and shorter until finally none of the old stuttering behaviors could be observed. The new strategy of slowly and progressively working through the motoric sequence of a feared word now became conditioned, not to the experience of actual fixation or oscillation, but to its expectancy. Prior to the moment of speech attempt, the stutterer deliberately seemed to revise his old motor planning. He would

simply set himself in advance to use the new kind of fluent stuttering as a replacement for his old responses. Early in this learning process, these replacements occurred only occasionally. They appeared to be almost unconscious and automatic, the stutterer showing surprise when they occurred. The cues which led him to expect that he would have considerable difficulty now were followed by a form of utterance which, though slightly different than normal speech, impeded the forward flow of communication very little and evoked very little negative reaction from his listeners. When the stutterers expected severe unpleasantness and then found little or none, their fears decayed in intensity very rapidly. As they became reduced, the frequency and severity of his stuttering began to lessen and this too was powerfully reinforcing. Some stutterers achieved very fluent speech as a result of this *automatic* acquisition of new preparatory sets.

One of the difficulties we experienced in working with these stutterers who learned to use the new fluent form of stuttering spontaneously and almost unconsciously was that they were often quite unaware of what they were doing or had done. There were always some of them who could use the new form rather consistently when the fears were low but when the fears were intense, the older motor sets became dominant and then they stuttered in their old ways. Accordingly we felt that it was necessary to help them know vividly what they had to do and to be able to assume the new preparatory sets voluntarily rather than automatically. Also there were always some stutterers who did not show this spontaneous acquisition of the new behavior. In them the new slow-motion stuttering remained locked to the percep-

10 An interesting account of stuttering therapy based upon motor planning is provided by Frick (1965).

tion that they were blocking or repeating. These stutterers needed help in learning to use the cues signalling approaching stuttering as mandates or alerters to change their preparatory motor sets. They needed to discover how to use the period just prior to the speech attempt to prepare to utter the word in a more fluent fashion.

Motor planning: normal and abnormal. We must recognize that a motor plan or preparatory set comes into being as soon as some cue colored by stuttering is perceived. Prior to therapy, the stutterer gets set to experience abnormality on some fragment of the motor sequence. He gets set to stutter. Prehearing the kind of abnormality he expects, he tends to go through a covert motor rehearsal that would produce that abnormality. These abnormal preparatory sets are bound to interfere with the normal motor plans that usually precede a normal speech attempt. The interference is compounded because it seems probable that a normal speaker employs a motor plan for normal speech that is much more extensive than one which occurs under threat of stuttering. Such a speaker's motor plan is one which probably represents in truncated form the prosody of the entire phrase or sentence rather than the smaller segment of a word, syllable, or sound. But when a stutterer expects to have trouble producing a word or syllable or even an isolated sound (and this is often what the stutterer does expect) these more comprehensive motor plans so characteristic of normal speech are disrupted by the preparations specific to those feared fragments. For example, if all of one's attention is riveted on the possibility of complete closure on the plosive "p," or on the probability of no phonation on an initial vowel,

or if he feels certain that he will repeat over and over again the first syllable of a word, disruption of the motor planning for the larger prosodic sequences will tend to occur. Usually we are not very conscious of the way we prepare for this normal encoding of motoric speech; the process is almost automatic. We open our mouths and start talking, formulating, and organizing as we go and the motoric processing requires little awareness. But, for the stutterer, with the red flare of danger illuminating certain speech fragments such as the sound or syllable, these fragments become the focus of his attention, and also the foci of his motoric planning. Anticipating difficulty on one of these segments, he therefore prepares to avoid, struggle, or cope with it in one abnormal way or another and therefore most of the preparatory sets he assumes almost insure that he will have the trouble he expects.[11]

Many of the methods used in treating stuttering owe their temporary efficacy to distraction. We believe that these techniques work only so long as they are able to interfere with the stutterer's specific abnormal motor sets, i.e., only so long as the techniques are novel enough to shift the stutterer's attention away from feared sounds, syllables, or words and so to prevent the occurrence of the abnormal motor rehearsals sets pertinent to each. They do not replace these abnormal motor sets with better ones. They merely blot them out temporarily. Therefore as soon as the novelty wears off, and the distraction no longer distracts, the stutterer's fluency-fragmentation again becomes

[11] For a more extensive discussion of the role of preparatory sets in stuttering therapy see Van Riper (1937), Van Riper (1958), Luper and Mulder (1964), and Robinson (1964).

prepotent and he is back where he was before treatment began.

Some therapists have tried valiantly to build up the awareness of the longer prosodic patterns by teaching the stutterer to rehearse his sentences in advance, to speak in careful and conscious phrasing, hoping that by so doing the larger motor plans would become dominant over the smaller more fragmentary stuttering ones. To a degree this can be done and should be done. We use similar methods later in stabilization, in terminal therapy. But we must remember that the stutterer localizes his difficulty not in his inability to say a phrase or sentence but in his felt inability to emit a sound, syllable, or word. It is on these latter segments that the negative emotionality settles. These are what get colored by fear and frustration; these are what carry the cues which indicate approaching stuttering. It is on sounds, syllables, and words that the stutterer feels he has had his past troubles thousands and thousands of times. Somehow we must find some ways to keep these cue perceptions from generating the specific abnormal motor sets that inevitably lead to unnecessary abnormality in utterance. Admittedly, the linkage is very strong after years of stuttering, and so we need competing preparatory sets *specific to these segments.* For example, after almost 40 years of saying the word "degree" pretty fluently, the author still finds his tongue automatically assuming an incorrect trigger posture whenever he even reads this word silently. He has revised this abnormal motor pattern many thousands of times and has not stuttered in his old way on the word for years, yet the tendency toward assuming the old abnormal motor set of the "d" of this word is still strong for it was very strongly conditioned long

ago. It does not extinguish; it does not go away. (If it did, the author would probably miss it.) He can now *automatically* reject this old motor plan and substitute a better one and he does. This little example makes the point we wish to stress: somehow we must provide the stutterer with competing preparatory sets and condition these to the same cues if we hope to reduce the inevitability of stuttering in the old fashion.

Bloodstein (1969) has a clear description of these abnormal motor sets that need replacement by better ones:

First, the stutterer establishes an abnormal focus of tension in his speech organs. Second, he prepares himself to say the first sound of the difficult word as a fixed articulatory posture rather than as a normal movement blending with the rest of the word. Third, he may adopt this unnatural posture of his speech organs appreciably before he initiates voice or airflow, resulting in a silent "preformation" of the sound. Having done all of these things, it is apparent that he has effectively destroyed his chances of saying it normally. (p. 33)

How then do we teach the stutterer to assume a different motor set when he approaches a feared word or sound? First of all, we help him have a clear *motoric* model of the new behavior, one which might if necessary be rehearsed prior to the speech attempt; secondly, we need to link this rehearsal with the precipitating cue; and thirdly, the speech attempt should follow directly on the heels of the rehearsal. We have already discussed in our account of cancellation and pull-outs how this new model of fluent stuttering can be developed and we must remember that even during the identification stage of therapy, the stutterer has occasionally recognized samples of these fluent slow-motion stutterings in his speech. But there is still a very real need to get the model very vividly in mind and mouth and to associate it with the stimuli which ordinarily trigger the old abnormal stuttering motor sets.

We have explored many possible ways of accomplishing this goal and we find that perhaps the most effective one is to get the stutterer to introduce the new behavior into his normal speech. We ask him to try to fill his communication, with facsimiles of these fluent stutterings at least two or three to a sentence. When he does so, he discovers that they create little interference with his communication. His listeners do not seem to object. Indeed, if the new kind of stuttering is done well, often his listeners do not even seem to recognize it as stuttering. Gregory (1968) gives a brief glimpse of this state of affairs in narrating his successful therapy with a 23-year-old female stutterer:

Cora was feeling increasing good about her new speech pattern as she used cancellations, pull-outs, and new preparatory sets. She worked on phrasing, increased oral activity (she had a tendency not to open her mouth sufficiently, resulting in slurred speech), inflection, etc. She reported the changed speech pattern was beginning to come naturally. In talking with a male friend about her stuttering and the reason why she would not go into teaching, she found this friend was not "impressed" by her stuttering problem and did not see why it should prevent her from being a teacher. (p. 44)

Admittedly the speech is slowed down somewhat by using these preparatory sets but the messages get through. Therefore at first we ask the stutterer to insert these models only on nonfeared words since our purpose is to make sure that the motor patterns of the new slow-motion behavior are thoroughly mastered. If the stutterer does find himself stuttering, on other words that he really does fear, he then uses the pull-outs and cancellation as before, thereby gaining the experiences that make vivid the models we seek, the models he needs for his motor planning. We have found it important that the stutterers stay in this phase of therapy for some time, certainly until they are able to communicate easily despite the presence of many of these deliberate insertions of slow-motion stuttering.

What usually occurs as a result of these experiences is that very soon the stutterer begins to use these new ways of attempting his feared words (as well as his nonfeared ones), with the change occurring spontaneously. Indeed this often occurs despite our instructions to the contrary or even despite the stutterer's own intention. This seems to be due to the fact that by flooding his speech with these new models, the stutterer is bound to have used the new fluent form of stuttering on many words and sounds that had potential cues for older forms of stuttering. After the stutterer has used the new smooth, slow, easy kind of pseudostuttering on many nonfeared words beginning with an "m" sound for example, he will naturally tend to use behaviors similar to it also when he perceives an m-word approaching that he mildly fears. There are gradients involved in these stuttering-colored stimuli, and if the new competing response-set is introduced far out on the gradient, it will tend eventually to generalize, dominate, and inhibit the older one. Something of the sort does seem to occur for soon we find the stutterers tending to use the new kind of fluent stuttering when attempting words which in the past elicited marked expectancy of stuttering. Sometimes, of course, the old motor sets win out and, as we have said, the person begins to stutter in his old way but this merely provides another opportunity to modify or to cancel the old behavior. In such an instance, we must remember that some progress is still being made whether the new preparatory set fails or not. In any event, the old form of stuttering is not being reinforced by communicative consummation. The tight linkage of the old struggle and avoidance behaviors with the same anticipatory cues is now stretched, strained, or broken. The vicious circle of self-maintenance that characterizes the disorder is now under hard attack.

Once these spontaneous attempts to substitute new preparatory sets for old ones begin to occur on the feared words with some consistency, we move to a new step involving the direct confrontation of choice. Now we ask the stutterer to seek out his most feared words in his most feared situations and attempt to substitute the new form of stuttering for the old. To facilitate this, we have the stutterers hunt for trophies, a trophy being a very feared word on which he overtly goes through a pantomiming [12] of the old form of stuttering, then pantomiming the new form of stuttering, then immediately to the

12 Brenner (1969) showed that voiced rehearsal of feared words yielded less stuttering than whispered, pantomimed or silent rehearsal thus indicating that the motor plan was aided when all the features of utterance were rehearsed. While this may be true for the conditions of his experiment, we feel that it is wiser to provide a hierarchy of approximations that begins with pantomimed rehearsal when teaching the stutterer new preparatory sets.

uttering of the word aloud in the new slow-motion way. Again, if he tries and fails, he pulls out of that old behavior, or failing that, cancels it, or failing even that, uses the same word again in some other sentence to provide some final opportunity to make progress. The reader will recognize here the parallel between this training in the use of new preparatory sets and the manner in which the stutterer earlier learned to cancel the words on which he stuttered involuntarily. Once again, the stutterer will find the listener's respect whether he wins or loses. Once again, he will find that eventually his successes will become more frequent than his failures.

Our next step in the therapy sequence at this stage is to get the stutterer to omit the overt pantomiming. First he omits only his pantomiming of the old kind of stuttering, and then later he omits both the old and new. Rehearsals now are covert and the therapist must be careful to determine that the stutterer actually rehearses covertly in the short pause before the feared word so that the pause is not used merely as a postponement. Then finally we ask the stutterer to omit any rehearsal of the old kind of stuttering and to confine his covert rehearsal only to the new fluent form of stuttering when he expects difficulty and to try to do this rehearsal as swiftly as possible. A few stutterers at this point temporarily fall into one of two traps. Either they use the slight pause prior to speech attempt not for rehearsing the new fluent form of stuttering but instead as a postponement trick or else they try to assume the new preparatory set while covertly rehearsing the old abnormal one. A knowledgeable therapist will counter by reinforcing swifter covert rehearsals and by suggesting that the stutterer come to a state of rest just before the rehearsal thus preventing what some have termed the "prephonational tonus." Most of our stutterers have not experienced these difficulties and they learn very soon to assume the motor sets for fluent stuttering almost automatically which of course is what we desire.

About this time there usually occurs a great surge of fluency. The stutterer has conquered his personal demon—so he thinks. He has learned that he can be very fluent even though he stutterers. His fears melt away. Often he goes on a talking jag, drunk with verbosity. Instead of avoiding, he hunts for tough speaking situations and feared words and discovers that now they are difficult to find and when found do not seem as formidable as before. One stutterer exulted, "I feel almost as though I were in love. In love with myself. I'm riding high." Hope soars; so does self-esteem. At such a time, the competent therapist will keep his fingers crossed and show them to the stutterer. He knows that there is more to be done but surely he will not begrudge nor soil this good moment of triumph.

Bibliography

ADAMCZYK, R. (Use of instruments for the production of artificial feedback in the treatment of stuttering), *Folia Phoniatrica,* 11 (1959), 216–18.

ALLPORT, F. H., *Theories of Perception and the Concept of Structure.* New York: Wiley, 1955.

BASILI, A. G., *An Electromyographic Study of Stuttering Tremor and its Relation to Isometric Contraction Tremor,* Doctoral Dissertation, Purdue University, 1971.

BLOODSTEIN, O., *A Handbook on Stuttering.* Chicago: National Easter Seal Society for Crippled Children and Adults, 1969.

BOHR, J. W. F., The effects of electronic and other external control methods on stuttering: A review of some research techniques and suggestions for further research, *Journal of South African Logopedic Society,* 10 (1963), 4–13.

BRENNER, N., *Effects of Types of Rehearsal on Frequency of Stuttering.* Doctoral Dissertation, University of Southern California, 1969.

BRYNGELSON, B., A method of stuttering, *Journal of Abnormal Social Psychology,* 30 (1935), 194–98.

————, M. E. CHAPMAN, and O. K. HANSEN, *Know Yourself—A Workbook for Those Who Stutter.* Minneapolis: Burgess, 1944.

BUTLER, R. R. JR. and P. E. STANLEY, The stuttering problem considered from an automatic control point of view, *Folia Phoniatrica,* 18 (1966), 33–44

CAMERON, N. A., Role concepts in behavior pathology, *American Journal of Sociology,* 55 (1950), 464–67.

CURLEE, R. F. and W. H. PERKINS, The effect of punishment of expectancy to stutter on the frequencies of subsequent expectancies and stuttering, *Journal of Speech and Hearing Research,* 11 (1968), 787–95.

DAMSTE, P. H., E. J. ZWAAN, and T. J. Schoenaker, Learning principles applied to the stuttering problem, *Folia Phoniatrica,* 20 (1968), 327–41.

DRINKWATER, B. L., T. CLELAND, and M. M. FLINT, Pilot performance during periods of anticipatory physical threat stress, *Aerospace Medicine,* 39 (1968), 994–99.

ELLIS, A., *Reason and Emotion in Psychotherapy.* New York: Stuart, 1962.

FESTINGER, L., *A Theory of Cognitive Dissonance.* Stanford, Calif.: Stanford University Press, 1957.

FIBIGER, S., *Stuttering Explained as a Physiological Tremor.* Stockholm: Department of Speech Communication, Royal Institute of Technology, 1971.

FRENCH, J. D., The reticular formation, in J. Field, H. W. Magoun, and V. E. Hall (eds.), *Handbook of Physiology*, vol. 2., Washington, D.C.: American Physiological Society, 1960, pp. 1281–1305.

FRICK, J. V., *Evaluation of Motor Planning Techniques for the Treatment of Stuttering*. Final Report Grant 32–48–0720–5003, U.S. Department of Health, Education, and Welfare, Office of Education, 1965.

GOLDIAMOND, I., Stuttering and fluency as manipulatable operant response classes, in K. Krasner and L. P. Ullman (eds.), *Research in Behavior Modification*. New York: Holt, Rinehart & Winston, 1965.

GOULD, E. and J. SHEEHAN, Effect of silence on stuttering, *Journal Abnormal Psychology*, 72 (1967), 441–45.

GREGORY, H., A clinical success: Cora, in H. Luper (ed.), *Stuttering: Successes and Failures in Therapy*. Memphis: Speech Foundation of America, 1968.

————— (ed.), *Learning Theory and Stuttering Therapy*. Evanston, Ill.: Northwestern University Press, 1968.

HARVEY, O. and G. BEVERLY, Some personality correlates of concept change through role playing, *Journal of Abnormal and Social Psychology*, 63 (1961), 125–30.

HAROLDSON, S. K., R. R. MARTIN, and C. D. Starr, Time-out as a punishment for stuttering, *Journal of Speech and Hearing Research*, 11 (1968), 560–66.

HEFFERLINE, R. F., Learning theory and clinical psychology—an eventual symbiosis, in A. J. Bachrach (ed.), *Experimental Foundations of Clinical Psychology*. New York: Basic Books, 1962, pp. 97–138.

HILGARD, E. R. and R. C. ATKINSON, *Introduction to Psychology*, 4th ed. New York: Harcourt Brace Jovanovich, 1967.

HOFFER, E., *The Ordeal of Change*. New York: Harper & Row, 1968.

JANIS, I. L. and J. B. GILMORE, The influence of incentive conditions on the success of role playing in modifying attitudes, *Journal of Personality and Social Psychology*, 1 (1965), 17–27.

JANIS, I. L. and B. T. King, The influence of role playing on opinion change, *Journal of Abnormal and Social Psychology*, 49 (1954), 211–18.

LAZARUS, A. A., Behaviour rehearsal vs. nondirective therapy vs. advice in effecting behavior change, *Behaviour Research and Therapy*, 4 (1966), 209–12.

—————, Behaviour therapy, incomplete treatment, and symptom substitution, *Journal of Nervous and Mental Diseases*, 140 (1965), 80–86.

—————, The results of behavior therapy in 126 cases of severe neurosis, *Behaviour Research and Therapy*, 1 (1963), 69–79.

LENNON, E. J., *Le begaiement: Therapeutiques modernes*. Paris: Doin et Cie, 1962.

LOTZMANN, G. (On the use of varied delay times in stammerers), *Folia Phoniatrica*, 13 (1961), 276–310.

LUPER, H. L. and R. L. MULDER, *Stuttering Therapy for Children*. Englewood Cliffs, N.J.: Prentice-Hall, 1964.

MACKAY, D. G., To speak with an accent: Effects of nasal distortion on stuttering under delayed auditory feedback, *Perceptual Psychophysics*, 5 (1969), 183–88.

McKENZIE, F. A., A stutterer's experience in using an electrolarynx, in W. Johnson (ed.), *Stuttering in Children and Adults*. Minneapolis: University of Minnesota Press, 1955.

MAIER, N. R. F. and P. ELLEN, The prophylactic effects of "guidance" in reducing rigid behavior, *Journal of Abnormal and Social Psychology*, 47 (1952), 109–16.

MARTIN, J. E., The signal detection hypothesis and perceptual defect theory of stuttering, *Journal of Speech and Hearing Disorders*, 35 (1970), 252–55.

MILLER, N. E., Some implications of

modern behavior therapy for personality change and psychotherapy, in P. Worchel P. and D. Byrne (eds.), *Personality Change.* New York: Wiley, 1964.

MYSAK, E. D., *Speech Pathology and Feedback Theory.* Springfield, Ill.: Charles C Thomas, 1966.

————, Servo theory and stuttering, *Journal of Speech and Hearing Disorders,* 25 (1960), 188–95.

NESSEL, E., Die verzögerts sprachruckkopplung (Lee-effekt) bei der stotterern, *Folia Foniatrica,* 10 (1958), 199–204.

OSGOOD, C. E. and P. H. TANNENBAUM, The principle of congruity in the prediction of attitude change, *Psychological Review,* 62 (1955), 42–55.

PERKINS, W. H. and R. F. CURLEE, Clinical impressions of portable masking unit effects in stuttering, *Journal of Speech and Hearing Disorders,* 34 (1969), 360–63.

QUARRINGTON, B. and E. DOUGLASS, Audibility avoidance in non-vocalized stutterers, *Journal of Speech and Hearing Disorders,* 25 (1960), 358–65.

RINGEL, R. C., and F. D. MINIFIE, Protensity estimates of stutterers and nonstutterers, *Journal of Speech and Hearing Research,* 9 (1966), 289–96.

ROBINSON, F., *An Introduction to Stuttering.* Englewood Cliffs, N.J.: Prentice-Hall, 1964.

SARBIN, T. R. and V. L. ALLEN, Role theory, in G. Lindsay and E. Aronson (eds.), *Handbook of Social Psychology.* Reading, Mass.: Addison-Wesley, 1968.

SHANNON, C. E., Prediction and entropy of printed English, *Bell System Technical Journal,* 30 (1951), 50–64.

SHEEHAN, J. G., Conflict theory of stuttering, In J. Eisenson (ed.), *Stuttering: A Symposium.* New York: Harper & Row, 1958.

————, *Stuttering: Research and Therapy.* New York: Harper & Row, 1970.

SODERBERG, G. A., Delayed auditory feedback and stuttering, *Journal of Speech and Hearing Disorders,* 33 (1968), 260–66.

————, Delayed auditory feedback and the speech of stutterers, 34 (1969), 20–29.

STROMSTA, C., Experimental blockage of phonation by distorted sidetone, *Journal of Speech and Hearing Research,* 2 (1959), 286–301.

STURM, I. E., The behavioristic aspect of psychodrama, *Group Psychotherapy,* 18 (1965), 50–64.

THIBAUT, J. W. and H. H. KELLEY, *The Social Psychology of Groups.* New York: Wiley, 1959.

TROJAN, F. A., A new method in the treatment of stuttering: The Kinetic discharge therapy, *Folia Phoniatrica,* 17 (1965), 195–201.

TROTTER, W. D. and M. M. LESCH, Personal experiences with a stutter-aid, *Journal of Speech and Hearing Disorders,* 32 (1967), 270–72.

TRUAX, C. B. and R. B. CARKHUFF, *Toward Effective Counseling and Psychotherapy.* Chicago: Aldine-Atherton, 1967.

VAN RIPER, C., Study of the thoracic breathing of stutterers during expectancy or occurrence of stuttering, *Journal of Speech Disorders,* 1 (1936), 61–72.

————, The preparatory set in stuttering, *Journal of Speech Disorders,* 2 (1937), 149–54.

————, Experiments in stuttering therapy, in J. Eisenson (ed.), *Stuttering: A Symposium.* New York: Harper & Row, 1958.

————, *Speech Correction: Principles and Methods,* 4th ed. Englewood Cliffs, N.J.: Prentice-Hall, 1963.

————, Clinical use of intermittent masking noise in stuttering therapy, *Asha,* 7 (1965), 381.

————, Dave. A clinical success, in Speech Foundation of America, *Stuttering: Success and Failures in Therapy.* Memphis, Tenn.: Fraser, 1968.

————, *The Nature of Stuttering.*

Englewood Cliffs, N.J.: Prentice-Hall, 1971.

WEBSTER, L. L. and B. B. LUBKER, Masking of auditory feedback in stutterer's speech, *Journal of Speech and Hearing Research,* 11 (1969a), 219–23.

————, Interrelationship among fluency producing variables in stuttered speech, *Journal of Speech and Hearing Research,* 11 (1968), 754–66.

WELSH, J. J., *Stuttering Tremor: An Exploration of Methodologies for Recording and Analysis.* Unpublished Master's Thesis, Western Michigan University, 1970.

WINGATE, M. E., Calling attention to stuttering, *Journal of Speech and Hearing Research,* 2 (1959), 326–35.

————, Effect on stuttering of changes in audition, *Journal of Speech and Hearing Research,* 13 (1970), 861–73.

WISCHNER, G. J., Experimental approach to expectancy and anxiety in stuttering behavior, *Journal of Speech and Hearing Disorders,* 17 (1952), 139–54.

WOLPE, J., *Psychotherapy by Reciprocal Inhibition.* Stanford, Calif.: Stanford University Press, 1958.

YATES, A. J., Delayed auditory feedback and shadowing, *Quarterly Journal of Experimental Psychology,* 17 (1965), 125–31.

————, Recent empirical and theoretical approaches to the experimental manipulation of speech in normal speakers and in stammerers, *Behaviour Research and Therapy,* 1 (1963), 95–119.

————, The relationship between theory and therapy in the clinical treatment of stuttering, in B. B. Gray and G. England (eds.), *Stuttering and the Conditioning Therapies.* Monterey, Calif.: Monterey Institute, 1969.

YOUNG, E. H., The motokinesthetic approach to the prevention of speech defects including stuttering, *Journal of Speech and Hearing Disorders,* 30 (1965), 269–73.

Stabilization

For many reasons which we shall seek to make clear, we have found it important to insert into our overall design of therapy a definite period devoted specifically to the consolidation and stabilization of the new behaviors which the stutterer has now learned in responding to the threat or occurrence of stuttering. We reject any temporary solution of the stutterer's problems. Were a short interval of fluency our goal, we could quickly and easily produce this through palliative methods. We could use suggestion, relaxation or timing tricks. We could put the stutterer into a laboratory booth and use contingent punishment. We could have him sing his way to better speech or hypnotize him. But our aim, instead, is to help the stutterer so that throughout the rest of his life, he will no longer need to live with a twisted tongue or a warped personality.

In our extensive review of the literature on stuttering therapy, we have found many reports of relapse but very little information concerning the steps taken by therapists to consolidate the gains made by the stutterer. Perhaps very little has been done. Once the therapy makes the stutterer fluent, he is dismissed and hopefully does not return. The operant therapists, however, have recognized the need for building a maintenance phase into their programs, and Ryan (1968) describes one of them as follows:

For Stan, the maintenance program included weekly meetings with the speech therapist near his home, weekly tape recordings made with his family and sent to the University Clinic for analysis, and periodic visits to the University Clinic. These visits totalled 45 hours over a nine month period. The tape recordings revealed a gradual increase in stuttering rate up to 8 stuttered words per minute. He and his parents also reported that his speech was even less fluent in natural situations than it was during the tape recording sessions and that some situations were still extremely difficult for him. As a result, we saw him again the following summer for an additional 95 hours of instruction. Throughout many varied speaking situations, including a speech to a meeting of over 100 speech therapists, he demonstrated fluency at a rate of less than .5 stuttered words per minute. In the following year, the maintenance program included tape recordings twice a week, telephone calls, periodic visits to the University Clinic, and no more local speech therapy. These activities were then faded out toward the end of the year. Altogether, there were 13 hours of tape recording and 29 telephone calls. This new low rate continued in a wide variety of speaking situations, including debating, leading prayers in church, etc., and has continued for the last 6 months. The present maintenance program consists of monthly post card and yearly clinic visits.

Stan's program was a little different from the program described in this chapter because Stan was one of the first people whom we put through the entire program, and we did not know at that time what steps were necessary, how long to keep him at various steps, and so on. Altogether, more than 225 hours were devoted to Stan's program, and we are not through yet. (p. 74)

Our own maintenance program is much more varied than the operant one just described and, as will become apparent, does not require the extensive use of "booster sessions."

The need for a stabilization phase of therapy

Once the stutterer has undergone the course of treatment we have been describing, he becomes very fluent. When fears again arise, he no longer is helpless or resigned but he has the tools to cope with them. If occasionally he stutters, he is not traumatized for he knows how to use these stutterings as opportunities to make further progress. Often for the first time in his life he really enjoys talking and he does a lot of it. He feels better about himself as a person. At such a time therapists are often tempted to terminate treatment prematurely—and so are the stutterers. They feel that the battle for self-understanding and self-mastery has been won; surely now it is time to retire from the therapeutic milieu. Unfortunately this does not seem to be the case. There is more to be done for we must consolidate our gains. Unless both the therapist and his case understand clearly the reasons for the stabilization stage of therapy, neither will willingly undertake the work it entails. Therefore we will try to clarify its rationale.

There is a very old law in psychology (Jost's law) which can be stated as follows: if two learned responses are of equal strength today, the older one will be stronger tomorrow. We have repeatedly stressed the fact that most of the abnormality of stuttering consists of learned responses to the expectancy or occurrence of temporally distorted words. By now our therapy has established new responses to these experiences but we have not repealed the laws of learning. These new and more adaptive responses have been built carefully and in the contexts of anxiety and frustration so that they could compete successfully with the old abnormal ones. However, when we deal with an adult stutterer, we are confronted by avoidance and struggle reactions that have been powerfully reinforced for years. We cannot expect that they will have been reduced to zero strength even when they do not appear to affect the stutterer's communication. We cannot expect that some spontaneous recovery will not occur and if these old responses to the threat or experience of fluency failure beget a renewal of the stutterer's old morbid attitudes, we can expect some relapse. The former struggle and avoidance responses lie latent, ready to arise. Slice as we will, there is a tendency for the hydra of stuttering to sprout a new head. The whole history of psychological investigation tells us that anxiety-conditioned avoidance responses have always proved remarkably resistant to complete extinction. Though we have continuously insisted that the stutterer do his therapy not solely in the safe little island of the clinic but out in the traumatic world, it is never possible to condition the new responses to all the old cues to which the stutterer may tend to respond by avoidance and struggle. There are always limits to the amount of generalization we can hope for. Under conditions of great stress or under fatigue, or in those periods when the stutterer's self-esteem is low, the latent strength of these old reactions is very likely to manifest itself. Having plenty of it himself, the author has a great respect for human frailty. No one can always do what he knows he should do.

There are other forces, too, that necessitate this stabilization stage of therapy. Self-concepts do not change overnight nor overyear. Though the experience is very pleasant, it often is also strange and unsettling to be speaking very fluently when one has stuttered throughout a lifetime. As one of our stutterers said, "It's almost as though a stranger were inhabiting my skin and doing my talking for me." Sheehan (1970) points up the problem in this bit of advice to the stutterer:

You may be astonished that fluency is anything to which you would have to adjust. Yet it is a central problem in the consolidation of improvement. Just as in the early stages of therapy, you had to accept your role as a stutterer, so in the later phases, you have to accept your role as a more normal speaker. The second adjustment is sometimes bigger than the first one. You have to overcome the feeling that all fluency is false and undeserved. (p. 294)

Moreover, old acquaintances may show pleasure when they observe the new fluency but in many ways they react as though the person were still the stutterer they have always known. They talk for him. They wait for him to talk. Their attitudes show that they constantly expect stuttering and are surprised when it is not apparent. Moreover, when the stutterer finds himself no longer handicapped by impeded speech, no longer having any excuses for not accepting the challenges that social living always presents, there will be times when he feels almost overwhelmed by these new demands and will almost wish he were stuttering again. Some secondary gains always attach themselves to the most unpleasant disability and the stutterer will tend to miss those small profits which had accrued to his stuttering.

Also, at this time, the stutterer often shows a change in personality. The formerly quiet and reserved person may now become highly verbal and aggressive, and his wife may prefer the shy man she thought she married. Parents perhaps find the stutterer no longer dependent but rebellious. Groups in which the stutterer had been able to find a secure place because he was a good listener or very acquiescent now are disrupted because he insists on challenging the leadership and talking too much and too long. Having had to be relatively silent for years, the stutterer often has an urge to dominate all conversation. There are many other such patterns but these illustrations make our point—that in this transitional period of adjustment to the new-found fluent tongue—the stutterer needs the security and insights that further therapy can provide.

At this time, new problems also arise that focus directly upon speaking. In the first fine flush of his new-found fluency, the stutterer discovers that it is very difficult to monitor his speech. He doesn't want to think about stuttering; he just wants to talk and talk and talk some more. Often too, the rate of his speech increases to the point where, if moments of expectancy or actual occurrence of stuttering ensue, these are disregarded. Without a prior period of stabilization training, miniature facsimiles of the old avoidance and struggle responses may appear in his speech with greater and greater frequency yet not be noticed until they result in an instance so abnormal that the confrontation cannot be denied and then he will become very anxious. At times, the stutterer will notice these little avoidances and struggles (or even some that are very marked) but he may then actively repress them, a process which inevitably rebuilds their strength. Coiled springs when compressed have more potential force than when they are not. Or the stutterer may want to protect his new fluency and so become unwilling to do the work which must be done. It is easier to pretend to himself that he is not fearful of an approaching situation or a feared word. It is more convenient to doubt the probability that he may indeed be likely to stutter than it is to prepare himself to tackle it in a different way. The new motor sets at this time are often far from becoming the general and automatic ones that eventually will insure appropriate preparation for any wisp of expectancy that may suddenly present itself. For a time, they still must be voluntarily assumed. Later on, as a result of our stabilization training, they do become general and automatic and, when they do, they no longer demand the alertness and labor that they required earlier.

The therapist and stutterer must also recognize that the newly found freedom in speaking brings other problems. For one thing, increased fluency means less stuttering and less expectancy. Therefore there will be fewer opportunities to discriminate the cues or to practice the newly learned responses to fluency failure. The more the stutterer speaks fluently, the less opportunity there will be to reinforce the new ways of responding to the threat or occurrence of stuttering. The old behaviors have a long history of reinforcement; the new ones have not. Somehow we must program some overlearning into our therapy design so that when reduced reinforcement results in some decay in the strength of the new fluent stuttering, the latter will still be strong enough to withstand the competition of the old.

Another need for stabilization training may be seen in the kind of *normal* speech shown by the stutterer after he has become more fluent. Rarely does a severe stutterer move directly from his old faltering, broken speech to anything like the relatively smooth flowing utterance of the normal speaker. One can often discern gaps and holes in his sentences where the stuttering had previously been. For years, the severe stutterer has felt lucky just to say a phrase or two before he blocked or had to repeat and now he continues to talk brokenly even though he is not stuttering very much or very abnormally. Indeed such a stutterer hardly knows how to say a good clean sentence and a long narration or explanation will be more than he can manage with any degree of fluency. Beebe (1957) and others have insisted that stutterers are deficient in "sentence mindedness," in the ability to express themselves in supra-morphemic units. They simply do not have a very good feel for normal prosody.[1] Stuttering, like nature, abhors a vacuum and it will fill those holes in the stutterer's speech unless countermeasures are taken. Hypersensitive as he is to pauses and to silence, his old stuttering behaviors will seep in to fill the gaps. Almost unconsciously, the stutterer often responds to these breaks by using retrials or accessory vocalization, or the postponement mechanisms that he has always employed to cover up the pauses in his speech. To counter these influences he needs to learn now how to integrate, not just the sounds, syllables, and words, (the fragmentary components of speech) but also the larger utterances, the phrases, sentences, and even larger sequences. Training in this integration of supra-morphemic sequencing is vital if regression is not to occur.

In most of the stutterers we have treated we have found no conversion reactions. A few of them developed headaches, backaches, other ailments; some of them got into trouble with their wives or employers or developed financial worries. (Usually these were the individuals with other neurotic complaints besides stuttering.) Most of the cases with whom we worked learned to handle their other anxieties and self-defeating behaviors during the course of their speech therapy. The carefully programmed exposure

[1] Wingate's (1966, 1967) experiments concerning the prosodic deficiencies of stutterers tend to support the statement.

to anxiety-producing stimuli and the constant opportunities to verbalize and ventilate their concerns in the relative safety of the individual conferences or the group sessions helped teach them how to live as well as talk. Though the stutterers had previously spent their lives in almost constant anxiety, much of this had been worked through by the time they entered the stabilization stage of therapy. Nevertheless, we found that as they became very fluent and knew that soon they would be leaving treatment, a surge of separation anxiety was evidenced by most of them. Every farewell is a little death and all therapists know that termination of therapy should not be sudden or abrupt. For all of these reasons then, and many more, we have found it wise to have the stutterers undergo a period of stabilization therapy before they leave us.

Activities of the stabilization period

We begin this stage of therapy with an individual conference or two in which we carefully explain to the stutterers those needs for stabilization training we have just been describing, and in our discussion, we help the stutterer to verbalize his feelings about the new work which must be still done. We also acquaint him with a change in the structure of the therapy. The individual conferences with the therapist will now be held less frequently; the group sessions will include many visitors. Depending upon the individual requirements, certain days devoted to intensive stabilization therapy will be alternated with other days when he should do no therapy at all. The concept of nucleus situations is also presented: the stutterer is not to attempt to work on his speech continuously but to confine his self-therapy to certain previously designated situations—certain persons, a specified time or place, a certain topic of conversation, and the like. Provision is made for the keeping of logs or diaries of his stuttering and emotional experiences. Inventories are provided to help him assess objectively the state of his speech and the state of his self. The therapist now becomes even more of a consultant than he has been before; the stutterer now becomes even more his own therapist, analyzing, prescribing, checking, reflecting, problem solving, applying appropriate rewards and punishments. It is often well to preface this structuring with an objective review of past therapy and progress, a review in which the stutterer's strengths, weaknesses and characteristic reactions to therapeutic tasks are clarified. Through these discussions, the stutterer comes to understand what being a good therapist requires. Though throughout the therapy he has always had much responsibility for the designing of his therapeutic activities and much responsibility for their carrying out and evaluation, the new work of stabilization is presented as a proving ground to assess and promote his competence as a self-therapist. This, more than anything else, is the basic goal of the stabilization phase of therapy.

Reconfiguring fluency

To overcome the tendency to speak in small segments and to eliminate the holes and gaps in his speech where the stuttering had been, we ask the stutterer to design programs that will take care of them. We acquaint him with some of the ways that other stutterers have solved this problem. For example, we may have him read the reports of stutterers who trained themselves intensively in continuous free association for increasingly longer periods of time. We tell him of the payoffs that resulted from this training: that these former cases became able to speak more continuously without the gaps, that their word-finding difficulties were eased, that practice in free association seemed later to help them to formulate their verbalized thoughts more fluently. The therapist can demonstrate the manner in which this verbalized free association was done but it is now up to the stutterer, as his own therapist, to design how he would proceed to master it, to overcome its difficulties, and to discover how much of this training he needs.

Shadowing in stabilization

The same sort of procedure is employed in introducing shadowing as another way of learning to speak in less fragmented ways. Again the therapist confines his role to demonstration and explanation, the responsibility for acquiring facility in shadowing again being placed squarely on the stutterer. Learning to shadow another person's speech, to echo it almost simultaneously as it unfolds, is a skill which is not always mastered easily.[2] When the stutterer reports his difficulties and failures in learning to shadow, or to do these other things, there is always the temptation for the therapist to assume his old role and to reflect the feelings, ease the frustration, and help the stutterer overcome the hurdles. We have had to work hard to resist this temptation

2 However, Sergeant (1961) showed that shadowing skill could be mastered to a remarkable degree by normal speakers and Cherry, Sayers, and Marland (1955) as well as Kelham and McHale (1966) have applied it as the major vehicle of stuttering therapy.

and to maintain our new role as consultant at such a time. Since our goal is to set the stutterer free from us, we simply affirm our faith in his ability to achieve what seems impossible and stay by him until he does so. This is a ticklish but necessary phase of treatment and how the therapist handles it may determine the prognosis. Shadowing by itself is no panacea. It does help the stutterer to get the knack of normal prosody, to speak as normal speakers speak, to know how it feels to be fluent but, in our experience, its major value is to focus the resistance that always arises in any weaning process. Some stutterers of course find little trouble in learning to shadow or, for that matter, in assuming the therapist's role, but for those who do, the mastery of these various stabilization techniques provides the opportunity they need for working through the emotionality that always accompanies separation and unwanted self-responsibility. In all of the activities that comprise the stabilization training, some of this interaction between therapist and stutterer tends to occur.[3] No matter how careful the therapist has been throughout the previous therapy to make the stutterer an active and responsible partner in the process, he should expect in this last phase of treatment to confront some emotional storms.

Prosody and formulation

Other useful ways of integrating the larger sequences of speech may be mentioned. Instead of cancelling individual words on which he stutters, the stutterer now should cancel whole phrases or whole sentences. Or he may practice the narration or exposition

[3] We hope that we have illuminated the psychodynamics of stabilization by this example so that we need not repeat ourselves.

of the same material to different listeners until he can do it very smoothly and continuously. The telling of jokes seems to be one of the favorite methods for accomplishing this. We have probably been the target of more shaggy dog stories and Dutch jokes than any other person in history. (We even know the one about the left-legged baboon.) Some of our college stutterers have found it valuable to employ immediate oral paraphrasing after they silently read material from their textbooks. They thereby not only improve their study habits but also learn to speak in larger wholes. Some of our group meetings have been structured about the finishing of unfinished sentences, each person in turn having to provide the first part of the sentence and to call upon his successor to repeat it again immediately and then to complete the sentence without faltering.

Continuous speaking

Some of our stutterers have explored the use of oral reading with the pauses and the phrasing having been previously marked in the material but they report little carry-over from such activities. The transfer from reading to spontaneous speech is seldom very strong. Others gave themselves experiences in continuous extemporaneous talking using a series of cue cards, each with a topic inscribed thereon. In contrast to the oral reading, they found these activities very valuable. In learning to speak continuously they usually set time limits that gradually increased in duration as they progressively mastered the art of impromptu speaking. Much of this was done alone at first but aloud, then later in the presence of a listener. Some of our cases developed extraordinary skill in in this extemporaneous speaking without faltering. We remember one young man who talked continuously for 87 minutes from five topic cards he had never seen before. He made a lot of sense and his speech was extremely smooth flowing even though some automatic slow-motion stuttering was often quite apparent.

Increasing the rate

We have also found that training the stutterer to increase his maximum rate of talking tends to automatize the new preparatory sets especially if masking noise or other means are provided to increase proprioceptive or visual feedback at the same time. Few severe stutterers really know how fast they can talk. Using memorized material or repeating sentences after the therapist as he seeks to increase his rate often surprises the stutterer. We do not, of course, recommend that he do all of his speaking at swifter speeds though many of our cases have gradually come to do so as they find that such speaking is possible. Often we ask the stutterer to insert many small, deliberate facsimiles of his fluent stuttering as he does this swift talking practice since this seems to greatly facilitate the creation of generalized sets. Yet there seems to be something else in this practice of fast talking that is therapeutic. Perhaps it is hinted at in the experiments of MacKay (1968) who found that "the slower a subject's maximum rate of speech, without feedback delay, the greater the tendency to stutter" when he was exposed to DAF. All we are sure of is that this training in increasing the maximum rate of the stutterer's speech is a useful tool in stabilization.

Reflecting

Many of our cases discover the usefulness of reflecting the thoughts of others in learning to use the larger configurations of speech. At first we wondered whether they had all been reading Carl Rogers' books. However the reason became clear when one of them volunteered the information that this reflecting in one's own words the things someone else had said had always been one of his old ways of coping with his disfluency. "I could never begin a conversation with a friend or stranger and I didn't like to answer their questions because I'd always stutter so I found very early that if I just said again what they'd been saying, they thought I was really understanding them and they liked and accepted me for it." Whatever the reason, the ability to transform into one's own words the feelings that one's conversational partner is expressing seems to help the stutterer to speak less fragmentally. During the stabilization period, we find that the stutterers exchange such discoveries of useful ways of integrating their speech and we have been surprised at the ingenuity and inventiveness they show. We have learned much from our stutterers.

Automatization of sets and strategies

Another major goal of stabilization is to free the stutterer from the necessity of having to deal specifically with each individual threat or experience of stuttering. No stutterer can be constantly alert to all the cues which may trigger the old preparatory sets to struggle or avoid. If all we could offer him would be a lifetime sentence to constant vigilance and hard labor we'd find some other kind of therapy. Fortunately, it is not necessary that the stutterer must forever get set to react appropriately to each individual signal of approaching or occurring difficulty. Though, in first learning how to stutter fluently, he must indeed go through a deliberate process of rejecting the old and planning the new behavior, eventually this process becomes automatized and can take place even at a low level of awareness. Consider the typist or pianist. They too, at first, must do their motor planning with care and perform the movement sequences with voluntary deliberation. They too will make their mistakes and cancel them. But eventually, the motor sequences become automatized and can be run through swiftly and precisely in an automatic fashion. The specific movements become organized into larger patterns governed by general sets. Much the same sort of thing tends to occur in stutterers. At first they must prepare for and react carefully to each specific instance of stuttering. It is hard, demanding work and we doubt whether any stutterer would be willing to continue modifying his stuttering were he always to have to watch his speech so vigilantly. But, as with typing, or piano playing, or driving a car, general motor sets replace the specific ones and when they do, the stutterer's burden is greatly relieved. One of the goals, then, of stabilization therapy is to facilitate the acquisition of these generalized sets.

The creation of a generalized set requires a state of readiness to perceive a cue or stimulus and also a readiness to carry out a specified behavior when that cue appears. In driving we automatically turn the wheel to the left when the car has been suddenly swerved to the right by some hump in the pavement. We perform the compensatory movement unthinkingly, hardly realizing that we have done so. How then can we help the stutterer to achieve this same automaticity in his speech? As we have said, it tends to occur as the result of

many conscious experiences in behaving appropriately but surely there must be other ways of facilitating the process. The following are some of the activities which our stutterers have devised for this purpose. They have constructed passages loaded heavily with the words and sounds which previously they feared and then they have read them or recited them from memory over and over again, beginning slowly, and carefully preparing for any possible difficulty. After many such practices they can speak these passages with surprising rapidity and when they do, generalized sets replace the specific ones. Or the stutterers may write down the actual sentences on which they had experienced some stuttering during the day, then speak them many times in the same fashion. Some of the stutterers take these materials, do some preliminary practice in working through the difficult words, then say the whole set of sentences with a burst of speed which prevents any possibility of specific preparation.[4] In achieving general sets for certain troublesome sounds, individual words have been presented serially on rapidly flipped cards or exposed on a memory drum or flashed on a screen and the stutterer speaks instantly only those that begin with that "hard" sound, and using the fluent form of stuttering. By speeding up

---

[4] Mysak (1966) makes a strong case for this sort of training since he views the dysautomatization in stuttering as due in part to oversensitive auditory monitoring servo-systems. He says, "Such an oversensitive monitoring channel may create feedback tonal flow error signals which are so small that they would ordinarily be disregarded. This excessive back-flow of inconsequential error signals overactivates the corrector device and hence speech automaticity is disturbed." Accordingly he recommends training in practicing the larger motor sequences of speech.

the exposure of these words, the person in advance has to prepare a general motor plan and to hold it in readiness, since though he may know that he must respond instantly to all "B" words, he never knows just which one will be presented. Sentences may also be exposed word by word sequentially in the same manner.

But there are other general sets, or preparatory instructions to react in certain ways, which the stutterer may adopt. He may plan, prior to utterance, to say all of his beginning stop consonants with loose contacts. With enough practice, he will find that soon he will be doing this automatically and even when he does not specifically command himself to do so. Since many of the tremors are triggered by the pressure of overtight contacts, he will thereby be able to escape many moments of fixation that might otherwise occur. Or he may plan in advance to speak with strong slow movements on all *accented* syllables without regard to whether the word is feared or not. The discriminating cue here is not the expectancy of stuttering on a specific word or sound but instead it is a feature common to all speaking. If he so sets himself, and certain stuttering-colored cues appear, the generalized set will often be sufficient in itself to insure that abnormality will not occur or that, at least, it will tend to facilitate the assumption of more appropriate specific preparatory sets and responses. By training himself to focus his attention on proprioception, the stutterer first will prepare himself to scan the smaller fragments of syllables and words but very soon he finds that he can assume a general set that will enable him to monitor his speech primarily through proprioceptive feedback. One of our stutterers said, "It's as though I turn on a little valve in my head. Once I do it, everything's all set and I'm talking slowly and strongly and fluently. My stutterings seem to handle themselves and I don't have to do anything. Just turn that valve."

Preparing for contingencies

While the present state of learning theory leaves much to be desired concerning the manner in which newly learned responses become stabilized, there is plenty of evidence that two memory storage systems exist, one dealing with short-term retention and the other with long-term retention. Since we are interested here in building stable new responses it is the latter form of retention that we seek. At least three factors seem to be involved in the transfer from short-term to long-term storage; somehow, the momentary responses or strategies may be transformed and coded symbolically (when new perceptions and behaviors are verbalized they tend to resist fading better than those which are not so coded); somehow we must make sure that the new perceptions and responses are attached to as many cues as possible (generalization); and finally, the sheer massing of practice in the new behaviors tends to promote consolidation and more permanent retention.

In all of our therapy we have constantly sought to encourage the stutterers to verbalize their experiences. In both the individual and the group sessions, they transform into words their new discriminations and newly found ways of responding to the threat or occurrence of stuttering. During the stabilization phase of therapy, we encourage this verbalization in every way possible. We ask them to set up hypothetical problems of various kinds and then to verbalize their solutions.

Here are only a few of those that they have invented: "What should I do if I find myself trying to say the word 'Hello' while holding my breath?" "How should I respond when I recognize that I substituted an easier word for one that I suddenly expected to have trouble saying?" "How can I shift from a prolonged 's' into the rest of the word?" "What should I do if my listener keeps interrupting me?" "I find myself in an unexpected lip tremor: how shall I extricate myself from this?" "I foresee a difficult situation approaching three days hence and find myself rehearsing some stuttering; what would be appropriate here?" The therapist will find that stutterers can invent hundreds of similar questions and also that they become able to verbalize in their own words the appropriate strategies that are required. We have found that this training in the verbal coding of the new responses not only seems to improve their stabilization but also that it relieves much of the residual or latent anxiety. In addition we also now encourage, even more than we have previously, the use of oral self-commentary on new experiences that concern speaking—the successful as well as the unsuccessful. Because stutterers have long been prone to repress unpleasant speaking experiences or even the pleasant ones (because of their fear that false hopes will arise only to be later deflated and because they have little facility in verbalizing anyway) we feel it very important during this stabilization period to teach them to put their insights into words. Stutterers must learn not only to talk to others but to themselves.

Generalization

Another major goal of the stabilization stage is to insure that the new responses become attached to a large number and wide range of stimuli. Though we have constantly sought to have the stutterer do most of his work outside the therapy room there will always be some communicative situations and conditions which remain untouched by the new learning. We therefore make a real effort at this time to define these and to do what we can to make the stutterer less vulnerable to their influence. Our stutterers have called this project "Operation Mop Up." First of all in the group sessions they review together their old memories of instances in which they remember stuttering severely. The advantage of doing this in the group is that one stutterer's recollections tend to evoke similar experiences in the others. One reported, for example, how once after having to stand in line waiting to purchase a ticket, he had stuttered very severely and this in turn reminded another how often he stuttered while waiting to recite in school as the teacher went through the class role in alphabetical order. Or one will tell of his traumatic experience of being quizzed by the judge at the traffic court and this may lead to accounts of difficulty in other situations involving confession or authority. Just the verbalization of these old memories seems to have some value for the stutterers report feelings of relief after the mop-up sessions. By deliberately using the new slow-motion stuttering as they say again what they said so stutteringly, some real gains are achieved.

In some instances, especially when, in the retelling, some stuttering expectancy occurs (and this is not uncommon), the group may turn to a bit of psychodrama, assuming the relevant roles and acting out the old traumatic situation. Or, more usually, the stutterer will deliberately try to create a facsimile situation; e.g., he may stand in line at the bus station and then ask the clerk a question concerning a ticket to some destination as one of his fellow stutterers observes. Admittedly not all of the old traumatic experiences can be so relived but many of them are. Much of this ventilation and reexperiencing evidently owes its usefulness to the suggestion that the stutterer has thereby laid to rest the old ghosts of his unhappy past. As one of our cases said, "It feels good to know that I erased a few of them anyway and that if I have some more in the future I can erase them too in the same way. It's almost like the good feeling I have when I cancel a stuttered word. I think of it as cancelling old bad situations."

Extinguishing fears

Another group of activities focuses on the further extinguishing of fears of words and sounds. First, the stutterers replay some of their earlier recordings and list the words on which they had stuttered, analyzing them in terms of the severity of stuttering and the sounds on which the stuttering occurred. They also carry around with them a portable tape recorder for a day or two to determine the loci of the remaining stuttering. The corpus thus obtained serves as the material used in extinction training with those sounds and words, which appear most frequently or generated most severity, being given special attention.

The principles of adaptation and extinction are employed in this training. The selected word, for example, is first repeated over and over again in isolation as many as a hundred times beginning with the old form of stuttering on the first few repetitions, then changing to the slow-motion kind of stuttering for the bulk of the trials and ending with the word being

spoken normally several times. To insure that the majority of these words were spoken slowly and carefully, some stutterers wrote out the first letter of the word simultaneously with its utterance, beginning to speak the word's first sound with the first stroke of the pen. Simultaneous talking and writing is an old technique, originally devised by Bringelson and Travis to associate speaking with a unilateral lead as required by the cerebral dominance theory. A description of its methodology will be found in Van Riper (1958, pp. 279–80). We use it, not for this purpose, but primarily to insure sufficient pairing of the old conditioned stimulus (the first sound of the word) with the new rather than the old response.

In the beginning we distrusted this sort of massed practice, anticipating that it might lead to an increase in fear of stuttering on the words and sounds thus segregated. However, the stutterers who invented the technique knew better than we did for no increment in word fear ensued. Evidently the massed repetitions of the word, especially when most of them are spoken in the slow-motion fashion, drain all the fear out of the word and if enough words are used in this practice, they are seldom remembered, or if they are, they are recalled as having been spoken fluently. We also wondered whether the effects of this practice on isolated words could have any real transfer. So did the stutterers and accordingly they followed this practice in isolation by using the same word in a series of sestences usually cast in terms of mand or egocentric speech or emotional expression. Often the words thus practiced were finally incorporated into sentences which were used in telephoning or speaking to strangers. Elsewhere we have shown (Brown and Van Riper, 1966) that speech serves many functions:

display of self, social control, formulation of thought, expression of emotion, and communication of messages. In the stabilization phase of therapy, we make sure that the stutterers have ample opportunity to use all of these kinds of speaking. If we hope for generalization and transfer of the clinically acquired fluent stutterings, we must make certain that the stimuli inherent in each of these speech modes are associated with the new responses.

While our stutterers at this stage in treatment had lost most of their phonemic fears, they of course remembered having them and so they designed methods for "wiping out the residuals," as one stutterer put it. What they did was to practice the formerly feared sound in nonsense syllables and nonsense words. For example, if a stutterer remembered that the "k" had been greatly feared in the past, he might invent and practice a series of syllables and nonsense words in which the "k" was used with all the vowel and blend combinations. To insure proper coarticulation, he would silently preform the succeeding vowel, then say the syllable. Or he might slightly prolong an aspirated "kh" to the first sound of the syllable if he remembered the tight contacts that had so often led to tremors. Or he might concentrate on the timing or strength or speed of the associated jaw movement. As we have said, the syllables bearing the feared sound were then incorporated into nonsense words of indescribable variety. In the group sessions the stutterers challenged each other with such combinations as "Kusizitch" and "oclithmaris." They said them slowly and then swiftly. They inserted them into otherwise meaningful sentences: "If you ask me, I think you're full of Kilchum." It was interesting to observe that these

unfamiliar combinations often triggered ambivalence and verbal approach-avoidance conflicts and offered some opportunity for their resolution. One of the stutterers reported that this practice helped him greatly—that he had long feared all unfamiliar words or strange names and now had found ways of overcoming his hesitancy.

As with the isolated words, the principle of massed practice was used. Some of the stutterers repeated these syllables thousands of times; others practiced only a few token ones. They devised their own assignments and occasionally we suspected that in the role of therapist the stutterer was being rather punitive with his case.

While we have no doubt that this massed practice had some real effectiveness for many of the stutterers, we are not sure that the effects were always due to deconditioning. Certainly, the new models were reinforced and to some extent the old cues lost some of their ability to precipitate stuttering as a result of the work done by the stutterers. It is our impression that those stutterers who did a lot of this practice seemed to show fewer of the unnoticed tiny blockings in their subsequent speaking than those who did not. Perhaps the sheer boredom of the practice sessions acted as a counterconditioner. Perhaps, by this work, anxiety was allayed or penance was done. All that we can say is that at the very least, the stutterers learned to discipline themselves, and eventually to be more willing to terminate therapy.

Nucleus situation in stabilization

To prevent the basic strategies of cancellations and pull-outs from growing dim due to lack of enough opportunity to use them, pseudostuttering is again employed. Certain nucleus situations are designated for each of the days devoted to therapy and, as these are experienced, the stutterer fakes enough of his old kinds of stuttering until he is satisfied that he can assume the behaviors without upheaval or distress, much as he did during the desensitization phase. Then he fakes several more of these former stutterings but follows them with careful cancellation. Next he "throws himself into some real stuttering," and uses the pull-out behaviors. Finally in the same situation he inserts some very brief, smooth, fluent stutterings and concludes by emphasizing the proprioceptive monitoring of essentially normal speech. Even if only two days a week are devoted primarily to therapy, the use of nucleus situations in this way has a very potent effect in stabilizing these important strategies. Different situations are chosen on different therapy days. For example, one stutterer, confronted with Monday as a therapy day, selected a certain girl whom he was sure to meet several times as the nucleus person, the noon meal as the nucleus time, the library as his nucleus place, and athletics as his nucleus topic. Whenever he was in each of these situations, he did the pseudostuttering, cancellation, pull-out, and monitoring sequence. This stutterer's next therapy day for that week was on Thursday and for that day an entirely different set of nucleus situations was designed. A different person, place, topic, and time were chosen but again he used the same sequence of therapeutic activities. It should be evident that this sort of programming insures that the stabilization training will have widespread effects. Within a month or so, most of the stutterer's communication will have felt its impact.

Buffering

Stabilization training also includes the building of higher barriers against the kinds of communicative stress to which the stutterer is especially vulnerable. Much of this is done in the group sessions. For example, if a given stutterer has tended to find more disruption when being interrupted or hurried, he may address the group on some topic and seek to maintain his calmness and continuity despite the deliberate heckling of the other members. If he is vulnerable to overpraise for his fluency, the group floods him with it. If he has trouble speaking over noise, the group creates a pandemonium. Or, if he is especially vulnerable to listener loss, he is to keep on talking even though the others turn their heads or get up and walk away. If suddenly accosted by a question, he learns to use a delay before answering. Bryngelson (1966) describes one of the "razz sessions" he uses as buffering experience:

At this point in the therapeutic program, the patients and the clinicians are putting themselves to the test of whether or not they can stand harsh criticism, name calling, jeering, etc. They must build into their emotional set an impenetrable wall against trigger or irrational responses to a somewhat cruel world. Seat your patients in a circle and tell them to "kid the hell" out of each other. They must open their emotional eyes to a burlesqued onslaught of names, imitations, and harsh, derisively spoken words. (p. 144)

Several of our stutterers reported triumphantly that since they had usually experienced more trouble when somewhat intoxicated they had got together with two bottles of whiskey and worked on their speech successfully despite the alcoholic intake. And they had the tape recordings to prove it.

The world outside the clinic also contains many individuals whose characteristic behaviors can create special stresses on the stutterer and these people can be located and used to facilitate the buffering process. The consistently angry man, the sarcastic clerk, the impatient policeman on the corner all are available and we have collected quite a stable of these characters against whom the stutterers can pit themselves. By deliberately entering these stressful contacts and winning more skirmishes than they lose, the stutterers become very toughened. Moreover, they come to consider these conditions of communicative stress as challenges rather than as threats.

Resistance therapy

In this terminal stage of treatment we have found it useful to help the stutterer to resist actively the suggestion that stuttering is inevitable when he perceives certain situational or phonemic stimuli that indicate its probability. When the stutterer first comes to us, he has only two choices when stuttering threatens: he may avoid the situation or word or he may stutter. Our therapy has thus far been devoted to giving him a third choice —a way of attacking the utterance so that little interruption or abnormality will result even though he does stutter. Now we provide a fourth alternative—to resist the suggestive influence of the stuttering-colored cues and to say the word normally despite them. In another text (Van Riper, 1971) we have shown that the correlation between stuttering expectancy and stuttering occurrence is not at all as great as the stutterer thinks. Some of the words on which he anticipates he will stutter will be spoken normally despite that anticipation. Moreover, every adult stutterer that we have ever

known has testified that occasionally he has had the surprising experience of summoning up his powers and refusing to let himself stutter, that occasionally he can "rise to the occasion." He usually cannot tell us how he does this but in the instances that we have observed there seems to be more energy in the speaking act—as though the servosystem amplified the signal over the noise of emotion. They almost seem to *will* not to stutter, to exhort and command themselves to speak fluently despite all odds. We cannot explain this phenomenon in terms of our present knowledge though possibly some biochemical facilitation of cortical integration may be involved. Perhaps it is due merely to a shift of attention or to countersuggestion. At any rate the fact that this ability to resist the threat of stuttering does exist is clinically evident and we should find ways of using it in therapy.

We have devised several methods of doing so and we're sure there must be others. The first of these employs speaking in unison or shadowing but not in the usual way. The therapist and the stutterer, or two stutterers, read the same material *together* or recite in unison a memorized passage composed of difficult words. As we have seen, this unison reading ordinarily produces marked fluency but we have also found that if one stutterer exhibits some stuttering its effect will be to cause the other stutterer also to have difficulty. This is found even more commonly when shadowing or echo speech is involved. What we do therefore is to prepare the stutterer in advance to determine to resist this empathic response tendency. If the therapist is doing the joint reading, for example, he will insert into his speaking some instances of stuttering. The stutterer does not know when these will occur but he gets set to resist their influence whenever they do. Usually some reciprocal stuttering does appear in his speech at first but with further training, he will become able to prevent their occurrence. If he is very vulnerable, the therapist inserts a form of stuttering which is very much unlike that usually shown by the stutterer and more infrequently. By carefully programming the number of instances of stuttering and their similarity to the stutterer's own behavior patterns, and making sure that the stutterer has more successes than failures, any stutterer can finally learn to resist. We also use old audio or video tapes of the stutterer's own speech for shadowing practice in resisting stuttering. Our cases like this resistance therapy very much and have reported a good deal of transfer. As one of them said, "I always thought that if I thought I would stutter, I had to stutter. I now find I don't—that I can fight and not surrender."

Another type of resistance therapy employs self-suggestion. Before entering a feared situation, or one that he had previously feared, the stutterer deliberately verbalizes aloud or to himself the suggestion that he will have some severe stuttering. In so doing, he duplicates all of the old forms of negative suggestion which he formerly employed. He rehearses the sentence, picks out the hard words, tells himself that he will be sure to "get stuck for a long time" that he will feel helpless and struggle in his old way. He will imagine the worst kinds of listener reaction. And then he will try to reject all this negative self-suggestion and speak as well as he can. Initially, the stutterers are dubious about undertaking this sort of experience. "I don't want to awaken my old abnormal ways of thinking," one of them protested. However, we have found this activity highly salutory. Though occasionally the negative suggestion will dominate and the stutterer will stutter just as he had told himself he would, he can always pull out or cancel, and with repeated experiences every one of our stutterers had eventually been able to do this resisting of their own negative self-suggestion very successfully. Indeed, we have found that such training does much to allay that anxiety which tends to flare up when the stutterer does find himself anticipating difficulty or thinking in his old morbid ways.

In the stabilization phase of our therapy we also use the delayed feedback apparatus to create cybernetic stress that the stutterer can resist. Some of this training is much the same as that used in the modification stage to enhance proprioceptive monitoring and the bypassing of the auditory self-scrutiny to which stutterers seem to be so prone. We find the delay time that seems to produce maximal disruption, for the individual stutterer, then using reading, monologue and conversation or paraphrasing, we intermittently switch from direct to delayed feedback, the stutterer seeking to keep speaking in exactly the same way under the delay as he does when it is not present. By simultaneously tape recording this practice session [5] and then listening to the samples produced, the stutterer can find out if he is truly resisting the delay.

DAF is also especially useful in resistance therapy with primarily clonic stutterers, those with compulsive runaway behaviors. Following the lead provided by Chase (1958) who found

---

[5] We find the Edison Voice Mirror most helpful in this practice since it provides an immediate replay without rewinding.

it very difficult to resist the delay and to stop repeating voluntarily when repeating syllables under DAF, we have these stutterers practice syllabic repetition at progressively faster speeds but stopping instantly when the therapist's signal is given. At first these stutterers tend to overrun, just as Chase, a normal speaker, did and the repetitions continue long past the signal but later they become able to "beat the machine." Some of these stutterers, by giving themselves a tactual signal to stop repeating (pressing the forefinger against the thumb) have said that its effectiveness seems to transfer to the occasional real clonic stutterings that they experience. They claim that after this training they can stop the compulsive recycling of syllables that characterized their old way of stuttering.

Reintegrating the self-concept

As we have mentioned, one of the problems experienced by stutterers in terminal therapy concerns the self-concept. For years he has defined himself as a stutterer, a deviant. For years, he has suffered a split in personality. His body image has been distorted; his roles constrained. How can we put Humpty Dumpty together again and what will he look like when he is assembled? The mild stutterers seem to have little difficulty in this regard but the severe ones usually experience some intense conflicts when they find themselves fluent. They can't believe that they can be the same person and speak so easily. When other persons, whom they have long known, marvel at the change, such a stutterer is likely to feel that he is masquerading, that the new self he is showing is really a sham. When he finds himself accepted by new acquaintances as a normal speaker, he tends to doubt

their acceptance and worries about what might happen if he showed his "real stuttering self" again. It is therefore mandatory that we do something in our stabilization therapy to aid the stutterer to cope with these and the other problems related to the revision of his self-concept.

We have intensively studied the changes in self-concept of the stutterers who passed through our clinic. They began this change by first solving the conflict between the stuttering self and the very fluent imaginary self of their fantasies and then by accepting the role of a stutterer undergoing treatment. They gave up their "Demosthenes complex" for the more realistic definition of themselves as individuals who had a remediable disorder of speech. Once this was accomplished and repeatedly demonstrated to others through their cancellations and pull-outs and other modifications, they next came to view themselves differently. They were stutterers who had formerly been severely handicapped by their disorder but were no longer. "I used to be a very bad stutterer but I'm doing pretty well now." The next shift in self-concept resulted in a self-definition as a "fluent stutterer." He was still a stutterer but a very fluent one. The next transition was to the self-concept which can best be described as the "person who occasionally stutters." Then there appeared the view of self as "a person who occasionally speaks stutteringly." As we have seen earlier, such a concept is common even among many of us. Most of our adult stutterers rarely get beyond this self-concept but a few finally manage to forget or to disregard the fact that they ever had stuttered. These persons consider themselves completely normal speakers. It should be mentioned that these changes seldom progress in a linear fashion. The stutterers oscillate back and forth, up and down the progression. At first, each new view of self is unstable and precarious and regression is frequently apparent but eventually it becomes consolidated and serves as a stepping stone for the next revision.

Our therapy, unlike many others, is designed to promote these changes. We do not try to convince the stutterer as did Froeschels, Fernau-Horn, Wendell Johnson, and many others, that he is no stutterer but merely a normal speaker who speaks stutteringly. When a listener or the person himself interprets the presence of broken words as indicating that he is a stutterer, it is very difficult for him to maintain the contrary. Consider the person who is regarded by all his acquaintances as an alcoholic and whose behavior all too vividly corroborates this impression yet who insists that he is only a social drinker! Even if, as Froeschels [6] insists, stuttering is the product of an error in logic, that it develops as a result of his own misdiagnosis of normal disfluencies, the sad fact of the matter is that when others see the person as a stutterer, so does he. While we are fairly certain that some stutterers acquire their disorder by learning abnormal responses to situational and phonemic cues, we are convinced that once the stutterer accepts the evaluations of his culture and defines himself as a stutterer, there is little clinical value in pretending that this concept of self does not exist. Let us instead accept the self-concept of a stutterer as a fact and then proceed to modify it.

It is during the stabilization period that many of the later changes in self-

concept take place. By this time the stutterer is at least defining himself as a stutterer who formerly was severely handicapped but is no longer so troubled. Indeed, most of our cases are now viewing themselves as very fluent speakers though still stuttering at times. How can we stabilize this self-concept and also facilitate even better self-concepts to come? How can we insure that the oscillatory swings in self-definition will move in the direction of being a fairly normal speaker? [7]

Although his fluency is confirmed every time he speaks, we have found it important to give the stutterer opportunities to display this fluency in formal speaking situations. Long ago Heltman (1941) held that the one factor he had been able to isolate as contributing most to permanent "cure" in his cases was that those who finally attained the status of normal speakers did a lot of public speaking. Being connected with a university, it has been easy for us to provide such formal speaking opportunities. In line with our belief in the necessity for a progressive modification in self-

---

[6] See "Imitation Stuttering," in E. Froeschels, *Selected Papers of Emil Froeschels* (Amsterdam: North Holland, 1964), pp. 95–101.

[7] The author of this text, formerly a very severe stutterer, was fortunate enough to have some good advice from Bryng Bryngelson shortly after he had acquired excellent fluency by modifying his own stuttering behaviors. Bryngelson suggested that, for a period of six weeks, the author, in a new life situation, pose as being a severe stutterer during the hours from 8 A.M. to 6 P.M., and then thereafter until he went to bed try to speak as well as he could. Reluctantly we acceded to this Cinderella therapy and followed the program quite thoroughly. It was very hard to do pseudostuttering so many hours a day when we knew we could speak fluently and we welcomed the clock striking six. Nevertheless, the program resolved our identity conflicts and no relapse occurred. In passing, we may say that we have never been able to get one of our own stutterers to carry out such a project.

concept, we make sure that each stutterer early in treatment has a chance to demonstrate himself as a severe stutterer and then later as one who has greatly improved but is still working hard on his problem. When he reaches the stabilization period, we give him several experiences before a friendly group in which he is to handle any residual stutterings so well that the audience does not recognize them or seems surprised when he points them out. At these times he exhibits the self-concept of the very fluent stutterer and his listeners agree. Finally we make arrangements so that he can speak to audiences of strangers who do not know that he has been a stutterer and he endeavors (without avoidance) to get them to accept him as a somewhat nonfluent normal speaker. By filming or videotaping these performances and viewing them repeatedly some remarkable changes in self-definition become evident. Even audio-recording has strong impact. Again he sees himself as others see him but now he is a different person. The screen and sound tell him so.

We do not, of course, expect that such display experiences will be sufficient in themselves to change the self-concepts of our stutterers. Rather they corroborate in a very vivid way the new perceptions which have gradually evolved from hundreds of person-to-person contacts. Early in therapy, he finds himself evaluated by the therapist, his fellow stutterers, and all the people he meets, as a stutterer and he learns finally to accept that reality. Next, as he begins to work on his stuttering behaviors, he discovers that others recognize and respect the fact that he is trying to cope with his disorder. As he improves, his acquaintances reflect that improvement by their attitudes and comments. Their

evaluations affect his own and he sees himself differently. Then, when he is able to speak very fluently despite some intermittent and minor stuttering, his friends marvel again at the change. Again their reactions almost force a shift in self-definition. And finally, in his contacts with those who had never known him before, he comes to realize that they view him as a normal speaker. Thus both the individual contacts and the display experiences join to alter the stutterer's self-concept.

Throughout therapy, we find ourselves asking these questions over and over again: "What exactly did your listener see and hear?" "How did he react?" "What sort of judgments about you do you think he made?" We ask these questions to help the stutterer free himself from his distorted perceptions but we find also that his answers always reflect the way he defines himself. During this stabilization period, we suggest to the stutterer that he collect and classify the differing ways in which his listeners view him. How many of his listeners saw and judged him to be a severe stutterer, or a stutterer hard at work on his speech problem, or a very fluent stutterer, or a person who occasionally speaks stutteringly, or even as a normal speaker? Of course he cannot always be sure how they felt, but what were their probable impressions? When he does check, does he find that his judgment has been correct? Sometimes for an entire day, the stutterer thus evaluates every listener to his speech and by the end of several weeks he cannot help but realize that he has undergone a sea change. He may find one or two individuals in his listener collection who probably did view him as a stutterer, albeit a mild one. He may also find a few who judged him to be a stutterer working on his speech. But there will be many more who will think him to be either a very fluent stutterer or a normal speaker who occasionally speaks stutteringly. What is most important about this sort of assignment is that it provides a vehicle for future reassessments as well. Once a stutterer, always a stutterer? We find little logic or virtue in such a defeatist position. What therapist dare set limitations upon human potential? We are quite content if the stutterer leaves us with the self-concept of a fluent stutterer but we prefer to have him oscillating between this role and that of the normal speaker. We once believed that a severe confirmed adult stutterer could never pass into the culture of the fluent world, and never attain the role of a normal speaker, but some of our cases have shown us that we were wrong. At least we should try to facilitate this end result rather than erect obstacles in its path.

Much anxiety accompanies each shift in self-concept. It seems as though there is an almost homeostatic protest against these fundamental changes in self regard. Stutterers have had their old poses of being a normal speaker punctured so often and so traumatically that they actively resist the therapist's invitation to find out if indeed they can be one. They now know the dangers of avoidance and pretense so they fear that they may be tempted to use these defenses again. They do not want to hope too much lest those hopes be dashed. At each new step along the road to better speech we find some protest or resistance because the stutterers fear their hopes. When they have falteringly confessed these feelings we have told them: "Let us explore. Let us see. Expect the worst if you must but let's find out how far you can go. The self is a bundle of roles about a body image. You have many sides to self, not just one. It is possible to be a fluent stutterer at one moment, and a normal speaker at another. You may even see yourself again as a severe stutterer when your frailty meets great stress and you surrender to it. The important thing is to help the desired roles to develop as far as they can grow. You will fluctuate back and forth but you have already seen that most of the time now you regard yourself differently than you once did. Perhaps finally you will find that being a fluent stutterer is the most predominant of these roles and that this is as far as you care to go. All right, let's see." We suspect that such reassurances are always more reassuring to the therapist than they are to the client but our stutterers seem to need some such guidelines at this time. One of our cases responded to something like the above by saying, "You mean it's OK to be a part-time normal speaker. I'll buy that but I'm not going to shoot for full time. Not yet. Maybe never." We felt that was fair enough.

Terminating therapy

"Everything has an end and a woman has two—and my Uncle Toby could never tell the one from the other," said Lawrence Sterne's Tristram Shandy. The therapist should know when to end therapy and how to end it. Usually the stutterer will tell him in many subtle or obvious ways when that time has come. He fails to show up for an appointment or two; he becomes impatient with his fellow members in the group sessions; he even appears bored with stuttering and with himself. He's not even very excited about his fluency but takes it for granted. It is time to terminate.[8]

If we can discern these signs before they become too obvious we may be able to prevent the sudden unexplained departure that may create some guilt. The therapist can space his conferences further apart. He can break up the large group into smaller ones. He can take a short vacation but suggest that the group meet without him and review their progress and discuss their feelings about ending treatment. Then finally, he arranges an individual conference in which he and the stutterer in the role of co-therapists explore the matter. Is this joint case of theirs really ready to leave? Does he need any continuing contact with therapist now? The therapist expresses his faith in the stutterer's ability to cope with any future problems; he verbalizes some of the feelings which other stutterers have had at such a time. He reviews the progress which has been accomplished. He says nothing about the stutterer's continuing weaknesses nor does he exhort or warn.[9] The conference is low keyed, almost casual. The therapist assures the stutterer that he will be available for consultation whenever an urgent need exists but that the formal therapy is concluded. The earlier commitments for yearly follow-ups and written and telephone reports are mentioned. The conference ends on a mutual note of relief. They have both done what they could do.

We have known therapists who found it hard to surrender their cases because of the counter transference or Pygmalian effect. When one has invested much of himself in another human being, has come to know him intimately, has been with him in both good and bad moments, the inevitable moment of farewell often seems to come too soon. There is always some unfinished business in the best of therapy but a healthy respect for the law of diminishing returns and a keen realization of the potential all of us have to heal ourselves—and without continuing help—will make the leave-taking easier. Besides there are others who need us too.[10]

[10] For an account of the author's successes and failures during a twenty-year period in which he continuously experimented with differing approaches in developing the therapeutic program outlined here, see his section in Eisenson, J. (ed.), *Stuttering: A Symposium* (New York: Harper & Row, 1958), pp. 275–390. For a later detailed case account of a clinical success and a clinical failure, see: *Stuttering: Successes and Failures in Therapy* (Memphis, Tenn.: Speech Foundation of America, 1968).

[8] Long ago, Thorne (1950) had some wise words to say about terminating therapy. First of all, he insists that the decision to terminate should be the therapist's responsibility though it should be based upon his assessment of the client's progress and accomplishments. Secondly, he warns against overtreatment as tending to reinforce the client's dependency needs.

[9] An illuminating account of the principles of case termination (after psychotherapy) can be found in pages 204–8 in Brammer, L. M. and E. L. Shostrom *Therapeutic Psychology* (Englewood Cliffs, N.J.: Prentice-Hall, 1960).

Bibliography

ALLPORT, G. W., *Becoming*. New Haven: Yale University Press, 1955.

ATKINSON, J., *The Psychology of Motivation*. New York: Van Nostrand, Reinhold, 1967.

BEEBE, H., Sentence mindedness, *Folia Phoniatrica*, 9 (1957), 44–48.

BLANK, L., and H. P. DAVID (eds.), *Source Book for Training in Clinical Psychology*. New York: Springer, 1964.

BROWN, C. T. and C. Van RIPER, *Speech and Man*. Englewood Cliffs, N.J.: Prentice-Hall, 1966.

BRYNGELSON, B., *Clinical Group Therapy*

for Problem People: A Practical Treatise for Stutterers and Normal Speakers. Minneapolis: Denison, 1966.

CHERRY, E. C., and B. M. SAYERS, and P. MARLAND, Experiments in the complete suppression of stuttering, *Nature,* 176 (1955), 874–75.

CHASE, R. A., Effect of DAF upon the repetition of speech sounds, *Journal of Speech and Hearing Disorders,* 23 (1958), 583–90.

EKSTEIN, R. and R. S. WALLERSTEIN, *The Teaching and Learning of Psychotherapy.* New York: Basic Books, 1958.

FINN, M. H. P. and F. BROWN, *Training for Clinical Psychology.* New York: International Universities Press, 1959.

FROESCHELS, E., *Selected Papers of Emil Froeschels.* Amsterdam: North Holland, 1964.

HELTMAN, H. J., History of recurrent stuttering and recovery, *Journal of Speech Disorders,* 6 (1941), 49–50.

HUNT, H. F. and J. E. DYRUD, Commentary, perspective in behavior therapy, in J. M. Shlein (ed.), *Research in Psychotherapy.* Washington: American Psychological Association, 1968, pp. 140–52.

JOURARD, S. R., *The Transparent Self.* New York: American Book Co., 1964.

KELHAM, R. and A. McHALE, The application of learning theory to the treatment of stammering, *British Journal of Disorders of Communication,* 1 (1966), 114–18.

KRAMER, E., *A Beginning Manual for Psychotherapists.* New York: Grune & Stratton, 1970.

KRASNER, L., Verbal conditioning and psychotherapy, in L. Krasner and L. Ullman (eds.), *Research in Behavior Modification.* New York: Holt, Rinehart & Winston, 1965.

LAZARUS, A. A., The results of behavior therapy in 126 cases of severe neurosis, *Behavior Research and Therapy,* 1 (1963), 69–79.

LILYWHITE, H. S., Toward a philosophy of professional behavior, *Asha,* 3 (1961), 39–42.

MACKAY, D. G., Metamorphosis of cortical interval-age-linked changes in the delay in auditory feedback that produces maximal disruption of speech, *Journal of Acoustical Society of America,* 43 (1968), 811–20.

MYSAK, E. D., Servo-theory and stuttering, *Journal of Speech and Hearing Disorders,* 25 (1960), 188–95.

————, *Speech Pathology and Feedback Theory.* Springfield, Ill.: Charles C Thomas, 1966.

PANDE, S. K. and J. J. GART, A method to quantify reciprocal influence between therapist and client in psychotherapy, in I. M. Shlien (ed.), *Research in Psychotherapy.* Washington, D.C.: American psychological Association, 1968, pp. 395–414.

ROGERS, C., *On Becoming a Person: A Client's View of Psychotherapy.* Boston: Houghton Mifflin, 1961.

RYAN, B. P., An illustration of operant conditioning therapy for stuttering, in *Conditioning in Stuttering Therapy.* Speech Foundation of America, Publication 7, Memphis, Tenn.: Fraser, 1968.

SERGEANT, R. L., Concurrent repetition of a continuous flow of words, *Journal of Speech and Hearing Research,* 4 (1961), 373–80.

SHEEHAN, J. G., *Stuttering: Research and Therapy.* New York: Harper & Row, 1970.

THORNE, F. C., *The Principles of Personality Counseling.* Brandon, Vt.: Journal of Clinical Psychology Press, 1950.

VAN RIPER, C., Experiments in stuttering therapy, in J. Eisenson (ed.), *Stuttering: A Symposium.* New York: Harper & Row, 1958.

————, A clinical success and a clinical failure, in M. Fraser, *Stuttering: Successes and Failures in Therapy.* Memphis, Tenn.: Speech Foundation of America, 1968, pp. 99–129.

————, *The Nature of Stuttering.* Englewood Cliffs, N.J.: Prentice-Hall, 1971.

WINGATE, M. E., Effect of stuttering on changes in audition, *Journal of Speech and Hearing Research,* 13 (1970), 861–73.

―――――, Prosody in stuttering adaptation, *Journal of Speech and Hearing Research,* 9 (1966), 550–56.

―――――, Slurvean skill in stutterers, *Journal of Speech and Hearing Research,* 10 (1967), 844–48.

WOLPE, J., Behavior therapy in complex neurotic states, in J. M. Shlien (ed.), *Research in Psychotherapy.* Washington, D.C.: America Psychological Association, 1968.

Treatment of

the Beginning Stutterer:

Prevention

We now turn our attention to the treatment of the child who is stuttering but who has not been stuttering very long. Although less has been written about the problems of the beginning stutterer than about those of the confirmed adult stutterer, there still is a wide literature to review. We do so primarily because in many parts of the world the stuttering child of preschool age is worked with very directly. This is an approach rarely used in this country but one that, from the published reports, has been highly successful. This direct approach is also one that we ourselves have now adopted though we do not use the sort of training these other workers advocate. In this chapter we will first describe the behaviors and problems characteristic of the beginning stutterer and the ways that other therapists have

coped with them and then we will present our own approach.

As we have seen in our discussion of the development of the disorder (Van Riper, 1971), the majority of these children show excessive syllabic repetitions, though some few begin with hard blockages. The disorder is usually cyclic, periods of complete fluency alternating with times when there are so many volleys of repetitive interruptions that communication is truly impeded and listener rejection or concern are evoked. The disorder in its initial phase is usually oscillatory in that the symptomatic patterns may change from the easy, effortless syllabic repetitions to occasional blockages with struggle and then the process may reverse itself. These children usually show little evidence of awareness or situation and word fears.

Their speech may be markedly broken but, in general, they do not react to their interruptions with expectancy or struggle. In Froeschel's (1952) terminology, we are speaking of the treatment of "physiologic stuttering," Bleumel's (1932) phrasing, "primary" as contrasted with "secondary" stuttering, and, in terms of Bloodstein's (1961) developmental concepts, the population discussed here is composed of those in the first two of his phases. A review of the literature makes very clear that many therapists feel that these children should be treated quite differently than "confirmed" or "advanced" or "secondary" stutterers, those who view themselves as "stutterers" and who have built up elaborate habituated behaviors to the anticipation or experience of interrupted communication.

Review of the literature

In reviewing the literature the first thing that strikes our attention is a general unanimity of opinion, especially in the United States, about how to manage beginning stuttering. Most of our therapists believe that the stutterer or the stuttering itself should never be worked with directly. Treatment tends to be very indirect and to be focused primarily on removing or reducing the stressful conditions which presumably precipitate the disfluency. Its major rationale is preventative, the therapists generally seeking to keep the child from developing awareness of stuttering or fears of speaking so that the disorder will not progress. Many workers, for example, feel that all their effort should be concentrated on altering parental attitudes, the family milieu and the conditions of communicative stress, with absolutely no interaction with the child himself. We find this emphasis

on indirect therapy very prevalent. In Israel, Zaliouk and Zaliouk (1965) say:

We, as most therapists, agree on an indirect approach, i.e., to try to handle the child's environment in such a way as to remove all the pressures affecting the healthy development of his personality. We undertake to create a harmony in the mutual relationship between the child and his parents, and the child and his environment. Of course, we stress a complete attitude of non-intervention in the speech. (p. 439)

In Holland, Damste (1968), states:

Children who are not yet clearly aware of a disorder of the speech should preferably not be given any logopedic treatment; the time saved in this manner is better spent in counseling the parents.

Also representative of this position is this American quotation from Eisenson and Ogilvic (1957):

The primary stutterer should be given no direct speech therapy or any other form of therapy that he can relate to his speech. Nothing should be done or said to the child that suggests that his speech is in any way in need of change. (p. 217)

At one time we felt much the same way as these authors but we have changed our beliefs and practices as the section describing our own therapy with the beginning stutterer will testify. While we still feel it unwise to work directly to modify the stuttering behaviors of such a child, we do work directly with him to facilitate his fluency and to *prevent* the growth of avoidance and struggle. This preventive aspect of therapy seems to be universally accepted. As Williams (1971) writes:

The emphasis in therapy cannot be the same for a child . . . as it is for an adult. Ordinarily, major attention in adult therapy is directed toward (1) reducing, modifying and in a sense breaking down the person's embarrassments and fear reactions toward speaking, and (2) reshaping the distorted interpersonal relationships that developed during his years of growing up. In the child, however, these faulty beliefs and related reaction patterns are just beginning to develop. One of the major purposes of therapy, therefore, is to *prevent* them from spiraling in intensity and complexity until they reach a level at which a child feels he can no longer cope with them. (p. 1075)

We insist, however, that preventive therapy should not be equated with a hands-off policy so far as the stuttering child is concerned.

Another observation concerning the literature on the treatment of beginning stuttering is that the research is practically nil. Most of the literature consists of theory, case observations, or general statements of policy. There also does seem to be a general agreement everywhere that the prognosis for the beginning stutterers is excellent and that their treatment is easier and less time consuming than for the adult stutterer. Let us see what others have said about how we should treat the child who has just begun to stutter.

Calling attention to beginning stuttering

All workers feel that one of the basic goals of therapy is to reduce the communicative stress felt by the child and most of them insist that no attempt be made to correct him when he does stutter.[1] As long ago as 1898 Gutzmann called attention to the unfortunate consequences of scolding or

[1] Tomkins (1916) was one of the few to disagree with this policy: "The only way to eliminate stuttering is to stop it. Society must refuse to listen to stuttering. Tell the stutterer to keep quiet until he can talk and then talk (p. 154)."

striking a child because he stuttered, and ever since that time most of the lists of "don'ts" given to parents include an injunction never to punish their children for stuttering. A few quotations may be representative: Spencer Brown (1949) writes:

If the child is showing little or no tension in his moments of non-fluency, the parents are advised that such interruptions are within or close to normal limits, and are in no sense a cause for alarm. Strict injunctions are given against expressing any sort of disapproval of non-fluency.

Morley (1957), the British therapist, says, "In the handling of the speech difficulty the mother is asked to refrain from impatience, and a desire to correct, assist or advise the child, and to insure that his speech is not ridiculed. She is asked to accept the child's hesitant speech as a temporary phase in his development and, as far as possible, to avoid any emotional reaction on her part towards it (p. 366)." Her colleague, Brook (1957) is even more emphatic:

Parents and others who seek 'to interfere imprudently or comment on clonic and tonic blockages in any way, are providing the precipitating factor which may lead to a real stammer developing. . . . Noticing that their child hesitates in his speech, many parents act upon foolish advice and try to put a stop to the "stammering." This is a most dangerous procedure, as it often introduces fear and shame into what was previously a fairly healthy situation. The child must not be allowed to suspect that there is anything unusual about his speech (p. 25)."

Punishment for beginning stuttering

Modern permissive practices in child rearing have pretty well eliminated the older use of punishment though the author well remembers several times during his boyhood when strangers slapped him across the face for having stuttered. They did not do it meanly but rather in the belief that stuttering was a nasty, dirty habit and that any listener had the moral obligation to break it as soon as possible. Some of these beliefs still exist among the lower socioeconomic classes or rural areas and they may be more common than one might expect. For example, Glasner and Rosenthal (1957) showed that over 70 percent of the parents they studied had used some active correction or punishment such as the following: "told him to speak more clearly, made him repeat, made him stop and say it over, said the word for him, reminded him not to stutter, got angry, etc." Moreover, these investigators found that despite (or because of) these practices a substantial number of the child stutterers corrected in this way became fluent. A similar point of view was shown by Albright and Raaf (1954):

> Well meant advice such as "Stop and think about what you want to say," "Say that over more slowly," and "Take a deep breath before you speak" are excellent aids if they are spoken with calmness, tenderness and friendliness on the part of the person giving the advice. However, these same aids make such practices unwise when stated with a tone of irritation or undue concern, and give the child feelings of embarrassment and fear. He will become ashamed of his speech and, in time, will give up trying to talk. (pp. 9–10)

The trouble with advice such as this is that parents tend to remember only the cautionary sentences they are supposed to say to the beginning stutterer and they forget the "calmness, tenderness, and friendliness." And even if they did say them tenderly, the child will soon become aware that he is having difficulty in talking. Luchsinger and Arnold (1965) express the opposing view that is commonly accepted by most workers: "All causes of excitement should be removed; the general management of the child should have a calming influence. Nothing will be achieved by punitive measures, forbidding orders or excessive sternness (pp. 759–60)."

The basic reason why punishment for *beginning stuttering* is not advised by any writer in the literature of whom we have knowledge (and this includes the operant conditioners) is that all of us wish to prevent the child from becoming aware of the interruptions in the flow of his speech. If he can be kept unaware of them, he will probably not develop the avoidance and struggle reactions which complicate the problem and are so difficult to extinguish. But we should recognize that there are other routes to this awareness besides ridicule, mockery, corporal pusishment, or rejection. The parents' evident anxiety and concern may send out signals so vivid that no child could fail to notice them. If they do, he will recognize that they occur at the moment when he is repeating or blocking. And he may even want that concern! He may be a child to whom, at a given moment in time, any attention is better than inattention.

Sheehan (1958) has pointed out that the initiation of a speech attempt is often the locus of any approach-avoidance conflict, and, as we have seen, more normal hesitancy and more stuttering occurs on the first words of an utterance than on any of the other words. If then a child begins to talk, merely desiring to attract attention by some opening verbal gambit such as "Mommy . . ." "I-I-I-I-" or "Ah . . . eh . . . uh . . ." and finds that he can capture his mother's ears more readily when he repeats than when he does not, that repeating will get strong reinforcement and will tend eventually to make him aware of what he is doing. Heltman (1955) puts it this way:

Children hesitate and repeat for the same reasons as adults. When a child starts to speak—that is, "makes as if" to speak—but instead hesitates or repeats, or both, the first sound, syllable, or word he enunciates is a *signal*. It is a signal which the over-anxious parent interprets from experience as an indication that the child is going to say something. To the child, on the contrary, this initial vocal act, when it is followed by excessive hesitation or repetition leading to the parents' diagnosis of stuttering, is but a device which he has discovered is effective in drawing attention to himself. (p. 39)

Such a child will soon learn to notice the antecedents of such a consequence. Shames and Sherrick (1963) make much of this:

An example might be the parent who delays immediate reinforcement of a child's first utterance because of inconvenience. The child may then repeat the utterance several times until the repetition becomes undesirable to the parent. Then the parent finally provides positive reinforcement for the child's demands, perhaps unaware that he is not only doing something for the child but also teaching him to repeat. (p. 6)

And eventually to be aware of his repetitions!

Even when the mother does not overtly respond to the child's speech hesitancies, she may be calling his attention to the *speech* (if not to his stuttering) in other ways. If she does, and the child becomes speech-conscious, sooner or later he will come to notice his fluency breaks. Thus, when a child is more nonfluent than

his brethren, most of us feel it wise to make no attempt to correct his grammar or his articulation or his pronunciation. With appropriate models, he will master these skills anyway and we are concerned about the possible spin-off from the awareness of one kind of error to those which could develop into severe stuttering.

There is special danger when the correction is done in the manner described by Rand, Sweeny, and Vincent (1962):

Laughing at the child's cute accent or his imperfect pronunciation is particularly dangerous since children are unable to discriminate kinds of laughter and do not always know the laughter of indulgent amusement from that of mockery. . . . Self-consciousness or fear of ridicule as a rule produces one of two results: either it discourages effort and tends to produce silence or it provides one of the commonest causes of stuttering. (p. 192)

We would add to their statement that any correction, however benign, tends to call attention to speech and may cause difficulty in the sense that Tomkins (1916) wrote about long ago:

The stammerer unfortunately makes an *effort* to talk. But since he does not know how he talks, the effort conflicts with his normally automatic words and so he stammers. In other words, stammering is a conflict between normal automatic speech and a misdirected conscious effort to speak.

Fifty years later, Jensen (1966) almost echoes Tomkins:

These reactions (by parents) presumably serve to create awareness by the child of the occurrence of disfluencies in his speech. He tries then to speak without them but this only leads to further complexity in the speaking act and, therefore, a potentially greater risk of disfluency. Thus, whereas his approach to speaking previously was largely "automatic" it is now becoming deliberate and effortful. This may, of course, lend confirmation to the parents' concern which may be expressed in more demonstrable form by further unsuccessful attempts at compliance by the child. (p. 89)

Several writers have also pointed out the folly of penalizing the stuttering child for his use of tabooed words and expressions. One of the first of these was the eminent psychologist Dunlap (1917). He felt that parental reactions to vulgar expressions were the basic cause of the disorder in that approach-avoidance conflicts were thus created which led to ambivalence in speech attempts. Barbara (1956) also stresses the effect of rejecting the child for unacceptable language. With rare exceptions, most American writers agree that it is unwise for parents to punish a stuttering child for any kind of unacceptable speaking. So do we.

Reducing the fluency disruptors

There is also general agreement everywhere that communicative stress must be reduced when a child begins to stutter. Often, the main effort of the therapist is directed toward the elimination of those pressures that tend to disrupt fluency in all of us since the beginning stutterer seems to be especially vulnerable to them. Among these pressures are listener loss, interruptions, competition for the conversational floor, the cross-examination kind of questioning, demands for display speech when we do not desire to be exhibitionistic, the demand for confession, having to talk under conditions of strong emotion such as guilt, fear or anger, or when fatigued or distracted. These are just a few of the fluency disruptors which seem to precipitate more stuttering in the child. The literature shows clearly that most therapists feel that they should be reduced or eliminated. The assumption, of course, is that if the people who talk to the stuttering child will endeavor to prevent these disrupting stresses, he will then stutter less and therefore be less likely to become aware of his speech interruptions as noxious.

Listener loss

Successful communication always involves a receiver as well as a sender of messages and there is a constant flow of feedback signals—visual, verbal or gestural—which tell the sender that he is being heard and understood. When these signals cease or do not seem appropriate, fluency breaks and hesitations tend to appear. In a booklet prepared by a group of American authorities on the prevention of stuttering (Murphy, 1962) we find the following:

Too often we listen in an indifferent, detached kind of way until that to which we are half listening stops; then we move on with whatever serves our own interests. The train whistle blows, and we wait until it stops blowing; the kettle whistles, and we interrupt our activity until the kettle is removed from the burner; a jet airline roars overhead, and we pause until it passes. This is listening which amounts to little more than waiting. The sounds are regarded as "noises," intrusions. This kind of listening may be appropriate for train whistles, kettles, and jet aircraft, but it is hardly appropriate for children. And yet we often regard the child's chatter as annoying noise; we listen only enough to recognize when the chattering stops, so that we can get on with more important matters; perhaps in order to resume our own chatter.

After repeated experiences of this kind, what must a child think? "They're not interested in what I have to say. I want them to know what I just did, what I just thought. I want to let them know how I feel—it's so good or so bad, but they don't want to know. They are not interested. Maybe I don't have anything interesting to say. Else why wouldn't they listen? Why keep trying to say things? Why try at all?" (p. 32)

Wendell Johnson (1949), in his "Open Letter to the Mother of a Stuttering Child," which has probably been viewed by more parents of stutterers than any other publication, gives priority to the reduction of listener loss. He says,

First of all, and above all, try to be the kind of listener your child likes to talk to. You know how to be this kind of listener, but it may be that no one has ever helped you to realize how tremendously important it is to your child—and to you, and to the two of you together—that you be such a listener whenever he talks to you.

Heltman (1955) is a bit more specific. He admonishes parents to listen to the child for what he has to say, rather than the way he says it. "Listen carefully enough so that when he has finished speaking you know what he has said. Listen with consideration for the fact that, if a child is to speak freely, he has to do it his way, not the way you think he ought to do it."

Interruptions and competition

All of us have met the verbal vulture who hovers impatiently, ready to pounce down and seize the conversation as soon as we pause or stop for a breath. It is always difficult to be fluent when speaking to such a person. Throughout the literature we find many cautions and injunctions insisting that we should free the stuttering child from *any* interruptions. Such an admonition, of course is quite impos-

sible to fulfill and can only make parents feel guilty. Any therapist who says something of the sort to a parent should have his frontal lobes examined. But parents can and should reduce the number of excessive interruptions in the interest of the child's precarious fluency. Schuell (1949) gives a pertinent excerpt from a parental interview: "Sara's trouble is that she never gets a chance to say anything. The rest of us talk all the time, and she can't get anyone to listen to what she wants to say." We too have known such blithe flowing parents. One of them was particularly resistant until we invited her to a group session with a number of very severe stutterers and had them verbalize their feelings about those who constantly interrupted them.

Time pressure

Related to interruption and competition is the influence of time pressure. A pertinent bit of research was performed by Beebe (1944) who asked normal adults to talk and read aloud as fast as possible. Almost all of her subjects, even those who were not able to talk any faster despite the instructions, showed fluency breaks. Doubtless, the common experience which most of us have had in trying to talk when under time pressure accounts for the familiar advice given stutterers "to slow down, to take it easy, to stop talking faster than you can think." Though such commands probably do no good and tend to make the stutterer even more frustrated, they reflect the basic nature of stuttering as a disorder of time. Throughout the history of stuttering, some slowing down of the speech of stutterers has been constantly recommended by a wide variety of theorists and practitioners. Many of the techniques used such as time beating, drawling, insertion of extraneous sounds, relaxation, use of visual pacers, even DAF, have worked, perhaps, because they did get the stutterer to speak more slowly. With a child who is relatively unaware of his fluency interruptions, however, it seems wiser to work more indirectly by reducing the number of times he meets an impatient listener each day, or by organizing his living so he does not need to hurry constantly, and above all by providing models of speech which are not exorbitantly swift.

Display speech

Sprinkled through the literature are many suggestions to the effect that parents should be counseled to reduce the amount of display speech required of the stuttering child. He is not to be encouraged to give recitations, to say the grace before meals, or even to recite his prayers. He is not to have approval for saying big words such as the names of the various dinosaurs. He is not to be encouraged to use long sentences. As Boome, Baines, and Harris (1939) wrote long ago, "It is a great temptation to show off the child to friends and relatives, to prove his superiority to other children by making him go through his linguistic paces, but it is a temptation which should be resisted." Some research seems to indicate that parents of stutterers do tend to be rather demanding and perfectionistic. Goldman and Shames (1964), for example, conclude that "the parents of stutterers set higher goals for their children generally, and higher speech goals specifically, than do parents of nonstutterers." Darley (1955) found that "the parents of stuttering children appeared to possess high standards generally and rather distinctively high

standards regarding speech behavior in young children." Moncour (1952) also found much the same pattern in his study of parental domination. These conclusions however, as Seligman (1966) has shown, must be viewed with some caution.

Nevertheless, in clinical practice, we do find many beginning stutterers who, through demand or excessive approvals, seem to suffer overload. Too often we have had to persuade certain parents not to teach their three year old child tongue twisters, or to insist that he recite the Lord's Prayer correctly or to go into ecstasy when he said "pumpernickel" or "indubitably." We feel it unwise to pull an onion to make it grow. Given good models and half a chance, children will learn to speak adequately without such coaching in exhibitionism. Speech is primarily a tool, not an ornament. One might reasonably assume that parents of a markedly disfluent child would have the good sense to cut down on the opportunities for such speech display and certainly not to encourage it, but unfortunately in far too many instances this is not the case. The speech therapist should always explore the possibility that, because of parental pressure, the beginning stutterer, as Wendell Johnson (1959) put it, is far too often "trying to talk over his head." Johnson continues:

The child is simply reacting to the beginnings of his doubt about his ability to speak "well enough" and of anxiety over the consequences of not doing so—by trying to speak better than he is able to under the circumstances, and at his stage of development. When a child begins to feel that he must do better than his best to gain his parents' approval, the resulting sense of insecurity is quite different from the less upsetting feelings he has when he is disapproved for something he can readily correct. (p. 23)

Demand speech

Less obvious but just as disruptive to fluency are the more subtle pressures represented by questioning, accusation, and other similar demands. Most of us, even as adults, tend to falter under cross examination. The instructor's sudden, unexpected question has caused many a student to give a garbled hesitant reply. When an answer is not immediately forthcoming, gaps tend to appear in our speech and we pause and repeat ourselves. If such interrogation can break up an adult's long stabilized fluency, how much more disruptive must it be for the little child?

We have observed thousands of verbal interactions between mothers and children and the amount of questioning which takes place just before volleys of stuttering occur is surprisingly great. We have no direct research on this but an examination of daily logs kept by parents in which they reported the characteristics of the communicative situation which yielded the most fluent and the least fluent responses shows clearly that parental questioning preceded stuttering in an impressive number of instances whereas only rarely did it precede a markedly fluent response.

It was also evident that at the time the child was questioned, the question had little to do with the activity in which he was then engaged or else it was a question for which no reasonable reply could be made. Examples of the latter are: "Why do you always have to keep picking your nose?" or "What are you going to do when Grandma comes?" or, "My, but aren't you a big boy now?" Any child who would really try to answer any of these would find difficulty. One mother kept track of the 132 questions she had asked her four-year-old son in a single day and concluded that 97 of them were stupid and most of the rest unnecessary. When questions are interruptions of the child's play activity, and have no bearing on the play, they always tend to provoke a reluctant or hesitant reply. Some of the worst ones, in terms of stress are those which demand that the child confess his wrong doing or relive a most unpleasant moment. "Why did you cut your finger?" "What did that bad dog do to you?" Surely, sufficient unto the moment is the evil thereof. Why ask a little child to put into his mouth words which recreate his hurt or shame? Why make speech painful? Confession may be good for the soul but it's bad for the child with fluency problems.

Emotionally disruptive influences

There are many other emotional conditions besides guilt which seem to evoke disfluency when the child attempts to speak while under their influence. When "things go thump in the night" and the child tries to tell his mother about them, his terror does not aid his fluency. The literature is full of such accounts and so are our case histories. Even novelists like to use repetitively broken words to indicate frightened speech, so commonly accepted is the idea that fear can impair fluency. Although no parent can possibly shield the child from all such experiences, we would not feel it wise to take a young stuttering child to a horror movie or to let him watch a television program rife with violence or to try to scare him out of his stuttering (as some parents have done).

Most children have fears enough without deliberately creating them. Schönhärl (1964) has a good sentence in this connection: "It could be said that the young stutter because they are anxious and the old are anxious because they stutter." Some parents seem to find it always necessary to get the child to verbalize his fears when they do arise. It would be better to have the mother do the verbalization herself if she knows the source of the fright, or, if she does not, to confine herself to comfort and reassurance. The same policy is useful in expressions of frustration, anger, or grief. If the mother can say what the child wants to say, he will not feel the terrible disrupting urgency and moreover, he then knows that she understands. The emphasis here is of course in talking *for* the child rather than talking to him when he is suffused with emotion. The Danish therapist, Forchammer (1964) points out the dangers of talking *to* the child when he is on the verge of tears or is actually crying. Sobbing is repetitive enough to trigger the recycling of syllables.

Excitement

A very common parental statement is that the child stutters more when he is excited or overstimulated and this, in our experience, seems to be true. In many homes, this overstimulation can be prevented with proper parental counseling but there is always the occasional visiting adult or child who can disrupt the precarious calm of the household. Often we have had to help parents find new playmates for their stuttering children to prevent this situation and we tell the parents what Blanton (1936) said so long ago: "Exclude ruthlessly from the child's environment those adults who overstimulate!" Unfortunately this may mean the impossible banning of a father, too.

Even pleasurable excitement can produce volleys of stuttering at times. Orchinik (1958), for example, de-

scribes from a psychoanalytic view the traumatic effect of tickling upon fluency. A child who attempts to protest while being tickled or played with roughly, or flung in the air and caught, or wrestled on the floor by a growling father may enjoy all of these activities immensely but his speech will often be the worse for them. Perhaps such interactive play helps release many emotions and promotes closeness between the child and his parent but it doesn't help his fluency. There is something to be said for a calm living environment when one is a young child trying to adjust to a demanding and complex world. Johnson (1949), in his "An Open Letter to the Mother of a Stuttering Child," summarizes the common advice of many writers in one sentence: "In general, try to avoid situations which are unduly frustrating, exciting, bewildering, tiring, humiliating, or frightening to the child."

Improper speech models

Children try to learn to speak the way that adults do and much of this learning process is indirect. The linguists tell us that the capability for grammatical and prosodic mastery is inborn and innate but that the models provided by the associates of the child in his early years soon become internalized and provide the templates by which his speech becomes organized.

In his book, *The Nature of Stuttering* (1971) the author has described the development of stuttering as generally following four discernable tracks. It would therefore seem reasonable to expect that therapy should be varied according to the differing features shown by these different children at onset. We do this by emphasizing certain kinds of therapeutic practices for certain children while still insisting that nonfluent children of all types can be helped by reducing fluency disruptors in the environment or by facilitating the fluency they already possess. In the next several sections of this chapter we discuss the methods used by workers in our own and foreign lands to help the child organize his speech and to help him formulate and express his thoughts. When done in such a way as to prevent the child from becoming anxious about how he talks, this sort of therapy would probably be good for all beginning stutterers but especially valuable for those with a cluttering component in their behavior picture.[2]

Stuttering usually begins at the very time that great advances in sentence construction occur and it seems tenable that when the speech models provided by the parents or siblings of the child are too difficult for him to follow, some faltering will ensue. In another book (Van Riper, 1961), we said this:

Consider for a moment what choices are open to a child whose parents set for him speech models which are too fast and too complex. He can either imitate the fast flow and talk jabberingly or else he can speak his consonants correctly and falter hesitantly. If he takes one path he may stutter; if he takes the other he will have a disorder of articulation. If only parents would blaze the third trail of easy simplified speech, we speech therapists would pretty well be put out of business. But they do not know the third trail and no one has told them about it. (p. 51)

This of course is not a new idea. Bleumel (1957) wrote:

Attention should be given to normal speech development. Speech in the home

[2] We have described these children as those following Track II (Van Riper, 1971, pp. 108-11).

should be clear, quiet and concise. Words should be simple, such as the child would choose for himself. . . . Not only should words be simple, but the sentences should be short, and the speech should be calm and unhurried. (p. 108)

An example of the sort of speech models which are very conducive to fluency is provided by Wyatt (1959):

The teacher began to describe the things that happened to the cat in the pictures. The objects and events in the book were on the child's level of interest and experience and the teacher used "early relational language" to describe the pictures, namely simple sentence structure with chain-like linking together of one short phrase to another. "And what does the kitty do here? He is getting out of his box, see—out of his box—and here, here he climbs over the box, over the box —here—and here, he jumps down, down into the grass." From time to time Betsy spontaneously fell in with the teacher: "out of the box . . . over the box . . ." and, laughing out loud, ". . . jumps out of the box. . . ."

Teacher and child thus demonstrated the ideal learning situation: both speech partners were attuned to each other and reciprocal identification between the speech partners was established through acts of mutual imitation. From time to time the teacher also participated in the child's motions and gestures as well as in her speech and, in addition, she communicated with the child on the pre-linguistic level through mutual body closeness and touch. (p. 6)

Some of the strain on the child's acquisition of fluency may be due to exorbitant parental expectations. Certain parents seem to create disrupting pressures by their urge to have their children speak unfaltering too soon. We have often found this in the situations of first born or only children and especially when a child has been a little slow in talking. These parents want the child to use adult speech as soon as possible and some of the things they do are often incredible. We have watched them reject perfectly good simple sentences and rephrase them in highly complex forms, then insist that the child say them their way. Nim (1965) has stressed that these unrealistic parental expectations are among the major reasons for the development of stuttering. Certainly the many reports of stuttering beginning when a child with delayed speech and language finally starts talking show that this may be true. As the author has written elsewhere (Van Riper, 1971):

One of the factors contributing to the onset of stuttering in these cases seems surprisingly to be the parents' delight in the newly attained speech. Often they overpraise and overencourage the child once he begins to talk and demand more and more verbal facility. Many times we have been able to eliminate the stuttering merely by reducing these parental expectations and demands. (p. 87)

We find this emphasis upon eliciting slower and simpler speech throughout the literature. To cite some examples: Rumsey (1937) in England writes: "I have personal knowledge of many cases in which a stammer was averted at its onset by the efforts made by the parents; no mention of the stuttering has been made, but the parents have spoken slowly, with the happiest results (p. 42)." and Daskalov (1962) in Bulgaria says, "Success in also determined by systematic training of parents in quiet and correct speech." We feel that Daskalov makes a very good point. It is easy enough for the therapist to tell the parent to talk slowly or simply but we have found few who seemed to be able to do so without some *training*. Altering the rate of one's speech is very difficult for any-

one to do consistently and without abnormality. Indeed we have found some parents who spoke so artificially when advised to talk slowly (a change which usually appeared suddenly and dramatically and immediately after the child has a volley of stuttering) that their abnormally slow speech immediately called attention to the stuttering. Instead we prefer to talk with the stuttering child to show the parents how to do it. We train them to lengthen their pauses, occasionally to hold a vowel a bit longer and especially how to speak simply and in shorter sentences. One mother who spoke so swiftly as almost to possess a tachylalia was completely unable to speak slowly until we showed her how to monitor her speech by proprioception. Usually, if a mother will merely try to speak simply and in short sentences, she will speak slowly enough.

Reading to the child

The literature is replete with suggestions that the parents should read to the stuttering child very frequently. We do not agree with this fairly common prescription. Though the reading situation usually provides a warm, close relationship, we have found too many parents reading so fluently that the model thereby presented was far beyond the child's ability to follow. Also, in such a situation the child often tries to interrupt and is unable to do so. Too often, such sessions end in mutual communicative frustration. We have found it wiser to have the parents paraphrase what they read, or talk about the pictures in the book, or make up stories of their own. The parental speech models thus presented tend then to be more natural and less complex and they will be much slower if only because of the burden of formulation and invention which these activities require. In this vein, Lennon (1962) suggests retelling familiar stories about the shared family life and reviewing the activities of the day while speaking slowly and calmly. We are certain that some parents can read to some children in a manner that will not create the difficulties mentioned but many of them cannot. For those few who can, perhaps Johnson's (1949) advice would be pertinent:

Read to him whenever you can. In reading or speaking to Fred, enunciate clearly, be interested in what you are reading, and avoid a tense voice. Make this reading fun and companionable. Do some of it every day, preferably just before bedtime if possible.

Creating and reinforcing fluency

While much of the current therapy for the beginning stutterer consists of the identification and elimination of the pressures and practices which seem to precipitate the child's disfluency there are also many positive things which can be done to facilitate and reinforce his normal speech. One of the most useful of these is that which takes advantage of the cyclic nature of beginning stuttering. On his "good days," when little stuttering occurs, it is wise to create many opportunities for the child to speak and to keep speaking; on his "bad days," and quite without his knowledge, parents can arrange things so that there is very little opportunity for him to need to talk. We have seen this single prescription cure many young stutterers and we use the word "cure" to mean normal fluency. But even on the days when the child is very nonfluent, there will be certain situations or conditions in which he will tend to be relatively fluent. These too can be identified and used. Thus one child

spoke very well while chewing gum, while another was always fluent at bedtime just before going to sleep. Certain conversational partners also seem to evoke remarkably good fluency. Speaking to dolls, or the cat, or dog, if these produce fluency can be encouraged. Many young stutterers speak very well when assuming a role in play activity or when wearing a mask, or when giving commands. If parents will concentrate their attention on the situations which produce more fluency instead of those which elicit stuttering, they usually find ways of creating more of the former kind. They can be trained also to find ways of discreetly reinforcing the fluent speech by occasional approvals or the immediate granting of attention. Bar (1971) describes how he used this approach with 48 child stutterers, 44 of whom became normal speakers. Both the therapist and the parents gave social approvals for fluent utterances first in the easy, nonstressful situations and then gradually applied them sequentially to other situations progressively more difficult in the hierarchy as the child improved.

Direct fluency training in Europe

Although, as we have seen, there are many who feel that no formal training in speech improvement should be given the beginning stutterer, this opinion is far from universal. In France, Pichon and Borel-Maisonny (1937) recommended that young stutterers be given direct drilling in combining words into phrases, often accompanied by rhythmic body movements, and done in unison with the therapist. They considered stuttering to be a language disorder, often stemming from delay in language maturation, and they insist that the child hesitates and falters because he has not learned how to organize his language linguistically or motorically. As Goldman-Eisler (1967) and Mahl (1957) and others have shown clearly, much of the hesitation in normal speech seems to be due to formulative difficulties. We even have some research by Weuffen (1961) that suggests that stutterers generally are deficient in word-finding ability. Certainly some of them are, though in our experience not many. Those who do have formulation difficulties could doubtless profit much from some of the procedures that Black (1960) saw in Russia:

Children as young as two years are given direct speech lessons. The generally accepted method includes removing children from their homes for a three-month period. The stutterers go to a residential school which specializes in speech work. The temporary separation of the child from his family is an effort to create a favorable psycho-physical environment for his speech development. Although direct speech therapy is rather formal, with directions for training for fluency by repeating sentences, by memorizing sentences, by narration of picture stories, by questions and answers, by independent narration, and finally by conversation regarding every day affairs, constant emphasis is placed on pleasant and challenging experiences rather than on a training routine. The *logoped* must have a large variety of didactic and illustrative material and be instructed to be friendly but firm and consistent. (p. 4)

Preobrajenskaya (1953) provides an outline of this direct therapy which was said to take about six months. The logoped (speech therapist) began by teaching the children to sit quietly, hands on the table, and to pay attention. Then the children practiced saying simple sounds beginning with the vowels, then to prolong them, much of the recitation being done in unison. Then short phrases and sentences, spoken without pausing, were uttered first in unison then alone. Next verses were recited as a group exercise and then individually. Group and solo singing were also used at this stage. Then fairy tales were told and retold and questions were asked about the content. Finally, arithmetic problems were posed which had to be solved verbally. Parents and teachers were also instructed to carry out the program. Preobrajenskaya reports "perfect speech" in eight children, "poor speech" in four, and "good speech in school but poor speech outside" for fifteen others.

Despite the possible dangers of calling attention to the speech by doing direct therapy of this sort or bringing stutterers together in groups, we find many other European authors advocating some of this training. Rhythmic and unison or echo-speaking experiences are generally recommended practices. Children, assembled in groups, first recite material together, then one child after another drops out until only a single child is speaking. In England, some of the older workers such as Behnke (1947) and Kingdon-Ward (1941) had child stutterers first relax, then memorize and recite in unison with the therapist, emphasizing vocal expression and inflections. Influenced by Cherry's (1957) cybernetic research we find Pauline Marland (1957) using shadowing techniques for young children as well as adults. Patterson (1958) also recommends shadowing and also "phrase copying," in which the therapist reads phrases, then pauses while the child repeats. Kelham and McHale (1966) found that younger children benefited more from shadowing than older ones. Although Froeschels (1952) feels that breath chewing with vocalization can be employed with children as young as five years, he suggests that for younger stutterers the parent or therapist look at picture books together and repeat the comments made about them meanwhile prolonging the vowels and thereby slowing the speech.[3]

The current belief so prevalent in this country that no therapist should work directly with a child who has just begun to stutter is probably based on the equating of direct therapy with punishment. This is a mistake; it is possible to deal directly with the child's speech in many ways without hurting him or focussing on stuttering as an evil. The direct training of young preschool stutterers in many European clinics is devoted primarily to the reinforcement and development of normal speech. In this we should remember Bluemel's (1957) insistence that stuttering is basically a disorder of unorganized or disorganized speech and thinking.

For many years the Russians have felt that the solution to the problem of stuttering was to reach the stuttering child early and to work with him immediately rather than wait until many abnormal conditioned responses had been built up around the disorder. Sikorski (1891), who insisted that stuttering should be treated as soon as it appeared in the very young child, has had a profound influence on all Russian workers. Rau (1953) protested the "false" belief that direct speech therapy with the beginning stutterer was necessarily harmful and recommended that the child be separated from his family, placed in a healthy speech environment, and given intensive therapy to reintegrate the

broken speech. A comprehensive review of the Russian literature on the treatment of stuttering in children is provided by Cheveleva (1967) and it indicates clearly that one of the basic aims of Russian therapy is to aid the child to develop fluent verbal *formulation*. Much of this teaching is done through the use of modelling with transitions from simple to more complex forms in imitative and memorized speech being practiced by the children and strongly reinforced by the therapist. Cheveleva, who feels that stuttering is the result of a deficit in "the child's ability to formulate his thoughts without the support of direct visual observation or clear-cut visual representation," an ability that develops gradually in all children, describes the therapeutic program as follows:

Since the greatest developmental progress is achieved under conditions of child activity, we came to the conclusion that our principles could be successfully utilized in speech training during the process of manual work. Communication while doing manual work permits the possibility of introducing the speech material with greater graduality. By gradually decreasing the amount of concrete visual stimulation and increasing the complexity of the speech models accompanying this manual work, we slowly help the children's speech to become more complex, thus creating the gradual transition to more abstract expressions, to unfolding explanations and finally, to the detailed narrative stories from which all direct visual support is eliminated. In this way we help the child to lean upon verbalization alone. By having all the children do manual activity together, the children learn to express in words their thoughts and actions. Thus, manual work can develop all the mental operations of children (analysis, synthesis, comparison, and generalization). (p. 6)

Other Russian workers, though

[3] One of the few American advocates of direct speech training was Edna Hill Young (1965) who utilized the motokinesthetic method with stuttering children as young as two and a half years.

they may not use manual activities as the vehicle of therapeutic interaction, or Cheveleva's transitions from situational (visually dependent) to contextual verbal formulations, do seek to improve the young stutterer's ability to formulate and express his thoughts in ever-increasing complexity. Thus Vlassova (1962) begins by concentrating on phrase and sentence building based upon pictures, drawing, rhythms, singing, dancing and other activities. An excerpt from one of her articles may be illuminating:

As we are dealing here with the developing function of speech and as the main part in its development is played by the auditory and visual analyzers, all logopaedic work in the speech re-education of the stuttering child is based on the activity of these analyzers. In the first place, this calls for a great variety of pictures, from those representing single objects to those representing long sentences which are built up step by step. The logopaedic work with stuttering children aims not only at teaching them to speak fluently, but also at enriching their vocabulary and teaching them to build sentences correctly, etc. All these things aid the development of the child's whole personality. This shows not only in their speech, but also in their play and mainly in their drawings. (p. 31)

Levina (1968) is another Russian worker who stresses the need for the stuttering child to be assisted in shifting from concrete to conceptual speech, and we find this emphasis on developing the skills of formulation and expression in other Iron Curtain countries as well. Thus Petkov and Iosifov (1960) and Daskalov (1962) incorporate direct training in progressing from simple to more complex utterances as part of the "total-push" treatment in the Bulgarian stuttering colonies.

We should emphasize that no direct attention is called to stuttering in the kind of speech therapy we have been describing. The concentration is instead upon procuring and reinforcing normal speech. As our excerpts have indicated, much of the therapy occurs in groups and much of the speaking by any one child is done in unison with the others. Transitions from singing to speaking are provided and the whole atmosphere is one of pleasant, organized activity. Moreover, the reported number of cures is very impressive. Perhaps one reason for these successes is that the stuttering children are usually given a completely new environment. They may attend logopedic kindergartens or live in remedial colonies or camps or be placed in hospitals where all their activities are supervised so as to facilitate good speech. As long ago as 1834, Smirnova insisted that treatment for the stutterer should begin early and be done in special schools and kindergartens and we find Katsovskaia (1960) and other east European authors maintaining the same point of view today. Wullfert (1964) describes such a logopedic kindergarten for child stutterers aged two to four and Vlassova (1961) tells of a six-year-old stutterer who stayed in a residential clinic for 18 months.

We do not wish to leave the impression however that all stuttering children in the Iron Curtain countries are taken away from their homes. Indeed certain workers, such as Lepsova (1965) in Czechoslovakia, protest that placement in special logopedic schools may hurt the child. She writes, "The Phoniatric School (Prague) recommends interruption of school attendance with the child being hospitalized during the course of the treatment (for stuttering). I found, in my work that during these weeks the child loses contact with the school and develops feelings of sickness and abnormality." Lepsova instead devised a camping stuttering program for vacation periods. Svend Smith (1955) also objects to the segregation of stutterers in special schoolrooms: "The children should not, in my opinion, enter a kindergarten for stuttering children, because then the child would be classified as a stutterer."

Nevertheless when we remember all the kinds of fluency-disrupting influences that may occur in certain homes and considering how often we find disordered family relationships, surely something may be said for the provision of a controlled therapeutic environment. It may well be that, even in our own country in years to come, day nurseries, preschools, and kindergartens specially designed to facilitate the acquisition of normal speech will be provided for all children with speech problems. There parents may come for counseling and training. There the parents and teachers of beginning stutterers could see how good speech can be created and maintained. Stuttering should not be permitted to grow abnormally if it can be prevented. We should not really have to treat adult stutterers at all. For them, the therapy must always be more complicated, laborious, and time consuming. In our own treatment of the beginning stutterer, which we will describe in a later section of this chapter, we also try to create such a new environment for the child and to train his parents, but unfortunately we usually have the child for only a brief time each day. Though for most beginning stutterers this is sufficient, for some others a "total push" in a completely therapeutic environment would be most helpful.

Counseling the parents of the beginning stutterer

There also appears to be widespread agreement in the literature that much of the treatment of the young stutterer should involve his parent and associates. The title to a subsection of the booklet "Toward Understanding Stuttering," by Wendell Johnson (1959) asked the question "Problem, Problem, Who's Got the Problem?" and he answered it by saying in effect that the parents are the ones who have the problem rather than the child. Johnson insisted that the problem of stuttering is due basically to parental misperceptions and misevaluations of the child's fluency difficulties and that these in turn lead the parents to behave in ways that only make the disfluencies more frequent and more severe.

Changing unwise parental practices. We have already described many parental practices which seemed to be definitely unwise in the handling of a young stutterer. Now we turn to a discussion of the ways through which a therapist can reduce or eliminate these unfavorable influences. In trying to provide a familial environment that will be likely to promote fluency rather than stuttering there exists a very wide range of therapist-parent interactions. They vary all the way from having a trivial sheet' of mimeographed advice mailed to otherwise uncontacted parents, to intensive parental counseling sessions, or even to parental psychoanalysis.

Generally, the therapist's view of the nature of the disorder seems to determine the way he structures his interactions with the parents of the beginning stutterer. For example Glauber (1958), a psychoanalyst, feels that the mother should have psychoanalysis or psychotherapy. A brief excerpt may illustrate:

The first task in the therapy of the mother was to work through her acceptance of her mixed feelings about her own need for treatment, a need that became more apparent in the discussion of her relationship to her own mother. Next in importance was the exposing and working through of her pent-up anger and anxiety connected with unresolved deep disappointment and frustrations at the hands of her mother. She became aware of these emotions in discussions regarding her separation from her mother and also from her stuttering child. . . . (p. 113)

Gertrude Wyatt (1969), a psychodynamically oriented therapist but not a psychoanalyst, views stuttering as resulting from a developmental crisis in the verbal interaction between mother and child. Accordingly, her parent counseling is based upon observation of parent-child and therapist-child interaction.

Thus the therapist teaches the mother, first through explanation and analysis of her own behavior and communication patterns; second, through demonstration of communication patterns appropriate for interaction with young children. Finally, the therapist helps the mother understand her own feelings for the stuttering child, which are intimately connected with her ability or inability to communicate successfully. (Wyatt and Herzan, 1962, p. 651)

Both these views differ from each other and even more different is the approach of workers such as Schuell (1949), Bloodstein (1958) Sander (1959), Williams and Roe (1960) and, of course, Wendell Johnson himself, all of whom feel that parental counseling is the treatment of choice. In this approach, a series of interviews is arranged in which the therapist explores the parents' attitudes toward the stuttering child and his speech

and then seeks to persuade them, through an analysis of their perceptions and evaluations, to view the disfluencies in a less morbid fashion. These therapists also provide parents with information and advice usually based upon the Iowa theory and research which indicates that what they and the child misevaluate as stuttering is no more than perhaps excessive but essentially normal disfluency. They stress that this normal disfluency is probably produced by communicative stress due to the perfectionistic parental demands upon the child.

The workers of the Iowa school rarely advocate any deep psychotherapy for parents since they consider them also to be essentially normal. They are viewed as individuals who have just failed to understand how speech develops, how it is affected by stress, or how disfluent it can be and yet be normal. A typical expression of the position of these Iowa trained therapists is found in this quotation from their main advocate, Johnson (1959):

Any problem is best approached by finding out first whose problem it is. So long as the problem affects the parents primarily, it is the parents who need information and counseling. Indeed, until the child gives definite evidence that he is disturbed about his own speech there would seem to be little or no justification for applying any therapy to him. The kind of information the parents need meanwhile is by and large the kind which this booklet contains. They need to know the basic facts about the way children learn to speak, and particularly they need to understand what they can reasonably expect of a child so far as speech fluency is concerned. They need also to be aware of the kinds of conditions or circumstances under which a child tends to speak more easily and smoothly, or with more hesitancy and unsureness. (pp. 31–32)

Since this point of view essentially puts the blame for the child's speech problem squarely on the parents, most of its adherents stress the need to allay the guilt feelings thus aroused or thereby augmented. Thus Bloodstein (1958) says:

Any effort to change some of the parent's behavior must start with the removal of guilt about the child's stuttering. The mother who brings her stuttering youngster to the clinic is likely to have a crushing sense that she herself was somehow implicated in the development of his speech difficulty. "What did I do wrong?" is a question which is one form or another she may ask as anxiously as "Will he outgrow it?" While she must be helped to accept a sizable share of responsibility for the child's speech improvement, there is hardly a more effective way of intensifying her anxieties than to corroborate her suspicion that his stuttering resulted from abnormalities in her relationship with him. On the other hand, our confidence in her basic adequacy as a parent will leave her better able to accept suggestions for specific changes in her behavior. We may not be able to tell her with conviction that she had nothing to do with her child's stuttering. But we can, in the author's opinion, truthfully tell her that stuttering seems to be brought about by a combination of many factors or conditions varying somewhat from case to case, and we can truthfully tell her that stuttering children appear to be found in every conceivable type of family environment, not excluding some which seem in many ways unusually wholesome and favorable. (p. 60)

The therapist in this type of counseling plays a role somewhat like that advocated by Albert Ellis (1958). He questions, elicits the attitudes and opinions of the parent, contradicts at times, and always submits the parental responses to analytical scrutiny. Brown (1949) suggests that the child should always be seen while interacting verbally with the parents so that his behavior and theirs could be assessed since the basic goal of therapy is to "alter the attitudes and behavior of the parents to that stuttering child and to his speech." Bloodstein (1958) speaks of the process as a "systematic discussion," beginning with the eliciting and accepting of the parents' guilt feelings, next in persuading them to remove the speech pressures, and finally in helping them to decrease their demands upon the child. Schuell (1949) felt that the parent counseling could usually be done "informally" in four interviews devoted to discovering parent-child relationships, and to uncovering adverse parental attitudes and practices, and the answering of questions about stuttering and the formulating of parental home assignments.

It also appears that another group of American workers feels that parental counseling need not be long-term nor intensive. These therapists organize groups of parents of stutterers to share their feelings with each other and also to receive the necessary information. Indeed, Wood (1948) describes these parents' meetings as "classes" with the therapist playing the role of lecturer, but Murphy and Fitzsimons' (1960) comment may be appropriate here: "The procedure of arranging talks or lectures by the staff or consultants is often interesting and bolstering to the ego of the speaker, but its effectiveness in developing parental understandings remains doubtful (p. 427)." Or perhaps we might add this remark of Zelda Wolpe (1957):

The term parent counseling has the unfortunate connotation of a therapist giving advice to the parent, having the answers at his disposal, being an advisor for all the complexities of human interpersonal relationships. This is a far cry from getting the parent to find for himself the answers to his problem, to understand his behavior, to determine the areas in which he has been blindly groping. A critical attitude in relationship to the parent can be no more productive than a critical attitude in relationship to the child in a therapeutic process. Whether child or adult, the patient feels himself in a threatened position or he would not need to develop defenses against his anxiety. (p. 1017)

Another group of therapists feels that many of the communicative pressures which disrupt speech in the child reflect basically disturbed parent-child relationships. Thus we find Baurand and Striglioni (1968) in France attributing the hesitant speech to ambivalent attitudes and practices in the interaction of the mother and child. From Russia (Vlassova, 1961), we find this little vignette about such a child:

Irene began to stutter at the age of four; she had hardly spoken at all before she was three, but with speech came also stuttering. Her parents, particularly the father, were in panic and turned for help from one doctor to another; and following one physician's advice they completely isolated the girl from any contact with other children. Irene was growing utterly capricious and spoiled. The father was obeying, to keep her from crying, every one of her whims; the mother, trying to moderate Irene's demands, was not even permitted to educate the child. Stuttering increased to the point when the question arose whether she should go to school at all. . . .

In our country, as Rotter (1942) has very vividly shown, such pampering and yielding to a controlling child can create the fundamental ambivalence in interpersonal relationships which can manifest itself in stuttering. Glasner (1949) also makes this point: "A calm and consistent house-hold, even though it may be unduly strict or even harsh, is far less likely to produce stuttering than a household where the atmosphere is indecisive and capricious." Gondairo (1960) in Japan describes his work with a young stutterer and his mother. Play therapy was used with the child and counseling with the mother. The problem was complicated by the fact that the boy had a deformed hand of which the father was so ashamed he would not be seen in public with the child. Gondairo writes:

I felt that this is a problem of the parents more than of T.K. (the child). They feel complete responsibility for T.K.'s deformity. Because of their sense of guilt, he is not permitted to play with other boys his age. Therefore I felt that in order to treat T.K. properly I must also treat his parents as well.

The treatment procedures that we are now describing, essentially forms of psychotherapy in the larger sense, seem to be especially useful for the kind of beginning stutterer whose onset and developmental features are those of the children on Track III (Van Riper, 1971, 111–14). In these children the stuttering appears rather later than usual and begins very suddenly with dramatic blockages. Awareness and frustration reactions are shown almost immediately. These beginning stutterers need special reassurance, a nontraumatic environment relatively free from stress, and an opportunity to act out their frustration in play therapy. Parents must understand the child's feelings of helplessness at this time and must not augment them by showing their own concern. Unfortunately the therapist rarely has the opportunity to treat the child early enough to prevent the fear or struggle reactions from developing and gaining strength. However, when we find a child showing his first stuttering in the form of silent fixations and an inability to produce vocalization, we try to intervene as soon as we can. We work directly with the child and do not confine our efforts to parental counseling or advice.

Children who show a sudden onset and severe blockages from the first require emergency measures and no therapist should fail to start therapy immediately. Long ago Bleumel (1935) recognized the seriousness of this kind of onset and prescribed some drastic treatment:

If the stammering begins suddenly, the child should be treated as though nervously ill and should be put to bed under medical care. Sedatives should be given in sufficient amounts to induce sound sleep throughout the night and occasional naps during the day. There should be no visitors, and no stimulation or excitement. Conversation should be kept at a minimum. Meanwhile the patient should not be made conscious of his speech; if an explanation is required for these procedures, it can be given to the child in terms of his nervousness. Bed rest and isolation should be continued in this manner for several days or weeks, according to medical judgment. A regimen of partial rest should follow, the child resuming his accustomed activities gradually.

With a young child who is not well disciplined, it may be difficult to enforce absolute bed rest, for the child may get up to play with his toys or to look out of the window. It would be inopportune to make an issue of the child's conduct at this juncture, for the situation might result in emotional reaction with increased nervousness. Under the circumstances it would be better to let the child profit from isolation and from whatever additional rest he may obtain. As a rule it is inadvisable to place a young child in a hospital in order that strict bed rest may be observed, for separation from home may cause emotional stress with conse-

quent aggravation of nervous symptoms.

Sometimes the effect of bed rest and tranquillization is immediate. Catherine S., 13 years old, was seen two days after she had developed marked stammering, accompanied by general nervousness. No history of shock was elicited, but the child complained of a lump in the throat (globus hystericus) and a feeling of shaking or jerking inside the body. She was put to bed and was kept drowsy for a few days with phenobarbital. Stammering disappeared in twenty-four hours and did not return. (pp. 154–55)

The same sort of treatment has also been used in Russia. According to Clark (1959), "They suggest that the child be put on silence for two or three weeks. If the stammer develops from shock, the use of sleep and silence is employed." Heavy dosing with tranquilizers has also been employed. We ourselves have not used any of these procedures, preferring instead to create a nontraumatic environment in which we can prevent the growth of fear and struggle responses.[4]

Limitations of advice and persuasion. Even if our own clinical experience were not sufficiently corroborative, the literature has enough accounts of similar problems to convince us, not only that direct intervention may be needed, but also that the therapist's interactions with parents of many beginning stutterers should include more than the provision of information, reassurance and advice. Quite apart from the problem of causation, we must recognize that once the parents become concerned about the child's speech and feel the silent accusation of the culture, they need some real opportunity for examining their lives and feelings. If they are pampering or punishing

[4] An account of therapy with one of our young stutterers with this type of onset will be found on pages 402–4.

the child, it is not enough to tell them not to do so. They should know why they need to react in such a way. If they continue to show wincing, scolding, interrupting, cautioning, labeling, and other punishing behaviors, these may flow from dark springs deep within. If the home tempo is hectic, or the mother's speech is too fast to serve as an appropriate model for the child, and they cannot be changed, there may be reasons often unrecognized. If the child falters in his speech, may he not be trying to seek contact and hesitantly to touch with words a parent whose responses he cannot predict? Does he hesitate because he senses covert maternal rejection as Kinstler's research (1961) indicated? Is his speech broken because he feels a broken relationship with his parents? Is he responding to an overdominating, perfectionistic parent with the same hesitancy that most of us show in a similar situation? Do his repetitive syllables reflect a need to return to an earlier and more satisfying sort of babbling communication as Stein (1949) and others have believed? We hold no brief for any of these interpretations and speculations. It is enough to know that once the parents have an opportunity to ventilate their feelings in a permissive, understanding situation, they often alter their attitudes toward the stuttering child and the ways they treat him.

Most of the parents we have thus counseled have not been highly disturbed or maladjusted individuals. They did not appear to need any deep psychotherapy but they did need some chance to complain and explain and wonder and wish. They needed someone to share their hopes and fears and troubles *before* they could change their management of the stuttering child or alter the environment in which he had to exist and communicate. When they have had this opportunity, we find that the spin-off produces marked gains in the child's fluency, as Glasner and Dahl (1952) mention:

> After the history is obtained and the child is examined, the problem in general is discussed with the parents. An attempt is made to help the parents understand the dynamics in the case stripped of the emotional coloring that generally confuses and prevents them from dealing adequately with the situation. In some cases, after the parents have had opportunity to discuss the problem in this setting, they are able to recognize the source of the difficulty without much help from us. In a few cases at the second interview the therapist is informed by the parents —"the child doesn't stutter any more!" Obviously the pressures and tensions have been removed from the environment and the stuttering has disappeared. More generally, marked improvement is noted. (p. 1114)

The person unfamiliar with beginning stuttering might view these remarks about such a sudden remission with some skepticism. We do not. We have repeatedly witnessed the dramatic cessation of stuttering and disfluent behavior in these children. Often it seems as though all one needs is to remove just one stick of the overload that has caused the child to falter in the gait of his communication and lo! he can walk again. Moreover, it can be almost any stick. We have seen instances when such children regained their fluency when a mother just stopped asking him questions, or just gave him more rest, or stopped fighting with her husband, or (in one instance) gave him medication which relieved him of worms. We have seen such a child become fluent when he acquired a puppy or had his father take him fishing. This is why the prognosis is so good in beginning stuttering and why usually therapy need not take long. Let us remove the pressures and especially those to which the child's fluency seems most vulnerable. Often we need only to reflect our understanding of the parents' feelings, answer some of their questions and the child stops stuttering. Over the years we have listened to a long procession of parents (usually the mothers) as they talked about their anxieties, guilts, angers, frustrations, quarrels, insecurities, disciplining, tensions, burdens, and hopes. Rarely have we had to offer much advice or counsel. We listen and share. Parents usually already knew how they should be responding to the child and his speech difficulties, and after they had done enough talking to us they changed their ways so that the child became fluent. Murphy and Fitzsimons (1960) whose book contains not only what is probably the best presentation of the personality dynamics of stuttering but also some excellent transcripts of actual parent counseling interviews, have this to say about what happens:

When a parent experiences a period of therapy, he finds himself better able to work through some of the troubling feelings which have resulted in his oppressive demands upon the child for unrealistic achievement, including speech and language accomplishments. The parent finds that he is able to accept his child's nonfluency. He has faith that some of his child's repetitions are to be expected in the course of normal language development. He feels able to react to his child's communicative speech attempts with respect and understanding rather than with correction and criticism. The parent becomes able to use therapy to neutralize anxieties and to effect needed changes in relations between himself and his child. He is able to create a relationship which rests upon acceptance, faith, love, respect, and understanding. (p. 424) [5]

Parents differ widely in their reactions to the opportunity for such counseling. Some greet it with alacrity; others come reluctantly if at all. It is especially difficult to get the fathers involved and the therapist is likely to get a distorted view of the family situation unless they are. One strategy which has proved effective is to ask the parents to have evening conferences in which they report to each other their observations of the child's speech and behavior. The following letter from a mother (Van Riper, 1961) will illustrate:

Dear Sir: You asked me to put down in a letter some of the things I told you we had done, and are still doing at home to help Bill overcome his stuttering. As I said, he now seems to have stopped it completely. Oh, once in a while he hesitates but no more than I do. You know how you hesitate when you aren't sure of what you're going to say but nothing unusual. I mean he talks fine and straight now just like anybody else. I've been waiting for another siege of it to come but it's been over three months now since any showed up so I really think it's gone. You asked me to tell you about our family talks after Bill went to bed. Well, they had to do with some of the things you mentioned when you told me that afternoon that your waiting list was so long and you couldn't promise us an appointment for a long time. I just couldn't bear to wait the way Billy was stuttering so I sat my husband down every night and we took a look at ourselves. It was kind of hard at first but it got interesting after we broke the ice. Every night we would

5 From A. T. Murphy and R. M. Fitzsimons, *Stuttering and Personality Dynamics.* Copyright © 1960, The Ronald Press Company, New York.

ask ourselves ten questions. Here they
are:

1. Are we irritated or sore at each other
   or with Billy? How and why?

2. Are we talking too complicated, too
   much, too fast or too long so he thinks
   he has to talk like that too?

3. Are we putting the pressure on him to
   talk, asking him too many questions,
   wanting him to tell us too much?
   Lord, we were always doing this, we
   found. Over and over again in spite of
   good intentions.

4. Were we breaking up his speech by interrupting, nodding our heads before
   he's finished, not paying attention,
   leaving him to do something else while
   he was talking? There was plenty of
   this that we had to stop.

5. Were we making sure he knew we
   loved him, that he was awfully important to us? I guess we hadn't done
   enough along this line.

6. Had we been criticizing him too much,
   punishing him too much or making
   him feel he wasn't good enough? Every
   day we found some of this at first.

7. Did we let him blow off steam enough,
   get mad, or even be a baby? We found
   we'd been bottling up that poor kid
   more than we knew.

8. Had we cut out the excitement or anyway cut it down? We discovered that
   unplugging the TV helped and there
   were plenty of other ways to get a
   calmer house.

9. Had we been expecting too much of
   the kid? We had, every day, almost
   every hour.

10. Could the boy see that we were upset
    when he stuttered? This was the hard-
    est of all to change but we changed it.

These were the questions we asked ourselves every night and I think this was the
most important thing we did. Oh, I guess
we also began to talk more slowly and
quietly ourselves. I know I didn't talk as
much or as fast and that was hard to
change too. And we started listening, like

you told us, to his good speech. At first
there wasn't too much of it but it kept
growing and soon that's all there was.
Funny thing, too, we're all a lot calmer
and happier. Anyway he's stopped so you
can take his name off your waiting list.
(pp. 110–11)

Child psychotherapy

There are always a few cases of beginning stuttering in which the disorder seems to be the outward manifestation of a rather deep seated emotional conflict. These are the children
we have described as showing the
Track IV kind of onset and development (Van Riper, 1971, pp. 114–16).
These children begin to stutter very
suddenly or dramatically and usually
in a situation of great emotional
stress. The stuttering behaviors are
usually stereotyped and symbolic of
the conflict and often they emerge
from mutism. They are usually highly aware of their difficulty in talking
immediately. These are the children
for whom psychotherapy is required.

Play therapy. Psychotherapy for
children necessitates a different approach than that used with adults for
many reasons. The child often has little motivation for seeking treatment;
he does not have the verbal facility
to introspect or to report his feelings.
Basically dependent upon his parents,
he has little sense of choice or responsibility for his behavior. It is often
difficult for the therapist to achieve
the usual parental kind of transference relationship which makes so
much difference in the healing of an
older person. Symbolic interpretations
have little effect; and finally, the
child's main interests revolve about
exploration and play.

Accordingly, the child psychotherapist usually begins by attempting to
create a strong rapport and close sup-

porting relationship so that the child will like and respect him. The therapist accomplishes this by engaging in the child's activities and play, supporting him, being useful, and above all behaving toward him in an accepting and nonpunitive manner. When such a relationship is to be established, materials are provided (clay, doll family figures, paints or crayons, etc.) that can provide for some expression of the child's emotional feelings and the conflicts which the therapist may then identify and try to resolve. In this psychotherapeutic play the child is usually encouraged to talk about what he is doing. Various roles are assumed by both the therapist and child in the games and play, especially those which offer an opportunity for acting out the basic conflicts. In these, the therapist often serves as a parent or sibling surrogate.

Some therapists confine themselves to providing opportunities for completely free and permissive play, using the information thereby gained to modify the parents' inappropriate behaviors. Other workers structure the play very carefully so that it will be conducive to the resolution of apparent conflicts. Some therapists comment and question; others are content to participate and observe.[6] Although the cathartic expression and release provided by therapeutic play clearly relieves some of the child's inhibited tension and anxiety, it appears that the rewarding relationship with an accepting parent figure is of greater importance. We usually find also that once a child feels secure in his new relationship with us, he tends to regress to earlier infantile levels, babbling, sucking, and smearing, some-

times to test us or perhaps so that he can begin over again the long climb up the precarious ladder to emotional maturity. Brunner (1936) provides a case report of this regression:

A two-year-old boy was cured of his stuttering by the following method. Apparently his condition was caused by regression, since during his suckling period he had been seriously ill and now had a poor appetite. It was arranged to allow him to return to this previous level by supplying him with candy suckers. After a few days this return was so complete that he had discarded his previously acquired habits of cleanliness but had ceased stuttering. Three months later he had acquired bladder and bowel control again, his appetite had improved, and his speech control had become perfect. (p. 362)

Stein (1949) recommends that this rhythmic sucking, laughing and babbling be encouraged even in adult patients. Plätzer (1954) says "In treating child stutterers, it is valuable to begin by having them make the characteristic movements and sounds of animals like the fox, frog and dog, first the simpler animals, then the monkeys, and first singly and then in family situations. This frees them from tensions in talking." One of our students visited a clinic in Hamm, Germany, where young stutterers and other children with mutism or delayed speech spent hours each day as monkeys in a contrived jungle environment. They swung from tree limbs, scratched themselves, made faces, were fed bananas, and were forbidden to speak except in cries and "monkey talk." The results were reportedly excellent.

As these accounts from various sources have shown, play therapy seems to be a fairly common method-

[6] For an excellent review of a variety of therapeutic approaches with children, see the reference by Haney (1971).

ology for the treatment of beginning stuttering.[7] In Japan, play therapy with the child is generally accompanied by parental counseling. Thus Tamai, Dendo, Kobayashi, and Umegaki (1962) concentrate their counseling on the mothers who were said to be well-to-do, overprotective, interfering, and overdemanding but they also utilize individual play therapy with the child as well. Takeuchi and his coworkers (1962) used a play therapy modelled after Axline's (1948) approach. One unusual variant is that reported by Gondairo (1964) who assembled a group of infant stutterers and gave them play therapy together.

Play therapy works better when a suitable playroom and materials are provided. The former should be a gay, colorful place, with one way mirrors

[7] Since the references on play therapy are scattered, we append this bibliography of works that we have found especially useful: Alschuler, R. H. and L. Hattwick, *Painting and Personality: Study of Young Children*. Chicago: University of Chicago Press, 1947. Arlow, J. and A. Kadie, Fingerpainting in the psychotherapy of children, *American Journal of Orthopsychiatry*, 16 (1946), 134–46. Axline, V. M., *Play Therapy*. Boston: Houghton Mifflin, 1947. Brammer, L. M. and E. L. Shostrom, *Therapeutic Psychology*. Englewood Cliffs, N.J.: Prentice-Hall, 1960. Bender, L. and A. C. Woltmann, The use of puppet shows as a psychotherapeutic method for behavior problems in children, *American Journal of Orthopsychiatry*, 6 (1936). Levy, D. M., Release therapy in young children, *American Journal of Orthopsychiatry*, 9 (1939), 383–90. Mann, L., Persuasive doll play, a technique of directive psychotherapy for use with children, *Journal of Clinical Psychology*, 13 (1957), 14–19. Moustakas, C. E., *Children in Play Therapy*. New York: McGraw-Hill, 1953. Murphy, A. T. and R. Fitzsimons, *Stuttering and Personality Dynamics*. New York: Ronald Press, 1960. Pollaczek, P. P. and H. D. Homefield, The uses of masks as an adjunct to role playing, *Mental Hygiene*, 38 (1954), 299–304. Shaw, R., *Finger Painting*. Boston: Little, Brown, 1934.

to permit observation by parents if the need for this arises. Cupboards out of reach of the children should contain a variety of toys, masks, doll figures of parents and siblings, nursing bottles, crayons and paper, toy toilets, stuffed monkeys, alligators, dragons or monster-figures, rubber mallets, finger paints, modeling clay, sand, and water. Some therapists use a playhouse already fitted but we prefer to create our own. We like to have a sandbox available in the room. Some therapists (Axline) insist upon free choice of materials and free play. Others (Levy, 1939) prefer to control the play materials and so do we.

The basic principles underlying play therapy are well known and we see no need to describe them in detail here. Instead we provide some excerpts that will illustrate the sort of activities and dynamics involved. The first account is a transcript of a bit of play therapy from the first session with Joel, a four-year-old with numerous repetitions of initial sounds and syllables accompanied at times by head banging.

Joel: I'm tired. I'm going to sleep in my house (crawling under a table, curling up and closing his eyes).
Therapist: You're so tired and you're going to sleep in your house.
J: (Snoring . . . pause. . . .)
J: (Snoring some more) I'm snoring.
T: Uh huh.
J: (Getting up and going to the nursing bottle) Jay-Jay has these. Jay-Jay is my little baby.
T: Jay-Jay is your baby and he has bottles like these.
J: Me-baby Joel (sucking on bottle).
T: You feel like a baby.
J: (Taking the bottle and going under the table, stretching out under the table, sucking on the bottle) Me, baby Joel.
T: You're baby Joel.
J: (Spending approximately ten minutes under the table, stretching out under

the table, sucking and chewing on the bottle) Me, baby Joel.

T: You chew on it just like a baby.

J: (Chewing vigorously) I chew hard.[8]

We must understand what happens in this therapeutic play. Essentially the child assumes the roles and performs the activities that enable him to handle his anxieties and solve the problems he encounters in being a small pigmy in a land of powerful giants. Wolpe (1957) has a fine passage:

In his play he relives over and over again his anxieties, for through the replaying of such anxiety scenes does he tend to diminish the intensity of his anxiety. His play is not the mere projection of fantasy. It is, along with this, the child's attempt at objectifying his anxiety, of releasing his hostility in safe areas, namely, on play objects or pretend characters, of identifying with authoritarian figures, and finally of setting his limits in terms of reality-testing. It becomes evident, then, that what might appear humorous to the adult may be a very threatening situation for the child, and the therapist's participation in the play must therefore be in accordance with the child's seriousness and direction. (p. 998)

Our next account comes from a very illuminating article by Harle (1946) in which she describes sequentially her psychotherapy with Patty, a three-and-a-half-year-old stutterer. The stuttering had started suddenly after a spanking and the girl had numerous other emotional problems:

A great deal of Patty's activity at the clinic centered around her toilet interests as shown in her messing play with paint and water, and in toilet rituals. At first

8 From A. T. Murphy and F. H. Fitzsimons, *Stuttering and Personality Dynamics.* Copyright © 1960, The Ronald Press Company, New York, p. 248.

there was a great deal of inhibition; on several occasions she refrained from touching the paints, saying that Mommy had told her she must not paint. When this happened she was restless and frustrated. She would say, "I wish I can't paint," meaning apparently "I wish I didn't want to paint." On one of these occasions she wet herself. As time went on, however, she became free to engage in the messing. She would slop the water and paint around, put thick blobs of paint on the paper or table and rub it around with her hands, smear it thickly on her arms and legs, and jump up and down with glee in a puddle of water. It was obvious that she derived intense sexual pleasure from these activities. She was absorbed, dreamy, and blissful as she caressed and patted the globs of paint, delighted as she splashed. She cooed with pleasure as she smeared it on her legs, murmuring "It feels good—it feels cold." It was obvious that this type of play also served as an expression of defiance against her mother. On several occasions she had insisted on wearing her best dress, volunteering to mother that she was not going to paint today. Then, at the clinic, she would go about almost systematically getting the dress messed up, remarking as she did so that Mommy thought she wasn't going to paint.

Associated with this messing play were activities around going to the toilet. At first she was secretive and timid. If anyone were in the bathroom she would come out and wait until they had gone, complaining "they 'sturb me." As her messing play became freer, so did her toilet activities. She began openly to show her pleasure in her bowel movement, and would leave it on display. She became more and more exhibitionistic about it, shouting "Peek-a-boo Fanny!" as she took down her pants, and "Ping! Ping! Ping!" as the feces dropped into the bowl. She agreed enthusiastically that it felt "good." She would play an exhibitionistic game as she sat on the toilet behind the swing door, "Can you see my foot?" "Can you see my pants?" "Can you see my underpants?" "Can you see my hand?" Not until after 23 hours of play consisting al-

most exclusively of activities around messing and the toilet, was Patty able to abandon it. About this time the mother reported that Patty was no longer consti-
pated. (p. 159)

Expressions of hostility are commonly encountered during play therapy
with young stutterers perhaps because
they vaguely feel the frustration of
their interrupted communication but
also perhaps because they feel some
need to express their resentment
against the irritation and rejection
shown by many parents when a young
child stutters too frequently. The following is a fragment of a recorded
play session with one of our own
cases:

B: Don't close door!
T: You don't want me to close the
door. All right.
B: What this here?
T: House.
B: What in here? (Points to toy cab-
inet.)
T: Chimney.
B: Why?
T: So smoke come out.
B: Why?
T: Smoke from fire go out there.
B: Yeah. What this here?
T: Bedroom.
B: What this? (Picks up mother doll.)
T: That mommy doll.
B: Why?
T: Just is.
B: Why?
T: You like to have me tell you things,
don't you.
B: No!
T: (Silent but accepting.)
B: Hey. Sizzo. See I cut finger (cuts
fingernails).
T: Uh-huh.
B: I cut dolly hair.
T: You want to cut the dolly's hair.
B: (Does so. Looks at therapist close-
ly.) See. I cut her.
T: You like to cut her.
B: Yeah. I cut you now.

In all of these exchanges we find the
child giving expression to feelings that
had been troubling him, feelings that
usually had no other outlet except
in situations where their acting out
had been punished. For these special
stutterers whose difficulties seem to reflect real emotional conflicts, such a
psychotherapeutic approach seems desirable. With the warm, permissive acceptance and understanding of the
therapist, his unacceptable feelings
find outlet other than in stuttering.
Interpersonal conflicts are worked
through and the child, in this special
environment, finds no need to inhibit
his utterance of the unspeakable. He
does what he wants to do and he says
what he wants to say. In his play he
not only recreates many of the stresses
that formerly disrupted his life and
his speech but he also masters them.
As he talks to the doll figures or answers the puppets, as he explains glee-
fully why he scribbled all over the
snapshot of his father, as he smashes
the playhouse or smears himself with
clay, the child loses much of his hesitancies and stuttering. Speech becomes
free when such a child becomes free.
Nevertheless, we wish to repeat again
that only a few of our young stutterers seem to need this kind of therapy.
For those that do, it should be available.

Our own treatment of the beginning stutterer

In this section we describe how we
work with a child who has not been
stuttering very long. It will be obvious
that we are not content with indirect
methods. While we seek, as others do,
to create an environment that is conducive to fluency by working with
the significant persons in the child's
life space, we also work directly with

the child himself. This is not to say that we work directly with his stuttering however. We always try and manage to keep that stuttering from becoming a stimulus or the source of struggle or avoidance. We do not want to start the vicious spiral to swirling. Many clinicians are so fearful that this might occur that they refuse to accept their professional duty to do many things that can facilitate fluency and minimize the stuttering. Like Pontius Pilate washing his hands, they content themselves with giving some superficial advice to the parents and thereby absolve themselves of unwanted responsibility. If the child grows worse, the parents have all the blame, and if he gets better, the therapist can claim the credit.

The basic program

Although we recognize the reality of these clinicians' fears, we do not feel they justify a hands-off policy. It is quite possible to interact with a young stutterer without calling attention to his stuttering or punishing it. Indeed the therapist may be the only person in the child's life space who can relate to him in this way. That child may need very badly, if only as an antidote, such a conversational partner when his parents or playmates continue to be anxious or rejecting. A skilled clinician can create a relationship which is so supportive that it will counteract many evil influences. By exploiting this relationship he can perform at least seven important functions:

1. He can make the child's speaking pleasant again;
2. He can stimulate the child with models of fluency that are within the child's reach, models which, when imitated, will increase the child's own fluency;
3. He can provide activities that integrate and facilitate the smooth flow of utterance;
4. He can program schedules of rewards and reinforcements for fluency that will enhance it;
5. He can desensitize the child to those stimulus conditions which tend to disrupt his fluency;
6. He can countercondition other anxiety inhibiting responses to the same fluency disruptors;
7. He can prevent the moments of stuttering from acquiring the stimulus value which so often leads to avoidance and struggle.

Surely, with all these opportunities to ameliorate the problem, it seems unwise to delegate all the responsibility to the parents. Therapists are trained to do these things; parents are not. We must remember also that many children overcome their initial stuttering despite adverse conditions. Indeed, it has been our experience that most of these children need only a little help to begin to speak normally. It is as though they have been so overburdened they cannot talk smoothly. Repeatedly we have been surprised to find how small a portion of that burden need be removed to give them fluency. We feel that the clinician's fear that he will harm the child is unrealistic. The child needs help; we should not ignore his silent cry. Besides, as the research has shown, four out of five beginning stutterers overcome their disfluency without professional help. Where else are the chances of doing successful therapy so favorable?

Making speech pleasant

Although most children, when they begin to stutter, seem quite unaware of their repetitions and prolongations we have frequently observed those little signs of generalized frustration that reflect the felt interference with communication. After a bout of stuttering these children often become irritable; they tend to act out and fling out. It is almost as though they have dimly sensed the interruptions without really recognizing their loci or nature. Some beginning stutterers then reduce their speech output; others respond by rapid compulsive talking. It is almost as though the keys on their speech typewriters or pianos stick irritatingly. A vague restlessness appears in their other motor behavior. They get "nervous;" they fidget. This unpleasant coloring of speech must somehow be reduced and speaking must become fun again. Parents will have to do most of this making speech pleasant but often the therapist must show them how by working directly with the child.

Our own approach as we will demonstrate in the case of Johnny (pages 402–4 has usually involved the use of free and directed play since young children are already experts in this activity. Each clinician, of course, has his own style, his own set of gambits for creating an initial relationship with a child. We have developed several of these approaches from which we choose the one that seems most appropriate to the child we are seeing perhaps for the first time. With an outgoing, highly verbal, active child we stress exploration of the clinic environment as our opening move. If the child on the contrary appears more passive and perhaps fearful, we may begin by using finger painting or showing him some of the pictures and clay figures that other children have created for us, then make it possible for him to draw or mold some of his own. Shaw (1934), Laczkowska (1965), and many others have demonstrated how helpful such art therapy can be in creating a favorable relationship and in facilitating the release of hidden emotions. Another approach uses commentary on projective drawings. The Travis Story Pictures, as described by Travis and Sutherland (1971), provide an excellent vehicle for establishing rapport and eliciting speech under emotion. For some children, the role of "helper" provides the only relationship in which the child can feel secure. By busying ourselves and casually requesting some help that he can give easily. ("Now, where did I put my pencil? Oh, thanks. Now let's see, I've got to plug this in. Mind helping me? Put it over there. Yeah, Thanks.")

One of our own favorite approaches with the shy child is through the use of two boxes of toys, one for the child and one for the clinician. Sitting on the floor, we open our boxes and take out the toys. In this play we usually program our interaction so that it progresses in an oscillating fashion through a series of stages. First the clinician—and the child—concentrate primarily on *solo play,* each concerned with his own activities. Next, the clinician occasionally makes contact with the child or his activities. He arranges the situation so that his toys occasionally touch or bump one of the child's playthings or invade some of his playing space. We have termed this *tangential* play. At this stage there is an intermittent sharing and intersecting of activities, momentary bits of cooperation, which gradually increase in frequency and duration depending upon the child's tolerance. Finally, we achieve a cooperative play relationship.

The progression from solo through tangential to cooperative play is seldom linear. As we have said, it oscillates because the clinician must always be alert to the child's acceptance or rejection of his contacts. Thus the clinician immediately returns to an earlier stage whenever the child shows signs of rejecting the relationship. With such a design in mind, we have rarely found it difficult to achieve the necessary interaction. Of course all children do not need so careful an approach, some being able to play cooperatively from the first, but the clinician is always alert to the possibility that he must return to a lower level of interaction when resistance is shown. We have enjoyed this sort of therapy. It's good to learn to play again.

Since our basic therapeutic aim is to make utterance pleasant rather than painful or frustrating, the skilled therapist gradually introduces speech into these progressive play activities. At first he plays silently, then accompanies his activities with vocalization, noises, grunts, interjections, then makes one word commentaries on what he is doing, perceiving, or feeling. Then he changes to short phrases or sentences. As the relationship shifts from solo to contact to intersecting and finally to unison activities, the amount of vocalization and verbalization also increases and changes in character and complexity. Once the clinician and child can play cooperatively, it is not too difficult to make speech itself the vehicle of play. And this is of course our target if we seek to make speech pleasant.

If the child does not become too excited by the make-believe, the playing of different roles also seems to create more fluency. Geraldine Siks (1958), in her book on Creative Dramatics makes the same observation: "A child is at ease when he's playing and seldom stutters or gets a 'block' while his mind is entirely off himself (p. 278)." We have often used fantasy with certain children most effectively in creating basal levels of fluency. Never-never lands can be invented where all is well and no evils

exist except The Long-Nosed Hoo whom we together can always outwit for he's outrageously stupid. Tries to talk out of his nose while holding his nose. Or we act out the tale of how to teach the little frog who had never learned to jump, or the little fish who woke up one morning and had forgotten how to swim. Any therapist with a touch of whimsy and some remnants of his own childhood can use such fantasy to make speech pleasant and create real fluency.

With very young children who show very marked disfluency we cannot use these little dramas of spontaneous fantasy but instead we return to more basic forms of play utterances such as animal or machine noises. The stuttering child will usually respond to the therapist's modeling of these by using them in his own play. When the child does so, the therapist can then join him, adding variety as the mutual imitation proceeds. We then move to babbling and baby talk, parrot talk, echoing each other, or using magical incantations to open jumping-jack boxes and doors. We put our own nonsense into a paper bag and listen to it and tell each other what we've heard. We put on masks and talk "Scamboolian," that lovely, nutty, nonsense language, accompanied by the gestures that carry the message. It is impossible here to list the hundreds of ways in which the clinician manages to give to utterance the sheer pleasure which all very young children know—and which perhaps they have forgotten. It is fun to make noises with the mouth; it is fun to talk; we must make it fun again.

Case report

As we have mentioned several times, there are some children who begin to stutter very suddenly and very hard from the first, the disorder usually arising in an intense conflict situation and characterized by silent fixations and an apparent inability to get started. When this occurs, the therapist must do everything he can to overcome the swiftly generating fears and to give the child the experience of speaking without struggling. We now present an account of how we helped such a child.

Johnny's stuttering began, according to his mother, after a traumatic incident at the age of six. The family lived on a farm in a house on a hill above a pond. The father had cautioned Johnny and his younger brother *not* to go near the pond or that they'd "get it good" from him. One afternoon Johnny appeared wet and breathless and the mother gave him the devil as soon as she saw him and his father spanked him hard while he was breathlessly trying to explain that he had just pulled his brother out of the water of the pond and that he thought the latter was dead.

The parents reported that after the scolding and speaking, Johnny had suddenly become almost mute. He would "open his mouth but nothing would come out." His first grade teacher reported the same phenomena in the classroom though she had heard the boy saying some sentences fluently on the playground. She said he seemed to be afraid to talk in class though before this time he had been very verbal and "a happy outgoing sort of child."

When I saw him, two months after the reported onset, Johnny was talking a little but his "stuttering" showed the following features. Whenever he began to speak, he would open his mouth wide with an accompanying tremor of the jaw and he seemed unable to produce vocalization or airflow. Then he would suddenly interrupt this silent laryngeal fixation by an inspiratory gasp. Often he would have to make four or five of these abortive attempts before he could begin to speak. Once he had begun, however, he could continue very fluently until some

pause occurred whereupon the same silent fixation and gasping appeared again. The behavior was very consistent in its patterning—a gasping, sobbing kind of utterance always manifested after a pause. Johnny at times also showed some speaking on the end of the breath as though reluctant to have to stop and reexperience the trauma of having to begin again. He was a very shy child and I found it very difficult to get him to talk to me during that first exploratory interview.

Accordingly, I felt my first task was to achieve a relationship which would involve little verbal communication. This I managed by assuming a role as his adult playmate—a rather silent one. We each had boxes of interesting toys. I played with mine; he played with his. First we played solo; then occasionally tangentially; then intersectingly; and finally cooperatively. I also worked out a progression in my own utterance: first silence; then a whispered noise or interjection; then a soft noise, then a meaningless tune, then a whispered word, then phrase; then a soft but vocalized word, then a simple sentence. All of these were merely self-talk, not communication. I asked him nothing; I did not speak to him. We just played imaginatively with our toys. Finally we began to play cooperatively though at first silently. Finally he began to talk to me but always with the same gasping attack on the first word of everything he said. Finally after we had reached the cooperative play stage we began to play with sounds and real speech.

I chose the following generalization gradient for the first utterances: whispering, singing, speaking. I also arranged it so that his utterance would come only as an ending to mine, with first words being whispered or sung or spoken first by me and with Johnny chiming in only at the end. The first utterances of this sort were "Open Sesame!" speech, magical speech. I had various toys such as Jack-in-boxes with secret releases which only I could set off. The things we whispered, or sung, or said were the magical incantations that made the Jack-in-the-box pop out. For example, I might whisper at first: "Jacky-Jacky, here you *jump*." It took two of us to *whisper* that last word before the box would pop open. Even despite this care, Johnny at first still gasped a little (but very little) as he joined me on "jump." I was not concerned because I knew something about conditioning, and so we did it again and again, and pretty soon, the gasping response on this whispered word was extinguished. Then Johnny was shown that he had to join me in whispering not just the last word but on the whole phrase: "here you jump." Again the gasping reappeared at first but soon extinguished. Finally, he could say the whole sentence in a whisper, first with me, and then alone without the gasping.

We then moved up the gradient from whispering to *singing*, using a toy cannon that shot a cork, one that was also operated by a hidden switch. Again he joined me on the final word of our sung incantation, then in speaking other words and finally, after repeatedly wearing out the gasping on each new modification, he was able to sing other songs not only in unison but alone. This series went much faster. Spontaneous recovery often reoccurred at the beginning of a new session but a few returns to earlier types of successful utterance soon took care of this. It was at this point that Johnny's mother reported that he was beginning to sing to himself and also to her and that she had noticed that no gasping occurred several times when he spoke to her in an offhand manner. I felt he was then ready to be desensitized to vocalized speech.

For this stage, I used a puppet with large lips and mouth which could be manipulated by my hand, or Johnny's hand, when it was inserted into the puppet's neck. I told Johnny that only the puppet could give the magical incantations—and he needed our help. So first we whispered, to the puppet, then sang, then began to speak first softly, then more loudly, then finally when shouting. As before, we began backwards, Johnny joining in on only the last words. Soon he was able to operate the puppet so it could rage or complain or express its fears—and his.

About this time I set up a model for a new way of talking: "Say it three times." This game was a "Boss me" game, deal-ing with demands. I had to carry out the demands made first by the puppet and then by Johnny alone (one day when the puppet was conveniently lost) but only after he had said or sung or whispered the command three times. I used this to reduce the time pressure and to desensitize him to the initiation of utterance on the first word. Again, a few gaspings occurred but soon they were gone. Then we played "Say it twice" and finally "Say it once." As I remember, we were able to extinguish all gasping speech in these demands in only two play sessions. At this time, his mother reported, and so did his teacher, that Johnny was talking much more at home and at school and that he was only gasping occasionally. Most of these gaspings seemed to occur mainly when he had to answer questions so I asked them to stop any questioning of the boy at home and school until I could work on that. I didn't want any intermittent reinforcement to bring back the strength of that gasping. I think they cooperated pretty well because soon Johnny was talking to me fairly often though I did not at first encourage this, nor did I talk much to him.

Instead I began to make comments on what I was doing, perceiving, or feeling. This self-talk commentary was at first whispered and then spoken softly, then normally. Then, since Johnny began to do some self-talk too, and with a marked decrease in gasping, I turned to parallel talking. I verbalized what the boy was doing, perceiving or feeling. Then Johnny first used the puppet to tell what I was doing, and then told me himself without the puppet. When an occasional gasping occurred, we went back to an earlier kind of speech until it was gone. Then I tackled the questioning, following the same procedure. Once more there was some occasional gasping. It was slower to extinguish but finally did.

I also felt that we must extinguish the gasping response to a listener's angry face since it had been part of the original traumatic situation. As part of our play, I drew angry faces on the blackboard and he erased them; then he drew them and I changed them to smiling faces; then he did too. Then we made faces in the mirror and Johnny, first through the puppet, then by himself, gave me commands about how to change my angry countenance. At times he would whisper these commands and directions even though I had not asked him to do so. But soon he was even shouting at me. Then I would say unpleasant things as I made my angry faces first toward the puppet, and finally to Johnny. I taught the puppet to tell me what he thought of my angry and unreasonable behavior then handed the puppet over to the boy. He loved this game but I had to handle it pretty carefully at first because it could make him gasp. I also used some masks, one of a woman, and after some interaction I scolded Johnny pretty hard for not doing some unreasonable thing I'd demanded (I think it was a command to climb up the wall.) This generated some emotion in him but there was no gasping, and I felt pretty triumphant. After a few sessions of this sort of thing it was apparent that Johnny's gasping was about gone. He was speaking well at home and at school and speaking a lot. His mother said, "He's a happy little boy again, always talking or singing." I began to space our play sessions further apart and to have his mother join our play. I began to consider dismissal.

As I reviewed the situation and therapy, I recalled that we had done nothing much to cope with another feature of the original traumatic situation: trying to speak when he had been running and was out of breath. So we did some whispering, singing, and talking after running upstairs in the clinic. One weak bit of gasping occurred, then it disappeared. I also had the puppet do a lot of bad things and had Johnny spank him as I held it. I made the puppet laugh the harder it was spanked. We also took turns beating up Bozo the Clown, a large life-sized inflated toy who, in my disguised voice, kept protesting that we were unfair and bad and dirty mean people, that he was a good boy, and why were we hitting him. Johnny loved that game.

Johnny never "stuttered" again until he was a sophomore in high school when he had a recurrence. The same type of silent blocks and gasping behavior occurred. This stuttering began suddenly when he was swimming in the YMCA pool and had failed to get out when the swimming instructor ordered him to do so. (He hadn't heard him.) The teacher gave him a good scolding and a "slight swat" for disobeying and he sternly demanded an explanation. So I worked with him in the pool, desensitized him, and in three days the stuttering disappeared and has not returned in twenty years. Perhaps we are wrong, but it is our impression that all this labor was not wasted. Perhaps Johnny's "stuttering" might have disappeared by itself. We do not think so. The behaviors were very strong. We are always concerned when the disorder begins in this sudden way for we have seen other similar cases who ended up as being very severe stutterers, very resistant to therapy.

Creating suitable fluency models

We have previously said that when the young child is presented with speech models that are too difficult for him to match, he tends to become hesitant. Accordingly we always try, in our interaction with the young stuttering child, to use a natural but very simplified form of speech. Thus in his play with the child the therapist begins first to use single words, then phrases, then short simple sentences as he comments on what he himself is doing or perceiving or feeling. Natural tempos are used but the speech is greatly simplified. The therapist does not speak in the long chains of complex sentences which characterize the child's ordinary speech partners. Instead, he speaks in short phrases or sentences with plenty of pauses and silence. As the play shifts from solo through contact to intersecting play, the therapist also shifts from self-talk to parallel talking and then to communicative interchanges. In parallel talking the therapist verbalizes what the child may be thinking or feeling and always he makes his commentary very simply and without hurry, using the child's language whenever he can. As the play becomes cooperative, unison or echo speech can be employed. Incantations can be uttered in unison. Puppets can be made to repeat what has been said to them, but again they should be made to speak very simply. We need to bombard the child's ears with simple phrases and shorter sentences, all unhurried and fluently spoken.[9]

Eventually a relationship develops which permits normal communicative interaction. The therapist and child then talk back and forth, making statements, asking and answering questions, and here again the therapist is careful to provide simple models of fluency that are easily within the child's reach. Bombarded by this sort of talking, the child responds in much the same way, and when he does his fluency improves remarkably. Through observing us in these sessions the parents also soon come to recognize the necessity for such simplified models. If, as Wendell Johnson claimed, stuttering begins in the parent's ear, then we might also say that fluency begins in the ear of the

child. We must not overload any system on the verge of oscillation. Let us provide simple models for him to imitate if we desire fluency rather than gluency.

Integrating and facilitating fluency

One of the most important of the many observations we can make about the beginning stutterer is that the motor sequencing of his speech seems to be highly vulnerable to disruption. This is so obvious that its implications for therapy are often overlooked. There are things we can do that seem to be able to stabilize his motor control system, and to render it less susceptible to momentary breakdown.

Under enough stress, any complicated sequence of motor movements tends to lose its integrity and speech is no exception. Indeed it is probably more sensitive to stress than most motor skills. The prosody of certain individuals is like steel; of others like cast iron; and of still others like clay tile. The fragility differs. Impacts that are easily resisted by some children can be devastating to others. Doubtless there are many reasons for this state of affairs but certainly it would seem wise to strengthen the stability of the motor sequencing systems of the young stutterer if it can be done.

Use of rhythmic timers

There is ample evidence in the literature that the fracturing of the flow of speech as represented by stuttering can be dramatically decreased by various techniques and as we have seen earlier, one of these is that which employs rhythmic timing. The very severe adult stutterer seems to be able to speak with remarkable fluency when he taps his finger or swings his arm to time the utterance of a syllable

---

[9] Froeschels (1952) recommends Liebmann's method of having the child imitate the therapist or parent as they speak simply but drawlingly:

The child is told stories from picture books three to five times a day for ten minutes each time, about three times weekly by the therapist, the other times by a person in charge of the child. The vowels should be pronounced drawlingly and the child should be asked to repeat phrases in the same way. (If a whole phrase cannot be remembered by the child, a phrase should be offered to him in parts.) Conversations should be performed also with drawled vowels. (p. 218)

or word with the accompanying movement. He can speak in unison with another speaker if he follows the other's lead. He sings with little difficulty. He can echo or shadow another person's speech with incredible ease if he does so automatically. He can do simultaneous talking and writing with little interruption if he uses the dominant stroke of the first letter of the word as a signal. It almost seems as though his own timing mechanism is faulty, that he needs an accessory timer, a model which he can use as a pacer.

Various explanations for this marked decrease in stuttering exist though we have not found any to be entirely satisfactory. It is possible that the timing movement increases the energy in the approach gradient of an approach-avoidance conflict. Or perhaps the effect is due merely to the distraction, the attention being shifted from his morbid perception of approaching difficulty. Yet even the young stuttering child who shows no signs of avoidance or fear seems to become much more fluent when such techniques are used. It may be that gross movements integrate the finer ones, or that the timing device serves as an accessory prime-mover, a bit of behavior which organizes the whole sequence of muscular contractions that comprises a syllable or word, as the pianist's nod integrates the whole sequence of flying fingers. There are many more such explanations but the important thing to remember here is that these techniques do facilitate fluency and reduce stuttering.

As we have said earlier, we have not found rhythmic timers to possess any major utility in the treatment of the confirmed secondary stutterer who has learned complex avoidance and struggle behaviors. But in the child whose speech is characterized by sim-

ple syllabic repetitions or phonemic prolongations and who shows no sign of fear and awareness, we have found these timing methods very valuable. They seem to show the child that he need not stumble, that he can speak smoothly. The same techniques, which in the adult yield only a temporary remission from stuttering and which show little transfer effect to old traumatic situations, can often result in complete and permanent freedom from stuttering in the child. To use an inexact analogy, these timers seem to serve similarly to the electronic-pacer stimulators used with heart patients to reintegrate and to stabilize a circulatory mechanism that has become dysrhythmic. Some of these young stuttering children seem to have lost the feel of smooth ongoing utterance. They have begun to speak a broken English, almost a stuttering language, one which, when rewarded by communicative consummation, even comes to feel natural to the beginning stutterers. But we must remember that they have not been speaking this way very long. Often all these children need to regain their former fluency (and most of them have had this fluency before they began to stutter) is some vivid experiences in speaking smoothly. We see no reason why we should not help them have them, providing that these timing methods are experienced not as direct therapy for the stuttering but merely as another interesting form of speech play, another game. Having been victimized by many charlatans and quacks who used these methods on us in our youth, we found it hard at first to employ them with beginning stutterers and only our very successful experience permits us to recommend them now.

We will describe only a few of these timing techniques. Perhaps the most common one is that which consists of tapping the finger or hand or foot, or even using body sway as the timer. The clinician in his speech play sets the model by saying each syllable of his utterance simultaneously with the accompanying movement. At first the syllables are regularly spaced but later on the timing movement can approximate the temporal intervals of normal speech. Also at first, intonation and accent are minimized, the person speaking in a monopitch or chanting fashion, but as facility is acquired the normal melodic patterns take over. Similarly, a progression can be created wherein, at first, the accompanying movement *times* the syllable, then later the word, still later the phrase and finally the sentence. Always the clinician shares in the play, the basic initial approach being that of do-it-together or follow-the-leader. When we have used these procedures with young stutterers we make sure that we do not confine ourselves to a single timer but to a wide variety of them. We are not trying to teach these young stutterers a new and admittedly artificial way of talking. We do not ask them to talk this way except in their speech play with us. Our aim is simply to give them repeated experiences in integrated, smooth-flowing speech so they can know what it feels like. We have not found that these children continue to speak this way in other situations; we have found only that they speak more fluently.

Other methods for facilitating fluency. Another group of techniques seems to owe its effectiveness to the integrating effect of other motor activities which themselves are highly integrated. If a child, for example, plays Indian and talks while rhythmically clapping his hand against his mouth, few repetitions or prolonga-

tions will occur. If he has learned to skip around the room, he will stutter very little when skipping continuously and speaking simultaneously as he does. The same holds true when speaking while strongly chewing as Froeschels discovered long ago. Thus we may play a game wherein the clinician (or in turn the child) uncovers his ears and listens only when he sees his partner chewing grossly, and covers them up again when he does not. There are many other such activities which can be used in speech play.

Often an increase in sensory feedback other than the auditory one seems to increase the child's fluency. Using Halloween masks with a large mouth hole, the therapist and child can "watch their mouths moving" in a mirror while speaking first in unison or echoing and then just talking. This activity seems to yield much smoother speech. We have also had stuttering children speak into a microphone and then watch the pilot light of the tape recorder flicker syllabically, or had them talk through a tube held near a candle to see it sway with the pulses of airflow. By holding a magnifying glass in front of the mouth and, in a mirror watching their gigantic lips and tongue and jaw move, the children always slow down and speak freely and enjoy the experience greatly. They also find speaking with an electrolarynx, first in pantomime, then in whisper, then while singing and then while speaking, to be most intriguing and we have never had a child stutter while doing so. Again, by having the child rest his chin on his hand and with his elbow on a table, the movements of the jaw are experienced very vividly and the child speaks more slowly and very fluently. We have also used various kinds of masking noise but most children seem to have a low tolerance for pure tone or white noise though the masking helps them speak fluently.[10] Instead, we have them do trumpet or horn talk, or speak while blowing a harmonica, or play "Guess what I'm telling you to do" while turning on the noise generator themselves. Tape loops of loud laughter seem to be the best masking noise but we have also used infant babbling and animal or machine noises for this purpose.

Another variety of speech play which seems to contribute to the same goal is that which stresses the rehearsal of the prosodic patterns of planned utterance. Couched in the form of "Guess what I'm going to say" play, the clinician and then the child hum the prospective sentence without articulating it while the partner tries to guess what is being hummed. We prefer to use commands for this. Thus: "mmm mm mm mmmmm" complete with inflections and emphases but merely intoned may represent the child's command to "Sit on the floor!" At times the clinician can guess what is meant by the child's other behavior but if not, he asks for more clues, and the child says "Sit mm mm mmmm!" And so on. We have many variations. In one of them, the command is spoken silently into a paper bag. The therapist then puts his ear at the opening and tries to guess what was in the bag. "You'll have to say it a bit louder. I can't hear it yet." The child puts the louder speech in the bag, and with

each rehearsal the prosody becomes more stabilized. We have also recorded commands on tape and played them back to the child very faintly at first, then gradually more loudly until he guesses what is said. The temporal patterning of speech seems to be perceived long before the actual message. Certainly when the child does finally say it, he says it fluently.

This emphasis upon integrated prosody can also be accomplished by games in which the child and therapist tap out all the syllables or words of a sentence before saying it in unison and then alone. Thus "We're going to eat a peanut now" would require seven or eight taps and the temporal patterning of the taps can be controlled by the clinician to ensure its naturalness. Omitting the taps, and after the therapist whispers the words of the prospective utterance, both child and his partner can say it in unison, then alone, before carrying out the act. We have also used a wide-mouthed puppet, manipulating its jaw to represent the motor planning before speaking. We also play puppet ourselves, the child manipulating our mouth for each word *he* speaks. If the child stands behind the therapist but watches the therapist's mouth in the mirror as he moves it in time to the words spoken by the child, the illusion of the therapist as a puppet is enhanced. We have never had a child put stuttering into our silent but moving mouth in such a game. The feel of integrated utterances can also be facilitated by many different games involving echoing, shadowing or unison speech. Often we introduce these by using strange voice qualities, different pitches or even odd changes in loudness on certain words, and then imitate each other. Children love this imitative talking and do it very easily.

---

10 Neimark (1968), the Russian therapist who recommends the use of "muffling" (masking with a tone of 100 Hz.) for adult stutterers, writes, "The use of muffling is not advisable in early childhood in view of the necessity for the natural training of speech habits and because of the possibility of an unfavorable effect upon the child's auditory apparatus which is still in an unstable state (p. 335)."

Reinforcing fluency. As we have indicated, taking advantage of the days when the stuttering child is very fluent to evoke much more speech, or decreasing communicative opportunities when the child is showing more stuttering than usual have often been enough to eliminate the disorder in a surprisingly large number of the beginning stutterers with whom we have worked. But in the interaction between the therapist and the child there arise many other opportunities for reinforcing the occasional fluency which all these children show upon occasion. Most important of the reinforcers is the therapist's attitude. By intermittently and casually showing more attention and appreciation of the child's fluent communication but only ordinary acceptance of his stuttering speech, we have been able to get marked gains in fluency by this simple procedure and without the child's conscious awareness of the contingency.

We also use the child's pleasure in controlling an adult as a reinforcer. Playing the game called "Boss me!" wherein the child gives commands which the therapist obeys, it is possible to program resistance and obedience to the commands so that the latter is contingent upon the child's fluency. This must be introduced gradually and carefully so that the child's stuttering gets no stimulus value. Children are usually more fluent in mand speech than they are, for example, in responding to questions. If the clinician will play the role of slave to the child as master, opening the window, falling down, standing up, putting his feet in the wastebasket, barking like a dog, but doing so promptly only when the child has given the command fluently, a powerful reinforcement is brought into play. If stutter-

ing occurs, the therapist occasionally lags or resists or appears distracted.

We have also used escape rewards, taking turns being in jail (a chalked circle on the playroom floor), having to stay in a pretended bed, wanting to leave the dinner table, being untied, etc. In each of these role situations we beg to be released and our captor asks "Why?" and we have to tell him. Whatever the child says when he is in turn confined, if he says it fluently, brings immediate release but not if stuttering occurs. He still gets released but he may have to beg harder and longer and give more reasons until one of them is fluent.

We also use other reinforcers such as food or surprises. A favorite game of all our stuttering children has been "Say the Magic Word." In this the child tells what he is seeing out of the window or in a picture book or telling what happened at home or in school and if he happens to say the magic word, a gong is rung, a jack in the box pops up, and he is told where to find the previously hidden jelly bean. Needless to say, the therapist has no specific magic word in mind. He gives the reward only after the child has been unusually fluent and then selects one of the words as the magical one. We also have an empty black reward box and have learned to palm a salted peanut into it to reward fluency, though the child seldom is aware of the contingency. All he knows is that when the therapist says, "I'll bet there's another peanut in that empty box now. Let's open it and see." There always is, and there is nothing satiating about a single salted peanut. Theorists might object that the child should know why he gets the peanut. We suspect that he may have a dim awareness that his fluency is what brings the reward but, if wisely programmed, we get the increased fluency without such conscious awareness.

Counterconditioning

In our interaction with children whose repetitive but pronounced stuttering did not seem to be accompanied by awareness, avoidance or struggle, we have been impressed by the similarity of the fluency disruptors in different children. The same communicative features appear as antecedents to stuttering time after time. Moreover, the reports of parents, when we routinely request them to assess the communicative stresses that seem to precipitate given moments of stuttering, also indicate that these parents find the same ones that we do. Their children stutter more frequently when answering questions or responding to peremptory demands for speech, or when hurrying their verbalizations because of time pressure. Disapproving or rejecting responses from their listeners evoke more disfluency. These children experience more trouble when they are interrupting or being interrupted. They stutter more when trying to get the attention of a listener as they begin their utterance and also when they sense listener loss during it. More complex formulations seem to generate more stuttering than simpler ones. The greater the uncertainty in encoding the more the disfluency. There are more prosodic breaks in speech offerings that express the negative emotional states. Not all young stuttering children show all these vulnerabilities, and some of them have others uniquely theirs, but all of them will show some of those we have mentioned.

We have two major ways of coping with such disturbing influences. We use the desensitization procedures outlined in our next session and we take steps to establish other competing responses to the same cues. These beginning stutterers, as we have mentioned, seem to have more difficulty in replying to questions than in making assertions. Questions are essentially demands for speech responses; they involve time pressure; they insist upon precedence over those other activities which the child may at the moment be engaged in performing. He may, for example, be much more interested in filling a bottle with sand than answering the question "Where's your little brother?" If questions have repeatedly led to faltering speech, the interrogatory inflection itself seems to serve as a cue to speech disruption. Somehow, we must change this situation.

We have found that by associating a pleasant integrated response to questions, the child becomes less vulnerable to their disrupting influence. In our speech play, for example, we have often found the following procedure to be effective. We have a little box containing a handful of peanuts, each individually wrapped in gaily colored paper. Playing the game "You can't catch me!" we demonstrate that either of us can have a peanut if the other person asks a question. But the rule of the game is that we must surrender the peanut if we begin to answer the question before chewing and swallowing it. By engaging in some interesting exploratory activity, and making sure that the child wins more than he loses, and that he often can make us surrender our own peanuts, the question as such becomes less disruptive, not only in our own interaction but in communication with others. This is but a single illustration of many similar activities that may be incorporated into speech play to reduce the strength of communicative stressers.

Similarly, in another "Can't catch me" game we train the child to respond to interruptions by rewarding him with a toy (or a poker chip token which he can later use to buy any one of a tray full of trinkets or toys) whenever he finishes his sentence after the interruption but finishing it slowly, not rapidly. In this, we also encourage the child to interrupt us and, when either we fail to finish our utterance, or finish it too rapidly, he wins the game and gets the reward. Again we make sure that he wins more than he loses.

We also condition verbal responses to various kinds of communicative stress. We reward the child whenever he responds to listener loss by saying "You aren't listening to me" or "Please, can I finish?" If the clinician will observe the child closely, he will discover that most children have already found certain verbal strategies for handling listener loss or the threat of it. By rewarding, perhaps only by the therapist's immediate attention, those which appear most successful, i.e., are integrated and effective, the child can be made less vulnerable to listener loss. For example, one of the children with whom we worked hard and long and who usually stuttered whenever we even looked away or showed any lack of attention occasionally would say, "What I mean is . . ." and then speak fluently. By reinforcing this response with immediate attention, and failing to respond to his increases in rate, pitch, and loudness or stuttering after listener loss, we soon had the child using the phrase very consistently and when he did, his stuttering was greatly reduced.

Attention-gaining devices (gambits)

can be taught in the same fashion and quite without the child's ever being aware of what has occurred. If the child stutters severely on the opening words of his utterance, we give him our attention only after some delay, but give it immediately if, by chance, he happens to say some signalling phrase such as "You know what?" or even "Umm" or "Say." All of us use gambits preparatory to utterance. Many of these are postural or patterned movements.[11] But some gambits are also verbal. By discriminating those which the child uses most successfully (i.e., with the least stuttering) and rewarding them with our immediate attention, their frequency can be made to increase remarkably. Since much stuttering occurs on the first words of the child's utterance, the successful use of such gambits brings immediate gains in fluency.

Communicative stress may also be felt by the child when his utterance is loaded with anxiety, guilt or hostility or when it carries messages which the listener might reject. We try to teach him that this sort of verbalization need not always 'be followed by punishment. To get him to express these feelings, we use unison speech, or echoing, or any of the other previously mentioned ways that have proved to be especially successful in promoting fluency. From his observation of the child, or from what the child or the parents have told him, statements are prepared by the clinician which reflect the disturbing feelings. These then are spoken, chanted or sung in unison, echoed, put into the mouths of puppets, uttered in Indian or animal talk, and so

11 For example, the author knows when his wife is going to say something to him in bed: she always wiggles her toes first.

on. Often after the therapist has demonstrated that he can say these things, the child will take over enthusiastically and lead the therapist in a surprising number of vivid emotional expressions. One of our child stutterers got behind us, put his arms around our neck and his hands over our mouth, then insisted that I say the following: "I'm bad . . . I'm a bad boy . . . My daddy don't like me . . . I spank my daddy . . . I kill him good . . . And my mommy and me. . . ." That was all but it was obviously a very pleasant experience for him and he was completely fluent for the remainder of the session!

Another child, a very fearful little boy with much stuttering and faltering speech, became very relaxed and fluent after daily sessions of harmonica talk. In this play, he echoed the things, which we said for him, by talking through the harmonica as he sounded it. Here is a brief excerpt from one of our recordings of such a session:

When I was a little boy . . . I used to be scared . . . I used to be scared to go to bed . . . and strange things . . . and monsters . . . and big boogie men . . . who might get me . . . but now I'm getting bigger . . . and I scare them . . . and I make noises like this (big howling) . . . and I'm big and bigger . . . big as a house. (In each of the gaps, we both inserted harmonica laughter and we remember this session especially because he insisted on ending that game by leading me in the following:) I'm a big man . . . and nice . . . and I like Tommy . . . and Tommy likes you.

We have also used "Talking in the Sleep" games in which we and the child, while relaxed and speaking very slowly and dreamily, express these feelings.

Desensitization

Although we always seek, through counseling the parents and associates of a young stuttering child, to reduce the communicative pressures that play so large a part in the precipitation of stuttering, and to make them less disrupting through counterconditioning, we strongly feel that it is necessary to toughen the child to their impact. Children are not hothouse plants existing in a controlled environment. Try as we will to reduce the environmental pressures and stresses, some will remain. Moreover, we have seen instances in which parents drastically changed the home atmosphere so that it suddenly had very little communicative stress only to find that the child became increasingly vulnerable to lesser amounts of that stress, amounts that formerly he could withstand. Drastic changes in communicative relationships often do more harm than good. When a child's world suddenly changes—even for the better —uncertainty increases. Accordingly it is often necessary to apply desensitization procedures designed to make the child more able to resist communicative stresses of all kinds.

These procedures of course are brought into play only after the child and therapist have achieved a warm friendly relationship and they can talk together easily. The therapist by this time knows how to create conditions so that the child can be temporarily fluent for at least a few minutes of continuous speech. This we call the *basal fluency level*. When this fluency has been achieved, the therapist then deliberately but gradually introduces increasing amounts of a specific fluency disruptor that previous observation has shown to be especially productive of stuttering. If, for example, the child is especially vulnerable to interruptions, the therapist will gradually begin to interrupt him, first only occasionally, then more frequently. Or he may at first interrupt the child almost at the conclusion of his utterance, then gradually insert it further forward. Whatever the fluency disruptor being employed, it is necessary that the dosage be increased gradually, and that it be terminated if possible just before it triggers some stuttering. A skilled clinician will soon discover the behavioral signs which indicate that this threshold is being approached. Though these threshold signals differ with each child, usually we note that when they occur, his fluency begins to become less freeflowing, more gaps appear, inflections decrease or the words may come in spurts even though no stuttering has yet appeared. Another child may show that he is approaching the stuttering threshold by becoming fidgety and restless; obvious tension may appear in his postures or movements. The alert therapist soon comes to recognize that when these signs appear it is time to cease his deliberate insertion of the communicative stress and return immediately to the basal fluency level. Then, after some further minutes of easy fluency, the disturbing influence is again applied and gradually increased until once again the threshold is approached. Then once again the basal fluency level is reinstated and the desensitization session is terminated.

It must be understood that at first the therapist will not alway be able to program the increasing amounts of the stress appropriately enough to be able always to keep below the stuttering threshold. Occasionally some stuttering will result. If it does, there is no great tragedy involved. The child has merely demonstrated one more

moment of stuttering and this certainly is much less, proportionally, than he usually shows. At this stage of the disorder's development the child has little or no awareness of its occurrence so there is no harm done. The therapist has merely learned a bit more about the child's tolerance of a particular sort of communicative stress and he will be more skillful in the future in measuring out his dosages.

We find, however, that many therapists are very reluctant to do desensitization therapy. They cannot bear to take the chance of *deliberately* precipitating a single moment of stuttering—as though one more such instance really mattered. Many, as Wingate (1971) has so eloquently shown, are secretly afraid of working with stutterers because they fear they may make the disorder worse. They fail to understand that most stutterers are pretty tough, that they have lived with communicative frustration for a long time. The fact that these stuttering children have probably had the disorder for many months or even years without even becoming much aware of it should reassure the therapist that exceeding the threshold a few times does not mean catastrophe. It's a part of the therapist's diagnostic process. He must test the stress tolerance to know the child's limits. He should also increase that tolerance.

What is most important is that this sort of desensitization is very effective. One often finds dramatic changes in the child's speech, not only in the therapy situation but at home, at play or in school after a series of desensitization sessions. We have often had parents say to us, "I don't know what you did today but he is speaking much better." The child doesn't know, either, so far as we can tell. As the desensitization sessions continue, the effects seem to summate—the child seems to be able to handle more and more of the stress before the signs of threshold appear. Basal fluency levels are also easier to achieve. In an early session we may be able to use only one or two desensitization sequences or "pushes;" in a later one we can use several more. Moreover, we can even combine fluency disruptors in applying the stress, i.e., interrupting with a question and showing impatience at the same time. One can almost see the perceptual calluses developing.

Many of our colleagues and students who have observed us doing this sort of desensitization have been surprised to find that the basic warm relationship between the therapist and child is not jeopardized in the least by such procedures. We do not find it strange. All of us experience stresses in our relationships with significant others. It's part of living. The important factor is how we resist those stresses. The art of the therapist lies in helping his client to adapt appropriately to communicative stress. This kind of desensitization is a technique and an art that can be learned.

Preventing stuttering from becoming a stimulus

Another major aim of therapy with young children who stutter is to keep the stuttering response from becoming a stimulus. We want to prevent the vicious spiral that so often characterizes the development of the disorder. We don't want the child to learn avoidance and struggle reactions. We have enough clinical evidence indicating that if we can keep the child from reacting to his moments of disfluency with frustration or anxiety, stuttering tends to disappear. Conversely, we know that when the child learns to react to his stuttering with frustra-

tion or fear, and their consequences, avoidance or struggle, the disorder tends to increase in frequency and severity. Among the major responsibilities of the clinician is that he must do all he can to prevent the child's stuttering from being its own maintaining cause.

We have studied the development of awareness of stuttering in many children. Initially this awareness is intermittent. On occasion, the child's eyes will widen when he stutters or he may stop talking for an instant. There may be a quick intake or holding of breath or he may even tell us "I can't say it!" However he usually continues, more interested in his listener's comprehension of his message than in its fluency characteristics. It is as though at first the awareness is vague, faint, and transitory. There is no real color of concern. As a stimulus, beginning stuttering usually possesses low intensity. It is easily forgotten or disregarded.

There seem to be several ways in which stuttering does become a noxious stimulus. In one of these, even when the child's listeners do not respond unfavorably or show any concern, the frustrating experience of interruptions in the flow of his speech may bring the behavior to his attention. Summation may also occur for, even if forgotten, several repeated moments of subliminal awareness may finally result in a moment of vivid recognition. As an observer we have repeatedly been impressed by the high barriers to awareness which most beginning stutterers possess. We have seen children repeat a syllable as many as eighteen times without ever showing any signs that they knew they had done so. It is the total communication which holds their attention. When they do become aware of the interruption to the forward flow of speech, beginning stutterers seldom recognize it in process; the recognition seems instead to come afterward. It is after the stuttered word has finally been spoken that they stop, or show signs that something strange has happened to them. In the developmental diagnosis, the therapist should always scrutinize the temporal loci of this recognition. When a child shows it *during* the repetitions or prolongations, we sense more danger than when it appears only after the word has been spoken. The therapist should also know that as the frequency and consistency of these recognitions increase, the probability of frustration and fear reactions also becomes greater. Another factor to be evaluated is the vividness of the awareness and the intensity of the reaction. If a child responds to a moment of stuttering by weeping or refusing to talk for some time or, for example, by shouting or spitting at his listener, such an experience is likely to be remembered longer and to have a greater effect than simple pausing or faltering.

When the growing awareness of stuttering seems to be attributable primarily to the sheer frequency of its occurrence or to its interference with the consummation of communication, there are several steps which can be taken immediately to reduce the danger of further development. One of the most obvious of these is to lessen the amount of talking the child needs to do. As we have said earlier, bed rest for several days was prescribed long ago by Bleumel (1940) and more recently by some of the Russian therapists along with medication to make the child drowsy enough to tolerate the isolation. An excellent general account of the Russian use of sleep therapy can be found in the English translation of Andreev's book, *Sleep Therapy in the Neuroses* (1960) and the application of sleep therapy to stuttering therapy is thoroughly reviewed by Pavlova-Zahalcova (1962). We find this approach being used very widely in Bulgaria and Russia. The administering of sedatives and tranquilizers at the onset of stuttering has caused some argument. On the one hand we find Luchsinger and Arnold (1965) cautioning us against administering potent drugs to child stutterers, and, on the other, Bibik (1966) reporting that when preschool children were given Benactyzine, four out of five of them became free from stuttering within six weeks. We personally have not used these procedures, feeling that there are better ways.

Without resorting to such measures, parents can simply reduce the child's opportunities to talk when he is showing a marked increase in disfluency. We must remember that beginning stuttering is usually episodic. Periods of pronounced stuttering are followed by relatively long periods of completely fluent speech. As we have mentioned in another context, by increasing the opportunities to speak on the good days or weeks and reducing those opportunities when the child shows a drastic increase in repetitive speech behavior, the possibility that stuttering will become a self-stimulus is minimized.[12] When bad days occur, it is wise for the therapist and the parents to redouble their efforts to achieve basal fluency levels no matter how brief they may be. We have often felt

---

[12] We have also been impressed by the effect of a change of environment at these times. Often a family trip to some other location, a vacation visit to the seashore or to some relative brings a cessation of stuttering especially if the changed relationships reduce the communicative stress. On the other hand, as Fitzsimons (1962) has shown in her *A New Boy on Hillside Street*, there are situations when adjusting to a new environment can be highly traumatic.

we were able to abort some of the evil effects of the volleys of stuttering at these times by seeing the child more often for the sort of fluency facilitation we have described earlier in this chapter. Our task is to prevent awareness, to keep the child from becoming conscious of his stuttering during these times of marked disfluency.

Other young stutterers first become aware of their interruptions in situations where the urgency for communication becomes very great. In these crisis situations the interference and the delay produced by the repetitions can be felt very vividly. Parents and stutterers frequently report instances of this sort and they are also to be found in the literature. Indeed, sooner or later, if the stuttering continues, some such situation can be expected to arise. The dog has been run over by a car and the parents must be told immediately. The barn is afire. He must say goodbye to the father running to catch the bus. Most of these situations involve a great deal of time pressure and emotion. All children experience them at one time or another but when a child finds that his stuttering prevents him from saying what he must say immediately, then stuttering tends to emerge as an unpleasant stimulus.

At such a moment, the parent's role should involve distracting the child's attention from his speech if this is at all possible and reassuring him if it is not. Some of the parents of the stuttering children with whom we have worked have become very skillful in using these distraction techniques. They casually accept or ignore the child's momentary distress and then change the subject or find something else more interesting for him to do. Most mothers have had many earlier experiences in this shifting of the

child's attention and they find this easy to do. If the impact of the traumatic experience persists, however, and the child shows his hurt and bewilderment, parents should pass the matter off by quietly remarking that all of us get tangled up sometimes when we have to talk too fast or can't think what we want to say. We do not, of course, recommend that parents tell the child to slow down or to rehearse his speech. Our aim is to prevent the fixation of the child's momentary awareness of his stuttering, not to prescribe a remedy which he cannot swallow anyway. To help the child accept the presumed normality of the experience, we may even ask selected parents casually to fake a little easy stuttering occasionally and to comment good naturedly on the fact that they had been tangled up in their talking again. Appropriately done, this too can be very reassuring.

Another method for reducing the stimulus value of the early stuttering involves a technique we have called *restimulation.* Following a moment of stuttering to which the child apparently reacts with startle or vivid recognition, *and after the completion of the utterance,* the parents (and the clinician) should calmly reflect what the child was attempting to communicate, by saying the same thing over again. Thus if the child had a long moment of stuttering on the word "candy" in the sentence: "Jimmy took my c-c-c-c-c-candy," and he showed some concern, the listener should respond by saying "You say he took your candy? That wasn't very nice of him, was it? Oh well, we'll get you another piece of candy." By restimulating the child with the same word spoken normally but quite casually, the memory of unpleasantness subsides swiftly. Sometimes, as Wray (1962) has recommended, all the parents should do is to keep the child talking until he has had a substantial period of fluency. To terminate the conversation hastily whenever stuttering appears would not appear wise since it would tend thereby to acquire stimulus value yet many parents seem to follow this policy. Restimulation, distraction, and parental attention to the message rather than the stuttering are more appropriate responses. Children forget swiftly.

Perhaps the quickest way to make a child become aware of his moments of stuttering is to have someone else call it to his attention. No surer way of giving stimulus value to stuttering has ever been invented. Somehow there always seems to be some ignorant but well-meaning person in the child's environment who will comment on it derogatorily, or demand that the child stop stuttering, or that he relax or speak more carefully. Such persons apply the stuttering label with gusto. We must also recognize that other children may mock the child who begins to stutter—often very cruelly. Strangers may even take it upon themselves to correct him on the spot. A brother or sister will tease him about it. A child with a lot of disfluency runs a gauntlet of many clubs and some of the harder blows he tends to remember. If parents are wise, they will do everything possible to protect the stuttering child against such onslaughts. They may have to restrict the child's outside contacts, educate friends and relatives, and create a home environment in which the siblings will have no need to bedevil. At the same time, parents should not feel that catastrophe inevitably descends if certain of these trauma occur. As Glasner (1949) and others have shown, many young stuttering children eventually become fluent despite home policies that admittedly vi-olate all these principles. Nevertheless, our job is to shape the odds in the child's favor so far as we can. Calling attention to the stuttering is not wise in the early stages of the disorder.

Once the parents understand the dynamics of the disorder's development these overt negative reactions to stuttering can apparently be prevented more easily than the covert ones. It is another matter when mothers react to the child's stuttering with ill disguised anxiety or fathers with impatience and disgust. The fawn always knows when the doe stiffens and becomes immobile. Postures and facial expressions can be far more eloquent than words. We have not found that cautions to disguise basic feelings have much effectiveness. Children know how their parents feel. The answer to this problem lies in the counseling process.

Removing other stresses

We must not forget that the child's hesitant speech may reflect stresses other than those directly connected with communication. We have known children to begin stuttering while ill and then to regain fluency when well. We have found separation from a beloved parent or playmate to trigger the disorder. We have even seen a child begin to stutter when his dog was run over by a car and to become fluent again when a new puppy was provided. There are a host of such accounts in the world literature and we shall content ourselves with two from the Japanese. Nishimura (1932) tells of a sudden cessation of stuttering when medication eased an eye disease and Koga (1940) reports the case of a seven-year-old child who developed stuttering and a boil on his tongue at the same time. One week after surgery, the stuttering disappeared. Without belaboring the point further let us remind all therapists that often we can help the child regain fluency by helping him solve problems other than those connected to speech.

Our parent counseling

In our culture, parents of a young stutterer come to the speech therapist with a multitude of concerns and attitudes and it is important that the therapist know what they are if his counseling is to have any effectiveness. Some parents are certain that the stuttering is merely a temporary aberration of development, that the child is sure to outgrow it eventually. Others view it as a bad habit like thumb sucking, to be broken as quickly as possible. When one of the parents or other members of the family possess it, the disorder may be viewed as a family curse to be endured or contained. Some see it as a social disgrace, a future occupational disability or merely as an irritating nuisance to communication. Many parents come to us with a profound sense of guilt, believing that somehow they have caused the child's difficulties and are directly responsible for its continuance. We also find a wide variety of anxiety and hostility reactions of various degrees of intensity. Unless the therapist is able to understand and to cope with these parental attitudes he can hardly hope that his counseling will have any value. Far too often the clinical counseling of parents consists of advice alone. In our experience we have not found that giving them a smug barrage of do's and don'ts changes the child's situation except for the worse. They only make the parents feel more guilty.

Our own clinical strategy calls for a preliminary interview in which we first concentrate on the gathering of information about the child and his family. When the parents insist, as they usually do, on our telling them immediately what the cause and cure of the stuttering may be, we reflect their concerns but tell them that these items must wait until after we have had an opportunity to see and work with the child, and also after they have been able to help us gather more information. We tell them that we are not so much interested in the original causes of the disorder as we are in those that are causing it to persist. We always try to give parents some immediate absolution for any communicative sins of the past. However, we do insist that they help us by observing the child in his daily activities and attempting to ascertain the communicative situations in which he is very fluent or very nonfluent. We ask for a written report to be compiled daily and sent to us before the next conference with them. We give them some information about the nature of communicative stress so that they will know what to look for but we emphasize that we are even more interested in the conditions which seem to result in momentary fluency.

This session is also used to provide basic information about the nature of stuttering and to inform them about the overall course of the treatment. We state that we will desire to work with the child alone at first, then next to have the parent observe us, then we will ask the parent to participate with us in therapy, and finally we hope that the parent will work with the child while we observe. We let them know that after each of the observation and participation sessions there will be an opportunity to discuss what was done and the reasons for doing so.

Most parents respond to this outline of the planning with profound relief. Their guilt and anxiety decrease since someone else is accepting and sharing the responsibility. They also have something specific to do. Accordingly, when the time comes for the discussion of the observation and participation sessions, they are usually both curious and receptive. In some instances, special sessions may be scheduled for intensive counseling if the interpersonal conflicts of the parent are such that this is needed. In this case we usually prefer to use other personnel of our own clinic, or referrals to psychiatrists, psychologists, or social workers since we prefer to focus our own efforts upon the child's problem rather than upon that of his parents. This, of course, is not always possible or even advisable. We have brought many disrupted families together by uniting them in the solution of the child's problem but we view ourselves primarily as speech therapists, not psychotherapists. Our basic task in the parent counseling we do is to diminish the forces that are precipitating stuttering and to increase those that increase the child's fluency. We do what we can with what skills we have and with the opportunities present themselves. For the rest, we generally prefer to use referrals.

The actual counseling interviews with the parents are so structured that their main emphasis is upon seeking to discover the influences in the child's environment that are still maintaining the stuttering, and to explore ways for ameliorating them. We explore and experiment. We suggest new approaches to the many problems which arise in daily living and then discuss their results. Among some of these problems are those which focus on feeding, sleeping, quarreling, sibling rivalry, overstimulation, tickling, separation anxiety, marital and financial worries, exorbitant demands and aspirations, discipline, broken promises, other fears, deprivations, dependency needs, threats and scolding, odious comparisons, teasing, the expression of hostility. It is impossible to give a complete list but these are at least a few of the topics which parents have discussed with us in their search for possible maintaining causes for their child's stuttering.

For some problems there are no solutions; all we can hope to do is to contain them or counteract them. Nevertheless we have been impressed by the frankness and willingness of most parents to make important changes in their way of living when they realize that their stuttering children are being hurt by such stresses. If the therapist focuses upon problem solving and not on guilt, shows no interest in past evils but only on present influences which make communication hesitant, these parents make better homes for their children. Sometimes we have to tell them how other parents have solved similar problems. Occasionally we have to show them other ways of responding. Often we have them join groups of parents of other stutterers or arrange to have a mother of a former stutterer visit their home to tell her story of what she did that helped so much. We do not preach to these parents. We let them discover the do's and don'ts for themselves. We do try to educate them to the realization that stuttering is lawful, not awful, that certain types of communicative stress increase it and so do penalty, frustration, anxiety, guilt, and hostility. We help them understand that whatever makes the child feel strong and loved and respected decreases the tendency to stutter. We demonstrate that his fluency can be increased.

As these parents scrutinize their patterns of living and their relationships and bring to us their discoveries of the precipitants of stuttering it is always important that we be accepting rather than accusatory. Our basic attitude is that of interest. We show our delight when they have pinpointed some new source of communicative stress and try to encourage their attempts to decrease its impact on the child but we often have to help them be realistic about the changes they plan to make. "My husband and I have agreed that we'll *never* argue in front of the children again!" When we hear such statements we try gently to suggest that it might be wiser just to decrease the amount or vehemence of the argument; that it is unwise to drastically and suddenly change a child's environment even for the better. Often parents come with a eureka "I have found it at last!" attitude and once again we try gently to help them see that usually there are several springs that feed the stream of stuttering, not just one. At the same time, of course, we show our appreciation for their discoveries and help them to make the necessary changes. It is difficult to describe the actual process of this counseling. It is a permissive, supportive, helpful relationship. As parental guilt and anxiety decrease, the child feels the change and his speech reflects it with new fluency. What is even more important, a series of these exploratory interviews seems to release parental energies which can be used constructively and positively.

For example, the same mother, who prior to the counseling seemed unable to simplify her own speech or even listen to the child with equanimity, now seems to be able to do it easily. Fathers begin to play with the boy again; they do things together. The daily tempo of living slows down; it becomes more organized. Parents are less demanding, more tolerant—and more consistent in their management. There is more evidence of love and consideration in the home, more sheer friendliness. Parents respond to the child's angry outbursts without immediate and severe retaliation. Standards are less rigid, more relaxed. The child stops stuttering.

In concluding this chapter we wish to state again that when a child can be given treatment soon after the disorder has begun to take hold, the prognosis is excellent. We fear that the sheer bulk of our exposition may have created the impression that the treatment of the beginning stutterer must be complex and time consuming. Actually, it is neither. The child often gains or regains complete fluency with very little therapeutic intervention. Often just removing one disturbing influence among many, or providing some facilitation of fluency, or solving one minor conflict is all that seems to be needed. We ourselves have been very successful with these beginning stutterers, and from all reports, others have been also. If our discussion has seemed unduly elaborate, it is because we felt it necessary to present most of the basic information and tools that a therapist needs to help these children. He will certainly not need to use all these tools with any single child but if he is to employ the few procedures that will be appropriate, he should know what most of them are. If we are ever to rid the human race of this age-old problem, we must not defer therapy until after the disorder has grown cancerous.

Bibliography

ALBRIGHT, A. and G. RAAF, *Stuttering: How Can Parents Help the Child*

Who Stutters. Milwaukee, Wis.: Marquette University, 1954.

ALSCHULER, R. H. and L. HATTWICK, *Painting and Personality: Study of Young Children.* Chicago: University of Chicago Press, 1947.

ANDREEV, B. V., *Sleep Therapy in the Neuroses.* New York: Consultants Bureau, 1960.

ARLOW, J. and A. KADIE, Finger painting in the psychotherapy of children, *American Journal of Orthopsychiatry,* 16 (1946), 134–46.

AXLINE, V. M., *Play Therapy.* Boston: Houghton Mifflin, 1947.

————, Some observations on play therapy, *Journal of Consulting Psychology,* 12 (1948), 209–16.

BAR, A., The shaping of fluency, not the modification of stuttering, *Journal of Communication Disorders,* 4 (1971), 1–8.

BARBARA, D. A., *Stuttering: A Psychodynamic Approach to Its Understanding and Treatment.* New York: Julian, 1954.

————, The classroom teacher's role in stuttering, *Speech Teacher,* 5 (1956), 137–39.

BAURAND, G. and L. STRIGLIONI, Importance du facteur parental dans le symptome begaiement, *Journal Francaise ORL,* 17 (1968), 209–16.

BEEBE, H. A., Auditory memory span for meaningless syllables, *Journal of Speech Disorders,* 9 (1944), 273–76.

BEHNKE, K. E., *Stammering, Its Nature Causes and Treatment.* London: William & Norgate, 1947.

BENDER, L. and A. C. WOLTMAN, The use of puppet shows as a psychotherapeutic method for behavior problems in children, *American Journal of Orthopsychiatry,* 6 (1936), 47–53.

BIBIK, V. A. (Experience with the use of tranquilizers in the treatment of stuttering), *Zhurnal Nevropatologii Psikhiatrie imeni Korsakov,* 60 (1966), 1089–90.

BLACK, M., Speech correction in the U.S.S.R., *Journal of Speech and Hearing Disorders,* 25 (1960), 2–7.

BLANTON, S., The treatment of stuttering, *Proceedings of the American Speech Correction Association,* 6 (1936), 23–31.

BLOODSTEIN, O., *A Handbook on Stuttering for Professional Workers.* Chicago: National Society for Crippled Children and Adults, 1969.

————, Stuttering as an anticipatory struggle reaction, in J. Eisenson (ed.), *Stuttering: A Symposium.* New York: Harper & Row, 1958.

————, Development of stuttering, *Journal of Speech and Hearing Disorders,* 25 (1960), 219–37 and 366–76; 26 (1961), 67–82.

BLUEMEL, C. S., Stammering and inhibition, *Journal of Speech Disorders,* 5 (1940), 305–8.

————, Primary and secondary stammering, *Quarterly Journal of Speech,* 18 (1932), 187–200.

————, *The Riddle of Stuttering.* Danville, Ill.: Interstate, 1957.

————, *Stammering and Allied Disorders.* New York: Macmillan, 1935.

BOOME, E. V., H. M. S. BAINES, and D. G. HARRIS, *Abnormal Speech.* London: Methuen, 1939.

BRAMMER, L. M. and E. L. SHOSTROM, *Therapeutic Psychology.* Englewood Cliffs, N.J.: Prentice-Hall, 1960, pp. 335–40.

BROOK, F., *Stammering and Its Treatment.* London: Pitman, 1957.

BROWN, S. F., Advising parents of early stutterers, *Pediatrics,* 4 (1949), 170–76.

BRUNNER, H., Beeinflussung des stotterns, *Zeitschrift Psychonalyses Padagogie,* 10 (1936), 360–65.

CHERRY, E. C., *On Human Communication.* Cambridge, Mass.: M.I.T. Press, 1957.

CHEVELEVA, N. A. (About Methods of Overcoming Stuttering: A Survey of the Literature), *Spetsial Shkola,* 3 (1967), 9–15.

CLARK, R., The status of speech correction and pathology in the U.S.S.R., *Cameo*, 26 (1959), 40–41.

DAMSTE, P. H., Het ontwikkelingsstotteren enzijn behandeling, *Nederlands Tijdschrift voor Geneeskunde*, 112 (1968), 886–89.

DARLEY, F. L., The relationship of parental attitudes and adjustments to the development of stuttering, in W. Johnson (ed.), *Stuttering in Children and Adults*. Minneapolis: University of Minnesota Press, 1955, pp. 74–152.

DASKALOV, D. D. (Basic principles and methods for the prevention and treatment of stuttering), *Zhurnal Nevropatologii i Psikhiatrii imeni S. S. Korsakova*, 62 (1962), 1047–52.

DUNLAP, K., The stuttering boy, *Journal Abnormal Psychology*, 12 (1917), 44–48.

EISENSON, J. and M. OGILVIE, *Speech Correction in the Schools*. New York: Macmillan, 1957.

ELLIS, A., Rational psychotherapy, *Journal of General Psychology*, 59 (1958), 35–49.

FITZSIMONS, R., *A New Boy on Hillside Street*. New York: Springer Publishing, 1962.

FORCHHAMMER, B. (My stutterers), *Nordisk Tidsskrift for Tale og Stemme*, 24 (1964), 94–99.

FROESCHELS, E., The significance of symptomatology for the understanding of the essence of stuttering, *Folia Phoniatrica*, 4 (1952), 217–30.

GOLDMAN, R. and G. SHAMES, A study of goal-setting behavior of parents of stutterers and parents of nonstutterers, *Journal of Speech and Hearing Disorders*, 29 (1964), 192–94.

GLASNER, P. J., Psychotherapy of the young stutterer, in D. A. Barbara (ed.), *The Psychotherapy of Stuttering*. Springfield, Ill.: Charles C Thomas, 1962, pp. 240–57.

———, Personality characteristics and emotional problems of stutterers under the age of five, *Journal of Speech and Hearing Disorders*, 14 (1949), 135–38.

——— and M. F. DAHL, Stuttering—a prophylactic program for its control, *American Journal of Public Health*, 42 (1952), 1111–15.

GLASNER, P. J. and D. ROSENTHAL, Parental diagnosis of stuttering in young children, *Journal of Speech and Hearing Disorders*, 22 (1957), 288–95.

GLAUBER, I. P., The psychoanalysis of stuttering, in J. Eisenson (ed.), *Stuttering: A Symposium*. New York: Harper & Row, 1958.

GOLDMAN-EISLER, F., Sequential temporal patterns and cognitive processes in speech, *Language and Speech*, 10 (1967), 131–40.

GONDAIRO, T., A case study of a boy with stuttering and physical malformation, *Japanese Journal of Child Psychology*, 1 (1960), 340–50.

——— (Psychotherapy for the infant), *Proceedings of Japanese Psychological Association*, Tokyo, 1964.

GORAJ, J. T., A report of three European speech facilities, *Asha*, 5 (1963), 860–64.

GUTZMAN, H., *Das Stottern: Eine Monographie fur Aerzte, Pedagogen, und Rehorden*. Frankford: Rosenheim, 1898.

HANEY, R., Child Therapy, in L. E. Travis (ed.), *Handbook of Speech Pathology and Audiology*. New York: Appleton-Century-Crofts, 1971, pp. 183–227.

HARLE, M., Dynamic interpretation and treatment of acute stuttering in a young child, *American Journal of Orthopsychiatry*, 15 (1946), 156–62.

HELTMAN, H., The nature of primary stuttering, *The Speech Teacher*, 4 (1955), 39–41.

JENSEN, P. J., Stuttering and iatrogenesis, *Ear, Eye, Nose and Throat Monthly*, 45 (1966), 86–87, 89.

JOHNSON, W., An open letter to the mother of a stuttering child, *Journal of Speech Disorders*, 14 (1949), 3–8.

————, *Toward Understanding Stuttering*. Chicago: National Society for Crippled Children and Adults, 1959.

KATSOVSKAIA, I (The problems of childhood stuttering), in *Third Session of the Institute of Defectology*. Moscow: Academy of Pedagogical Science, 1960, pp. 133–34.

KELHAM, R. and A. McHALE, The application of learning theory to the treatment of stammering, *British Journal of Disorders of Communication*, 1 (1966), 114–18.

KINGDON-WARD, W., *Stammering*. London: Hamilton, 1941.

KINSTLER, D. B., Covert and overt maternal rejection in stuttering, *Journal of Speech and Hearing Disorders*, 26 (1961), 145–55.

KNUDSEN, R., Behandling of talefijl i frankrig, *Nordisk Tidsskrift for Tale og Stemme*, 10 (1948), 48–66.

KOGA, D (A tongue boil and stuttering), *Dental Clinic*, 12 (1940), 610–12.

KOLODNEY, E., Treatment of mothers in groups as a supplement to child psychotherapy, *Mental Hygiene*, 28 (1944), 437–44.

LACZKOWSKA, M., Painting in stuttering children, *De Therapia Vocis et Loquellae*, 1 (1965), 367–69.

LENNON, E. J., *Le Begaiement, Therapeutiques Modernes*. Paris: Doin, 1962.

LEPSOVA, M (A holiday camp for stuttering children), *De Therapia Vocis et Loquellae*, 1 (1965), 479–82.

LEVINA, R. Y., Study and treatment of stammering among children, *Journal Learning Disabilities*, 1 (1968), 24–30.

LEVY, D. M., Release therapy in young children, *American Journal of Orthopsychiatry*, 9 (1939), 387–90.

LUCHSINGER, R. and G. E. ARNOLD, *Voice-Speech-Language*. Belmont, Calif.: Wadsworth, 1965.

MAHL, G., Disturbances and silences in the patient's speech in psychotherapy, *Journal of Abnormal and Social Psychology*, 42 (1957), 3–32.

MANN, L., Persuasive doll play: A technique of directive psychotherapy for use with children, *Journal of Clinical Psychology*, 13 (1957), 14–19.

MARLAND, P. M., Shadowing—a contribution to the treatment of stuttering, *Folia Phoniatrica*, 9 (1957), 242–45.

MONCOUR, J. P., Parental domination in stuttering, *Journal of Speech and Hearing Disorders*, 17 (1952), 155–65.

MORLEY, M. E., *Development and Disorders of Speech in Childhood*. Edinburgh: Livingstone, 1957.

MOUSTAKAS, C. E., *Children in Play Therapy*. New York: McGraw-Hill, 1953.

MURPHY, A. T. (ed.), *Stuttering: Its Prevention*. Memphis: Speech Foundation of America, 1962.

———— and R. M. FITZSIMONS, *Stuttering and Personality Dynamics*. New York: Ronald Press, 1960.

NEIMARK, E. I., The treatment of the stuttering neurosis on the basis of the physiological interpretation of its mechanism, in R. West (ed.), *Russian Translations on Speech and Hearing*. Asha Reports, No. 3 (1968), 332–35.

NIM, P. (Methods and goals in stuttering therapy for children), *Nordisk Tidsskrift for Tale og Stemme*, 25 (1965), 69–72.

NISHIMURA, M. (Stuttering and Eye Disease), *Diagnosis and Treatment*, 19 (1932), 271–72.

ORCHINIK, C. W., On tickling and stuttering, *Psychoanalysis and Psychoanalytic Review*, 45 (1958), 25–29.

PATTERSON, S. A., The stammering child, *Practitioner*, 180 (1958), 428–33.

PAVLOVA-ZAHALCOVA, A. (Complex sleep therapy for stutterers in logopedic rehabilitation), *Proceedings Institute of Defektology*, Prague, 1962.

PETKOV, D. and I. IOSIFOV, Our experience in the treatment of stuttering in a speech rehabilitation colony, *Zhur-*

nal Nevropatologii i Psikhiatrii imeni S. S. Korsakova, 60 (1960), 903–4.

PICHON, É. and S. BOREL-MAISONNEY, *Le Begaiement, Sa Nature et Son Traitment.* Paris: Maisson, 1937.

PLÄTZER, O. (Biodrama, a form of play therapy), *Zeitschrift für Psychotherapie und Medizinische Psychologie,* 5 (1954), 297–304.

POLLACZEK, P. P. and H. D. HOMEFIELD, The use of masks as an adjunct to role playing, *Mental Hygiene,* 38 (1954), 299–304.

PREOBRAJENSKAYA, V. D. (Work with preschool stuttering children), *Experiences in Logopedic Practice.* Moscow: Institute of Defectology, 1953.

RAND, W., M. E. SWEENEY, and E. L. VINCENT, *Growth and Development of the Young Child,* 3rd ed. Philadelphia: Sanders, 1962.

RAU, F. A. (Experience in logopedic work with young stuttering children), *Proceedings Institute of Defectology,* Moscow, 1953.

ROTTER, J. A., A working hypothesis as to the nature and treatment of stuttering, *Journal of Speech Disorders,* 7 (1942), 263–88.

RUMSEY, H. St. J., *Your Stammer and How to Correct It.* London: Muller, 1937.

SANDER, E. K., Counseling parents of stuttering children, *Journal of Speech and Hearing Disorders,* 24 (1959), 262–71.

SCHÖNHÄRL, E. (Age-connected changes in the structural picture of stuttering), *HNO,* 12 (1964), 152–54.

SCHUELL, A., Working with parents of stuttering children, *Journal of Speech Disorders,* 14 (1949), 251–54.

SELIGMAN, J., The personality, attitudes and behavior of parents of children who stutter, *Journal of the Ontario Speech and Hearing Association,* 2 (1966), 35–106.

SHAMES, G. and C. SHERRICK, A discussion of nonfluency and stuttering as operant behavior, *Journal of Speech and Hearing Disorders,* 28 (1963), 3–18.

SHAW, R., *Finger Painting.* Boston: Little, Brown, 1934.

SHEEHAN, J., Conflict theory of stuttering, in J. Eisenson (ed.), *Stuttering: A Symposium.* New York: Harper & Row, 1958.

SIKS, G., *Creative Dramatics: An Art for Children.* New York: Harper & Row, 1958.

SMIRNOVA, A. M. (Pathogenesis, treatment and prophylaxis of stuttering in children of school age), *Sovetsky Nevropathologie,* 3 (1934), 74–94.

SMITH, S. (Pedagogic Treatment of Stuttering), *Nordisk Larebog for Talepedagoger.* Copenhagen: Rosenkilde og Baggers Forlag, 1955.

SOLOMON, M., Incipient stuttering in a preschool child aged two and one half years, *Proceedings American Speech Correction Association,* 3 (1933), 38–44.

SSIKORSKY, I. A., *Über das Stottern.* Berlin: Hirschwald, 1891.

STECHER, S., Speech therapy techniques in germany, *Asha,* 6 (1964), 157–59.

STEIN, L., emotional background of stammering, *British Journal of Medical Psychology,* 22 (1949), 189–93.

TAKEUCHI, M. (An experience in applying psychotherapy to a stuttering child), *Childrens Mentality and Nerves,* 2 (1962), 59–63.

TAMAI, S., T. DENDO, I. KOBAYASHI, and M. UMEGAKI, Studies of stuttering children, *Japanese Journal of Mental Health,* 10 (1962), 72–83.

TOMKINS, E., Stammering and its extirpation, *Pedagogical Seminary,* 23 (1916), 151–74.

TRAVIS, L. E. and L. D. SUTHERLAND, Psychotherapy in public school speech correction, in L. E. Travis (ed.), *Handbook of Speech Pathology and Audiology.* New York: Appleton-Century-Crofts, 1971, pp. 911–49.

VAN RIPER, C., *The Nature of Stuttering.* Englewood Cliffs, N.J.: Prentice-Hall, 1971.

————, *Your Child's Speech Problems.* New York: Harper & Row, 1961.

VLASSOVA, N. A. (Value of the complex method of treatment of stuttering in children), *Folia Phoniatrica,* 16 (1963), 39–43.

————, (Prevention and treatment of stuttering in children in the U.S.S.R.), *Ceskoslovenska Otolaryngologie,* 11 (1962), 30–32.

————, Psychotherapy of child stuttering, in R. B. Winn (ed.), *Psychotherapy in the Soviet Union.* New York: Philosophical Library, 1961, pp. 98–104.

WEUFFEN, M., Untersuchung der wortfindung bei normalsprechen und stotternden kindern und jubendlichen im alter von 8 bis 16 jahren, *Folia Phoniatrica,* 13 (1961), 255–68.

WILLIAMS, D. E., Stuttering therapy for children, in L. E. Travis (ed.), *Handbook of Speech Pathology and Audiology.* New York: Appleton-Century-Crofts, 1971, pp. 1073–93.

————, A point of view about stuttering, *Journal of Speech and Hearing Disorders,* 22 (1957), 390–97.

———— and A. M. ROE, Teachers, parents and stutterers, *Education,* 80 (1960), 471–75.

WINGATE, M. E., the fear of stuttering, *Asha,* 13 (1971), 3–5.

WOLPE, Z. E., Play therapy, psychodrama and parent counseling, in L. E. Travis (ed.), *Handbook of Speech Pathology.* New York: Appleton-Century-Crofts, 1957.

WOOD, K. S., The parent's role in the clinical program, *Journal of Speech and Hearing Disorders,* 13 (1948), 209–10.

WRAY, E. C., Advice on stammering, *Journal of the Australian College of Speech Therapists,* 12 (1962), 22–24.

WULFFERT, N. F. (Recent work in Bulgaria on the treatment of logoneuroses), *Review Soviet Medical Sciences,* 1 (1964), 57–61.

WYATT, G., *Patterns of Therapy with Stuttering Children and Their Mothers.* U.S. Public Health Service, N.I.H., Small Grant No. M-2667, 1959.

————, *Language Learning and Communication Disorders in Children.* New York: Free Press, 1969.

———— and M. HERZAN, Therapy with stuttering children and their mothers, *American Journal of Orthopsychiatry,* 32 (1962), 645–59.

YOUNG, E. H., The motokinesthetic approach to the prevention of speech defects, including stuttering, *Journal of Speech and Hearing Disorders,* 30 (1965), 269–73.

ZALIOUK, D. and A. ZALIOUK, Stuttering: A differential approach in diagnosis and therapy, *De Therapia Vocis et Loquellae,* 1 (1965), 437–41.

Treatment of the Young Confirmed Stutterer

We now consider the clinical problems presented by the child who has begun to interiorize the problem, who calls himself a stutterer and who shows word and situation fears. Such a child may be feeling some shame about his breaks in fluency. He is now responding to the threat of approaching speech difficulty by avoidance and, when he experiences it, with struggling. We have worked with children as young as three years who fulfilled all these criteria but the majority of those who develop this picture of advanced stuttering do so after they enter school. In this discussion, we shall confine ourselves largely to those between the ages of 7 and 14 since youths older than this age can usually be treated in much the same way that we treat adults, while with children younger than 7 years, our therapy is a combination of that used with the beginning stutterer along with other procedures specific to the group we now discuss.

Differences between adult and child therapy

There are many important differences in the clinical problems presented by young confirmed stutterers that contrast with those shown by adults. Our therapy must therefore reflect these differences. First of all, we must remember that the child is brought to therapy; he seldom seeks it. For this and many other reasons, we cannot assume the same amount of motivation that we find in adults. The child, for example, has not suffered as much as has the adult nor for so long a period. He has not known the social and economic handicaps as vividly. Secondly, we cannot expect a young child to be as willing to undergo temporary unpleasantness for future payoff. To children, tomorrow is very far away. They tend to respond in terms of the pleasure or pain of the moment. Thirdly, it is very difficult for children to understand the rationale for treatment or to accept much responsibility for its implementation. We cannot expect them ever to be their own therapists. Since they have often been hurt by those who should have loved them, severe child stutterers are often reluctant to accept an intimate relationship with the therapist, another potentially unreliable or hurtful adult. Finally, because stuttering has become so unpleasant, they do not want to observe it, feel it, talk about it, or modify it.

On the other hand, the disorder is still not fully developed in the child. Its component behaviors have not had as long a history of reinforcement. They are not as fixed. The avoidance and struggle reactions are less complex. Morbidity is lower. Living primarily in the present, past trauma are less important in the design of therapy. The child stutterer forgets his unpleasant experiences more swiftly than the adult who often nurtures them. The child's fears also seem to be more transitory and his malattitudes less severe. The clinician finds that the child's resistances are more open and direct; we do not find the ingenious sabotage which often characterizes the adult stutterer. And perhaps most important of all, the child has not interiorized the stuttering role to the degree manifested by the adult. All these factors are advantageous.

Motivation

Even more than with adults, the establishment of a warm, close relationship with the young stutterer is cru-cial to the success of therapy. Unless this can be achieved, great difficulty will be experienced. No severely stuttering child will do very much to modify his behavior unless it is important to him that he desires to please you. An excellent example of how one therapist achieved such a relationship is found in the case report by Emerick (1968), as the following excerpt may illustrate:

Mark needed to identify with a male figure and I was able to fulfill for him the role of father or big brother This was perhaps the most important aspect of the therapy experience; indeed, solely by this positive bond with the clinician—which developed very rapidly from the first meeting—I feel that his stuttering problem would have been at least partly solved. There were several interesting and rather unique facets involved in Mark's identification with the clinician. The first aspect, and most probably the basis for the rapidity with which the relationship developed, was that we shared a mutual interest in the out-of-doors. We had an instant basis for communication since I am an amateur naturalist, hunter and fisherman. This leads to the second facet. The interests we shared could be enjoyed without verbal communication. Mark seemed to want deeply to just follow someone around, to do things with someone without talking, to just share and relate on a nonverbal level. As a stutterer I well remember the importance of this in my own life. My grandfather, a taciturn old Cousin Jack copper miner from the Upper Peninsula of Michigan, provided an island of silent safety in a frightening verbal world. Although he never would have admitted it and indeed dismissed all modern notions about child rearing as so much bloody balderdash (his language was more colorful), he seemed to sense what a little kid hurt in the mouth needed. We did many timeless and simple things together quietly, but most of all I remember the silent ritual performed each evening behind his cabin in the northwoods. Sitting side by side on a crude bench he had made with his own hands, we watched the sun slowly make its descent behind the trees and wash the pines with fingers of pale gold. He neither tolerated or desired chatter and all others were banished from this evening rite. Perhaps Mark's parents did not understand—at least at first—the silent hikes along the Buffalo River, the quiet fishing trips, but Grandfather would have understood and approved.

Grandfather would have also approved of the third facet of the identification between Mark and myself for he loathed sham or facade. I found that I really liked the kid and enjoyed doing things with him and I think he realized this very soon. We did many extra things together that we both enjoyed: we built models of birds and painted them; I taught Mark how to shoot a bow and arrow; and Mark taught me how to collect and classify insects. Why did I do all this? Perhaps because Mark reminded me so vividly of my own "ghosts of stuttering past," of the bewildered and belligerent second grader that I had been. Interestingly, because of the intense identification and extensive interaction, Mark was forced to drop his defenses. When one is with another person for such prolonged intervals of time, one cannot keep from revealing his real self. Thus, not only were we then able to directly confront the stuttering problem, but also Mark had the vivid experience of acceptance of his real self from another human being.

Specifically, how did I portray the role of father or big brother? Actually it was an evolving role. At first I was good old Dad in a wool shirt, warm and friendly, trustworthy, and smelling of pipe smoke and old leathers, sharing blocks and relating closely by nonverbal means. As Mark's speech improved and he derived satisfaction from this, and as his own father began to take over his heretofore abrogated role, I gradually withdrew and became a somewhat aloof patrician sort of pater, directing behavior by precept but not as intimately involved. (pp. 27–28)

We, too, have done similar things in establishing a close relationship

with our young secondary stutterers for many of them seem starved for such interactions with an adult. Often we have served as a substitute parent, one who shows no anxiety or rejection concerning the stuttering, one who is completely devoted to the child's welfare, one who understands his problems and can help. Therapists should expect a period of testing during which the child may show indifference and negativism or other forms of resistance before he surrenders and accepts them as surrogates but, once he does, half the battle is won. In this testing period, it is absolutely essential that the therapist show immediately, and over and over again, that the stuttering does not bother him. These children will scan you for the slightest signs of impatience or rejection or lack of understanding. The following excerpt from a booklet published by the Speech Foundation of America (1964) illustrates how the therapist revealed his accepting attitudes toward stuttering in the initial interview. It illustrates how the therapist revealed his understanding of stuttering and his lack of rejection: [1]

Hello. I suppose you're wondering what's going to happen today. You know that my job is to help you get rid of your stuttering. But you don't know what kind of person I am except that I'm a stranger and that you often have more trouble talking to a stranger. And you don't know how much I'll make you talk or how much stuttering you'll have. So you're probably a bit scared. You don't have to

[1] This excerpt, like others that follow, was taken from edited transcripts of recordings of the author's actual therapy with an eleven-year-old boy who stuttered severely. Some of these illustrations were previously published in a noncopyrighted pamphlet: *Treatment of the Young Stutterer in the School*. Memphis: Speech Foundation of America, 1964.

be, because today, I'm going to do most of the talking.

You probably noticed that I didn't ask you your name. That's because I know that saying your name is often one of the hardest things there is to do. How did I know that? It's because I've worked with other kids who've stuttered . . . a lot of them. And I've gone into stores and stuttered like this . . . (demonstrates) and like this . . . and like this . . . and many other ways, too. I know how it looked and how it felt. And at first, I was sure scared and embarrassed—especially when I had to do it on the phone or to some stranger. Sometimes my stuttering almost seemed to run away with me and I couldn't stop. So I think you'll find that I can understand how you feel when you stutter. I've learned how to help the stutterer and I want to help you. So let's get started. . . .

The first thing I've got to do is to know *how* you stutter. Let me give you some samples and ask you if you've ever had that kind of stuttering. How about this kind? (Therapist illustrates a very severe and unusual kind of stuttering.) You don't have that kind? Good! How about this kind? . . . Or this? . . . (Therapist gradually shows models of decreasing abnormality and unfamiliarity.) But I bet you've often had some like this, haven't you? (Illustrates.)

Well, I've got a vague idea about how you stutter, but I don't know how it feels, and I've got to know that. So look at this picture and tell me—after you put it down —what's happening in the picture. And if you stutter, fine! I can see what we've got to work with. Go ahead. . . .

You probably noticed that when you stuttered on those two words, that I was stuttering right along with you—but silently. I was trying to understand just what you were doing and trying to know how it felt. I don't think I quite got it but it was something like this. . . . On the word "boy" you pressed your lips together and off on one side . . . like this . . . and then they began to quiver as you forced . . . like this . . . and then you popped your mouth open like this . . . and the word came out. Let us get an-

other one to study. Say "Banana, banana, banana" very swiftly. . . . Ok. Same kind of stuff, eh? I bet you felt as though your lips were glued together. Let me try to see what it must have felt like. . . .

That's enough stuttering for today. Now let me outline for you exactly how we're going to work on this problem together. . . .

Another essential and difficult thing to do in motivating a young secondary stutterer is to help him understand what he should do differently when he fears or experiences stuttering. We cannot state the goals of therapy in abstract language. Instead we must use examples or metaphors based upon the child's own experiences. In the following therapy session we were seeking to help an 11-year-old child realize that his stuttering behaviors were not completely uncontrollable:

Good morning! Today we're going to try to tackle that feeling of yours that when you're stuck, you're helpless. I know it feels like that. I know your lips feel jammed together or your tongue is squeezed shut or your throat seems plugged up. Something seems to be stuck or else it seems to be running away with you. You feel your lips bouncing, almost by themselves—as though some mysterious power was in control of you. . . .

But look! I can do anything you can do. I can glue my lips together and push hard against them like this . . . (demonstrates) . . . just like you do. And I can get them bouncing too like this . . . (demonstrates). Let's watch ourselves in the mirror together as you tell me exactly how you go home from school. When you stutter, I'll do on purpose everything you do when you're feeling helpless. . . . (They carry out the task.) Now let's trade places. I'll tell you how I go home from school, and when I stutter on a word, you imitate me exactly. (Therapist uses a kind of stuttering different from that of the case.) Good! That looked like stuttering, didn't it? But I don't think it had the same feeling as some of your real stuff. It didn't because you knew you were imitating me, that you were doing it on purpose. But you were still doing it. When you stutter, it's *you* who squeezes your lips; it's *you* who makes your lips bounce. There's no one else here except you and me . . . no one else who is pressing your lips or making them bounce. It's you!

Now let's try to get the same idea another way. The other day you had a hard time saying my name. Let's say it over and over now until the stuttering stops and you are saying it all right. . . . Fine! Do it again! . . . No stuttering now, is there? Well, let's put some in. Let's see if you can do exactly what you did when you stuttered but this time, do it on purpose. Squeeze your lips tightly. . . . Press harder. . . . Ok, you did everything you do when you stutter . . . but you say you didn't feel you were stuttering? Why? Because you didn't feel you couldn't help it? But there isn't any mysterious magician making you stutter. It's just that you don't know that you're the one who's doing it. It's your mouth, and only you can make it move. When you stutter, you move it wrongly. . . .

Now let's make your fingers stutter. Press your thumb and forefinger together hard like this . . . (demonstrates). Now press extra hard until they vibrate. Now make them bounce just like your lips do. Now let's do the same thing but also use our lips as well as our fingers as we say "banana" . . . on the *b* sound. Press both your lips and fingers together at the same time. Get them vibrating. . . . Get them bouncing. . . . Good! Now let's do the same thing over again, but this time, when I press this buzzer, you have to stop instantly. . . . Fine! You can stop your lips from pressing or bouncing just as quickly as you can your fingers, can't you? Now, how about reading this sentence? I bet you five cents you'll stutter on that *b* word I've underlined and that you'll press your lips together hard like you did your fingers a moment ago. Well, when you do, and you hear me sound the buzzer, you've got to stop instantly. Stop everything. Here we go! . . . Good! You stopped the lip pressing instantly, didn't you? Why? Why could you? If your stut-

tering is so uncontrollable, how can you stop it so fast?

That's about all for today. But you've got some thinking to do about what happened this morning. It's *you* who are pressing your lips so tightly together . . . and you don't need to do it. You can do it on purpose and you can stop doing it instantly. You're the boss of your mouth. Why do the wrong things?

In the following example we were trying to get the boy to understand that it is unwise to avoid feared words and feared speaking situations. Note that the language is concrete and pictorial, that the point is made through anecdotes that are easily understood by a child:

I suppose you're wondering what we're going to do today. Well, first of all I want to show you those snapshots we took of ourselves last week. Here's the one of me stuttering on the word "banana" and in this other one I'm saying it ok. Look at the difference. And now here are two of you that I took when I held the camera. Here's the stuttering one on banana and here you are saying it all right. Quite a change, isn't there, especially when you didn't stick out your lips and squeeze them shut so tightly?

Now today I'd like to help you understand something awfully important about stuttering. It is this: *the more you run away from it, the worse it gets.* Let me tell you a story about my Aunt Emily. I've never seen anyone so scared of thunder and lightning. When a black cloud came up in the west, she'd start to shake. And then she would make her little nest under the front stairs. She'd take a mattress and put it there, and then she'd get a sheet and put it over her head and when the thunder came, she plugged her ears with her fingers and just lay there moaning with fear. I never saw anyone so scared of lightning. Aunt Emily lived with us then and at first she made me scared too, just to watch her. But then my Dad stepped in. He told me to come out in the rain with him and everytime it thundered, we'd holler as loud as we could . . . and look at the lightning . . . and then we'd come in all wet but we always had a big party, ice cream and everything, and lots of fun. Poor Aunt Emily never had any of it. She just lay there in her nest, shaking with fear. My Dad felt sorry for her but he always said that by running and hiding, she only made her fear worse, that the only way to get over a fear was to go out and look it in the face.

Well, stuttering is like that too. If you are scared to make a telephone call, or to answer the phone, and you let it ring until someone else answers it, you just make your fear bigger and the more you fear, the more you stutter. Say this with me: *"The more I fear, the more I stutter!"* Now let's yell it, so you'll remember that. . . .

Ok. Now there's something else we'd better say too. It's this: *"The more I run away from stuttering, the more stuttering I'll have later on."* Write that out on this card and keep it in your pocket. I'll ask to see it every time we get together. I want you to remember it. It's true. It's better to stutter hard than to say some other word instead of the one you fear. Every time you duck a feared word, you escape *that* stuttering, but you also put ten more stuttered words in your mind that will come out of your mouth later on. It isn't worth it. Remember that!

Look, here's a picture of a hoop snake. See how he's chasing the little boy. That's because the boy started running away. Hoop snakes (they're just imaginary ones, of course) chase anything that runs away. But now look at this other picture. See? Now the boy is chasing the hoop snake . . . and it's running away. Stuttering is just like the hoop snake. If you run from it, it chases you. If you go after it, it runs away! If you run away from stuttering, you just get more afraid of it, and then the fear makes you stutter more.

Now tell me about your favorite TV program and every time I see you running away from stuttering, I'm going to show you the picture of your face stuttering on banana, so you'll remember not to

do it. Or sometimes I'll show you the picture of the little boy chasing the hoop snake, if I see that you're going right into your stutterings without ducking them. You can't be like Aunt Emily all your life. You've got to stop making your fear worse. OK. Let's go! [2]

Identification

With the younger child we do not attempt to get him to identify the component stuttering behaviors with any precision as we do with the adult. Certain gross instrumental acts—such as eye closing, head jerking, pronounced lip protrusion, or gasping—may be brought to his attention as things he should try not to do when he stutters but any detailed analysis is quite beyond his powers. When caught in the throes of his stuttering, the child is mainly consumed by frustration. Immediately afterward, his awareness seems to be chiefly that of relief or, more rarely, embarrassment. Certainly he does not want to remember the unpleasantness he has just experienced. If we ask him what he just did, he will answer, "I don't know." He really doesn't know and doesn't want to know. If you ask him to watch his stuttering in the mirror, he will see only a miserable struggling child.

These observations refer primarily

[2] These transcripts unfortunately were taken under conditions in which only our own voice was being recorded and they may therefore give the erroneous impression that the child was merely a passive listener. This most certainly was not the case for he actively participated. His verbal responses (and ours to them) must therefore be imagined and we are sorry about this. In addition, we wish to state that these excerpts are illustrations, not prescriptions. We present them to show how we talked with one certain eleven-year-old stutterer. We have never said the same things to another one.

to the struggle and escape reactions. With regard to the avoidance, postponement, and sometimes starter reactions, a different situation exists. The child is quite aware of his tricks (many children use this word) for at this stage most of them are still used voluntarily rather than habitually. In the adult, these avoidance responses to the fear of stuttering have become automatized but the child is much closer to their origin and they have not been so highly reinforced or practiced for so many years. Thus we find that when the child substitutes easy for hard words, refuses to begin to talk, uses pauses or "um" or "ahs" to postpone, or employs starter retrials, or words and phrases, he is usually quite conscious of what he is doing. Through differential reinforcement procedures these behaviors can be identified, weakened, and eliminated. One of the best ways we have found for doing this is to have the child and therapist take turns trying to "catch" each other in the use of these behaviors. The interaction then becomes a game and we are able to bypass the unpleasantness which usually accompanies any such confrontation. Also we program rewards into the identifying process so that the child wins more often than he loses in this "catch me" game. The interplay also permits the therapist to share through demonstration the stuttering shown by the child, thus reducing some of its unpleasantness. During the identification period, we do not try to get the child to stop using his tricks. We merely want him to know when he uses them and also to understand that the therapist knows too. Nevertheless, as Wingate (1959) has shown, calling attention to the stuttering in the advanced stutterer seems to reduce its frequency and we have found this to be true

also with young children especially if it is done in a nonpunitive way.

A different situation exists, however when we tackle the escape and struggle behaviors. Most young children just cannot tolerate the confrontation of their facial contortions, jaw jerks, or other forms of struggling. Any attempt to get them to identify or analyze these behaviors will be greeted by profound resistance and defeat. About all we can do is to help the child to differentiate between "hard" and "easy" stuttering and this seems to be sufficient. Again we use the "catch me" game as the vehicle for this identification and discrimination. Even very young children (we have used this procedure successfully with several children who were only three years old) seem to be able to recognize the difference between hard and easy stuttering, not only when the therapist puts some of both into his speech, but also when evaluating their own performances. With older children, it is possible to get them to recognize the features which characterize their "hard" stuttering but only after they have shown themselves able to differentiate between the two forms. Fortunately, we have not found this to provide any major obstacle to treatment. Children respond more globally and less analytically than adults. Though they cannot tell you what they do when they stutter easily or hard, once they realize they have a choice, they learn eventually to choose the easier way.

With somewhat older children, those in adolescence or near it, more precise identification of the component stuttering behaviors is possible. Again, however, we eschew any abstract description but instead we show the person what he did and then give it a name. Cooper (1965) has addressed himself to the same problem in an excellent article from which this quotation is taken:

A method found to be useful both in identification of the behavioral components of stuttering and in structuring therapy for children involves the use of a graphic representation of the stuttering problem on the behavioral level. This graphic representation has been termed the "stuttering apple." The "stuttering apple" is created in the following manner: The therapist suggests to the child that the "core" of his problem is "getting stuck on words," (or another easily understood term or phrase meaning nonfluency). Most children will agree readily that this is the *basic* problem and will agree that their stuttering probably began with simple nonfluency (or in their vocabulary: "I couldn't get a word out"). A small circle is drawn on a paper and "nonfluency," "block," or simply "getting stuck" is written inside the circle.

Next, the therapist encourages the child to note "things I do because I stutter, and things I do when I get stuck." As the child (frequently with suggestions by the therapist) notes such behavior as "I block my eyes when I stutter," "my hand jerks when I get stuck," "I don't answer in class," etc., the therapist draws small circles attached to and surrounding the "core," writing in each circle that behavior which the youngster has noted.

This procedure is continued until the child, with the aid of the therapist, has put in the graphic display all those behaviorisms associated with the moment of stuttering (or block). Frequently, therapist and child may observe more stuttering behaviorisms as therapy progresses and these are added to the graphic display. It is explained that a circle can be drawn around the "core" and all the attached labeled circles, and a stem added to produce the "stuttering apple!" The completed stuttering apple represents the child's stuttering behaviorisms. (p. 76)

We do very little identification of the child's difficult words or sounds and feel it very unwise to do so. Though these young confirmed stutterers do fear certain words, and to a less extent certain sounds, usually it is the positional or "getting started" or semantic cues that determine which words are dreaded rather than the past history of stuttering upon them. The word and phonemic fears these young stutterers possess are often unstable and inconsistent. They vary markedly from day to day and from situation to situation. We therefore find no wisdom in asking the child to fix them in his awareness. We don't want him to become any more "word conscious" or "sound conscious" than he is already.

This is not true, however, for situation fears. We have found that the young confirmed stutterer is able to identify these with ease and that talking about them does not increase their intensity but instead diminishes it. This is probably due to the fact that the child has seldom had anyone else to whom he could freely confide his anxiety and dread. Those with whom he has attempted to verbalize these feelings have usually responded by telling him that there was nothing to fear about speaking to Mrs. Jones, or in giving a book report in class and so on, that such fears were silly and that he should not indulge himself by having them. Many such children consequently have had little opportunity for ventilation; they urgently need the relief. In the person of the therapist the child finds, perhaps for the first time, an adult who will not give false reassurance or disparagement. He has a confidant who can understand and accept these fears and feelings. The author has been privileged to have shared many of these childhood confidences and he knows how intense and real these speech-related anxieties can be.

We have also been able in many instances to help the child test the reality of his fears. When we get him to do so, rarely does the actual misery equal the unpleasantness he anticipated. Even as adults we rarely remember the times when our morbid expectations are *not* corroborated; we only recall those instances that confirm them. By encouraging the child to express his fears of speaking in certain situations and then having him tell us later what actually occurred, much of the chronic worrying begins to disappear. And when the feared speaking does occasionally produce much unpleasantness, at least the child has an opportunity to verbalize his feelings in a safe and healing situation thus preventing the repression and reverberation which only compound the evil. One of the criteria by which we measure the closeness of the relationship to be achieved with the little stutterer is the amount of this confiding he can do with us.

Desensitization

Since the fears, avoidance, and struggle which characterize advanced stuttering stem from its unpleasantness, an unpleasantness which tends constantly to grow stronger, no therapy can hope for success unless it seeks directly to reduce it. The simplest way to achieve this reduction, of course, would be to prevent the occurrence of any stuttering. If there were none, the child would then feel little frustration in communication, and he would not receive the penalties and rejection which create so much of his distress.

Unfortunately this is easier to conceive than to accomplish. We always try to increase the amount of fluency in these children and we want them to

feel it and recognize it when it does occur rather than to focus their attention only on the stuttering. As we have advocated for the beginning stutterer, when we work with younger children with advanced stuttering, we again may occasionally use various forms of timing devices, unison speech and other fluency-increasing techniques so that they can know again some freedom in speaking. By being a warm, permissive listener, we also create the basic conditions which facilitate fluency. By reinforcing the fluent speech when it does occur, we encourage it. But a sizable amount of stuttering will still be shown by these children and somehow we must find other ways to reduce its unpleasantness if we hope to teach them to speak without avoidance and struggling.

One of the most important measures which can be taken is to reduce or eliminate the penalties that the child is currently receiving. By making a careful survey of all the persons with whom the child is in contact, we usually find one or two who are mocking him, teasing him, or responding to his stuttering in ways which are highly unpleasant. A child's life space is fairly restricted and the sources of his hurt feelings can usually be determined.

In the adult, it is the past penalties more than the present ones which contribute most to his perception of stuttering as noxious and many of them cannot even be recalled. In the young child, however, the penalties he receives are more open and obvious. He is called names like "P-p-porky the p-p-pig," or "Stutter-cat" or "Putt-putt." He is admonished to "say it; not spray it" (Williams, 1971). Other children are fascinated by the stutterer's repetitions and contortions and imitate them empathically if not punitively. Besides these, there are other more subtle and covert rejections which the child feels keenly and often attributes to the stuttering. We have found that when we could reduce these penalties, the young confirmed stutterer usually began to stutter more easily and without his avoidance tricks. To illustrate: one boy who was stuttering severely began to show some school phobia, refused to go out to play at recess and often stayed for a half hour or so after school was out, saying he had to do his homework there. We discovered that one of his classmates was making his life miserable by constant mockery and by getting the other children to bedevil the child. The teacher suggested that she should probably give a little talk to her class stating in effect that "all children have some differences, that some are fatter than others, some are a bit more clumsy, that some may stutter a little and so no one should tease anyone else." For obvious reasons we vetoed the suggestion and asked her instead to call the ring leader in after school, to tell him that his teasing was making the stutterer much worse and might cause him to stop talking altogether, and finally to charge him with the responsibility for keeping the other children from teasing the boy. This prescription, together with some daily conferences with the little bully to check up, solved the problem. He liked the new authority and became the stutterer's protector. We have found that most children will discontinue their teasing if they believe that it is doing real harm.

It is also often necessary to give the little stutterer some verbal defenses against this teasing. We have taught them to say, "Ok, if you think it's funny, go ahead and laugh," or, "Yup, I stutter, so what?" or, "Better be careful or you might catch it," or merely to laugh along with the tormentors and leave. Without any such answering response to teasing, the child is completely vulnerable. It does not matter really what he says, but it is very important that he says something. There exists perhaps no better response to teasing than the old rhyme children have used from time immemorial: "Sticks and stones may break my bones, but names will never hurt me!" Most of the efforts made by adults to punish the teaser or mocker only make the matter worse. Out in the jungle of the school yard or playground, the child must cope as best he can and we should try to give him weapons, usually verbal ones. In a few instances we have even taught our little cases how to throw an effective punch to the nose. The best defense against teasing, however, is acceptance rather than aggression or withdrawal. The teasing usually stops when the child fails to respond by fight or flight and seems to disregard it.

It is probably the therapist who helps most to make the stuttering less unpleasant. His support, his interest, his help, coupled with a close and rewarding relationship focused directly on the stuttering behavior, probably does more to relieve the noxiousness of stuttering than anything else that can be done. By talking about the stuttering calmly, by putting it in his own mouth, by manipulating it, by examining it in a context of rewarding warmth, the therapist can erase much of its evil. As the therapist becomes more and more important to the child, the stuttering becomes less and less unpleasant. At the moment of stuttering most children feel terribly vulnerable, helpless, and alone, but not when they have an understanding supportive therapist by their side. Usually, too, the therapy sessions create not only relief from the usual amount of stuttering due to the therapist's skill, but also they inspire hope that the stuttering may diminish. The belief that one will not always stutter forever does much to reduce its momentary unpleasantness and the therapist's presence signals that belief.

Since some of the unpleasantness of stuttering resides in its mystery, we have also found it important to help the child understand something of its nature. This, of course, does not mean that we give lectures on the subject or go into the matter in any depth. We simply tell the child that just as there are some children who find it difficult to learn to ride a bicycle or to draw a picture well or to be a good batter of baseballs, there are some children who have a harder time than most in speaking smoothly. We tell him that he is not the only one who stutters, that there are more than two million people in this country who have the same difficulty, and that most everyone stutters once in a while. We tell him that his main trouble is in finding out how to say certain words smoothly, that sometimes he gets tangled up when trying to do so, but that with our aid he can learn how to unravel those tangles. We help him to understand that when he gets stuck or starts repeating, he can find an easier way of saying the word, and that we will help him learn how to do it. We tell him that most other people don't really understand what stuttering is and so they make a lot of suggestions that don't really help, but that we know what to do and have helped many other children who once stuttered and now are speaking very well. This is the general tenor of the information we provide but we do not feed it to the child all at once. Rather, we wait for the appropriate moments, for the times when he does

express his wonderment or bewilderment. Sooner or later all our young confirmed stutterers have brought up the topic with some comment or question and, when they have done so, our explanation, brief and simple as it may sound, seems to satisfy and reassure them greatly.

We have not found the usual Wolpean methods of systematic desensitization very effective with the young confirmed stutterer, especially those which involve the construction of hierarchies of stimulus situations either imaginary or real. In part this is due perhaps to our inability to create the appropriate hierarchies. Young children just do not have the analytical or verbal capacity to rank such situations in terms of expected difficulty. Also the variability of their stuttering in these situations seldom provides enough clues of importance. Their fears are determined more by the immediate circumstances of the speaking situation, or by their morale of the moment, rather than by the history of past unpleasantness. However, it is possible in the therapy situation to get these children to adapt to listener loss, or interruption, or to time pressure, provided they understand what the therapist is doing and when the activity is structured in game form.

The following excerpt from a therapy session with a ten-year-old boy may illustrate how a therapist tried to get him to be less vulnerable to interruption, a fluency disruptor which exploration had shown would almost always trigger some stuttering:

Hello again. Today we're going to have another battle, and I hope you win more than you lose, but you'll really have to fight me. I've been trying to find out what makes you stutter most often, and I think there are several things that really seem to throw you for a loop: The first is when the person to whom you're talking is always interrupting you, finishing your sentences, saying the stuttered word for you, or not paying attention to what you are saying and then talking about something else. It's hard for any of us to keep talking and not to hesitate when we meet an interruptor like that. They just aren't very polite . . . and the only way to handle them is to beat them at their own game.

See, here's a pile of M & M candies. You like M & Ms? . . . So do I. Well, every time that you can keep on talking . . . or even stuttering . . . *without giving up or hurrying* when I interrupt you, you can have a candy. But every time I interrupt and you stop talking or stutter hard and don't say it again easily, then I'm the one who eats the candy . . . and I'm sure hungry for candy. . . . Ready? Ok. Tell me what we're going to do. . . .

Stutterer: W-w-well, I've got to start t-t-t-t-. . . .

Therapist: (Interrupts) Yes, you've got to start talking about. . . . Ah, I caught you already (eats a candy with relish). Your job is to resist my interrupting you. If you had kept on and had said t-t-t-talking, and had finished what you were going to say, then you would have had the candy instead of me. Let's start over, and this time you beat me!

Stutterer: Well, I, I, I've got to start t-t-talking . . . talking (therapist begins to interrupt, but the boy continues) about something and, and, and if you in-in-terrupt I k-k-keep going on. . . . How's that? I b-b-beat you that time. Gimme the M & M. (Therapist does so, pretends to be disappointed and expresses his hunger, etc.)

Therapist: Tell me about that electric train set of yours you mentioned the other day. What's it like? . . . And remember that I'm going to heckle you and get the candy if I can.

(The rest of the session is spent in building up the stutterer's ability to resist various types of interruption, the sudden question, the finishing of the stuttered word, the finishing of the stutterer's sentence, etc. The therapist makes sure that the stutterer wins more often than he loses and that his ability to resist grows. He redefines the goal as needed. Later in the session, the therapist asks the stutterer to say all stuttered words three times and yet to continue talking without giving up. For this performance, five candies are given. If time permits, the roles are reversed and the therapist stutters while the boy interrupts. Again the boy gets more candies than the therapist.)

Therapist: Well, all the candies are gone. But I'll have some for you next time if you bring me, on a paper, the names of the people who interrupted you without making you give up. You can have three candies for every name.

We have also been able to use humor and assertive behavior as counterconditioners to negative emotionality when trying to get stuttering children to become less sensitive to the core behavior of repetitions and prolongations but we have had little success using relaxation. To ask a squirrelly little boy to relax is to ask a great deal; to hope that he can remain relaxed when stress is administered is to ask the impossible. We have rarely been unable to achieve a deep enough relaxation in most of our young secondary stutterers to make any progress. By having a few of them assume a "lazy man" role and creating some fantasy, we have procured some semblance of the relaxed state but usually it has been too transitory to serve as a counterconditioner. Perhaps the greatest utility of desensitization techniques is found in the same use we made of it with beginning stutterers, i.e., to create a basal level of fluency and then gradually to introduce fluency disruptors. This sort of desensitization does create fluent speech under stress and shows some real transfer.

Reducing frustration

Since much of the struggle behavior shown by these transitional stutterers seems to be the result of their feelings of communicative frustration we do everything we can to reduce this important factor. Frustration generates aggressive responses and we have found that the child's struggling with his speech can be markedly decreased by decreasing the overall number of frustrations which he is experiencing in his daily life. By deliberately providing opportunities for the release of aggression, and by desensitizing him to frustrations of various kinds, he tends to react less to his stutterings.

In this we need not and should not confine our efforts to the frustrations of speech alone. Over and over again we have found that by getting the parents to stop saying "No" or "Don't do that" (the negative speech which bombards the child almost every hour of his waking time), the stuttering becomes less forced and easier. It seems almost as though the amount of struggling shown in the child's speech directly reflects the cumulative amount of felt frustration he is experiencing in his daily living. However; we do not hold the conviction that children should be raised in a completely permissive environment. We have seen too often how the little controlling monsters, so created, have wrecked families, and become even more insecure. And we have seen such children traumatized when later they had to enter the real world. But we have also observed that when young stutterers are given more freedom from their usual demands and restrictions for a few weeks, the tension and struggle subsides. This is crisis intervention, not general or permanent policy, and parents can accept the recommended changes only when they understand this. In the therapist's interactions with the child, he too can do much to give the little stutterer some relief from the demands, time pressures, and prohibitions to which the latter is so thoroughly subjected.

However, it is also necessary to build frustration tolerance. Here we employ the procedures of our own desensitization therapy. After determining the kinds of frustrating stimuli to which the child is most vulnerable, we first create a situation in which the child feels completely free from any restraints, then gradually introduce the frustration evoking stimuli, constantly scanning the child to determine the threshold of his tolerance thereof. As soon as we see the first signs of aggressive reactions, we withhold our frustrating and return again to the permissive, freedom condition. A child, subjected to such a carefully administered program, soon becomes able to tolerate more and more frustration and, as he does so, the tension and struggle disappear from his speech. We have been able to reverse the course of the disorder's development in many children by concentrating our efforts on frustration reduction and frustration tolerance.

Reducing the unpleasantness of the stuttering

Basically, the source of the young stutterer's unpleasant awareness of his broken fluency seems to reside in the delay in communication that his stuttering interposes and in his momentary inability to find the motoric sequences which he needs. There is also, of course, the unpleasantness which comes from the listener's reactions to the fluency breaks which, when applied contingently, tend to color the stuttering uglily. Somehow we must find ways to help the young stutterer to insulate himself from the evil impact of these disturbing influences. If he can become aware of the stuttering behavior without feeling that it is unpleasant or traumatic, he will not force or struggle. If he can have listeners who will not interrupt or supply words or show impatience when he stutters, the delay in communication created by the stuttering will be quite bearable and he will not have to search so frantically for the necessary integrations. If he has already been subjected to the stigma represented by the labels "stutterer" or "stuttering" and has accepted them, we can also do much to make those terms less opprobrious.

One of the first things we do is to use the modelling approach by inserting into our own speech enough samples of easy, unforced, repetitive, and prolonged stuttering behaviors to make the child aware of them. We use these disfluencies only often enough to create this awareness, perhaps with the syllabic repetitions occurring regularly and at the tempo of the other syllables. We rarely repeat a syllable more than two or three times and in these repetitions we provide a model of the kind of searching for proper coarticulation and integration, a model which the child can use. Thus we might begin a sentence with "Wh . . . Whuh . . . Wheh . . . When," making sure that the airflow is continuous and the repetitions come closer and closer to the motoric sequence of the word we are trying to say. Or we may introduce a prolongation or two into our speech. "Wwwwwere you tired after your trip to the park?" making sure that the transition from the "w" to the rest of the word was done slowly and without tension. At the same time we desire to provide a model for the child's searching, one which he can and will emulate if he identifies with us. We do this sort of pseudo-stuttering very easily and casually. As he becomes aware of it in our speech he is bound to notice that we are not disturbed and that we do not force or

hurry. We merely work our way calmly through the repetitions and prolongations, then finally say the word, at times repeating it again as though correcting ourselves. Then, again casually, we continue with our communication. This can be done very naturally with a little practice and we have trained many students and parents to put these models into their conversation. It has been fascinating to observe how soon a child will begin to use the same behaviors after he has heard and seen them in the speech of his important listeners. We have reversed the course of stuttering in many children merely by using this technique. The child learns that since *we* do not seem to need to struggle when we stumble over a word, he need not either.

But for some children, putting these models into the child's ear is not enough; we must also put them into his mouth. We have therefore devised some guessing games to be incorporated into the speech play which we share with the child. These are expressly designed to take the pain or frustration out of the stuttering and at the same time to teach him better ways of integrating his speech. An example from a session with an eight-year-old boy might be appropriate here:

Therapist: See if you can guess what kind of animal I'm thinking of. If you can guess what it is before this little hand of my watch goes down to here (30 seconds), you get this salted peanut. If you don't, well, it's mine and I'll eat it. Ok, here we go. I'm thinking of a sh . . . a shi . . . a . . . sh . . . a shih . . . a shee . . . a shee . . . a sheep (imitates clonic stuttering). Well, you didn't guess it in time so I eat the peanut. Let's play another one. I'm thinking of a p . . . (silent prolongation of the bilabial), a pih . . . pih . . . pih . . .

Child: A pig.

Therapist: That's right—pig. You guessed it. Here's your peanut. Now you think of a word and say it like I was doing and see if I can guess it.

Child: Ok. Mmmm . . . muh . . . muh . . . muh . . . muuh . . . mun . . . monk . . . monkey.

The therapist deliberately fails to guess the word and the child keeps repeating easily for some time until the therapist gives up. The the child tells him the word and eats the peanut.

In such word play there are many things happening. The role reversal, the status change, the lack of time pressure, the experience of repeating and fixating under benign conditions and with reward, the gradual integration of the word's motoric sequence, the removal of noxiousness from the sound or feeling of broken words, and many other factors are involved in this deceptively simple interchange. We have found such activities extremely useful in reducing the unpleasantness and frustration which usually accompany the stuttering. We have seen many children shift from the old hurried, tense struggling, when they found themselves repeating syllables or prolonging sounds, to the more simple patterns provided by this activity. There also seems to be a change from involuntariness to voluntariness, from the almost automatic reverberation or sustained fixation to controlled repetitive behavior. Playing these games, the little stutterers learn to sound out their words, to move forward rather than recoil, to search for integration.

The illustration we have sketched does not indicate the many possible permutations and combinations of this guessing game technique. We can use larger units: phrases and sentences, mand speech and tacts. We can use something akin to Shannon's redundancy guessing technique, employing carrier phrases preceding the words on which repetition or prolongation occurs. For example:

Therapist: See if you can guess what I'm seeing in this picture I'm hiding from you. There's a gray pussy c . . . c . . . ca . . . ca . . . (*Child:* Cat!). Cat up in a t. . . tr . . . truh . . . tree and she's looking at a sssss . . . sk . . . skw . . . squirrel eating a nnnnnn . . . nnnuh . . . (*Child:* Nut!).

Therapist: This is a boss me around game. You are to give me hints like we played before about what I have to do. For example: Do what I tell you to do now. Sssss . . . sssih . . . sss . . . sssih . . . sit down on the ffff . . . fffluh . . . fffloor. Ok? Now you tell me what I have to do.

Child: Puh . . . puh . . . put your head in the wwww . . . wuh . . . waste basket and mmmmmm . . . mmme . . . meow like a ccc . . . cuh . . . cat!

He has put these previously unpleasant repetitions and prolongations into his mouth and found them to be without unpleasantness.

Another activity which we have found useful in removing the unpleasantness from the repetitions and prolongations of the young stutterer involves the speaking of strange, difficult, or nonsense words or sentences. The therapist and child take turns composing them and asking each other to repeat them as exactly as possible, and having three trials to do so. Thus the therapist may ask the child to say "statistics" or "alligochapeeda" or "unnamulamaitua" or even a foreign phrase such as "ou sont les neiges d'antan." These often produce some faltering and some repetitive or fixative behavior but very rarely will a child show any tension or struggle as he attempts them. Also when the child has his turn and composes some complicated nonsense utterance for the therapist to repeat, the therapist can deliberately insert some easy repetitions and even prolongations as he tries to duplicate what the child has said. Children love this word play and the hilarity which usually accompanies it certainly reduces the unpleasantness of the hesitancies thereby provoked.

In his chapter in Travis' *Handbook of Speech Pathology and Audiology,* Williams (1971) describes another approach. He interprets the stuttering behavior to the child as simply consisting of mistakes in talking and as being similar to the mistakes the child makes in learning to ride a bicycle, in learning to skate, or in mastering any other similar physical skill. He points out to the child that struggle behavior does not help in the acquisition of any skill, and that the child must learn to talk "easily rather than hard," that struggling doesn't help one eliminate mistakes. Other writers use various methods to convince the child that speech is easy and that his effortful reactions to blockage are unnecessary. By focusing upon the large amount of normal speech shown by the child, in the context of the therapist's reassurance that all is well, the child's tendency to struggle when he finds himself prolonging or repeating is weakened. Much of the direct therapy for the beginning stutterer is aimed at the same goal. We have not found much difficulty in treating very young confirmed stutterers successfully. Certainly, the therapy is much less difficult than when we have to work with an adult full of long-established fears and avoidances.

Removing the stigma

As we have mentioned earlier, many of these young confirmed stutterers have already felt the force of the culture's rejection of stuttering behavior. Even when the parents have abstained from overt correction or calling attention to his breaks in fluency, the child usually meets a playmate or two who will have imitated his stuttering mockingly or applied the stuttering label. These children will tell you that they stutter though they generally use the word to refer primarily to the repetitions of syllables rather than to the prolongations. Yet, at this stage, they do not seem overly concerned or anxious. They often still speak with spontaneity and without any sign of avoidance. When we meet this labelled awareness, we do not seek to convince the child that the label is wrong and that his parents and playmates are in error when they use it as some therapists have recommended. Rather, we reinterpret the label so that it becomes innocuous. We tell the younger child, usually at an appropriate moment when he brings up the matter, that yes, he did stutter just then, and that everyone stutters occasionally, especially when they get tangled up in their thinking or become emotional or hurried. But we tell him that there are two kinds of stuttering—the easy and the hard kinds —and we illustrate both. We help him understand that the easy kind is harmless and that children usually get over it. We show him that the hard kind is unnecessary, that it makes him feel stuck, that it makes it even harder to talk and that other people notice it more. Then we reward and reinforce the easy kind contingently and withhold the reinforcement from any stuttering which is accompanied by force or tension. When all this confrontation is done casually and with good humor, the child seems relieved and his speech usually becomes more fluent.

Modification

We now turn to the task of teaching the child to stutter easily and without struggling. Most of the children with whom we have worked find it very difficult to eliminate specific stuttering behaviors by simply being asked to do so. For example, if one asks the child to try to open his eyes *during* a moment of stuttering, he seems completely unable to manage this until after the moment of stuttering has terminated. The same situation exists if he is asked to change an abnormal mouth posture or to inhibit a gasp. Accordingly, we work more for replacement than for variation or modification. We try almost immediately to get the child to substitute a new pattern of easy stuttering for the old one of struggle and this he seems able to accomplish with an ease that often seems surprising to one who has worked mainly with adult stutterers.

Essentially, what we do is to *show* him how to stutter in the new way, not tell him. We now fill our own speech full of these new easy stutterings as we converse with him, making slow shifts from sound to sound, prolonging the word as a whole rather than any one phoneme, emphasizing slow smooth transitions without tension. When the child stutters, we stutter right along with him but differently, often saying the word several times in the new slow motion way while he is still struggling to emit it once. "Try to stutter this new way rather than your old way" is the basic charge we give him. Children are great imitators and they soon learn the new way of working through their hard words.

Once we have the new way of stuttering thoroughly identified and practiced, we set up appropriate reinforcement schedules to increase its strength. At first, using almost continuous reinforcement, we reward the child in various ways every time he uses the new kind of stuttering, then later we employ intermittent reinforcement as the new response becomes more consistent.[3] Always we simply ignore the old kind of stuttering and do not penalize it. If the therapist has achieved a warm relationship with the child, this interplay and programmed reinforcement produces very swift changes. We have had some children who changed the way they stuttered in only two or three sessions.

In their pell-mell hurry to communicate, most of these children find it very hard to cancel. However, if the process of cancellation is structured as correcting a mistake, or as an erasing of the stuttering that has just occurred, some of them can be brought to do enough of it to remove the built-in reinforcement which the furtherance and consummation of communication provides. If we can get the child to correct his moments of old stuttering behaviors by pausing, and then by stuttering in the new easy way, we do much to weaken the strength of the old behaviors but we must recognize that often we cannot get this correction. The following excerpt, from a session with a ten-year-old boy, may illustrate how we successfully introduced cancellation:

Hi, there! See this? I bet you've never seen so big an eraser, have you? Well, today we're going to erase stuttering. Let me have your finger. I'm going to draw a stuttering face on your fingernail like this. . . . Now erase it! Ok. It's gone. Think we could erase real stuttering as easy as that?

The trouble with real stuttering, Jimmy, is that it leaves an invisible mark on you. You can't see it once the word comes out, but it's there just the same. Let me show you. See here? I've got some invisi-

---

3 For a description of a rigorous operant conditioning approach suitable for these young confirmed stutterers, see the reference by Ryan (1971).

ble ink. (It's really only lemon juice but you can write with it and after it dries, it becomes invisible.) Look, here's a piece of paper on which I wrote something this morning when I was thinking about you. Can you read it? No, it really is invisible, isn't it? Now let's look what happens when I heat it up. (Therapist holds paper over a lighted match and the words "I stuttered hard" appear magically.)

I'll let you write with the invisible ink in a moment but first we've got some thinking to do. When you stutter hard, it's just like writing down that word in invisible ink inside your head. After the word comes out, it's gone . . . or you think it is but it's still there in your head . . . invisible . . . and when you get all hot with fear or excitement, there is is again . . . *unless you erase it!* You've got to learn how to erase your stuttering after it happens so it won't come out again when you get scared of talking. . . .

Ok, you want to write with the invisible ink. . . . All right. Every time you stutter hard when you're reading this geography book, stop after the word comes out and then I'll give you this pen and the lemon juice and you can write the word you just stuttered. . . . Understand? . . . No, you can't have it until you've stuttered and then you've got to stop and write down that word. (Boy reads and writes down the stuttered words as instructed.)

Now we've got to wait a bit until it dries and while it does, let me tell you something about how you can erase your stuttering so it won't come out again when you're scared. The best way is to stop right after the word comes out and to erase it right then. Don't wait until it soaks in. We've got to erase it right away. . . . How do you erase it? . . . You say the word again slowly, smoothly, and without forcing. Let me show you how I erase a stuttered word. I'll say "Barbara" and stutter on it until it comes out, then I'll stop, and then I'll say it the new, easy way (therapist illustrates).

Ok, should be about dry now. Yes, see! Those words you stuttered on have all gone away. You can't see them. But the stuttered words are still there. Let's try

heating it over another match. . . . Aha, there they come . . . look at them. . . . Every one is still there. . . .

Now let's do it again, the same way. But this time, on every other word, we'll erase it with this piece of wet blotter, if you'll do what I just showed you about stopping and saying it again smoothly. . . . First let's just stutter and not erase. . . . Oh, that was a hard stutter. Write down the word with the invisible ink. Now this next time you stutter, remember how to erase it by stopping, and then saying it again smoothly after you've written it down. . . . (Boy does so.) Good! You erased it fine but wait until it dries. I wonder which word will show up when we heat the paper. . . . You don't want to keep all those stuttered words inside of you. They'll keep coming out some other time. It's better to erase them right away. . . . Well, it ought to be dry now. . . . All right, this time you hold the match and heat it. . . . Aha, see . . . just like I told you. The first one is there but the one you erased is gone. . . .

From the workbook by Vette and Goven (1965) we quote another illustration showing how the therapist sought to explain the basic reasoning behind the cancellation process to an *older* child.

You have seen the word "cancel" several times in this manual. It means to erase. When you stutter on a word, the fear of stuttering keeps building up and leaves its mark on you. You cannot see it, but it is there. When you cancel, you erase this mark and strike it out.

Up to now, after you have stuttered on a word, you have run away from it the minute you were free of the unpleasantness of the stuttering. The free speech which follows the stuttering acts like a reward for your stuttering. It is like cheating on a test and getting an "A" on the paper. As long as you get away with it, you will probably cheat again, but if you are caught and have to do it over, you will think twice about cheating the next time. What usually happens is that after the block, you run as far away from it as possible and try to forget you stuttered. The struggle which got you through the word is rewarded by the good speech that follows. Later, when you get stuck again, you will try to break out of the block the same foolish struggling way because you remember that it worked before. Like the "A" the good speech rewards the wrong thing. If you do something about the block right after it happens by taking control and erasing the struggle, the control will then be rewarded. (p. 77)

Though, as we have said, it is easier for severe child stutterers to replace the old kind of stuttering by the new kind rather than to modify it while it is occurring, nevertheless, we have been able to show many of them how to pull-out of their blocks by simply duplicating their initial stuttering behaviors, then demonstrating how to ease out of their repetitions or blockages slowly and smoothly. After providing examples of these models, we then· join the child, duplicating his initial stuttering in unison but then we shift to the new form while he is still struggling. If the child is able to read, we often read along with him, feeding our voice into one ear as he cups his hand to hear himself with the other ear, and when he stutters, we do so too but use a pull-out to provide the necessary contrast. By timing our shift so that it first occurs at about the time the child can be expected to have his release, then moving the shift forward in time until it occurs almost at the beginning of his stuttering, we have found that the young stutterer soon masters the new release.

With older children, the pull-out technique can be taught more directly as the following interaction demonstrates:

Today we're going to try to show you how to work your way out of your blocks —out of your stuttering. About the only

ways you now have to do that is to force or jerk or back up and start again. Or sometimes you only keep on doing it. You just wait until it stops itself. There are better ways than those. . . .

When your mouth is jumping or running away with you, you feel pretty helpless. And when it feels frozen or glued shut, it's kind of scarey. And so you do all the wrong things. You get panicky and you hurry and struggle almost blindly. That really doesn't help. It only makes the stuttering worse. You've got to learn a different way—a better way.

Remember how I told you once that learning to lick your stuttering is like learning to swim? You've got to do just the opposite of what you first start to do. Instead of holding your head up high in the water, you've got to lie down in it. Instead of thrashing around and struggling and spanking the water with your hands, you've got to cup them like this in order to pull yourself forward. And you're scared of the water when you first learn to swim . . . and when you sink, your nose gets full and it's sure unpleasant. Instead of getting all tensed up and hurrying, you've got to relax and move slower. There's a knack to swimming and you don't learn it all at once. It's the same way with stuttering.

Now watch me. I'm going to stutter like you do and first I'll hurry and struggle and force and jerk—the wrong way. Like this . . . (demonstrates) and now I'll start the old way, the old wrong way, but then I'll work my way out of the stuttering nice and slowly and smoothly. Like this . . . (demonstrates). Did you see how I stopped forcing and hurrying? Did you see how I slowed down and made my mouth move so it made· the word come out easily? Let me give you some more samples of the hard way and the easy way to swim with your mouth (therapist demonstrates).

Now let's play follow the leader. You watch me and do exactly what I do. Let's do it the old way, the wrong way, first on the word "butter." Aha, you really did get into some real stuttering that time, didn't you? That's what happens when you do it wrongly. Now imitate me as I first get stuck, then work my way out of it easily and smoothly. . . . Came out pretty slickly, didn't it? Let's work on some other hard words together the same way (they do).

Now this time, suppose you take these pictures and tell me their names. I think I've picked out hard ones, haven't I? But we're going to do it a bit differently. You start to say the word and if you stutter, just keep on stuttering and let me finish the word. Let me show you how to pull out of your stuttering. You do the stuttering and I'll pull out of it and say the word. Don't you say the word. That's my job. I've got to show you how to work out of it so watch how I do it. . . . (They carry out the task.)

Fine! Think you've got the idea? Now this time, I'll do the stuttering and you show me how to work out of it. Show me. Don't tell me. All right, here we go. . . . (Therapist throws himself into a severe stuttering and boy joins him, but works his way out of it smoothly while the therapist continues to stutter.) Guess you'd better show me again. . . . (This time, the therapist follows the boy's demonstration of the pull-out.) Pretty good. I followed you that time, didn't I? You're a good speech teacher. Show me again on this word. . . . (They do several in this same fashion.) Now suppose you see if you can show yourself how to get out of your own stuttering the new easy way on these pictures. . . . (They work until the child has some real success.)

We have not found it feasible to attempt to teach young stutterers to assume new specific preparatory sets when approaching their feared words. We find that such scanning and preparation only increases the sound and word fears and that children react negatively to having to talk with such vigilance. Instead we rely primarily on the natural tendency for the new way of stuttering to move forward in time, from the cancellation to the pull-out and from that to an automatic preparatory set. This seems to occur without any formal training.

Stabilization

In contrast to the adult stutterer, children do not seem to require much stabilization of their new form of stuttering. Often the whole disorder melts away once the child begins to stutter easily. The smooth, slow-motion kind of stuttering readily transforms itself into normal speech since its motoric sequences are closely similar. At times we help the child by having him talk to us, deliberately using more of these new forms of stuttering than he needs to, but usually all we need to do is to arrange for some booster sessions at intervals and to be available whenever he wants to see us. Usually there are some few unfortunate experiences or crises to handle in the next few months following the gradual termination of therapy but they soom diminish in frequency. It is also necessary to have the parents and teachers understand that occasional lapses are to be expected. Nevertheless, our work with young severe stutterers has convinced us that therapy can be very successful when it is organized according to these principles. Moreover, it has been our experience that if the morbid course of the disorder's development can be reversed during these early years, the prognosis is excellent. These children need not, and should not wait until they are adults to receive intensive treatment. They need it now and will profit from it more than they will as adults. Again we stress the importance of working with stutterers as early as possible if the problem of stuttering is ever to have a satisfactory solution.

Environmental therapy

Although we have already mentioned several ways in which the parents and teachers of the young confirmed stutterer may help him, most of our exposition has concerned the interactions between the speech therapist and the child. We do not apologize for this emphasis. We feel that if a therapist can become a highly significant person in the child's life, his impact will be far more important than the limitations of time and contact might seem to indicate. Most of our lives are shaped by only a few key individuals. It is the therapist's mandate to be one of those in the life of the stuttering child.

Nevertheless it is obvious that if we can alter the impacts of other significant persons in the stutterer's environment so that they will contribute to the resolution of his communicative problems rather than to their evil growth, we should certainly do so. At this age the stutterer is largely under environmental control, his stuttering varying in severity with the amount of the communicative stress imposed upon him by his listeners. The influence of his teachers, parents, and playmates is paramount.

Environmental change

One solution is to provide the young stutterer with a controlled environment. On the continent of Europe and especially behind the Iron Curtain we find such children being placed in special schools or classrooms or even in hospitals. Thus Vlassova (1964) writes:

The modern method of composite treatment, evolved by speech therapists in collaboration with physicians, includes the following: general invigoration by medication and physiotherapy, psychotherapy, logopedic and logorhythmic musical exercises. In Russia this composite therapy is applied in special day hospitals, day nurseries and kindergartens, and in the logopedic departments of pediatric clinics. (p. 41)

Institutional treatment for stutterers was used for many years in this country in the last half of the last century and in the early part of this one. As we have described in earlier chapters, therapists brought stutterers into their own homes or had them live in their commercial institutes where almost total environmental control was possible. Norway has had a state supported special school for stutterers up in the mountains at Skrukli for decades, and even today in our own country there are some few residential clinics where stutterers may live and receive concentrated therapy. Some of these are summer camps where young stutterers can get intensive treatment during their school vacations and are specially designed to provide a more favorable environment. We find these camps all over the world (Biesalski, 1964; Lepsova, 1965; Masura, 1965; Clancy and Morley 1950; Gunderman and Weuffen, 1965; Higdon, 1968; Ward, Godfrey, and Jousse, 1968; Prins, 1970). Most of them report favorable results.

The home and school environments

Only a very few of our young stutterers will receive therapy in camps or institutions; they will be treated in the clinics or the schools. If we are to alter their environments so that they will be conducive to recovery rather than to the increase of stuttering, we must do what we can to alter the communicative conditions in these settings. We have found many instances in which a child's severe stuttering disappeared shortly after we had changed his environment and managed to remove some of the communicative stresses or to create conditions which were conducive to fluency. To ignore the fact that most of the child's time is spent in the home and school and to hope that a few weekly clinical sessions will be sufficient to solve his problems seems unrealistic.

In our chapter on the treatment of the beginning stutterer we have described in detail the things therapists can do to create a favorable home environment and we feel no need to repeat this information here. There are, however, two additional features which should be emphasized. First, it is now necessary to lay the cards on the table openly. The child knows that he stutters. He is receiving treatment for his stuttering. To ignore the disorder at this stage is the worst of folly for it will only give the child the impression that it is unspeakably evil. As Luper and Mulder (1964) say in insisting upon open discussion of the stuttering problem by parents and child:

It should be pointed out that the child may even progress more rapidly through the developmental stages of stuttering if he gets the impression that he must battle alone against the strange thing he thinks is happening to him when he talks. He may even conclude that he can never truly win or even deserve his parents' love unless he rids himself of his impediment. He may think along these lines: "I know that I am having an awful time talking, but strangely enough no one else seems to care. Maybe everyone else has given up on me. Maybe what I do is so bad no one dares mention it." (p. 73)

The same point of view is shared by Falck (1969):

To ask a parent to pay no attention to speech which is obviously nonfluent enough to be disturbing to the listener may be unrealistic. To expect a parent to show no reaction while the child struggles through a speech attempt is also unrealistic. (p. 45)

Our own policy is to make sure that the parents have an opportunity to see us working with the young stutterer, and to observe how we openly discuss the various tasks of therapy unemotionally and objectively. Sometimes we even hook the parents to a DAF apparatus so that they will understand how it feels to have one's speech disrupted. Showing the parents how to talk about the child's stuttering is much more effective than a 'lot of verbal counseling. Once the door to frank discussion has been opened, both the child and his parents seem much relieved.

Secondly, we seek to use the parents as observers and reinforcers. We explain and demonstrate the kinds of responses that we wish to discourage and to encourage. We ask them to be our eyes and ears, to provide the reports that we need. We describe our subgoals in language that they can understand. The parents' basic role in this cotherapy is to provide positive reinforcement for the behaviors we wish to strengthen but they are not to punish those we wish to weaken. The latter they simply observe and report to us.

Creating a favorable school environment. Martha Black (1964), in speaking to the public school therapist, writes:

First of all, remember that you are in a school, and to a degree (sometimes a very significant one) you may be able to manipulate the child's environment to produce situations from which he receives ego satisfaction and which he can communicate with a minimum of stress. . . . Your therapy room is a part of his environment in which the child spends the major portion of his waking hours. It is in school that the greatest demands are made on him for good speech.

It is, of course, the classroom teacher who plays the most important role in determining the characteristics of the school environment. Her policies with regard to recitation, her attitudes toward stuttering, and her concerns for the stutterer himself are vital. Some teachers run a very strict classroom, often calling upon the children in alphabetical order and insisting upon quick and correct answers to questions, a policy which is almost certain to produce more stuttering. Others excuse the child from all oral recitation. The author well remembers his feelings of isolation and deviance when subjected to this practice. Shapoff (1954), another stutterer, contrasts the emotional states he experienced when in a classroom with such a teacher and in another one who was more understanding. With the first, he felt rejected and resentful; with the second, he gained the esteem that led to successful mastery of his stuttering. Murphy and Fitzsimons (1960) have this passage:

The true thoughts of most stutterers about themselves in relation to the class setting and about their teachers seldom are aired directly, except perhaps in a confidential therapy situation, at which times such statements as the following are made: "Every time I stutter, she looks away, and that is the worst thing anybody can do to me." "She makes me so angry whenever she says the word for me—doesn't think I can get it out by myself—but I just take it." "I like her all right, except every time she says to slow down or speak more slowly, I just about bust." (p. 472)

Knudson (1939) reports that half of the stutterers she interviewed said that they had answered "I don't know" or had deliberately given the wrong answer in avoiding feared words when called upon to recite. (As a child, the author always made sure to misspell a word as soon as possible

when "spelldown" sessions were the order of the day. He even misspelled "cat" in the ninth grade when a suspicious teacher gave him a series of easier and easier words. Since his name began with "V," a letter near the end of the alphabet, and with teachers who called upon pupils in alphabetical order, the amount of panic that he experienced became overwhelming as inexorably the need to display his abnormality came progressively closer. On one occasion, tormented by anxiety beyond all measure, he picked up his Latin book and heaved it at the teacher's head. She had called, as usual, upon all of the students in the alphabetical order but on that particular occasion had skipped him.) Long oral reports for a severe stutterer are sheer murder. Not only do they torture the stutterer with serial frustrations but also they make his classmates irritable and impatient. It is not pleasant to have to sit and endure the long gaps and reverbatory struggles of a stutterer trying to make a long recitation. Knudson (1939) has some good advice:

Some students may not be able to give entire book reports or make long oral recitations until they have had more help with their speech. In severe instances it may not be wise or practical for either the student or the class. All stutterers, however, can give "yes" or "no" responses or very brief replies in order not to feel ignored or excluded from the group (p. 46)

When classroom teachers have asked us how they should handle this problem we suggest that it is usually wise to ask the stutterer himself or at least to offer several alternatives from which he can choose. Would he prefer to be called upon for long or short answers, or for answers that he perhaps knows as contrasted with those that he might not know? Would he prefer to be called on early or late in the class session? Will he ask his speech therapist how she should proceed? Would he prefer to be called on only when he raises his hand to volunteer?

The teacher should tell him that she knows he has some trouble talking because of his stuttering and that when he has a hard time saying a word, she won't hurry him or interrupt him or say the word for him but will always wait patiently. She helps him know that she recognizes his problem and is interested in helping him in every way she can. Eisenson and Ogilvie (1957) recommend that the young stutterer "should be told that everyone has some kind of speech trouble at some time just as all children stumble occasionally when they walk or run." They even suggest that "It might help considerably if the teacher, in a not too evident way, does some hesitating or repeating of her own. Beyond this, the teacher should explain to the class that teasing and name calling are not permitted and that some privilege will be denied to any offending member (pp. 227–28)." We would not agree with this latter advice. Public admonitions of this sort and the equating of stuttering with normal speech -hesitations will probably only make the stutterer feel that he cannot trust that teacher or that she does not really understand his difficulties. It would be wiser to deal with the mocker or teaser individually and privately as we have suggested earlier. Rather than try to get acceptance and tolerance by public command, it is better to provide a model which the children can follow. As West and Ansberry (1968) say, "The teacher's manner toward the child should be casual, unhurried and show no annoyance. This attitude will not only put him at ease but serve as a model for the other children in the room to follow (p. 351)." We have known many teachers who acted in this way as a model listener before the class and did much to ease the stutterer's burden. These teachers were also the ones who usually had created an opportunity to discuss the stuttering, not only with the therapist but also privately with the child himself. They had found out what the therapist was trying to do and the difficulties he and the child were encountering. Some teachers, in their ignorance, and despite the best of intentions, have done a lot of things that hurt. They have insisted that the child say a stuttered word over again and again and again until it was spoken fluently, a demand which could result in real trauma if adaptation does not occur swiftly. They have told him to sit down and relax until he could "think straight and talk straight." They have had all the other children in the class help him "say the word." They have been oversympathetic, almost maudlin in their evident pity, consoling with him publically about "his unfortunate impediment, poor little boy." There are still others who make no effort to talk to the child about his stuttering and who act as though it doesn't exist no matter how apparent the struggling may be. Few stutterers manage to stay emotionally healthy in such a classroom. Their stuttering becomes not only unmentionable but unspeakable. Teachers need the counsel of the speech therapist if they are to be forces for good rather than evil.

And they can be tremendous forces for good. Once they understand the special needs of the stuttering child, they can create not only the happy atmosphere which helps all children learn eagerly but also the special conditions that facilitate fluency. They can work a lot of unison oral reading and speaking into the program; they can create communicative situations in which little anxiety is evident. They find ways of increasing the stutterer's self-esteem. They help the child to find a rewarding place in one of the subgroups that always exist in a classroom so he has the feel of belonging and participation. They can provide positive reinforcement for any progress in attaining the subgoals outlined by the therapist, and even shape peer reinforcements in the same direction. We have known a good many master teachers who did much more for our child stutterers than we could do once they understood what had to be done.

Concluding remarks

Incredibly, we have a few more things to say as this book comes to a close. First and most important, we urge the support of basic research that may help us know what happens at the moment of stuttering that results in temporally distorted words. Clinicians stumble in the dark without this vital information. Secondly, we must work much harder with the child who has just begun to stutter. We should not wait until his fears and frustrations create habitual secondary behaviors. Stuttering is a disorder that requires an organized public health sort of program. Society has neglected stutterers too long. Thirdly, our clinicians need to be better trained if they are to help the desperate adults who come to them. Our present preparation of these workers is, with some exceptions, outrageously inadequate. Finally, we must make an all out attempt to scrutinize the kinds of therapy now being offered with a cold objective eye, to insist upon rigorous cri-

teria for all claims of success, and constantly to explore new and better approaches. And with this last suggestion, the author who has spent a lifetime in the vineyard of stuttering therapy will try hard to put down his hoe.

Bibliography

BIESALSKI, P. (Experiences with a youth hostel for speech therapy), *Zeitschrift fur Laryngologie, Rhinologie, Otologie und Ihre Grenzgebietl,* 43 (1964), 254–57.

BLACK, M. E., *Speech Correction in the Schools.* Englewood Cliffs, N.J.: Prentice-Hall, 1964.

CLANCY, J. N. and D. E. MORLEY, Summer speech and hearing programs, *Journal of Speech Disorders,* 15 (1950), 9–15.

COOPER, E., Structuring therapy for therapist and stuttering child, *Journal of Speech and Hearing Disorders,* 30 (1965), 75–79.

DASKALOV, D., Basic principles and methods of prevention and treatment of stuttering, *Nevropatolgii i Psikhiatrii imeni S. S. Korskakova,* 62 (1962), 1047–52.

EGLAND, G. O., *Speech and Language Problems.* Englewood Cliffs, N.J.: Prentice-Hall, 1970.

EISENSON, J. and M. OGILVIE, *Speech Correction in the Schools.* New York: Macmillan, 1957.

EMERICK, L., A clinical success: Mark, in H. L. Luper (ed.), *Stuttering: Successes and Failures in Therapy.* Memphis: Speech Foundation of America (1968), pp. 21–31.

————, Therapy for young stutterers, *Exceptional Children,* 31 (1965), 398–402.

————, Treatment for teens, *N.M.U. Journal of Speech Therapy,* 3 (1971), 4–5.

FALCK, F. J., *Stuttering: Learned and Un-*

learned. Springfield, Ill.: Charles C Thomas, 1969.

GUNDERMAN, H. and M. WEUFFEN, Uber den nutzen von stottererkursen, *Zeitschrift fur Laryngol. Rhinol. Otol.,* 44 (1965), 517–21.

HIGDON, H., Michigan's remarkable summer camp, *Today's Health,* 74 (May 1968), 34–37.

HIRSCHBERG, J. (Stuttering), *Orvosi Hetilap* (Hungary), 106 (1965), 780–84.

KATSOVSKAIA, I. (The problems of childhood stuttering), *Proceedings of the Third Session of the Institute of Defectology.* Moscow: Academy of Pedagogical Science, 1960, pp. 133–34.

KNUDSON, T. A., A study of the oral recitation problems of stutterers, *Journal of Speech Disorders,* 4 (1939), 235–39.

————, What the classroom teacher can do for stutterers, *Quarterly Journal of Speech,* 26 (1940), 207–12.

LEPSOVA, M. (A holiday camp for stuttering children), *De Therapia Vocis et Loquellae,* 1 (1965), 479–82.

LUPER, H. L. (ed.), *Stuttering: Successes and Failures in Therapy.* Memphis: Speech Foundation of America, 1968.

———— and R. L. MULDER, *Stuttering Therapy for Children.* Englewood Cliffs, N.J.: Prentice-Hall, 1964.

MASURA, S. (The results of vacation courses in the treatment of stuttering in children), *De Therapia Vocis et Loquellae,* 1 (1965), 473–76.

MURPHY, A. T. and R. M. FITZSIMONS, *Stuttering and Personality Dynamics.* New York: Ronald Press, 1960.

NEELY, K., Letters to the editor, *Journal of Speech and Hearing Disorders,* 16 (1951), 165–66.

PETKOV, D. and I. IOSIFOV, Our experience in the treatment of stuttering in a speech rehabilitation colony, *Zhurnal Nevropatologii i Psikhiatrii imeni S. S. Korsakova,* 60 (1960), 903–4.

PRINS, D., Improvement and regression in stutterers following short-term intensive therapy, *Journal of Speech and Hearing Disorders,* 35 (1970), 123–35.

RYAN, B. P., Operant procedures applied to stuttering therapy for children, *Journal of Speech and Hearing Disorders,* 36 (1971), 264–80.

SHAPOFF, I., A stutterer writes to a former teacher, *Journal of the National Education Association,* 43 (1954), 348.

VETTE, G. and P. GOVEN, *A Manual for Stuttering Therapy.* Pittsburgh: Stanwix House, 1965.

VAN RIPER, C. (ed.), *Stuttering: Treatment of the Young Stutterer in the School.* Memphis: Speech Foundation of America, 1964.

VLASSOVA, N. A. (Value of the complex method of treatment of stuttering in children), *Folia Phoniatrica,* 16 (1964), 39–43.

WARD, J. F., C. M. GODFREY, and A. T. JOUSSE, An intensive summer speech therapy program for children, *Canadian Journal of Public Health,* 59 (1968), 54–56.

WEST, R. and M. ANSBERRY, *The Rehabilitation of Speech,* 4th ed. New York: Harper & Row, 1968.

WILLIAMS, D. E., Stuttering therapy for children, in L. E. Travis (ed.), *Handbook of Speech Pathology and Audiology.* New York: Appleton-Century-Crofts, 1971, pp. 1073–93.

———— and A. M. ROE, Teachers, parents, and stutterers, *Education,* 80 (1960), 471–75.

WINGATE, M. E., Calling attention to stuttering, *Journal of Speech and Hearing Research,* 2 (1959), 326–35.

Author Index

Subject Index